D0769209

Acute Toxicology Testing

SECOND EDITION

NATIONAL UNIVERSITY
LIBRARY   SAN DIEGO

Acute Toxicology Testing

SECOND EDITION

Shayne C. Gad

Gad Consulting Services
Raleigh, North Carolina

Christopher P. Chengelis

WIL Research Laboratories
Ashland, Ohio

ACADEMIC PRESS

San Diego   London   Boston   New York   Sydney   Tokyo   Toronto

This book is printed on acid-free paper. ∞

Copyright © 1998, 1988 by ACADEMIC PRESS

All Rights Reserved.
No part of this publication may be reproduced or transmitted in any form or by any
means, electronic or mechanical, including photocopy, recording, or any information
storage and retrieval system, without permission in writing from the publisher.

Academic Press
a division of Harcourt Brace & Company
525 B Street, Suite 1900, San Diego, California 92101-4495, USA
http://www.apnet.com

Academic Press Limited
24-28 Oval Road, London NW1 7DX, UK
http://www.hbuk.co.uk/ap/

Library of Congress Card Catalog Number: 97-80232

International Standard Book Number: 0-12-272250-7

PRINTED IN THE UNITED STATES OF AMERICA
97 98 99 00 01 02 BB 9 8 7 6 5 4 3 2 1

*To Samantha, Katina, and Jake, who keep their Daddy
young and smiling. To Joyce, who will always be in
my heart.*
SCG

*To my father, Chris Chengelis, and the living memory
of my mother, Demetra Kapnistos Chengelis.*
CPC

CONTENTS

6 Photosensitization and Phototoxicity

7 Lethality Testing

8 Safety Considerations for the Administration of Agents by the Parenteral Routes

9 Systemic Acute Toxicity Testing

10 Routes, Formulations, and Vehicles

11 Considerations Specific to Animal Test Models

12 Statistical Analysis of Acute Toxicology and Safety Studies

13 Acute Inhalation

14 Problems and Issues

PREFACE TO THE FIRST EDITION

Acute toxicology testing constitutes the first line of defense against potentially dangerous chemicals—indeed, for many man-made chemicals, it is the only health effects assessment performed. The test designs are, at the same time, the oldest still in use and also the most likely to change over the next five to ten years.

The first (and most important) step in designing acute studies is developing a statement of the objective for the study—what question is to be answered and what depth of information is desired. The two major categories of acute studies, in terms of the nature of their objectives, are single-end-point studies (which assess dermal and ocular irritation and corrosion, sensitization, photosensitization, and lethality) and "shot-gun" (multiple-end-point) studies (which assess or identify systemic effects such as target organs and effect and no observable effect levels). In this book we present protocols for and review each of the common designs of these tests, their development and objectives, the types of data they generate, and the current status of alternative test designs and models. For each type of test, applicable U.S. and international guidelines are also presented. Also reviewed are the problems associated with study design and interpretation of the results, and some of the special concerns and problems associated with the techniques and animal models employed in these studies. At the same time, we have tried to present (in a critical manner) the alternative designs and models which have been or are being developed for conducting these tests in a manner that both meets society's needs as well as or better than the classical methods and reduces animal usage and discomfort.

Also presented and reviewed are (1) considerations for the formulation and selection of vehicles or dosage form; (2) the characteristics of the eight most commonly used laboratory animal species and the rationale for model selection; (3) a presentation of the basic principles and methods of statistics and experimental design applicable to acute toxicology, with special emphasis on the philosophy and methodology of screening in toxicology; and (4) sources and techniques for searching published (print and electronic) information sources to locate and identify existing acute toxicity data.

We hope that this book is a very practical, usable, and complete (as far as possible) handbook for the design, conduct, and interpretation of an acute toxicology testing system and, we hope, a view and path to the future of the field.

1988

PREFACE TO THE SECOND EDITION

It has been a distinct pleasure to bring the completely revised second edition of *Acute Toxicology Testing* into being. In the 10 years since the first edition was written (including the past 5 years, in which the book has been out of print), the discipline of acute toxicology has evolved tremendously, and the authors have learned more tricks of the trade in both the literature and the laboratory. The result is a volume much more valuable and useful than the first edition.

The field of alternatives to animals in toxicology testing has continued to have acute toxicology as its primary focus, and this is reflected in the second edition's broad coverage of alternatives in the framework of endpoint-directed testing. Regulations have also undergone a vast number of changes, and these new and revised requirements are presented in their current form throughout the book. A table at the beginning of the volume summarizes the sources of regulatory guidance for acute testing in the United States, Europe, and Japan.

New animal (*in vivo*) tests and models have not been overlooked, but are presented in parallel with traditional and alternative models. In addition, areas with special testing requirements, such as medical devices and biomaterials, have been given increased attention.

Finally, throughout *Acute Toxicology Testing,* typos and errors that appeared in the first edition have been corrected, and data and references have been updated.

The result is, we hope, a single-source volume that provides the basis for selecting, designing, conducting, and critically interpreting all of the acute toxicity tests required and/or commonly used to evaluate and manage the hazards posed by short-term exposures to chemicals.

1997

CHAPTER 1

Introduction

Acute toxicity studies, as defined in this book, are those which evaluate the short-term (less than 30 days) adverse biological effects of a single exposure (or a small number of exposures over a week or less) to a material or physical agent. Generally, such exposures occur at such large amounts or high concentrations that long-term repeated exposures would not occur at similar levels. These exposures, for materials other than cosmetics, medical devices, and pharmaceuticals, are most frequently the result of accidents. Such exposures could be the result of misuse of a consumer product, leaking containers, industrial accidents, transportation mishaps (truck accidents or leaks, train derailments, etc.), curious children or mislabeled containers, agricultural accidents, product tampering, or intentional suicide attempts. Cosmetics, medical devices, and pharmaceuticals exposures are both intentional and accidental, but concerns about their short-term effects are characteristically associated with larger exposures or doses.

Acute toxicity studies or evaluations are at once both the oldest (in several senses) and the most common of the toxicity or safety evaluations. They are the oldest in terms of being prehistoric in origin (the earliest such evaluation being man determining what was safe to eat by tasting plants or feeding them to others), of being the oldest formalized tests, and of having undergone only recent critical review and revision since the Second World War.

These tests constitute the front line of defense against chemicals and agents which have the potential to damage individuals in society. They are the first tests performed to begin to evaluate such potential hazards. Indeed, for the vast majority of new man-made chemicals (or biotechnology-derived materials) entering the marketplace and the environment, acute studies are the only health effect assessments performed. However, both the study designs and the methodologies employed date from 40 or more years ago and have only recently undergone critical evaluation and reform. This review and reform, presented as an integral portion of this book, is resulting both in alterations in the way traditional *in vivo* tests are performed and in the development of alternative *in vitro* tests which use no vertebrate animals or, indeed, no intact animals at all. Later in this chapter, we will present the rationales driving the development of alternatives.

Though acute toxicology tests are of critical economic and societal importance, their scientific importance has generally not been acknowledged by toxicologists, regulators, and the public. Professionals have historically placed emphasis on longer-term repeat-exposure studies which have been seen as providing definitive answers to health effect questions. The traditional wisdom was that one only sees extreme effects associated with extreme dosages or exposures in acute studies. Also, the longer-term studies are "big-ticket" items that are individually expensive in terms of time (representing 1 to several years of effort toward the development of any compounds which must be registered, such as drugs, food additives, and pesticides), money, and the utilization of available assets. Acute studies have been perceived as being cheap in terms of all these assets (when performed, it should be noted, in a manner that meets the objective of providing the "minimal necessary" information only, such as an LD_{50}) and could readily be repeated if poorly performed or failed to produce the required data.

At the same time, the general public and others, both in and out of the field of toxicology, have come to question both the relevance of these tests and their sensitivity in terms of detecting true potential hazards to humans. These questions arise due to some misrepresentations of what is done (in the popular press and in literature produced by animal rights groups), lack of understanding of the objectives of these tests (both by the public and by some of those who are in the field of toxicology), and some real problems in study design, conduct, and interpretation. Such tests, however, remain a regulatory requirement. The health effects testing guidelines published in 1996 by the EPA's Office of Prevention, Pesticides and Toxic Substances clearly states, "The Agency considers the evaluation of toxicity following short term exposure to a chemical to be an integral step."

As this text will hopefully establish, most of the legitimate concerns about acute tests arise from a lack of understanding of, and focus on, the objectives to be served. For those whose information needs end with acute studies, the requirement to get the maximum quality of information should be clear. For many others, acute studies are done as a step to generate data to improve (or often, even allow) the design and conduct of longer-term studies. When conducted as a preparatory step, acute studies can define doses to be used, organs to be closely scrutinized, and special tests or observations to be incorporated. Though the traditional wisdom has been that acute studies do not predict the results of longer-term studies and, in fact, they cannot generally predict true chronic effects, there are data in the literature covering large numbers of studies (Wiel and McCollister, 1963; Gad *et al.,* 1984) which establish that, when properly done, a short-term or acute study can predict target organs for long-term studies. It should be noted that such predictive value is increased markedly (indeed, may only exist) when the acute study is conducted at levels which are not lethal during the term of the test (generally, 2 weeks after dosing).

QUESTIONS OF RELEVANCE AND SENSITIVITY

The most critical questions about acute studies as they are currently conducted concern their ability to predict potential hazard to humans and the degree to which they either overpredict or are not sensitive enough to predict human effects, especially the former (that is, that the tests are too sensitive).

The first question that must be addressed is how well each of the acute study types predict the human case. We say "study types" because, as will be elaborated later, there are multiple types aimed at answering quite different questions. A problem with assessing relevance to humans is that there are generally very little human data where the essential factors which influence the severity of acute effects (dose, concentration, vehicle, and extent and duration of exposure) are described. As will be addressed in conjunction with each specific test type, there is, however, data such that some comparison of animal model and human sensitivities can be made. But, in general, there is not much "controlled" human data where both exposure factors and effects are described tightly enough to allow side-by-side direct comparisons to animals.

A factor which adds to the relevance debate arises from misconceptions and illusions on the part of both the general public and toxicologists. The former believes that there must be a direct point-for-point correlation in both structure and function for an animal model to accurately predict what happens in humans. Among toxicologists, on the other hand, there are widely held (but often unfounded) beliefs as to the existence of certain "best models for man." An example is the belief that the pig is the best model of dermal absorption in man—in fact, as will be shown in this specific case (and in most general cases), the best animal model to predict what happens in humans varies with the physicochemical nature of the compounds to be studied. The only universal model for humans—that is, one which would best predict what would happen at a given endpoint across the full range of chemical structures, concentrations, etc.—is other humans. It is clearly not ethically or morally acceptable to let people be our device to detect those compounds which present an unacceptable risk in the marketplace or environment. Human testing is only ethically acceptable when either the risk is negligible (patch testing for irritation or sensitization with low-risk materials) or there is reason to believe that there is a potential benefit that outweighs the risk.

The problem of relevance is further compounded by the fact that all such tests must use relatively small numbers of animals (or isolated tissues, cells, or whatever) to predict what would occur in a much larger and heterogeneous population at risk (that is, the human population which may be exposed). The level of an effect that would be unacceptable in a human population is dependent on the nature of the effect and the use for which the chemical is intended. But generally such risk levels are low enough that an animal study with sufficient animals to ensure, with statistical confidence, that such an effect is not present would have to be unacceptably large. Also, in general, human exposures will be at relatively low levels.

The solution to this quandary has, as its basis, the concept of dose–response. This concept, which is the single most fundamental principle in toxicology, holds that there are statistical and biological trends which accompany any trend in doses. As dose increases (above some minimum level, called threshold, below which there is no response to or effect from exposure to the agent), both incidence and severity of adverse effects will also increase. Incidence (statistical trend) means that, as dose increases, so does the proportion of animals suffering an adverse effect (Fig. 1). Severity (biological trend) means that as the dose increases, the extent of adverse effect seen in individual animals increases both qualitatively and quantitatively.

Dose–response is used to address the need for increased power in toxicology tests by conducting the tests (particularly in acute studies, in which test animal group sizes generally range from, depending on the test, 5 to 15 animals per group) at higher doses (the high end of the dose–response curve). This acts to increase both the statistical and biological incidence of effect. The problem is, of course, to not overly increase the doses to the point that either animals do not survive long enough to express effects or that the extreme high-dose effects are such that they mask effects that may otherwise be more relevant to the dose range in which we are truly interested.

Therefore, what this means is that, to provide maximum possible protection against potentially hazardous effects in humans, acute toxicity studies are

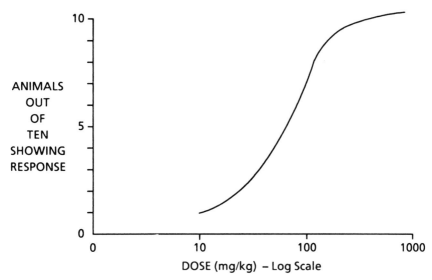

FIGURE 1   Dose–response curve with response being displayed as a quantal event.

conducted at high doses and concentrations and in such a manner as to generally maximize the response (and, therefore, the sensitivity of the test system). The ways of doing this, other than maximizing dose and/or concentration, will be reviewed for each study type. But it should be kept in mind that this is a basic objective and design feature of all the tests described in this volume. The application of the results to humans is performed by either severely limiting potential human exposure for materials found positive in single endpoint studies (as will be defined later) or by applying a safety factor (usually 10-fold from the highest observed no effect level or 100-fold from the lowest observed effect level) to project a "safe" dose (Weil, 1972).

How well do the current test designs serve to give results which predict potential human hazards. This will be looked at for each study type throughout this volume. The general consensus for all the study types is presented in summary in Table 1.

DEFINING TEST OBJECTIVES

The first (and most important) step in designing acute studies (or, indeed, any kind of study) is to develop a clear statement of the objective of the study—that is, what is the question to be answered?

TABLE 1   General Predictive Bias of Current Acute Toxicity Studies

	Overall predictive value of effects in humans		
Study endpoint	Over[a]	No bias	Under[b]
Rabbit eye irritation	X		
Rabbit skin irritation	X		
Rabbit skin corrosion	X		
Dermal sensitization	X		
Muscular irritation		X	
Photosensitization	X		
Phototoxicity	X		
Acute oral		X	
Acute dermal	X		
Acute inhalation		X	
Cytotoxicity	X		

[a]Overprediction, of course, leads to a higher incidence of "false positives." Overprediction is of both incidence and severity.
[b]Underprediction leads to a higher incidence of "false negatives." This is generally not acceptable.

Based on the broadest classification of tests in terms of focus of question asked, there may generally be said to be two major sets of objectives. The first leads to what can be called single endpoint tests. Single endpoint tests are those for which only one restricted question is being asked. Such studies, as will be shown below, are generally straightforward and generate relatively simple date.

Such tests and their objectives (the questions they ask) are detailed below.

A. Primary dermal irritation (PDI): Evaluate the potential of a single dermal exposure to cause skin irritation.
B. Primary eye irritation: Evaluate the potential of a single ocular exposure to cause eye irritation.
C. Dermal corrosivity: Determine if a single 4-hr dermal exposure will result in skin corrosion.
D. Dermal sensitization: Evaluate the potential of a material to cause delayed contact hypersensitivity.
E. Photosensitization: Evaluate the potential of a material to cause a sunlight-activated delayed-contact hypersensitivity.
F. Lethality: Determine if a single dose of a material, at a predetermined level, is lethal.
G. Cytotoxicity: Predict biocompatibility of a material in the body.

The second category contains the shotgun tests. The name "shotgun" suggests itself for these studies because it is not known in advance what the endpoints are. Rather, the purpose of the study is to identify and quantitate all potential systemic effects resulting from a single exposure to a compound. Once known, specific target organ effects can then be studied in detail if so desired. Accordingly, the generalized design of these studies is to expose groups of animals to controlled amounts or concentrations of the material of interest, then to observe for and measure as many parameters as is practical over a period during or following the exposure. Further classification of tests within this category is defined either by the route by which test animals are exposed or dosed (generally, oral, dermal, inhalation, intraperitoneal, or intravenous are the options here) or by the scope (or "level") of question being asked. Shotgun acute systemic tests attempt to address some portion of the following objectives:

Meet a minimal regulatory need or requirement.
Set doses for later studies.
Identify very or unusually toxic agents.
Estimate lethality potential.
Identify organ system affected.

Which of these objectives are addressed (or how many) depends on the level of the study. In acute studies, there are generally three distinct levels of type of answers sought and, therefore, of degree of effort merited in performing a study. The simplest level is the screen, which is designed purely to identify compounds which give such extreme results (such as lethality at very low dosage levels) that no data are desired on other aspects of toxicity. A subset of these are limit tests, which ask a pass/fail question at one dose level. The intermediate category is the probe, which is intended to give enough information to either perform a more definitive study or to be able to compare, rank, and order a set of compounds (prioritizing them for further study). The most complicated acute study is intended to provide as much information as is possible from an acute study and is frequently used when it is intended to be the "definitive" toxicology study for the foreseeable future.

Each of these three levels may actually occur in either of the two major categories of acute studies (in terms of the scope of questions asked). Thus, single endpoint studies (which assess dermal and ocular irritation and corrosion, sensitization, photosensitization, and lethality) and shotgun studies (which assess or identify systemic effects such as target organs and no-observable-effect levels) may be screens, probes, or full-blown evaluations, but the first two tend to only occur in shotgun-type studies. In this volume, we will review each of the common designs for these tests, their objectives, the types of data they generate, and some current alternative test designs and models. We shall also present some of the problems associated with test design and analysis.

To understand both the history and the current state of study design, it is essential to realize why such tests are being performed. For the purposes of this book, in which the major concern is chemicals in commerce (either currently or potentially) or the environment, there are four major reasons behind such testing.

1. *Good stewardship:* Before any product or material is introduced into the marketplace or people are potentially put at risk by being exposed to it (and allowed to find ways to use and misuse it), any moral person feels the need to ensure that no unreasonable risk is presented by the product. In many cases, we let the next two reasons (fear of litigation and regulatory requirements) stand for this moral requirement. And, often what satisfies one of these other reasons (particularly in the case of regulatory requirements) is confused with meeting the test criteria for the good stewardship reason for testing: Do I have sufficient information to be reasonably sure that my product will not harm anyone?

2. *Fear of litigation:* The first of the major reasons for acute tests to be performed by manufacturers or developers is to provide data to avoid (by not manufacturing or changing the conditions of use of a potentially dangerous product) being sued for adverse health effects caused by their product or to at least have a strong basis for defense should one be sued. Materials which injure or are widely perceived to injure people are litigens—they induce/ cause litigation.

3. *Regulatory requirements:* One of the social phenomena since 1960 has been an explosion in the number of agencies and regulations involved in seeking to protect individuals and the environment from the adverse effects of man-made materials. These regulations generally take the form of requiring certain tests, performed in accordance with a set of guidelines. These agencies and regulations are known (and will be identified in this volume) by an acronym (such as FDA for Food and Drug Administration), a list of (and key to) which is provided as Appendix A. Such regulatory requirements are precursors to development or marketing in some cases (pharmaceuticals, pesticides, and cosmetics, for example) and are a necessity to packaging and shipping in almost all. There is an increasing tendency for these testing requirements to take the form of a checklist. A real problem is ensuring that a test meets all of the relevant regulatory requirements, especially because some contradict each other. For each test type, we have presented a summary of relevant regulatory requirements as a table in the appropriate chapter. Table 2 presents a summary of current references for each of the testing requirements. This has led to an approach to the design and conduct of acute toxicity studies which, at least in common practice, has become very rigid and has not been subject to the sort of critical review which is frequently focused on proposed

TABLE 2 Summary of Acute Toxicology Major Guidelines Study Design Requirements

Regulatory body	Guideline	Acute dermal toxicity	Acute oral toxicity	Acute inhalation toxicity	Primary dermal irritation	Primary ocular	Dermal sensitization
U.S. Environmental Protection Agency (EPA FIFRA)	Pesticide Assessment Guideline Subdivision F: Hazard Identification; Human and Domestic Animals	Section 81-2	Section 81-1	Section 81-3	Section 81-5	Section 81-4	Section 81-6
U.S. Environmental Protection Agency (EPA FIFRA)	Health Effects Guidelines 40 CFR 798	798.1100	798.1175	798.1150	798.4770	798.4500	798.4100
U.S. Consumer Product Safety Commission (FHSA)	16 CHR, Chapter II	1500.40	None	None	1500.41	1500.42	None
U.S. Department of Transportation (DOT)	49 CFR 173	173.132	173.132	173.132	173.136	None	None
Organization for Economic Development and Cooperation (OECD)	OECD Guidelines for Testing Chemicals, Section 4, Health Effects	Guideline 402	Guideline 401, Guideline 420 (fixed dose), Guideline 423 (toxic class)	Guideline 403	Guideline 404	Guideline 405	Guideline 406
European Economic Community (EEC or EU)	Methods for the Determination of Toxicity, Directive 92/69, Adaption of 67/548/EEC, Annex V	Part B3	Part B1, Part B1 bis (fixed dose)	Part B2	Part B4	Part B5	Part B6
Japanese Ministry of Health and Welfare (JMOHW)	Guidelines for Toxicity Studies of Drugs Manual, January 1994	Guideline (1), p. 114	Guideline (1), p. 114	Guideline (1), p. 114	None	None	Guideline (6), p. 129
Japanese Ministry of Agriculture, Forestries, and Fisheries (JMAFF)	59 NohSan No. 4200 1985, Guidance on Toxicology Study Data for Application of Agricultural Chemical Registration	p. 20	p. 19	p. 22	p. 25	p. 23	p. 27

new study designs or test types. The changes made in the past 15 years have been largely restricted to using more animals and rigidly following a standard protocol. The first of these changes, in an attempt to increase the value of the information from such studies by increasing statistical power, is a crude approach to improving study design. The second change is meant to ensure the integrity of the data trail and documentation, but by its nature makes sensitive and efficient conduct of investigations more difficult. Clearly, use of some of the approaches described in Gad *et al.* (1984), Gad and Weil (1988), or the statistics chapter in this book (and more to the point, adoption of the underlying philosophy) would significantly reduce animal usage while increasing both the amount and the value of information gained.

4. *Research and development tool:* For many classes of chemicals, there are many "candidate" compounds or mixtures from which, after a lengthy and costly development process, one or a few products will actually be manufactured and will enter commerce. Acute toxicology tests can and should play a significant part in the process by which candidate compounds are eliminated, allowing resources to be efficiently employed on those compounds or mixtures with the greatest promise.

DISPLAY OF STUDY DESIGNS: THE LINE CHART

To make it easier to display and understand the design and conduct of studies presented and discussed in this volume, a common shorthand for presenting these facts has been adopted and will be used throughout this volume. This devise is the line chart.

The line in the line chart, with bars to identify discrete points or intervals in time (generally key events) during the interval of the study, is the starting point. As the first of several conventions for these charts, the first day any animal (or other test system) is dosed or exposed to a chemical will be designed Study Day 0 (SD 0) except in lethality and systemic oral tests (Chapters 7 and 9), where this is denoted as Day 1. Figure 2 as a simple example of such a line chart.

Note that the line charts also provide all the information on any special aspects of a study design [such as special measurements (histopathology in the example) and numbers of animals per group]. It should also be noted that the specific study designs presented in this book are only one way of performing the subject studies. There are other, equally appropriate, ways which vary in some manner or another.

A   **Acute Oral Toxicity Study Design**

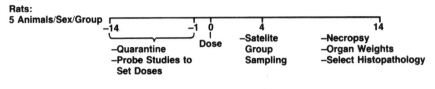

- Body Weights: Days –1, 0, 1, 4, 7, 11 and 14
- Clinical Signs Every Day After Dosing
- Neurobehavioral Signs: Days 0, 1, 4, 7 and 14
- Satelite groups may be for hematology, necropsy, or both

FIGURE 2A   Example line chart for study design and conduct. Shown is a diagrammatic display of the key events (and design features) of a supplemented acute oral toxicity study.

THEORY AND USE OF SCREENS, INNOVATIONS, AND ALTERNATIVES

As was stated at the beginning of this chapter, there are significant questions condemning current practices in acute toxicology testing and significant forces behind changing these practices. The questions include those of sensitivity, reproducibility, and relevance, while the forces for change are largely a result of increased concern as to both reducing the numbers of animals used in research and testing (or even eliminating their use altogether) and ensuring the use of the most humane methods possible in such testing.

Throughout this book, three approaches [to pursuing new and more effective (and efficient) ways to do necessary testing] will be presented or at least overviewed. These are screens, alternatives, and innovations. These approaches each have a separate set of assumptions, rationale, and necessary steps for development and general acceptance. These are addressed in the sections that follow.

SCREENS

One major set of activities in toxicology (and in pharmacology, for that matter) is screening for the presence or absence of an effect. Such screens are almost always focused on detecting a single endpoint of effect (such as mutagenicity, lethality, neural or developmental toxicity, etc.) and have a particular set of operating characteristics in common.

1. A large number of compound are to be evaluated so that ease of performance (efficiency) is a major desirable characteristic.

2. The screen must be very sensitive in its detection of potential effective agents. An absolute minimum of effective agents should escape detection—that is, there should be very few false negatives (in other words, the type II error rate or β, as defined in the statistics chapter, should be low).

3. It is desirable that the number of false positives be small (that is, that there be a low type I error rate or α level).

4. Items 1–3 are all to some degree contradictory, requiring the researchers involved to agree on a set of compromises. These typically start with acceptance of a relatively high α level (0.10 or more).

5. In an effort to better serve item 1, such screens are frequently performed in batteries such that multiple endpoints are measured in the same mode. Additionally, such measurements may be repeated over a period of time in each model.

In an early toxicity screen, a relatively large number of compounds will be tested. It is unlikely that one will stand out so much as to be statistically significantly more important than all other compounds. A more or less continuous range of activities will be found. Compounds showing the highest activity will not proceed to the next assay in the series and may be used as lead compounds in a new cycle of testing and evaluation.

Each assay can have an associated activity criterion. If the result for a particular test compound meets this criterion, the compound may pass to the next stage. This criterion could be based on statistical significance (i.e., all compounds with observed activities significantly greater than the control at the 5% level could be tagged). However, for early screens, such a criterion may be too strict, and few compounds may go through to further testing.

A useful indicator of the efficiency of an assay series is the frequency of discovery of truly active compounds. This is related to the probability of discovery and to the degree of risk associated with a compound. These two factors, in turn, depend on the distribution of activities in the test series and the probability at each stage of rejecting and accepting compounds with given activities.

Statistical modeling of the assay system may lead to the improvement of the design of the system to reduce the interval between discoveries. Preliminary results suggest that, in the early screens, it may be beneficial to increase the number of compounds tested, decrease the number of animals per group, and increase the range and number of doses. The result will be less information on more structures, but an overall increase in the frequency of discovery (assuming that truly active compounds are entering the system at a steady rate).

The design of each assay and the choice of the activity criterion should therefore be adjusted, bearing in mind the relative costs of retaining false positives and rejecting false negatives. Decreasing the group sizes in the early assays reduces the chance of obtaining significance at any particular level (such as 5%) so that the activity criterion must be relaxed, in a statistical sense, to allow more compounds through. At some stage, however, it becomes too expensive to continue screening many false positives and the criteria must be tightened up accordingly.

An excellent introduction to this subject is Redman's (1981) interesting approach which identifies four characteristics of an assay. It is assumed that a compound is either active or inactive, and that the proportion of actives can be estimated from past experience. After testing, a compound will be classified as positive or negative. It is then possible to design the assay so as to optimize the following characteristics:

"Sensitivity"—the ratio of the true positives to total actives
"Specificity"—the ratio of true negatives to total inactives
"Positive accuracy"—the ratio of true to observed positives
"Negative accuracy"—the ratio of true to observed negatives

An advantage to testing more compounds is that it gives the opportunity to generalize activity for structural classes of compounds, or study quantitative structure—activity relationships (QSARs). QSARs can be used to predict the activity of new compounds and thus reduce the chance of *in vivo* testing on extremely toxic compounds. It can increase the proportion of truly active compounds passing through the system.

In conclusion, it may be said that maximization of the performance of a series of screening assays requires close collaboration between the toxicologist, chemist, and statistician. It should be noted, however, that screening forms only part of a much larger research and development context.

Screens may thus truly be considered the biological equivalent of exploratory data analysis (EDA). EDA methods, in fact, provide a number of useful possibilities for less rigid and yet quite utilitarian approaches to the statistical analysis of the data from screens.

ALTERNATIVES AND INNOVATIONS: RATIONALE

There are three major sets of reasons behind efforts to develop either alternatives to *in vivo* tests (which do not use intact vertebrate animals) or innovative approaches (variations) on existing test designs. The first are questions about the adequacy of current *in vivo* designs. In assessing the adequacy of the currently employed test designs to fulfill the objectives behind their use, we must evaluate them in terms of (1) their accuracy (how well they predict the hazard to humans), (2) whether comparable results can be obtained by different technicians and laboratories, and (3) reproducibility and precision within any single laboratory (how well a single lab can repeat tests and accurately evaluate standard or "control" materials) (Fig. 2B).

The second reason concerns questions about the ethics of how animals are used, or indeed whether they should be used at all. The pressure of public opinion, exerted with variable intensity in different parts of the world, to reduce animal use in biomedical and toxicology research and testing has greatly stimulated the interest in "alternative methods." The latter term was defined in 1959 by Russel and Burch and implies the three R's: (a) the replacement of the use of animals; (b) a reduction in the number of animals needed in a particular test; and (c) refinements or improvements in technique such that the amount of suffering endured by test animals is reduced (Goldberg, 1985). The toxicologist must also keep in mind the fourth R—responsibility, which is to ensure that products entering the marketplace harm no one when used correctly.

The third major reason is the evolution of toxicology from a descriptive to a mechanistic science, and the impact of the economical and societal ramifications of these changes. Since 1960, the field of toxicology has become increasingly complex and controversial in both its theory and its practice. Much of this change is due to the evolution of the field. As in all other sciences, toxicology started as a descriptive science. Living organisms, be they human or otherwise, were exposed to chemical or physical agents and the adverse effects which followed were observed. But as a sufficient body of descriptive data was accumulated, it became possible to infer and study underlying mechanisms of action—to determine in a broader sense why adverse effects occurred.

		ACTUAL CASE	
B		**GROUPS DIFFERENT**	**GROUPS NOT DIFFERENT**
STATISTICAL TEST RESULTS	SIGNIFICANT DIFFERENCE	CONCLUSION CORRECT	TYPE I ERROR (P = α LEVEL)
	NO SIGNIFICANT DIFFERENCE	TYPE II ERROR (P = β LEVEL)	CONCLUSION CORRECT

FIGURE 2B   A table showing the possible interpretations of outcome of the statistical analysis of a biological study, including the two types of error.

As with all sciences, toxicology has thus entered a later stage of development—the mechanistic stage, in which active contributions to the field encompass both descriptive and mechanistic studies. In this mechanistic stage, we are coming to understand the general principles which dictate the nature of biological responses and the basis for these principles. Frequently, in fact, present-day studies are a combination of both approaches.

As a result of this evolution, studies must be designed and executed to generate increased amounts of data which are then utilized to address specific areas of concern (such as renal or cardiovascular effects). At the same time, the upwardly spiraling cost of everything involved in such studies (labor, equipment, supplies, test material, and animals) is exerting a significant pressure to be as efficient as possible; use no more of each of these components than are necessary to have reasonable expectation of answering the desired questions.

Innovations vary from alternatives in that they do not call for such radical departures from what has been done (and, therefore, what we know) and that there is no existing experience or database to guide us in solving problems with test systems and in interpreting what results mean. Innovations are more evolutionary than revolutionary and, therefore, offer fewer risks (and rewards).

REFERENCES

Environmental Protection Agency (EPA) (1996). Health Effects Guidelines UPPTS 870. 1000 Acute Toxicity Testng Background. EPA 712-6-96-189.

Gad, S. C., and Weil, C. S. (1988). *Statistics and Experimental Design for Toxicologist,* 2nd ed. Telford Press, Caldwell, NJ.

Gad, S. C., Smith, A. C., Cramp, A. L., Gavigan, F. A., and Derelanko, M. J. (1984). Innovative designs and practices for acute systemic toxicity studies. *Drug Chem. Toxicol.* 7(5), 423–434.

Goldberg, A. M. (1985). Integration of fundamental knowledge and *in vitro* testing strategies. In *Concepts in Toxicology* (F. Homburger, Ed.), Vol. 3, pp. 1–5. Karger, Basel.

Redman, C. E. (1981). Screening compounds for clinically active drugs. In *Statistics in the Pharmaceutical Industry* (C. R. Buncher & J. Tsay, Eds.), pp. 19–42. Dekker, New York.

Weil, C. S. (1972). Statistics vs. safety factors and scientific judgments in the evaluation of safety for man. *Toxicol. Appl. Pharmacol.* 21, 454–463.

Weil, C. S., and McCollister, D. D. (1963). Relationship between short- and long-term feeding studies in designing and effective toxicity test. *Agric Food Chem.* 11(6), 486–491.

CHAPTER 2

Acute Toxicology Program: Study Design and Development

The most important part of any toxicology evaluation program is the initial overall process of developing an adequate date package to define the potential hazards associated with the manufacturer, sale, use, and disposal of a product. This process calls for asking a series of very interactive questions, with many of the questions serving to identify and/or modify their successors. This book is designed as a companion and guide to the acute toxicity aspects of such a process, and this chapter is intended as a step-by-step guide to what should be the essential, accompanying process of question-asking.

In the product safety evaluation process, we must first determine what information is needed. This calls for understanding of the way the product is to be made and used and disposed of, with the potential exposures to humans associated with these processes. This step will be covered in this chapter and forms the basis on which a hazard and toxicity profile is outlined. Once such a profile is outlined (as illustrated by Fig. 3), one performs a search of the available literature to determine what is already known. With consideration of this literature information and of the previously defined exposure potential, a tier approach is used to generate a list of tests or studies to be performed.

			Component			Intermediate	Waste Material
	Mixture	1	2	3	4	A	B
1. Literature review							
2. Physiochemical properties							
3. Use/exposure hazard							
1. LD_{50} (Rat)							
(Mouse)							
2. LD_{50} (Rat)							
(Mouse)							
3, Dermal irritation							
4. Ocular irritation							
5. Skin sensitization							
6. Mutagenisis							
7. Teratology							
8. Reproduction							
9. Repeated exposure studies							
10. Carcinogenicity							
11. Metabolism							

FIGURE 3   Hazard and toxicity profile—A form of collecting and summarizing the essential data for understanding and managing the potential hazards of a material. Shown is a form set up for a mixture composed of four components, having one intermediate in its formulation, and producing in the end a single waste material to be disposed of.

This chapter seeks to develop an understanding of the principles on which such programs (and, more important, the studies composing such programs) are selected and designated.

What goes into a tier system is determined (as will be seen in later chapters) both by regulatory requirements imposed by government agencies and by the philosophy of the parent organization. How such tests are actually performed is determined on one of two bases. The first (and most common) is the menu approach: selecting a series of standard design tests as "modules" of data. The second is an interactive approach. In this interactive approach, studies are designed (or designs are selected) based on our needs and what we have come to know about the product. The test designs and approaches presented in the bulk of the chapters in this text address these particular testing needs in detail within the scope of acute toxicology.

Data structures should, of course, be customized to meet specific product needs.

DEFINING THE OBJECTIVE

The initial and most important aspect of an acute toxicity evaluation program is the series of steps which leads to an actual statement of problems or of the objectives of any testing and research program. This definition of objectives is essential and, as proposed here, consists of five steps: defining product or material use, quantitating or estimating exposure potential, identifying potential hazards, gathering baseline data, and, finally, designing and defining the actual research program. Each of these steps is presented and discussed in detail below. Identifying how a material is to be used, what it is to be used for, and how it is to be made are the essential first three questions to be answered before a meaningful assessment program can be performed. These determine, to a large extent, how many people are potentially exposed, to what extent and by what routes they are exposed, and what benefits are perceived or gained from product use. The answers to these questions are generally categorical or qualitative and become quantitative (as will be reviewed in the next section) at a later step (frequently long after acute data have been generated).

DEFINING EXPOSURE POTENTIAL

Starting with an examination of how a material is to be made (or how it is already being made), there frequently are several process segments which each represent separate problems. Commonly, much of a manufacturing process is "closed" (that is, occurs in sealed airtight systems), limiting exposures to leaks with (generally) low-level inhalation and dermal exposures of significant portions of a plant workforce and short-term higher level inhalation and dermal exposures to smaller numbers of personnel (maintenance and repair workers). Smaller segments of the process will almost invariably not be closed. These segments are most commonly either where some form of manual manipulation is required or where the segment requires a large volume or space (such as when fibers or other objects are spun or formed or individually coated or where the product is packaged—such as powders being placed into bags or polymers being removed from molds). The exact manner and quantity of each segment of the manufacturing process, given the development of a categorization of exposures for each of these segments, will then serve to help quantitate the identified categories.

Likewise, consideration of what a product is to be used for and how it is to be used should be used to identify who (outside the manufacturing process) will potentially be exposed, by what routes, and to what extent.

The answers to these questions, again, will generate a categorized set of answers but will also serve to identify which particular sets of regulatorily required toxicity testing may be operative (such as those for DOT, FDA, or CPSC). If a product is to be worn (such as clothing or jewelry) or used on or as an environmental surface (such as household carpeting or wall covering), the potential for the exposure of a large number of people (albeit at low levels in the case of most materials) is very large, while uses such as for exterior portions of buildings would have much lower potentials for the number of individuals exposed. Likewise, the nature of the intended use (e.g., as a pharmaceutical vs an industrial product) determines potential for extent and degree of exposure in overt and subtle manners. For example, a finish for carpets to be used in the home has a much greater potential for dermal and even oral (in the case of infants) exposure than such a product used only for carpeting in offices. Likewise, in general, true consumer products (such as household cleaners) have a greater potential for both accidental exposure and misuse.

THE DATA MATRIX

Once the types of exposures have been identified and the quantities approximated, one can develop a toxicity matrix by identifying the potential hazards. Such an identification can proceed by one of three major approaches:

Analogy from data reported in the literature
Structure–activity relationships (SARs)
Predictive testing

Larson *et al.* (1995) have detailed how to perform both rapid and detailed literature reviews. Such reviews can be performed either on the actual compounds of interest or on compounds which are by structure and/or use similar. Either way, the information from a literature review will rarely match exactly our current interests (that is, the same compounds being produced and used the same ways), but analogous relationships can frequently be developed.

The use of SARs has been presented elsewhere (Gad and Weil, 1988) and will not be addressed here. There are, however, nonmathematical analogy methods which are still used effectively. These methods are really forms of pattern recognition, starting with a knowledge of the hazards associated with similar or related structures. An example of such a scheme is that of Cramner *et al.* (1978), in which a decision tree based on structural features (or lack of them) is used in a decision tree approach to categorize potential hazards.

The third approach, which the bulk of this book addresses, is actual acute predictive testing. All the major forms of predictive testing for acute effects are addressed by one or more chapters elsewhere in this book. The next section sets forth a philosophy for test and test program design.

It should be noted, as pointed out in the Introduction, that each of these three approaches has the potential to evaluate hazards in one of two ways: The first way is to identify and/or classify existing types of hazards. If the potential for a hazard is unacceptable for the desired use of the material (such as a corrosive would be for a cosmetic), then this level of answer is quite sufficient. The second way (or degree to which) a category of potential toxicity may be addressed is quantitatively. Quantitative (as opposed to categorical or qualitative) toxicity assessments require more work and are more expensive. This principle will be stressed throughout this text. It should be recognized that the literature approach can really only categorize potential hazards, and that SAR approaches are most effective as screens to classify potential hazards. Only predictive testing is effective at quantitating toxicity, and testing may also be designed (either purposely or by oversight) so that it serves to screen or classify toxicities.

It should be noted that there is a major area of weakness in all three approaches. This is the question of mixtures. The literature, SAR methods, or our current testing methods are not effective at evaluating compounds other than pure compounds. This problem will be addressed in some detail at the end of this book.

TEST SELECTION AND DESIGN

The majority of the chapters in this book are devoted to the conduct and interpretation of actual tests and studies in toxicology. There are, however, general principles for the design of these tests. Before any tests are conducted at all, however, a program must be designed so that resources are employed in an efficient manner at the same time as all required information is generated.

As was pointed out at the beginning of this chapter, there are three approaches to selecting which tests will be included in a safety evaluation package: battery testing, tier testing, and the special case of SAR approaches to designing programs to test series of compounds. For all three approaches, one must first perform a review of existing data and then decide whether or not to repeat any of the tests reported. If the judgment is made that the literature data are too unreliable or incomplete, then a repeat may be in order.

The battery testing approach, which is not generally recommended or favored, except for acute testing, calls for performing a set of tests from an existing list. This approach has two advantages. First, it is the most practical and easiest to control for an operation testing as many compounds as possible (which is commonly the case in acute testing). Second, the results of such test packages are easy to compare to those of other compounds evaluated in identical packages. The main disadvantages are also compelling, however. First, battery programs use up more of every resource (animals, manpower, and test material, for example) except time. Second, the questions asked and answered beyond the acute tests by the battery approach are not as sharply focused because the test designs employed cannot be modified in light of data from lower tier tests.

The tier approach, which can have some application even to acute testing programs, arose in the 1970s when concern about health effects broadened in scope and there were insufficient testing capabilities available to do every test on every material of concern. These schemes are proposed as a means of arriving at and performing an appropriate level and efficient course of testing. The levels of testing, or information generation, are arranged in a hierarchical system. Each tier contains a number of suggested tests which can be chosen as needed to complete information gaps or to establish the appropriate information necessary for safe use or disposal of the material. Beck *et al.* (1981) have developed and published a tier approach system. They provide some valuable points of guidance as to criteria for proceeding to the higher (and more expensive) tier levels.

The last approach is for the special case when one is faced with evaluating a large series of materials which have closely related chemical structures and one seeks to rank them as to relative hazard. Frequently, time is a concern in completing such a program for these purposes, and efficiency in use of assets is very much desired. The SAR matrix approach calls for identifying and classifying the structured features of the compounds. These features frequently vary on a simple basis (length of carbon chain or number of substituent nitrogens, for example). One can select the compounds at either end of such a linear series (for example, the compounds with 5 and 18 carbon chains) and evaluate them in a series of acute and mutagenicity tests. From this, one should find out the endpoints (e.g., sensitization potential and dermal irritation) which are of the greatest concern for the compounds in their intended use. Each compound in the series can then be tested for only these endpoints. Those that are then selected for use or further development based on such a methodology should be evaluated fully in a tier approach system.

STUDY DESIGN

The most important step in designing an actual study is to firmly determine the objective(s) behind it, as presented in the first chapter. Based on the broadest classification of tests, there are generally two major sets of objectives. As previously discussed, these are single endpoint and shotgun tests. Acutes, for example, imply a single exposure or a short series of exposures over a brief interval (generally of 24 hr or less) period of dosing of test material. The other objective in designing studies is to meet various regulatory requirements. A complete review of this objective is beyond the intent of this chapter. As it pertains to specific test types, it is addressed in the majority of the other chapters. Also, Page (1986) has provided a good short overview of regulatory considerations and their complications.

Toxicology experiments generally have a twofold purpose. The first regards whether or not an agent results in an effect on a biological system. The second regards how much of an effect is present. Both the cost to perform research to answer such questions and the value that society places on the results of such efforts have continued to increase. Additionally, it has become increasingly desirable for the results and conclusions of studies aimed at assessing the effects of environmental agents to be as clear and unequivocal as possible. It is essential that every experiment and study yield as much information as possible, and that (more specifically) the results of each study have the greatest possible chance of answering the questions it was conducted to address. This process, aimed at structuring experiments to maximize the possibilities of success, is called experimental design.

We have now become accustomed to developing exhaustively detailed protocols for an experiment or study prior to its conduct. However, frequently such protocols do not include or reflect a detailed plan for the statistical analysis of the data generated by the study and, even less frequently, reflect such considerations in their design. A priori selection of statistical methodology (as opposed to the post hoc approach) is as significant a portion of the process of protocol development and experimental design as any other and can measurably enhance the value of the experiment or study. Prior selection of statistical methodologies is essential for proper design of other portions of a protocol such as the number of animals per group or the sampling intervals for body weight. Implied in such a selection is the notion that the toxicologist has both an in-depth knowledge of the area of investigation and an understanding of the general principles of experimental design because the analysis of any set of data is dictated to a large extent by the manner in which the data are obtained.

The four basic statistical principles of experimental design are replication, randomization, concurrent ("local") control, and balance. In abbreviated form, these may be summarized as follows:

Replication: Any treatment must be applied to more than one experimental unit (animal, plate of cells, litter of offspring, etc.). This provides more accuracy in the measurement of a response than can be obtained from a single observation because underlying experimental errors tend to cancel each other out. It also supplies an estimate of the experimental error derived from the variability among each of the measurements taken (or "replicates"). In practice, this means that an experiment should have enough experimental units in each treatment group (that is, a large enough N) so that a reasonably sensitive statistical analysis of data can be performed. The estimation of sample size is addressed in detail later in this chapter.

Randomization: This is practiced to ensure that every treatment shall have its fair share of extreme high and extreme low values. It also serves to allow the toxicologist to proceed as if the assumption of "independence" is valid. That is, there is no avoidable (known) systematic bias in how one obtains data.

Concurrent control: Comparisons between treatments should be made to the maximum extent possible between experimental units from the same closely defined population. Therefore, animals used as a "control" group should come from the same source, lot, age, etc. as test group animals. Except for the treatment being evaluated, test and control animals should be maintained and handled in exactly the same manner.

Balance: If the effect of several different factors is being evaluated simultaneously, the experiment should be laid out in such a way that the contributions of the different factors can be separately distinguished and estimated. There are several ways of accomplishing this using one of several different forms of design, as will be discussed below.

There are four basic experimental design types used in toxicology. These are the randomized block, Latin square, factorial design, and nested design. Other designs that are used are really combinations of these basic designs and are very rarely employed in toxicology. Before examining these four basic types, however, we must first examine the basic concept of blocking.

Blocking is, simply put, the arrangement or sorting of the members of a population (such as all of an available group of test animals) into groups based on certain characteristics which may (but are not sure to) alter an experimental outcome. Such characteristics which may cause a treatment to give a differential effect include genetic background, age, sex, overall activity levels, and so on. The process of blocking then acts (or attempts to act) so that each experimental group (or block) is assigned its fair share of the members of each of these subgroups.

We should now recall that randomization is aimed at spreading out the effect of undetectable or unsuspected characteristics in a population of animals or some portion of this population. The merging of the two concepts of randomization and blocking leads to the first basic experimental design, the randomized block. This type of design requires that each treatment group has at least one member of each recognized group (such as age), the exact members of each block being assigned in an unbiased (or random) fashion.

The second type of experimental design, the Latin square, assumes that we can characterize treatments (whether intended or otherwise) as belonging to clearly separate sets. In the simplest case, these categories are arranged into two sets which may be thought of as rows (e.g., source litter of test animal, with the first litter as row 1, the next as row 2, etc.) and the secondary set of categories as columns (e.g., ages of test animals, with 6–8 weeks as column 1, 8–10 weeks as column 2, etc.). Experimental units are then assigned so that each major treatment (control, low dose, intermediate dose, etc.) appears once and only once in each row and each column. If we denote our test groups as A (control), B (low), C (intermediate), and D (high), such an assignment would appear as follows:

Source litter	6–8 Weeks	8–10 Weeks	10–12 Weeks	12–14 Weeks
		Age		
1	A	C	C	D
2	B	D	D	A
3	C	A	A	B
4	D	B	B	C

The third type of experimental design is the factorial design, in which there are two or more clearly understood treatments, such as exposure level to test chemical, animal age, or temperature. The classical approach to this situation (and to that described under the Latin square) is to hold all but one of the treatments constant, and at any one time to vary just that one factor. Instead, in the factorial design, all levels of a given factor are combined with all levels of every other factor in the experiment. When a change in one factor produces a different change in the response variable at one level of the factor than at other levels of this factor, there is an interaction between these two factors which can then be analyzed as an interaction effect. This is most common in current acute studies.

The last of the major varieties of experimental design are the nested designs, in which the levels of one factor are nested within (or are subsamples of) another factor. That is, each subfactor is evaluated only within the limits of its single larger factor.

A second concept, that of censoring, and its understanding are essential to the design of experiments in toxicology. Censoring is the exclusion of measurements from certain experimental units, or indeed of the experimental units themselves, from consideration in data analysis or inclusion in the experiment at all. Censoring may occur either prior to initiation of an experiment (in modern toxicology, this is almost always a planned procedure), during the course of an experiment (when they are almost universally unplanned, resulting from such factors as the death of animals on test), or after the conclusion of an experiment (when data are usually excluded because of being identified as some form of outlier).

In practice, a priori censoring in toxicology studies occurs in the assignment of experimental units (such as animals) to test groups. The most familiar example is in the common practice of assignment of test animals to study groups, in which the results of otherwise random assignments are evaluated for body weights of the assigned members. If the mean weights are found not to be comparable by some preestablished criterion (such as a 90% probability of difference by analysis of variance) then members are reassigned (censored) to achieve comparability in terms of starting body weights. Such a procedure of animal assignment to groups is known as a censored randomization.

The first precise or calculable aspect of experimental design encountered is determining sufficient test and control group sizes to allow one to have an adequate level of confidence in the results of a study. This number (N) can be calculated using the formula

$$N = \frac{(t_1 + t_2)^2 S}{d^2}$$

where t_1 is the one-tailed t value with $N - 1$ degrees of freedom corresponding to the desired level of confidence, t_2 is the one-tailed t value with $N - 1$ degrees of freedom corresponding to the probability that the sample size will be adequate to achieve the desired precision, d is the acceptable range of variation in the variable of interest, and S is the sample standard deviation, derived typically from historical data and calculated as

$$S = \frac{1}{N - 1} (V_1 - V_2)^2$$

where V is the variable of interest.

A good approximation can be generated by substituting the t values for an infinite number of degrees of freedom.

There are several aspects of experimental design which are specific to the practice of toxicology. Before we look at a suggestion for step-by-step development of experimental designs, the following aspects should first be considered:

1. Frequently, the data gathered from specific measurements of animal characteristics are such that there is wide variability in the data. Often, such wide variability is not present in a control or low-dose group, but in an intermediate dosage group variance inflation may occur. That is, there may be a large standard deviation associated with the measurements from this intermediate group. In the face of such a set of data, the conclusion that there is no biological effect based on a finding of no statistically significant effect might well be erroneous.

2. In designing experiments, a toxicologist should keep in mind the potential effect of involuntary censoring on sample size. In other words, though a study might start with five dogs per group, this provides no margin should any die before the study is ended and blood samples are collected and analyzed. Starting with just enough experimental units per group frequently leaves too few at the end to allow meaningful statistical analysis, and allowances should be made accordingly in establishing group sizes.

3. It is certainly possible to pool the data from several identical toxicological studies. For example, after first having performed an acute inhalation study

in which only three treatment group animals survived to the point at which a critical measure (such as analysis of blood samples) was performed, we would not have enough data to perform a meaningful statistical analysis. We could then repeat the protocol with new control and treatment group animals from the same source. At the end, after assuring ourselves that the two sets of data are comparable, we could combine (or pool) the data from survivors of the second study with those from the first. The costs of this approach, however, would then be both a greater degree of effort expended (than if we had performed a single study with larger groups) and increased variability in the pooled samples (decreasing the power of our statistical methods).

4. Another frequently overlooked design option in toxicology is the use of an unbalanced design—that is, of different group sizes for different levels of treatment. There is no scientific requirement that each group in a study (control, low dose, intermediate dose, and high dose) must have an equal number of experimental units assigned to it. Indeed, there are frequently good reasons to assign more experimental units to one group than to others, and, as we shall see later in this book, all the major statistical methodologies have provisions to adjust for such inequalities, within certain limits. The two most common uses of the unbalanced design have larger groups assigned to either the highest dose, to compensate for losses due to possible deaths during the study, or to the lowest dose, to give more sensitivity in detecting effects at levels close to an effect threshold—or more confidence to the assertion that no effect exists.

5. We are frequently confronted with the situation in which an undesired variable is influencing our experimental results in a nonrandom fashion. Such a variable is called a confounding variable; its presence, as discussed earlier, makes the clear attribution and analysis of effects, at best, difficult and, at worst, impossible. Sometimes such confounding variables are the result of conscious design or management decisions, such as the use of different instruments, personnel, facilities, or procedures for different test groups within the same study. Occasionally, however, such confounding variables are the result of unintentional factors or actions, in which case it can also be called a lurking variable. Examples of such variables are almost always the result of standard operating procedures being violated, such as water not being connected to a rack of animals over a weekend, a set of racks not being cleaned as frequently as others, or a contaminated batch of feed being used.

6. Finally, some thought must be given to the clear definition of what is meant by experimental unit and concurrent control.

The experimental unit in toxicology encompasses a wide variety of possibilities. It may be cells, plates of microorganisms, individual animals, litters of animals, etc. The importance of clearly defining the experimental unit is that the number of such units per group is the N which is used in statistical calculations or analyses and critically affects such calculations.

The experimental unit is the unit which receives treatments and yields a response which is measured and becomes a datum.

A true concurrent control is one that is identical in every manner with the treatment groups except for the treatment being evaluated. This means that all manipulations, including gavaging with equivalent volumes of vehicle or exposing to equivalent rates of air exchanges in an inhalation chamber, should be duplicated in control groups just as they occur in treatment groups.

The goals of the four principles of experimental design are statistical efficiency and the economizing of resources. It is possible to think of design as a logic flow analysis. Such an analysis is conducted in three steps and should be performed every time any major study or project is initiated or, indeed, at regular periods during the course of conduct of a series of "standard" smaller studies. These steps are detailed as follows:

I. Define the objective of the study; get a clear statement of what questions are being asked.

—Can the question, in fact, be broken down into a set of subquestions?

—Are we asking one or more of these questions repeatedly? For example, does X (an event or effect) develop at 30, 60, or 90+ days and/or does it progress/regress or recover?

—What is our model to be in answering these questions? Is it appropriate and acceptably sensitive?

II. For each subquestion (i.e., separate major variable to be studied):

—How is the variable of interest to be measured?

—What is the nature of the data generated by the measure? Are we getting an efficient set of data? Are we buying too little information (would another technique improve the quality of the information generated to the point that it becomes a higher "class" of data?) or too much information (i.e., does some underlying aspect of the measure limit the class of data obtainable within the bounds of feasibility of the effort?)?

—Are there possible interactions between measurements? Can they be separated/identified?

—Is our N (sample size) both sufficient and efficient?

—What is the control—formal or informal? Is it appropriate?

—Are we needlessly adding confounding variables (asking inadvertent or unwanted questions)?

—Are there "lurking variables" present? There are undesired and not readily recognized differences which can affect results, such as different technicians observing different groups of animals.

—How large an effect will be considered biologically significant? This is a question which can only be resolved by reference to experience or historical control data.

III. What are the possible outcomes of the study—i.e., what answers are possible to both our subquestions and our major question?

—How do we use these answers?

—Do the possible answers offer a reasonable expectation of achieving the objectives that caused us to initiate the study?

—What new questions may these answers cause us to ask? Can the study be redesigned before it is actually started so that these "revealed" questions may be answered in the original study?

When considering the last portion of our logic analysis, we must start by considering each of the things which may go wrong during the study. These include, for example, the occurrence of an infectious disease, the finding that extreme nasal and respiratory irritation was occurring in test animals, or the uncovering of a hidden variable. Do we continue or stop exposures? How will we now separate those portions of observed effects which are due to the chemical under study and those portions which are due to the disease process? Can we preclude (or minimize) the possibility of a disease outbreak by doing a more extensive health surveillance and quarantine on our test animals prior to the start of the study? Could we select a better test model—one that is not as sensitive to upper respiratory or nasal irritation?

There are some common pitfalls that occur in the design of acute studies, proving that it is quite possible to design a study for failure. Some of these common shortfalls include the following:

1. Wrong animal model.
2. Wrong route.
3. Wrong vehicle or form of test material.
4. In studies in which several dose levels are studied, the worst thing that can happen is to have an effect at the lowest level tested (not telling you what dose in animals, much less in man, is safe). The next worst thing is to not have an effect at the highest dose tested (generally meaning that you will not know what the signs of toxicity are and it will invalidate a study in the eyes of many regulatory agencies).
5. Making leaps of faith. An example is to set dose levels based on others' data and to then dose all your test animals. At the end of the day, all animals in all dose levels are dead. The study is over; the problem remains.
6. Using the wrong concentration of test material in a study. Many effects (including both dermal and gastrointestinal irritation, for example) are very concentration dependent.

The vehicle for translating a study design into the finished product is the protocol. A good protocol details who will do what, when, where, and how. As such, it might well be considered to be like the itinerary for a long and complicated trip. Gralla (1981) has provided excellent guidance as to the do's and dont's of protocol preparation.

REFERENCES

Beck, L. W., Maki, A. W., Artman, N. R., and Wilson, E. R. (1981). Outline and criteria for evaluating the safety of new chemicals. *Regul. Toxicol. Pharmacol.* 1, 19–58.

Cramner, C. M., Ford, R. A., and Hall, R. L. (1978). Estimation of toxic hazard—A decision tree approach. *Fd. Cosmet. Toxicol.* 16, 255–276.

Gad, S. C., and Weil, C. S. (1988). *Statistics and Experimental Design for Toxicologists,* 2nd ed. Telford Press, Caldwell, NJ.

Gralla, E. J. (1981). *Scientific Considerations in Monitoring and Evaluating Toxicological Research.* Hemisphere, New York.

Larson, D. L., King, T. O., Nelson, R. P., and Gad, S. C. (1995). Information sources: Building and maintaining data files. In *Safety Assessment for Pharmaceuticals* (S. C. Gad, Ed.). Van Nostrand Reinhold, New York.

Lu, F. C. (1985). *Basic Toxicology,* pp. 68–95. Hemisphere, New York.

Page, N. P. (1986). International harmonization of toxicity testing. *In Safety Evaluation of Drugs and Chemicals* (W. E. Lloyd, Ed.), pp. 455–467. Hemisphere, New York.

Russell, W. M. S., and Burch, R. L. (1959). *The Principles of Humane Experimental Technique.* Methuen, London.

CHAPTER 3

Tests for Dermal Irritation and Corrosion

Evaluation of materials for their potential to cause dermal irritation and corrosion due to acute contact has been common for industrial chemicals, cosmetics, agricultural chemicals, and consumer products since at least the 1930s (generally, pharmaceuticals are only evaluated for dermal effects if they are to be administered topically—and then by repeat exposure tests, which will not be addressed here). As with acute eye irritation tests, one of the earliest formal publications of a test method (though others were used) was that of Draize *et al.* (1944). The methods currently used are still basically those proposed by Draize *et al.* and, to date, have changed little since 1944. Though (unlike their near relatives, the eye irritation tests) these methods have not particularly caught the interest or spotlight of concern of the animal welfare movement, there are efforts under way to develop alternatives that either do not use animals or are performed in a more humane and relevant (to human exposure) manner.

Among the most fundamental assessments of the safety of a product or, indeed, of any material that has the potential to be in contact with a significant number of people in our society, are tests in animals which seek to predict potential skin irritation or corrosion. Like all the other tests in what is classically called a range-finding, tier I, or acute battery, the tests used here are both among the oldest designs and currently undergoing the greatest degree of scrutiny and change. Currently, all the established test methods for these endpoints use the same animal model—the rabbit (almost exclusively the New Zealand White)—though some other animal models have been proposed.

Virtually all man-made chemicals have the potential to contact the skin of people. In fact, many (cosmetics and shampoos, for example) are intended to have skin contact. The greatest number of industrial medical problems are skin conditions, indicating the large extent of dermal exposure where none is intended.

Testing is performed to evaluate the potential occurrence of two different, yet related, endpoints. The broadest application of these is an evaluation of the potential to cause skin irritation, characterized by erythema (redness) and edema (swelling). Severity of irritation is measured in terms of both the degree of these two parameters and how long they persist. There are three types of irritation tests, each designed to address a different concern.

Primary (or acute) irritation, a localized reversible dermal response resulting from a single application of, or exposure to, a chemical without the involvement of the immune system.

Cumulative irritation, a reversible dermal response which results from re-peated exposure to a substance (each individual exposure is not capable of causing acute primary irritation). This is beyond the scope of acute toxicology and will not be discussed in this book.

Photochemically induced irritation, which is a primary irritation resulting from light-induced molecular changes in the chemical to which the skin has been exposed. This is discussed in Chapter 6.

Though most regulations and common practice characterize an irritation that persists 14 days past the end of exposure as other than reversible, the second endpoint of concern with dermal exposure—corrosion per se—is as-sessed in separate test designs. These tests start with a shorter exposure period (4 hr or less) to the material of concern and then evaluate simply whether tissue has been killed or not (or, in other words, if necrosis is present or not).

It should be clear that, if a material is found to have less than severe dermal irritation potential, it will not be corrosive and, therefore, need not be tested separately for the corrosion endpoint.

The adult human has 1.8 m^2 of skin, varying in thickness from 0.02 in. on the eyelids to 0.12–0.16 in. on the back, palms, and soles of the feet (Hipp, 1978). The epidermis, the outer portion of the skin, is several layers thick, covers the entire surface of the body, and is referred to as the horny layer or stratum corneum. It is the first line of defense against physical, chemical, and thermal exposure. The skin is host to normal bacterial flora consisting of

Micrococciae and *Corynbacterium,* which play an important role in the protection against infection. The melanocyte system, responsible for skin coloration, is located at the interface of the epidermis and the dermis. New cells are constantly being formed from the basal layer and slowly migrate to the surface, replenishing themselves approximately every 2 weeks (Monash and Blank, 1958; Matoltsy *et al.,* 1968).

A stylized typical cross section of skin is shown in Fig. 4. The dermis, or true skin, contains hair follicles, sebaceous glands, sweat glands, blood vessels, and nerve endings and is composed primarily of connective tissue. Hair follicles and sweat glands may also serve as a route of systemic entry (for highly polar materials).

Irritation is generally a localized reaction resulting from either a single or

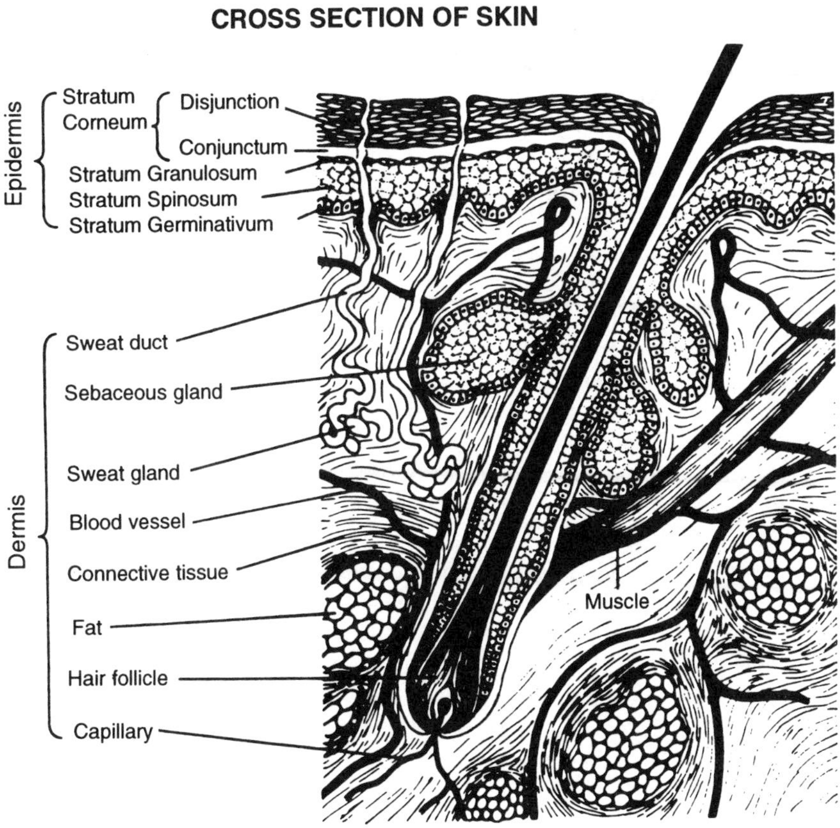

CROSS SECTION OF SKIN

FIGURE 4   Stylized typical cross section of skin, showing the common components encountered.

multiple exposure to a physical or chemical entity at the same site. It is characterized by the presence of erythema (redness) and edema and may or may not result in cell death. The observed signs are heat (caused by vessel dilation and the presence of large amounts of warm blood in the affected area), redness (due to capillary dilation), and pain (due to pressure on sensory nerves). The edema often observed is largely due to plasma, which coagulates in the injured area, precipitating a fibrous network to screen off the area, thereby permitting leukocyte to destroy exogenous materials by phagocytosis. If the severity of injury is sufficient, cell death may occur, thereby negating the possibility of cellular regeneration. Necrosis is a term often used in conjunction with cell death and is the degeneration of the dead cell into component molecules which approach equilibrium with surrounding tissue (Montagna, 1961).

There are three major objectives to be addressed by the performance of these tests. These are as follows:

1. *Providing regulator required baseline data*—Any product now in commerce must be both labeled appropriately for shipping [Department of Transportation (DOT), 1992] and accompanied by a material safety data sheet (MSDS) which clearly states potential hazards associated with handling it. DOT regulations also prescribe different levels of packaging on materials found to constitute hazards as specified in the regulations. Environmental Protection Agency (EPA) (under FIFRA) also has a pesticides labeling requirement. Similar requirements exist outside the United States. These requirements demand absolute identification of severe irritants or corrosives and adherence to the basics of test methods promulgated by the regulations. False positives (type I errors) are to be avoided in these usages.

2. *Hazard assessment for accidents*—For most materials, dermal exposure is not intended to occur, yet it will occur in cases of accidental spillage or mishandling. Here, we need to correctly identify the hazard associated with such exposures, being equally concerned with false positives and false negatives.

3. *Assessment of safety for use*—The materials at issue here are the full range of products for which dermal exposure will occur in the normal course of use. These range from cosmetics and hand soaps to bleaches, laundry detergents, and paint removers. No manufacturer desires to put a product on the market which cannot be safely used and will lead to extensive liability if placed in the marketplace. Accordingly, the desire here is to accurately predict the potential hazards in humans—that is, to have neither false positives nor false negatives.

Table 3 sets forth the current regulatorily mandated test designs which

TABLE 3 Regulatorily Mandated Test Designs for Dermal Irritation/Corrosion

Agency	Test material — Solid	Test material — Liquid	Exposure time (hr)	Number of rabbits	Sites per animal (intact/abraded)	At end of exposure	Scoring intervals postexposure	Note	Reference
Department of Transportation (DOT)	Moisten	Undiluted	4[a]	3[b]	1/0	Skin washed with appropriate vehicle	4 and 48 hr	Endpoint is corrosion in 2 of 6 animals	DOT (1992)
Environmental Protection Agency (EPA)	Moisten	Undiluted	24	6	2/0	Skin wiped, but not washed	24 and 72 hr; May continue until irritation fades or is judged irreversible	Toxic Substance Control Act test (TSCA) and FIFRA	EPA (1979)
Consumer Product Safety Commission (CPSC)	Dissolve in appropriate vehicle	Neat	24	6	1/1	Not specified	24 and 74 hr	Federal Hazardous Substances Act (FHSA)	CPSC (1980)
Organization of Economic Co-operation and Development (OECD)	Moisten	Undiluted	4[a]	3*	1/0	Wash with water or solvent	30–60 min, 24, 48, 72 hr or until judged irreversible	European Common Market	OECD (1992)

[a] If at 1 hr no serious skin reaction is seen in a single animal.
[b] But additional animals may be required to clarify equivocal results.

TABLE 4   Evaluation of Skin Reactions[a]

Skin reaction	Value
Erythema and eschar formation	
No erythema	0
Very slight erythema (barely perceptible)	1
Well-defined erythema	2
Moderate to severe erythema	3
Severe erythema (beet redness) to slight eschar formation (injuries in depth)	4
Necrosis (death of tissue)	+N
Eschar (sloughing or scab formation)	+E
Edema formation	
No edema	0
Very slight edema (barely perceptible)	1
Slight edema (edges of area well defined by definite raising)	2
Moderate edema (raised approximately 1 mm)	3
Severe edema (raised more than 1 mm and extending beyond the area of exposure)	4
Total possible score for primary irritation	8

[a]These scores are illustrated by the color prints in Fig. 5A.

form the bases of all currently employed test procedures. Though these designs vary somewhat in detail, they are by and large comparable.

All these methods use the same scoring scale, the Draize scale (Draize *et al.*, 1944), which is presented in Table 4. However, though the regulations prescribe these different test methods, most laboratories actually perform some modified methods. Here, two modifications (one for irritation and the other for corrosion) which reflect prior laboratory experience are recommended.

PRIMARY DERMAL IRRITATION TEST [FIGS. 5, 5A (SEE COLOR PLATES), AND 6]

A. Rabbit screening procedure
   1. A group of at least 8–12 New Zealand White rabbits are screened for the study.
   2. All rabbits selected for the study must be in good health; any rabbit exhibiting snuffles, hair loss, loose stools, or apparent weight loss is rejected and replaced.
   3. One day (at least 18 hr) prior to application of the test substance, each rabbit is prepared by clipping the hair from the back and sides using a small animal clipper. A size No. 10 blade is used to remove the long hair and then a size No. 40 blade is used to remove the remaining hair.

PRIMARY DERMAL IRRITATION STUDY DESIGN

Species: Rabbit
Strain: New Zealand White
Test Group: 6 Animals

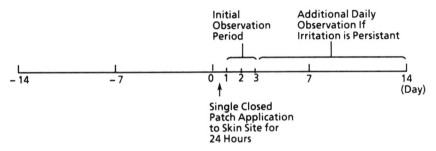

FIGURE 5   Line chart for design and conduct of primary dermal irritation study (PDI) in rabbits.

AREAS OF APPLICATION TO RABBIT SKIN

Skin Site:
1 Test Substance
2. Negative Control (Untreated Gauze Patch)
3. Positive Control (1% Sodium Lauryl Sulfate)
4. Vehicle Control

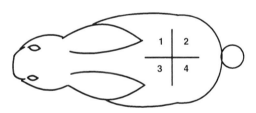

FIGURE 6   Areas of application of patch sites on back of rabbit for multipatched primary dermal irritation study. 1, test substance; 2, negative control (untreated gauze patch); 3, positive control (1% sodium Lauryl sulfate); 4, vehicle control.

4. Six animals with skin sites that are free from hyperemia or abrasion (due to shaving) are selected. Skin sites that are in the telogen phase (resting stage of hair growth) are used; those skin sites that are in the anagen phase (stage of active growth, indicated by the presence of a thick undercoat or hair) are not used.

B. Study procedure
   1. As many as four areas of skin, two on each side of the rabbit's back, can be utilized for sites of administration.
   2. Separate animals are not required for an untreated control group. Each animal serves as its own control.
   3. Besides the test substance, a positive control substance [a known skin irritant, 1% sodium lauryl sulfate (distilled water is used as the vehicle for sodium lauryl sulfate)] and a negative control (untreated patch) are applied to the skin. When a vehicle is used for diluting, suspending, or moistening the test substance, a vehicle control patch is required—especially if the vehicle is known to cause toxic dermal reactions or if there is insufficient information about the dermal effects of the vehicle.
   4. The four intact (free of abrasion) sites of administration are assigned a code number:
      1. Test substance
      2. Negative control
      3. Positive control
      4. Vehicle control (if required)
   5. The pattern of administration (illustrated in Fig. 6) makes certain that the test substance and controls are applied to each position at least once.
   6. Each test or control substance is held in place with a 1 × 1-in. square 12-ply surgical gauze patch. The gauze patch is applied to the appropriate skin site and secured with 1-in. wide strips of surgical tape at the four edges, leaving the center of the gauze patch nonoccluded.
   7. If the test substance is a solid or semisolid, a 0.5-g portion is weighed and placed on the gauze patch. The test substance patch is placed on the appropriate skin site and secured. The patch is subsequently moistened with 0.5 ml of physiological saline.
   8. When the test substance is in flake, granule, powder, or other particulate form, the weight of the test substance that has a volume of 0.5 ml (after compacting as much as possible without crushing or altering the individual particles, such as by tapping the measuring container) is used whenever this volume weighs less than 0.5 g. When applying powders, granules, etc., the gauze patch designated for the test sample is secured to the appropriate skin site with one of four strips of tape at the most ventral position of the animal. With one hand, the appropriate amount of sample measuring 0.5 ml is carefully poured from a glycine weighing paper onto the gauze patch, which is held in a horizontal (level) position

with the other hand. The patch containing the test sample is then carefully placed into position onto the skin by raising the remaining three edges with tape dorsally until they are completely secured. The patch is subsequently moistened with 0.5 ml of physiological saline.

9. If the test substance is a liquid, a patch is applied and secured to the appropriate skin site. A 1-ml tuberculin syringe is used to measure and apply 0.5 ml of test substance to the patch.

10. If the test substance is a fabric, a 1 × 1-in. square sample is cut and placed on a patch. The test substance patch is placed on the appropriate skin site and secured. The patch is subsequently moistened with 0.5 ml of physiological saline.

11. The negative control site is covered with an untreated 12-ply surgical gauze patch (1 × 1-in.).

12. The positive control substance and vehicle control substance are applied to a gauze patch in the same manner as a liquid test substance.

13. The entire trunk of the animal is covered with an impervious material (such as Saran Wrap) for a 24-hr period of exposure. The Saran Wrap is secured by wrapping several long strips of athletic adhesive tape around the trunk of the animal. The impervious material aids in maintaining the position of the patches and retards evaporation of volatile test substances.

14. An Elizabethan collar is fitted and fastened around the neck of each test animal. The collar remains in place for the 24-hr exposure period. The collars are utilized to prevent removal of wrappings and patches by the animals, while allowing the animals food and water *ad libitum.*

15. The wrapping is removed at the end of the 24-hr exposure period. The test substance skin site is wiped to remove any test substance still remaining. When colored test substances (such as dyes) are used, it may be necessary to wash the test substance from the test site with an appropriate solvent or vehicle (one that is suitable for the substance being tested). This is done to clean the test site to facilitate accurate evaluation for skin irritation.

16. Immediately after removal of the patches, each 1 × 1-in. square test or control site is outlined with an indelible marker by dotting each of the four corners. This procedure delineates the site for identification.

C. Observations

1. Observations are made of the test and control skin sites 1 hr after removal of the patches (25 hr postinitiation of application). Ery-

thema and edema are evaluated and scored on the basis of the designated values presented in Table 4.

2. Observations are performed again 48 and 72 hr after application and scores are recorded.

3. If necrosis is present or the dermal reaction needs description, the reaction should be described. Necrosis should receive the maximum score for erythema and eschar formation (4) with a (+N) to designate necrosis.

4. When a test substance produces dermal irritation that persists 72 hr postapplication, daily observations of test and control sites are continued on all animals until all irritation caused by the test substance resolves or until Day 14 postapplication.

D. Evaluation of results
  1. A subtotal irritation value for erythema or eschar formation is determined for each rabbit by adding the values observed at 25, 48, and 72 hr postapplication.
  2. A subtotal irritation value for edema formation is determined for each rabbit by adding the values observed at 25, 48, and 72 hr postapplication.
  3. A total irritation score is calculated for each rabbit by adding the subtotal irritation value for erythema or eschar formation to the subtotal irritation value for edema formation.
  4. The primary dermal irritation index is calculated for the test substance or control substance by dividing the sum of total irritation scores by the number of observations, 18 (3 days × 6 animals = 18 observations).
  5. A test/control substance producing a primary dermal irritation index (PDII) of 0.0 is a nonirritant, >0.0 to 0.5 is a neglible irritant, >0.5 to 2.0 is a mild irritant, >2.0 to 5.0 is a moderate irritant, and >5.0 to 8.0 is a severe irritant. This categorization of dermal irritation is a modification of the original classification described by Draize (1944): PDII = 0.0, nonirritant; >0.0–0.5, negligible irritant; >0.5–2.0, mild irritant; >2.0–5.0, moderate irritant; >5.0–8.0, severe irritant. Other abnormalities, such as atonia or desquamation, should be noted and recorded.

DERMAL CORROSIVITY TEST (FIG. 7)

This procedure is based on the Department of Transportation's Method of Testing Corrosion to Skin (CFR, 1984).

DERMAL CORROSIVITY STUDY DESIGN

Species: Rabbit
Strain: New Zealand White
Test Group: 6 Animals

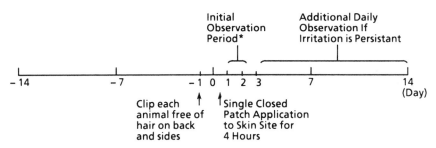

*Sites observed and evaluated at 4 and 48 hours

FIGURE 7 Line chart for design and conduct of dermal corrosivity study in the rabbits. *Sites observed and evaluated at 4 and 48 hours.

A. Rabbit screening procedure
  1. A group of at least 8–12 New Zealand White rabbits is screened for the study.
  2. All rabbits selected for the study must be in good health; any rabbit exhibiting snuffles, hair loss, loose stools, or apparent weight loss is rejected and replaced.
  3. One day (at least 18 hr) prior to application of the test substance, each rabbit is prepared by clipping the hair from the back and sides using a small animal clipper. A size No. 10 blade is used to remove the long hair and then a size No. 40 blade is used to remove the remaining hair.
  4. Six animals with skin sites that are free of hyperemia or abrasion (due to shaving) are selected. Skin sites that are in the telogen phase (resting stage of hair growth) are used; those skin sites that are in the anagen phase (active stage of hair growth) are not used.

B. Study procedure
  1. Separate animals are not required for an untreated control group. Each animal serves as its own control.

2. Besides the test substance, a negative control (untreated patch) is applied to the skin.
   a. If the test substance is a liquid, it is applied undiluted.
   b. If the test substance is a solid or a semisolid, it is applied as such.
   c. If information about the effects of moistening a solid or semisolid test substance is required, a third (optional) site can be added to the test.
3. The intact (free of abrasion) sites of administration are assigned a code number:
   1. Test substance
   2. Negative control
   3. (Optional) test substance moistened with 0.5 ml of physiological saline
4. The diagram shown in Fig. 3.3 (using only sites 1–3) illustrates the pattern of administration used in each study.
5. The test substance is held in place with a 2.5 × 2.5-cm square, 12-ply surgical gauze patch. The gauze patch is applied to the appropriate skin site and secured with 1-in. wide strips of surgical tape at the four edges, leaving the center of the gauze patch nonoccluded.
6. If the test substance is a solid or semisolid, a 0.5-g portion is weighed and placed on the gauze patch. The test substance patch is placed on skin site 1 and secured.
   a. When the test substance is in flake, granule, powder, or other particulate form, the weight of the test substance that has a volume of 0.5 ml (after compacting as much as possible without crushing or altering the individual particles, such as by tapping the measuring container) is used whenever this volume weighs less than 0.5 g.
   b. When applying powders, granules, etc., the gauze patch designated for the test sample is secured to the appropriate skin site with one of four strips of tape at the most central position of the animal. With one hand, the appropriate amount of sample measuring 0.5 ml is carefully poured from a glycine weighing paper onto the gauze patch, which is held in a horizontal (level) position with the other hand. The patch containing the test sample is then carefully placed into position onto the skin by raising the remaining three edges dorsally until they are completely secured with tape.
8. As an option, the effects of moistening a solid or semisolid can be investigated. If so, the test substance is applied to site 3 (as de-

scribed previously) and then the patch holding the test substance is subsequently moistened with 0.5 ml of physiological saline.

9. If the test substance is a liquid, a patch is applied and secured to skin site 1. A 1-ml tuberculin syringe is used to measure and apply 0.5 ml of test substance to the patch.

10. The negative control site 2 is covered with an untreated 12-ply surgical gauze patch.

11. The entire trunk of the animal is covered with an impervious material (such as Saran Wrap) for a 4-hr period of exposure. The Saran Wrap is secured by wrapping several long strips of athletic adhesive tape around the trunk of the animal. The impervious material aids in maintaining the position of the patches and retards evaporation of volatile test substances.

12. An Elizabethan collar is fitted and fastened around the neck of each test animal. The collars remain in place for the 4-hr exposure period. The collars are utilized to prevent removal of wrappings and patches by the animals, while allowing the animals food and water *ad libitum*.

13. The wrapping and patches are removed at the end of the 4-hr exposure period. When colored test substances (such as dyes) are used, it may be necessary to wash the test substance from the test site with an appropriate solvent or vehicle (one that is suitable for the test substance being tested). This is done to clean the test site to facilitate accurate evaluation.

14. Immediately after removal of the patches, each 2.5 × 2.5-cm square test or control site is outlined with an indelible marker by dotting each of the four corners. This procedure delineates the site for identification purposes.

C. Observations

1. After 4 hr of exposure, observations of the test and control sites are described. Observations are again made at the end of a total of 48 hr (44 hr after the first reading).

2. In addition, the Draize grading system for evaluation of skin reactions is used to score the skin sites 4 and 48 hr after dosing (Table 4).

D. Evaluation of results

1. Corrosion would be considered to have resulted if the test substance caused destruction or irreversible alteration of the tissue on at least two of the six rabbits tested. Ulceration or necrosis of the tissue at either 4 or 48 hr postexposure would be considered permanent tissue damage (i.e., tissue destruction does not include merely

sloughing of the superficial epidermis, or erythema, edema, or fissuring) (CFR 1984).

2. If a conclusive assessment of the extent of damage to the skin can not be made after 48 hr (it is difficult to determine whether or not permanent, irreversible damage is present), daily observations of the skin sites are made and recorded, either until a determination can be made about the extent of skin damage or until Day 14 after exposure. Photographs are taken at those time intervals after exposure that are most meaningful for documentation purposes.

3. If the test continues to Day 14 exposure, a final evaluation of the skin is made, resulting in a conclusive assessment of the test substance's potential to cause corrosion to skin. Scar tissue formation at this time is indicative of permanent tissue damage.

FACTORS AFFECTING RESPONSES AND TEST OUTCOME

The results of these tests (and particularly of the irritation test, which produces a graded response as opposed to the all-or-none response of the corrosivity test) are subject to considerable variability due to relatively small differences in test design or technique. Weil and Scala (1971) arranged and reported on the best known of several intralaboratory studies which clearly established this fact. Though the methods presented previously have proven to give reproducible results in the hands of the same technicians over a period of years (Gad *et al.*, 1986a) and contain some internal controls (the positive and vehicle controls in the PDI) against large variabilities in results or the occurrence of either false positives or negatives, it is still essential to be aware of those factors which may systematically alter test results. These factors are summarized as follows:

A. In general, any factor which increases absorption through the stratum corneum will also act to increase the severity of any intrinsic response. Unless these factors mirror potential exposure conditions, this may, in turn, adversely affect the relevance of test results.

B. The physical nature of solids must be carefully considered before testing and in the interpretation of results. Shape (sharp edges), size (small particles may serve to abrade due to being rubbed back and forth under the occlusive wrap), and the rigidity (stiff fibers or very hard particles will be more physically irritating) of solids may all contribute to enhancing an irritation response.

C. As the outline for the procedures of the corrosivity test design indicates, solids frequently give different results when they are tested dry rather than if wet. As a general rule, solids are more irritating if moistened (going back to Item A, this tends to enhance absorption). Care should also be taken as to what is used as a moistening agent—some (few) batches of USP physiological saline (used to simulate sweat) have proven to be mildly irritating to the skin on their own. Liquids other than water or saline should not be used.

D. Several older regulations require that some or all of the animals in a PDI test group have their test site skin abraded before test material application. This is based on the assumption that abraded skin is uniformly more sensitive to irritation. Experiments have shown this to not necessarily be true; however, some materials produce more irritation on abraded skin, whereas others produce less (Guillot *et al.,* 1982; Gad *et al.,* 1986b).

E. The degree of occlusion (in fact, the tightness of the wrap over the test site) also alters percutaneous absorption and therefore irritation. One important quality control issue in the laboratory is achieving a reproducible degree of occlusion in dermal wrappings.

F. Both the age of the test animal and the application site (saddle of the back vs flank) can markedly alter test outcome. Both of these factors are also operative in humans, of course (Mathias, 1983), but in these tests, the objective is to remove all such sources of variability. In general, as animals age increases, sensitivity to irritation decreases. Also, the skin on the middle of the back (other than directly over the spine) tends to be thicker (and therefore less sensitive to irritations) than that on the flanks.

G. The sex of the test animals can also alter study results, as both regional skin thickness and surface blood flow vary between males and females.

H. Finally, the single most important (yet also most frequently overlooked) factor which influences the results and outcome of these (and, in fact, most) acute studies is the training of the staff. In determining how test materials are prepared and applied and in how results are "read" against a subjective scale, both accuracy and precision are extremely dependent on the technicians involved. To achieve the desired results, initial training must be careful and all-inclusive. Importantly, some form of regular refresher training must be exercised—particularly in the area of scoring of results. Use of a set of color photographic standards as a training and reference tool is strongly recommended; such standards should clearly demonstrate each of the grades in the Draize dermal scale.

I. Limitations: It should be recognized that the dermal irritancy test is designed with a bias to preclude false negatives and, therefore, tends to exaggerate results in relation to what would happen in humans. Findings of negligible (or even very low-range mild) irritancy should therefore not be of concern unless the product under test is to have large-scale and prolonged dermal contact. Unlike the primary dermal irritancy test, the results from the corrosivity test should be taken at face value. There is some lab-to-lab variability and the test does produce some false positives (though these are almost always at least severely irritating compounds), but does not produce false negatives.

PROBLEMS IN TESTING (AND THEIR RESOLUTIONS)

Some materials, by either their physicochemical or toxicological natures, generate difficulties in the performance and evaluation of these tests. The most commonly encountered of these problems are presented below.

A. *Compound volatility*: One is sometimes required or requested to evaluate the potential irritancy of a liquid which has a boiling point between room temperature and the body temperature of the test animal; as a result, the liquid portion of the material will evaporate off before the end of the testing period. There is no real way around the problem; one can only make clear in the report on the test that the traditional test requirements were not met, though an evaluation of potential irritant hazard was probably achieved (because the liquid phase would have also evaporated from a human that it was spilled on).

B. *Pigmented material*: Some materials are strongly colored or act to discolor the skin at the application site. This makes the traditional scoring process difficult or impossible. One can try to remove the pigmentation with a solvent; if successful, the erythema can then be evaluated. If this fails or is unacceptable, one can (wearing thin latex gloves) feel the skin to determine if there is warmth, swelling, and/or rigidity—all secondary indicators of the irritation response.

C. *Wrong test*: Sometimes we find severe necrosis in a primary dermal irritation study or irritation (but no corrosion) in a corrosivity test. In the former, we can grade the material as a severe irritant but cannot make an evaluation as to its (as defined by regulation) corrosive potential. In the latter case, we can judge the material as not corrosive and to have irritating potential. The difference is, of course, in the length of the exposure period (though more recent EPA guidelines suggest making both tests of 4 hr in length).

D. *Systemic toxicity*: On rare occasions, the dermal irritation study is begun only to have the animals die very rapidly after test material application. Though it is not possible to evaluate potential irritancy in such cases, the results are even more important in the hazard evaluation process, and such findings should be rapidly communicated to those producing and handling the subject material.

E. There are occasions when the responses to questions asked about the dermal irritancy or corrosivity of a material are more complicated than a yes/no. These are generally when we know that the material at some concentration

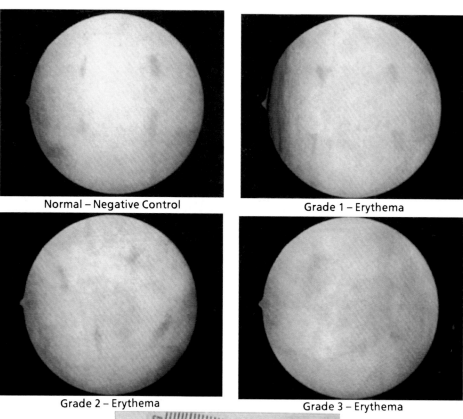

Normal – Negative Control

Grade 1 – Erythema

Grade 2 – Erythema

Grade 3 – Erythema

Grade 4 – Erythema with Eschar and Edema

FIGURE 5A Representative illustrations of skin irritation scores.

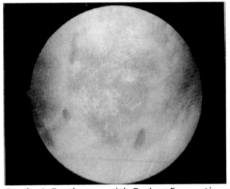

Grade 4–Erythema with Eschar Formation

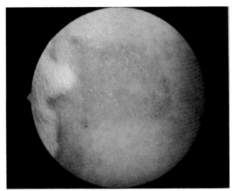

Grade 4–Erythema with Blanching

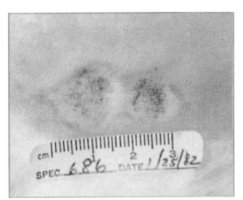

Blanching and Necrosis at 49 hours –
Corrosivity in the rabbit

FIGURE 5A (*Continued*)

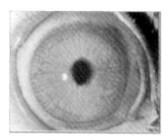

Normal Eye

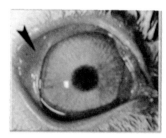

1 Redness

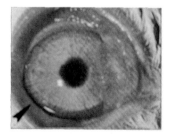

2 Redness

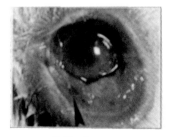

3 Redness

FIGURE 9A Representative illustrations of Draize eye irritation scores. (From CPSC, 1972)

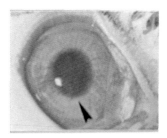

1 Opacity

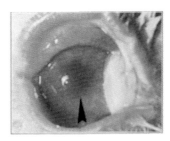

2 Opacity

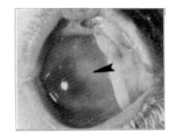

3 Opacity

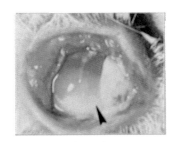

4 Opacity

FIGURE 9A *(Continued)*

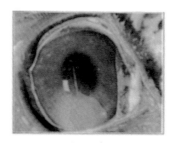

1 Opacity

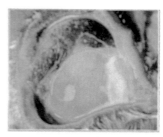

2 Opacity

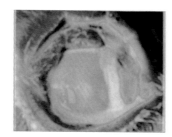

3 Opacity

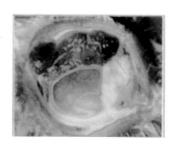

4 Opacity

FIGURE 9A (*Continued*)

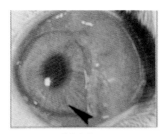

1 Iritis

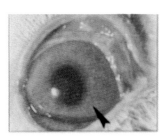

1 Iritis

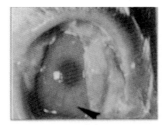

2 Iritis

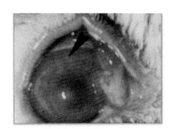

2 Iritis

FIGURE 9A (*Continued*)

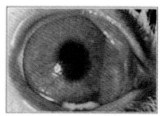

3 Chemosis

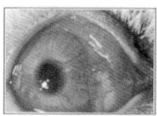

4 Chemosis

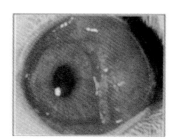

1 Chemosis

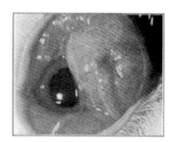

2 Chemosis

FIGURE 9A (*Continued*)

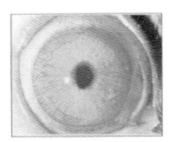

Normal Eye

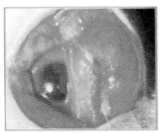

1 Hour
2-3 Redness   >2 Opacity
1 Iritis   4 Chemosis

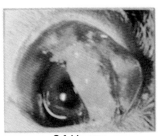

24 Hours
3 Redness   1 Opacity
2 Iritis   >3 Chemosis

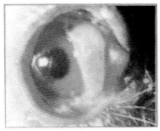

48 Hours
3 Redness   >1 Opacity
2 Iritis   3 Chemosis

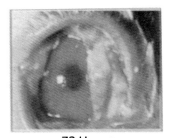

72 Hours
3 Redness   >1 Opacity
2 Iritis   >2 Chemosis

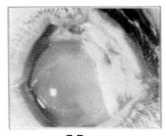

7 Days
3 Redness   4 Opacity
2 Iritis   2 Chemosis

FIGURE 9A (*Continued*)

has the effect and desire to know what a nonirritating or noncorrosive concentration might be.

For our first example, a polymer produced potentially for cosmetics use contains a certain level of unreacted monomer (such as acrylic acid) that is known to be irritating. At additional cost, the levels of residual monomer could be reduced. How much must monomer levels be reduced to make the polymer nonirritating? In this case, one would design and conduct a dose–response study in which irritation was examined at several different concentration levels (at different sites on the same animal). A single set of six animals could be used to evaluate as many as four concentrations, each animal being patched at four separate sites.

In a second example, the desire is to identify a level of exposure of a material that is not corrosive. Table 5 (from Derelanko et al., 1985) demonstrates an approach to this problem of defining exposure limits to a known hazard. Both

TABLE 5   Summary of Lesion Incidence in Rabbits Exposed to Dilute Hydrofluoric Acid (HF) Solutions or Distilled Water for Varying Periods of Time

Treatment/ exposure	Time (min)	No. of animals exposed	No. of animals with lesions	Mean no. of lesions per animal[a]	Size range of lesions (cm)
Distilled water	60	5	0	—	—
2% HF (neutralized)	60	5	0	—	—
2% HF	60	5	3	3.3 (2–6)[b]	0.4 × 0.4–3.5 × 1.0
2% HF	30	5	4	2.8 (1–6)	0.1 × 0.1–0.6 + 0.3
2% HF	15	5	3	2.7 (2–4)	0.1 × 0.1–1.3 × 1.0
2% HF	5	5	2	1.5 (1 + 2)	0.1 − 0.1–0.6 × 0.4
2% HF	1	5	0	—	—
0.5% HF	60	5	2	2.0 (1–3)	0.2 × 0.2
0.5% HF	30	5	1	4.0	0.1 × 0.1
0.5% HF	15	5	1	3.0	<0.1–0.2 × 0.2
0.5% HF	5	5	3	1.7 (1–2)	0.1 × 0.1–1.0 × 0.6
0.1% HF	60	5	1	1.0	0.5 × 0.5
0.1% HF	30	5	1	1.0	0.2 × 0.1
0.1% HF	15	5	2	1.5 (1–2)	0.1 × 0.1
0.1% HF	5	5	2	1.5 (1–2)	<0.1–0.1 × 0.1
0.01% HF	60	5	2	2.0	0.1 × 0.1–0.2 × 0.2
0.01% HF	30	5	0	—	—
0.01% HF	15	5	2	3.0 (2–4)	0.1 × 0.1–1.0 × 0.6
0.01% HF	5	5	2	2.5 (1–4)	0.1 × 0.1

[a]Animals with lesions.
[b]Range.

concentration and time of exposure can be varied to produce two sets of dose responses.

This particular study was performed because a manufacturer considered producing a household cleaner with between 2 and 20% hydroflouric acid in it, claiming it would be safe because of a lack of evidence to the contrary in the literature.

It is equally important to evaluate and consider the persistence or reversibility of observed irritation. Obviously, the degree of concern is considerably greater for a material whose effect does not fade quickly.

DESIGN ALTERNATIVES AND INNOVATIONS

In vivo alternative approaches to evaluating dermal toxicity are limited to one other dose site and two other species of small animals. These are the guinea pig, mouse ear, and rabbit ear tests. Gilman (1982) has previously presented a short overview of these three alternatives, but some additional information has since become available.

GUINEA PIG

The response of the guinea pig has been reported as being less severe and more like man (Nixon et al., 1975; Drill and Lazer, 1976), and there have been recommendations that it be the species of choice with the test being performed in the same manner as in the PDI. FIFRA guidelines, indeed, name the guinea pig as an alternative species for the PDI test. However, the rabbit is cheaper and its larger size makes multiple patching more practical than the guinea pig.

MOUSE EAR

The ear of the albino mouse has been proposed as an alternative test system (Uttley and Van Abbe, 1973). As originally proposed by these authors, the test was performed as follows:

Ten microliters (liquid) or 10 mg (solid paste) are applied to the dorsal aspect of one ear; the contralateral ear serves as a control.

Test material is applied topically, daily on 4 consecutive days.
Dermal reactions are used read on Day 5 as follows:
    0: No visible blood vessels or erythema.

2: Few blood vessels, barely visible; no erythema.

4: Main blood vessels visible on lower half of ear; slight erythema over lower third or base of ear.

6: Main blood vessels more obvious; suggestion of capillary network of tips of main vessels; slight or generalized erythema.

8: Main blood vessels extended to edge of ear; more extensive capillary network between main blood vessels; possibly internal hemorrhage; erythema more pronounced; ear may begin to fold back and lose suppleness.

10: Pronounced blood vessels and extensive capillary network evident; marked erythema; possibly "frilling" of ear margin.

12: Pronounced blood vessels and extensive capillary network extending to ear margins; severe erythema; frilling and thickening of ear margins; crusting more in evidence.

14: Pronounced blood vessels and severe erythema; obvious thickening of ear; possibly necrosis; crusting may extend over whole ear surface.

Daily differences between control and treated ears for each animal are added. A correction is given for any difference between the control and treated ears initially, divided by 5, and interpreted as:

0–9: Probably not irritating to human skin.

10–15: May be slightly irritating to some users.

Over 15: Likely to prove sufficiently irritating to elicit user complaints at unacceptable levels.

In 1985, Patrick et al. utilized the mouse ear model to evaluate dermal irritants and try to distinguish mechanisms behind irritation. Also, in 1986, Gad et al. published a paper in which a new method for evaluating dermal sensitization was described, but in doing so, also presented a substantial amount of dermal irritation data arising from a mouse ear model.

The mouse is cheaper than the rabbit and appears to give results analogous to those in the rabbit. The chief drawbacks to the model appear to be custom and the existence of a large database in the rabbit model.

RABBIT EAR

Over the years, several people have proposed a dermal irritation evaluation model based on the test material being applied to the inside surface of the rabbit ear. The advantages are that this site does not have to be shaved and may not overpredict results as much. Seemingly no formal evaluation of a method based on this site has been performed and published.

The reader should also be aware that there are a variety of cumulative irritancy test designs available, such as the guinea pig immersion test (Uttley and Van Abbe, 1973) and the 21-consecutive-day occluded patch test in rabbits (Phillips *et al.*, 1972; Steinberg *et al.*, 1975; Marzulli and Maibach, 1975).

IN VITRO ALTERNATIVES

Extensive progress has been made in devising alternative (*in vitro*) systems for evaluating the dermal irritation potential of chemicals since this author last reviewed the field (Gad and Chengelis, 1988). This is an effort that extends back to the early 1960s (Choman, 1963), but which saw little progress until the 1990s. Table 6 overviews 20 proposed systems that now constitute five very different approaches.

The first set of approaches (I) uses patches of excised human or animal skin maintained in some modification of a glass diffusion cell which maintains the moisture, temperature, oxygenation, and electrolyte balance of the skin section. In this approach, after the skin section has been allowed to equilibrate for some time, the material of concern is placed on the exterior surface and wetted (if not liquid). Irritation is evaluated by swelling of the skin (a crude and relatively insensitive method for mild and moderate irritants), by evaluation of inhibition of uptake of radiolabeled nutrients, or by measurement of leakage of enzymes through damaged membranes.

The second set of approaches (II) utilizes a form of surrogate skin culture comprising a mix of skin cells which closely mirror key aspects of the architecture and function of the intact organ. These systems seemingly offer a real potential advantage but, to date, the "damage markers" employed (or proposed) as predictors of dermal irritation have been limited to cytotoxicity.

The third set of approaches (III) is to use some form of cultured cell (either primary or transformed), with primary human epidermal keratinocytes (HEKs) preferred. The cell cultures are exposed to the material of interest, then either ectotoxicity, release of inflammation markers, or decrease of some indicator of functionality (lipid metabolism, membrane permeability, or cell detachment) is measured.

The fourth group (IV) contains two miscellaneous approaches—the use of a membrane from the hen's egg with morphological evaluation of damage being the predictor of endpoint (Reinhardt *et al.*, 1987) and the SKINTEX system, which utilizes the coagulation of a mixture of soluble proteins to predict dermal response.

Finally, in group V there are two structure–activity relationship models which use mathematical extensions of past animal results correlated with structure to predict the effects of new structures.

Many of these test systems are in the process of evaluation of their perfor-

TABLE 6 *In Vitro* Dermal Irritation Test Systems

System	Endpoint	Validation data?[a]	Reference
I. Skin patches			
Excised patch of perfused skin	Swelling	No	Dannenberg (1987)
Mouse skin organ culture	Inhibition of incorporation of [^{3}H]thymidine and [^{14}C]leucine labels	No	Kao et al. (1982)
Mouse skin organ culture	Leakage of LDH and GOT	Yes	Bartnik et al. (1989)
II. Surrogate skin			
Test skin—cultured surrogate skin patch	Morphological evaluation	No	Bell et al. (1989)
Cultured surrogate skin patch	Cytotoxicity	No	Naughton et al. (1989)
III. Cultured cells			
Human epidermal keratinocytes (HEKs)	Release of labeled arachidonic acid	Yes	DeLeo et al. (1988)
Fibroblasts	Acid release		Lamont et al. (1989)
HEKs	Cytotoxicity	Yes	Gales et al. (1989)
HEKs	Cytotoxicity (MIT)	Yes	Swisher et al. (1988)
HEKs, dermal fibroblasts	Cytotoxicity	Yes	Babich et al. (1989)
HEKs	Inflammation mediator release	No	Boyce et al. (1988)
Cultured Chinese hamster ovary	Increases in β-hexosaminidase levels in the media	No	Lei et al. (1986)
Cultured C$_3$ H10T$_{1/2}$ and HEK cells	Lipid metabolism inhibition	No	DeLeo et al. (1987)
Cultured cells			
BHK21/C13	Cell detachment	Yes	Reinhardt et al. (1987)
BHK21/C13	Growth inhibition		
Primary rat Thymocytes	Increased membrane permeability		
Rat periodontal mast cells	Inflammation mediator release	Yes (surfactants)	Prottey and Ferguson (1976)
IV. Miscellaneous biological systems			
Hen's egg	Morphological examination		Reinhardt et al. (1987)
SKINTEX—protein mixtuer	Protein coagulation	Yes	Gordon et al. (1989, 1990)
V. Mathematical models			
Structure–activity relationship (SAR) model	NA	Yes	Enslein et al. (1987)
SAR model	NA	No	Firestone and Guy (1986)

[a]Evaluated by comparison of predictive accuracy for a range of compounds compared with animal tests results. Not validated in the sense used in this chapter. NA, not applicable.

mance against various small groups of compounds for which the dermal irritation potential is known. Evaluation by multiple laboratories of a wider range of structures will be essential before any of these systems can be generally utilized.

PERCUTANEOUS ABSORPTION

Closely related to all aspects of evaluating dermal irritation and corrosion must be an understanding of what factors influence the absorption of materials through the skin, and also the bases of variation of such absorption due to species, sex, age, technique, etc. This topic is well beyond the scope of this text, being itself the subject of numerous books [such as Brandau and Lippold (1982) and Bronaugh and Maibach (1985)]. The reader should be aware, however, that this literature exists and that there are experimental systems for evaluating this property of a material.

INTRACUTANEOUS REACTIVITY (IRRITATION)

The intracutaneous irritation test is a sensitive acute toxicity screening test and is generally accepted for detecting potential local irritation by extracts from biomaterials (generally, materials used in medical devices) (USP, 1990). Extracts of material obtained with nonirritation polar and nonpolar extraction media are suitable, and sterile extracts are desirable.

INTRACUTANEOUS TEST

This test is designed to evaluate local responses to the extracts of materials under test following intracutaneous injection into rabbits.

TEST ANIMAL

Select healthy, thin-skinned albino rabbits whose fur can be clipped closely and whose skin is free from mechanical irritation or trauma. In handling the animals, avoid touching the injection sites during observation periods, except to discriminate between edema and an oil residue. Rabbits previously used in unrelated tests, such as the Pyrogen Test, and that have received the prescribed rest period may be used for this test provided that they have clean unblemished skin.

TABLE 7   Intracutaneous Reactivity Test

Extract or blank	Number of sites (per animal)	Dose (μl per site)
Sample	5	200
Blank	5	200

PROCEDURE

Agitate each extract vigorously prior to withdrawal of injection doses to ensure even distribution of the extracted matter. On the day of the test, closely clip the fur on the animal's back on both sides of the spinal column over a sufficiently large test area. Avoid mechanical irritation and trauma. Remove loose hair by means of vacuum. If necessary, swab the skin lightly with diluted alcohol, and dry the skin prior to injection. More than one extract from a given material can be used per rabbit if you have determined that the test results will not be affected. For each test sample use two animals and inject each intracutaneously, using one side of the animal for the test sample and the other side for the blank, as outlined in Table 7. (Note: Dilute each gram of the extract of the test sample prepared with polyethylene glycol 400, and the corresponding blank with 7.5 vol. of sodium chloride injection to obtain a solution having a concentration of about 120 mg of polyethylene glycol per milliliter.)

Examine injection sites for evidence of any tissue reaction such as erythema, edema, and necrosis. Swab the skin lightly, if necessary, with diluted alcohol to facilitate reading of injection sites. Observe all animals at 24, 48, and 72 hr after injection. Rate the observations on a numerical scale for the extract of the test sample and for the blank using Table 3.5. Reclip the fur as necessary during the observation period.

If each animal at any observation period shows an average reaction to the test sample that is not significantly greater than that to the blank, the test sample meets the requirements of this test. If at any observation period the average reaction to the test sample is questionably greater than the average reaction to the blank, repeat the test using three additional rabbits. On such a repeat test, the average reaction to the test sample in any of the three animals is not significantly greater than the blank.

REFERENCES

Babich, H., Martin-Alguacil, N., and Borenfreund, E. (1989). Comparisons of the cytotoxicities of dermatotoxicants to human keratinocytes and fibroblasts *in vitro*. In *In Vitro Toxicology: New Directions* (A. M. Goldberg, Ed.), pp. 153–167. Liebert, New York.

Bartnik, F. G., Pittermann, W. F., Mendorf, N., Tillmann, U., and Kunstler, K. (1989). Skin organ culture for the study of skin irritancy. Third International Congress of Toxicology, Brighton, UK.

Bell, E., Gay, R., Swiderek, M., *et al.* (1989). Use of fabricated living tissue and organ equivalents as defined in higher order systems for the study of pharmacologic responses to test substances. Presented at the NATO Advanced Research Workshop, Pharmaceutical Application of Cell and Tissue Culture to Drug Transport, Bandol, France, September 4–9.

Boyce, S. T., Hansbrough, J. F., and Norris, D. A. (1988). Cellular responses of cultured human epidermal keratinocytes as models of toxicity to human skin. In *Progress in in Vitro Toxicology* (A. M. Goldberg, Ed.), pp. 23–37. Liebert, New York.

Brandau, R., and Lippold, B. H. (1982). *Dermal and Transdermal Absorption.* Wissenschaftliche Verlagsgesellschaft, Stuttgart.

Bronough, R. L., and Maibach, H. I. (1985). *Percutaneous Absorption.* Dekker, New York.

Choman, B. R. (1963). Determination of the response of skin to chemical agents by an *in vitro* procedure. *J. Invest. Dermatol.* **44**, 177–182.

Code of Federal Regulations (CFR) (1984). Transportation, Title 49: Part 173, Appendix A— Method of Testing Corrosion to Skin, Revised; November 1.

Consumer Product Safety Commission (CPSC) (1980). Federal Hazardous Substances Act Regulations, CFR 150, 41.

Dannenberg, A. M., Moore, K. G., Schofield, B. H., Higuchi, K., Kajiki, A., Au, K., Pula, P. J., and Bassett, D. P. (1987). Two new *in vitro* methods for evaluating toxicity to skin (employing short-term organ culture). In *Alternative Methods in Toxicology* (A. M. Goldberg, Ed.), Vol. 5, pp. 115–128. Liebert, New York.

DeLeo, V. A., Midlarsky, L., Harber, L. C., Kong, B. M., and Salva, S. D. (1987). Surfactant-induced cutaneous primary irritancy: An *in vitro* model. In *Alternative Methods in Toxicology* (A. M. Goldberg, Ed.), Vol. 5. pp., 129–138. Liebert, New York.

DeLeo, V., Hong, J., Scheide, S., Kong, B., DeSalva, S., and Bagley, D. (1988). Surfactant-induced cutaneous primary irritancy: An *in vitro* model-assay system development. In *Progress in in Vitro Toxicology* (A. M. Goldberg, Ed.), pp. 39–43. Liebert, New York.

Department of Transportation Code of Federal Regulations (1992). Title 49, 173:137.

Derelanko, M. J., Gad, S. C., Gavigan, F. A., and Dunn, B. J. (1985). Acute dermal toxicity of dilute hydrofluoric acid. *Ocular Dermal Toxicol.* **4**(2), 74–85.

Draize, J. H., Woodard, G., and Calvery, H. O. (1944). Method for the study of irritation and toxicity of substances applied topically to the skin and mucous membranes. *J. Pharmacol. Exp. Ther.* **82**, 337–390.

Drill, Y. A., and Lazer, P. (1976). Prediction of skin irritancy and sensitization potential by testing with animals and man. In *Cutaneous Toxicity* (J. F. Griffith and E. Buehler, Eds.). Academic Press, New York.

Enslein, K., Borgstedt, H. H., Blake, B. W., and Hart, J. B. (1987). Prediction of rabbit skin irritation severity by structure–activity relationships. *In Vitro Toxicol.* **1**, 129–147.

Environmental Protection Agency (EPA) (1979). *Acute Toxicity Testing Criteria for New Chemical Substances* (EPA 560/13-79-009) EPA, Office of Toxic Substances, Washington, DC.

Firestone, B. A., and Guy, R. H. (1986). Approaches to the prediction of dermal absorption and potential cutaneous toxicity. In *Alternative Methods in Toxicology* (A. M. Goldberg, Ed.), Vol. 3, pp. 56–536. Liebert, New York.

Gad, S. C., and Chengelis, C. P. (1988). *Acute Toxicity: Principles and Methods.* Telfor Press, Caldwell, NJ.

Gad, S. C., Dunn, B. J., Dobbs, D. W., and Walsh, R. D. (1986a). Development and validation of an alternative dermal sensitization test: The mouse ear swelling test (MEST). *Toxicol Appl. Pharmacol.* **84**, 93–114.

Gad, S. C., Walsh, R. D., and Dunn, B. J. (1986b). Correlation of ocular and dermal irritancy of industrial chemicals. *Ocular Dermal Toxicol.* **5**(3), 195–213.

Gales, Y. A., Gross, C. L., Karebs, R. C., and Smith, W. J. (1989). Flow cytometric analysis of toxicity by alkylating agents in human epidermal keratinocytes. In *In Vitro Toxicology: New Directions* (A. M. Goldberg, Eds.), pp. 169–174. Liebert, New York.

Gilman, M. R. (1982). Skin and eye testing in animals. In *Principles and Methods of Toxicology* (A. W. Hayes, Ed.), pp. 209–222. Raven Press, New York.

Gordon, V. C., Kelly, C. P., and Bergman, H. C. (1989). SKINTEX, an *in vitro* method for determining dermal irritation. International Congress of Toxicology, Brighton, UK.

Gordon, V. C., Kelly, C. P., and Bergman, H. C. (1990). Evaluation of SKINTEX, an *in vitro* method for determining dermal irritation. *Toxicologist* **10**(1), 78.

Guillot, J. P., Gonnet, J. F., Clement, C., Caillard, L., and Trahaut, R. (1982). Evaluation of the cutaneous-irritation potential of 56 compounds. *Fd. Chem. Toxicol.* **201**, 563–572.

Hipp, L. L. (1978). The skin and industrial dermatosis. *National Safety News,* April.

Kao, J., Hall, J., and Holland, J. M. (1982). Quantitation of cutaneous toxicity: An *in vitro* approach using skin organ culture. *Toxicol. Appl. Pharmacol.* **68**, 206–217.

Lamont, G. S., Bagley, D. M., Kong, B. M., and DeSalva, S. J. (1989). Developing an alternative to the Draize skin test: Comparison of human skin cell responses to irritants *in vitro*. In *In Vitro Toxicology: New Directions* (A. M. Goldberg, Ed.), pp. 183–184. Liebert, New York.

Lei, H., Carroll, K., Au, L., and Krag, S. S. (1986). An *in vitro* screen for potential inflammatory agents using cultured fibroblasts. In *Alternative Methods in Toxicology,* (A. M. Goldberg, Ed.), Vol. 3, pp. 74–85. Liebert, New York.

Matoltsy, A. C., Downes, A. M., and Sweeney, T. M. (1968). Studies of the investigation of the chemical nature of the water barrier. *J. Invest. Dermatol.* **50**, 19.

Marzulli, F. N., and Maibach, H. I. (1975). The rabbit as a model for evaluating the skin irritants: A comparison of results obtained on animals and man using repeated skin exposures. *Fd. Cosmet. Toxicol.* **13**, 533–540.

Mathias, C. G. T. (1983). Clinical and experimental aspects of cutaneous irritation. In *Dermatoxicology* (F. M. Margulli and H. T. Maibach, Eds.), pp. 167–183. Hemisphere, New York.

Monash, S., and Blank, H. (1958). Location and reformation of epithelial barrier to water vapor. *Arch. Dermatol.* **78**, 710–714.

Montagna, W. (1961). *The Structure and Function of Skin,* 2nd ed. Academic Press, New York.

Naughton, G. K., Jacob, L., and Naughton, B. A. (1989). A physiological skin model for *in vitro* toxicity studies. In *Progress in in Vitro Toxicology* (A. M. Goldberg, Ed.), Vol. 7, pp. 183–189. Liebert, New York.

Nixon, G. R., Tyson, C. R., and Wertz, W. C. (1975). Interspecies comparisons of skin irritancy. *Appl. Pharmacol.* **31**, 481–590.

Organization for Economic Cooperation and Development (OECD) (1992). OECD guidelines for testing of chemicals, Section 404, Acute Dermal Irritation/Corrosion, adopted July 17, 1992, Paris.

Patrick, E., Maibach, H. I., and Burkhalter, A. (1985). Mechanisms of chemically induced skin irritation. *Toxicol. Appl. Pharmacol.* **81**, 476–490.

Phillips, L., II, Steinberg, M., Maibach, H. I., and Akers, W. A. (1972). A comparison of rabbit and human skin response to certain irritants. *Toxicol. Appl. Pharmacol.* **21**, 369–382.

Prottey, C., and Ferguson, T. F. M. (1976). The effect of surfactants upon rat peritoneal mast cells *in vitro*. *Fd. Chem. Toxicol.* **14**, 425.

Reinhardt, C. A., Aeschbacher, M., Bracker, M., and Spengler, J. (1987). Validation of three cell toxicity tests and the hen's egg test with guinea pig eye and human skin irritation data. In *Alternative Methods in Toxicology* (A. M. Goldberg, Ed.), Vol. 5. Liebert, New York.

Steinberg, M., Akers, W. A., Weeks, M., McCreesh, A. H., and Maibach, H. I. (1975). A comparison on test techniques based on rabbit and human skin responses to irritants with recommendations regarding the evaluation of mildly or moderately irritating compounds. In *Animal Models in Dermatology. Relevance to Human Dermatopharmacology and Dermatoxicology.* H. Maibach, Ed.), pp. 1–11. Churchill Livingstone, Edinburgh, UK.

Swisher, D. A., Prevo, M. E., and Ledger, P. W. (1988). The MTT *in vitro* cytotoxicity test: Correlation with cutaneous irritancy in two animal models. In Goldberg, A. M. (Ed.), *Progress in in Vitro Toxicology,* Mary Ann Liebert, New York, pp. 265–269.

United States Pharmacopeia (1990). Intracutaneous reactivity test, *United States Pharmacopeia XXII,* USP Convention, Rockville, MD, pp. 1180–1183.

Uttley, M., and Van Abbe, N. J. (1973). Primary irritation of the skin: Mouse ear test and human patch test procedures. *J. Soc. Cosmet. Chem.* 24, 217–227.

Weil, C. S., and Scala, R. A. (1971). Study of intra- and inter-laboratory variability in the results of rabbit eye and skin irritation tests. *Toxicol. Appl. Pharmacol.* 19, 276–360.

CHAPTER 4

Ocular Irritation Testing

The test methods designed and used to evaluate the potential to cause irritation or damage to the eye by a splash or other accidental occurrence hold a unique and ambivalent place in our society. On the one hand, the eyes represent a uniquely valuable and vulnerable asset to people; the sense of vision is critical for functioning in our world, and the responsible organs are delicate and relatively unprotected. At the same time, the traditional tests—and their misuse and misunderstanding of their use—have served as the rallying point for those concerned about the humane and proper use of animals. This has caused the field of testing for potential to cause irritation or damage to the eyes to become both the most active area for the development of alternatives and innovations and the most sensitive area of animal testing and use in research.

HISTORY OF OCULAR IRRITATION TESTING

Early in the 1930s, an untested eyelash dye containing *p*-phenylene diamine ("Lash Lure") was brought onto the market in the United States. This product (as well as a number of similar products) rapidly demonstrated that it could sensitize the external ocular structures, leading to corneal ulceration with loss of vision and at least one fatality (McCally *et al.,* 1933). This occurrence led to the revision of the Food and Drug Act, which became the Food, Drug and Cosmetic Act of 1938. To meet the provisions of this act, a number of test methods were proposed. Latven and Molitor (1939) and Mann and Pullinger (1942) were among those to first report on the use of rabbits as a test model to predict eye irritation in humans. No specific scoring system was presented to grade or summarize the results in these tests, however, and the use of animals with pigmented eyes (as opposed to albinos) was advocated. Early in 1944, Friedenwald *et al.* published a method using albino rabbits in a manner very similar to that of the original Draize *et al.* (1944) publication, but still prescribing the description of the individual animal responses as the means of evaluating and reporting the results. Though a scoring method was provided, no overall score was generated for the test group. Draize (head of the Dermal and Ocular Toxicity Branch at the Food and Drug Administration) modified Friedenwald's procedure and made the significant addition of a summary scoring system.

Over the 40 years since the publication of the Draize scoring system, it has become common practice to call all acute eye irritation tests performed in rabbits "the Draize eye test." However, since 1944, ocular irritation testing in rabbits has significantly changed. Clearly, there is no longer a single test design that is used, and there are different objectives that are pursued by different groups using the same test. This lack of standardization has been recognized for some time and attempts have been made to address standardization of at least the methodological aspects of the test (such as how test materials are applied and how scoring is performed), if not the design aspects (such as numbers and sources of test animals). For the purposes of this test, we have therefore replaced the term "Draize test" with eye irritancy testing.

The common core design of the test consists of instilling either 0.1 ml of a liquid or 0.1 g of a powder (or other solid) onto one eye of each of six rabbits. The material is not washed out, and both eyes of each animal (the nontreated eye acting as a control) are graded according to the Draize scale (Table 8) at 24, 48, and 72 hr after test material instillation. The resulting scores are summed for each animal. The major variations involve the use of three additional rabbits which have their eyes irrigated shortly after instillation of test material. There are, however, many variations of these two major design subsets (that is, with and without irrigation groups).

Even though the major objective of the Draize scale was to standardize scoring, it was recognized early that this was not happening, but that different people were "reading" the same response differently. To address this, two sets of standards (also called training guides, to provide guidance by comparison)

TABLE 8 Scale of Weighted Scores for Grading the Severity of Ocular Lesions[a]

I. Cornea
    A. Opacity–degree of density (area which is most dense is taken for reading)
        Scattered or diffuse area—details of iris clearly visible 1
        Easily discernible translucent areas—details of iris slightly obscured.............................2
        Opalescent areas, no details of iris visible, size of pupil barely discernible 3
    B. Area of cornea involved
        One-quarter (or less) but not zero 1
        Greater than one-quarter, less than one-half..2
        Greater than one-half, less than three-quarters...3
        Greater than one-half, less than whole area...3
        Greater than three-quarters up to whole area..4
            Scoring equals A × B × 5; total maximum = 80
II. Iris
    A. Values
        Folds above normal, congestion, swelling, circumcorneal ingestion (any one or all of
        these or combination of any thereof), iris still reacting to light (sluggish reaction is
        possible) 1
        No reaction to light, hemorrhage, gross destruction (any one or all of these)................2
            Scoring equals A × B; total possible maximum = 10
III. Conjunctivae
    A. Redness (refers to palpebral conjunctival only)
        Vessels definitely injected above normal..1
        More diffuse, deeper crimson red, individual vessels not easily discernible....................2
        Diffuse beefy red...3
    B. Chemosis
        Any swelling above normal (includes nictating membrane) 1
        Obvious swelling with partial eversion of the lids..2
        Swelling with lids above half closed..3
        Swelling with lids about half closed to completely closed 4
    C. Discharge
        Any amount different from normal (does not include small amount observed in inner
        canthus of normal animals..1
        Discharge with moistening of the lids and hair just adjacent to the lids 2
        Discharge with moistening of the lids and considerable area around the eye.................3
            Scoring (A + B + C) × 2; total maximum = 20

Note. The maximum total score is the sum of all scores obtained for the cornea, iris and conjunctivae.
[a]Representative examples of various scores are presented in Fig. 9A (see color plates). From Draize et al. (1994).

have been published by regulatory agencies through the years. In 1965, the Food and Drug Administration (FDA) published an illustrated guide with color pictures as standards (FDA, 1965). In 1974, the Consumer Product Safety Commission (CPSC) published a second illustrated guide (CPSC, 1974) which provided 20 color photographic slides as standards. The Environmental Protection Agency (EPA, 1979) also supported the development of a guide with color plates/slides, which is still available from NTIS (Falahee et al., 1981).

A second source of methodological variability has been in the procedure utilized to instill test materials into the eyes. There is a general consensus that the substance should be dropped into the cul-de-sac of the conjunctiva formed by gently pulling the lower eyelid away from the eye, then allowing the animal to blink and spread the material across the entire corneal surface. In the past, however, there were other application procedures (such as placing the material directly onto the surface of the cornea).

There are also variations in the design of the "standard" test. Most laboratories observe animals until at least 7 days after instillation and may extend the test to 21 days after instillation if any irritation persists (in fact, EPA labeling requires such an extension). These prolonged postexposure observation periods are designed to allow for evaluation of the true severity of damage and for assessing the ability of the ocular damage to be repaired. The results of these tests are evaluated by a descriptive classification scale (Table 9) such as that described in NAS publication 1138 (NAS, 1977), which is a variation of that reported by Green et al. (1978). This classification is based on the most severe response observed in a group of six nonirrigated eyes, and data from all observation periods are used for this evaluation. These will be examined more fully in the next section of this chapter. The U.S. EPA has promulgated a new categorization scheme (Table 10).

Different regulatory agencies within the United States have prescribed slightly different procedures for different perceived regulatory needs (Gilman,

TABLE 9   Severity and Persistence[a]

Inconsequential or complete lack of irritation—Exposure of the eyes to a material under the specified conditions caused no significant ocular changes. No staining with fluorescein can be observed. Any changes that do occur clear within 24 hr and are no greater than those caused by normal saline under the same conditions.

Moderate irritation—Exposure of the eye to the material under the specified conditions causes minor, superficial, and transient changes of the cornea, iris, or conjunctivae as determined by external or slit-lamp examination with fluorescein staining. The appearance at the 24-hr or subsequent grading of any of the following changes is sufficient to characterize a response as moderate irritation: opacity of the cornea (other than a slight dulling of the normal luster), hyperemia of the iris, or swelling of the conjunctivae. Any changes that are seen clear within 7 days.

Substantial irritation—Exposure of the eye to the material under the specified conditions causes significant injury to the eye, such as loss of the corneal epithelium, corneal opacity, iritis (other than a slight injection), conjunctivitis, pannus, or bullae. The effects clear within 21 days.

Severe irritation or corrosion—Exposure of the eye to the material under the specified conditions results in the same types as in the previous category and in significant necrosis or other injuries that adversely affect the visual process. Injuries persist for 21 days or more.

[a]From NAS (1977).

TABLE 10 US EPA Toxicity Categories for Eye Irritation

Category	Definition
I	Corrosive (irreversible destruction of ocular tissue) or corneal involvement or irritation persisting for >21 days
II	Corneal involvement or irritation clearing in 8–21 days
III	Corneal involvement or irritation clearing in ≤7 days
IV	Minimal effects clearing in <24 hr

Note. Berdasco et al. (1996).

1982). These are looked at in more depth later in this chapter. There have also been a number of additional grading schemes, but these will not be reviewed here.

CURRENT IN VIVO TEST PROTOCOLS

Any discussion of current test protocols (or of any proposed in vitro alternatives) must start with a review of why tests are done. What are the objectives of eye irritation testing and how are these different objectives reflected not just in test design and interpretation but also in the regulations requiring testing and in the ways that test results are utilized?

There are four major groups of organizations (in terms of their products) which require eye irritation studies to be performed. These can be generally classified as the pharmaceutical, cosmetic and toiletries, consumer product, and industrial chemical groups. There are also minor categories of use (which we will not consider here) such as for military agents.

For the pharmaceutical industry, eye irritation testing is performed when the material is intended to be put into the eye as a means or route of application or for ocular therapy. There are a number of special tests applicable to pharmaceuticals or medical devices which are beyond the scope of this volume because they are not intended to assess potential acute effects or irritation. In general, however, it is desired that an eye irritation test that is utilized by this group be both sensitive and accurate in predicting the potential to cause irritation in humans. Failing to identify human ocular irritants (lack of sensitivity) is to be avoided, but of equal concern is the occurrence of false positives. A subset of this group is the contact lens industry, which has both lenses and their cleaning/soaking solutions regulated as medical devices. As such, the products have extensive ocular contact and cannot have either acute or cumulative irritation potential.

The cosmetics and toiletries industry is similar to that pharmaceutical industry in that the materials of interest are frequently intended for repeated application in the area of the eye. In such uses, contact with the eye is common, though not intended or desirable. In this case, the objective is a test that is as sensitive (as that in the preceding paragraph), even if this results in a low incidence of false positives. Even a moderate irritant would not be desired but might be acceptable in certain cases (such as deodorants and depilatories) in which the potential for eye contact is minimal.

Consumer products which are not used for personal care (such as soaps, detergents, and drain cleaners) are approaches from yet a different perspective. These products are not intended to be used in a manner that either causes them to get into the eyes or makes that occurrence likely, but because of the very large population that uses them and the fact that their modes of use do not include active measures to prevent eye contact (such as the use of goggles and face shields), the desire is to accurately identify severe eye irritants. Agricultural chemicals generally fit in this category, though many of them are covered by specific testing requirements under FIFRA.

Finally, there are industrial chemicals. These are handled by (relative to consumer products) a smaller population. Eye contact is never intended, and, in fact, active measures are taken to prevent it. The use of eye irritation data in these cases is to prevent it. The use of eye irritation data in these cases is to fulfill labeling requirements for shipping and to provide hazard assessment information for accidental exposures and their treatment. The results of such tests do not directly affect the economic future of a material. It is desired to accurately identify moderate and severe irritants (particularly those with irreversible effects) and to know if rinsing of the eyes after exposure will make the consequences of exposure better or worse. False negatives for mild reversible irritation are acceptable.

The needs of these different groups (that is, their test objectives) are summarized in Table 11. To fulfill these objectives, a number of basic test protocols have been developed and mandated by different regulatory groups. Table 12 gives an overview of these as previously presented in part by Falahee *et al.* (1982). Historically, the philosophy underlying these test designs made maximization of the biological response equivalent with having the most sensitive test. As our review of objectives has shown, the greatest sensitivity (especially at the expense of false positive findings, which is an unavoidable consequence) is not what is universally desired. As we shall see later, maximizing the response in rabbits does not guarantee sensitive prediction of the results in humans.

Methodological variations that are commonly used to improve the sensitivity and accuracy of describing damage in these tests are inspection of the eyes with a slit lamp and instillation of the eyes with a vital dye (or, most commonly, fluorescein) as an indicator of increase in permeability of the corneal barrier. These techniques and an alternative scoring system, which is more comprehen-

TABLE 11   Matrix of Test Objectives vs Required Test

	Features			
	Desired sensitivity (lowest level of irritation that it is essential to detect)[a]	Need to evaluate recovery and effects of timely irrigation	Acceptable incidence of	
Organization (intended product use)			False positives	False negatives
Pharmaceutical	Moderate	None	None	None
Cosmetic	Moderate	Recovery–high; Irri-ation–none	Minimal	None
Consumer product[b] (personal use)	Moderate	Recovery–high; Irri-ation–low	Minimal	None
Consumer product (household use)	Substantial	Medium to high	Low	Low for moderates; none for substan-tials
Industrial chemical	Substantial	High	Low	Low for substan-tials; none for se-veres

[a]Categories from Table 4.
[b]Current FHSA regulations require that any consumer-use product (other than pharmaceuticals and cosmetics, which are regulated by FDA) must be identified as to its potential to cause irritation as defined earlier in this section.

sive than the Draize scale, are reviewed Ballantyne and Swanston (1977) and Chan and Hayes (1985).

Almost universally, the philosophy underlying these test designs equates maximization of the biological response with production of the most sensitive test. As our review of objectives has shown, the greatest sensitivity (especially at the expense of false positive findings, which is an unavoidable consequence) is not what is universally desirable.

OCULAR IRRITATION TEST

The primary eye irritation test is intended to predict the potential for a single splash of chemical in the eye of a human being to cause reversible and/or permanent damage. The basic study design for this test is shown diagramatically in Fig. 8. Since the introduction of the original Draize test some 50 years ago

TABLE 12 Regulatory Guidelines for Ocular Irritation Test Methods

	Reference								
	Draize et al. (1944)	FHSA (1972, 1979)	NAS (1977)	OECD (1981)	IRLG (1981)	CFR 16 (1981) (CPSC)	TOSCA (1982)	FIFRA (1982)[a]	Japan (MAFF, 1985)
Test species	Albino rabbit	Same	Same[b]	Same	Same	Same	Same	Same	Ng
Age/wt.	NS[i]	NS	Sexually mature/less than 2 yrs. old	NS	Young adult/2.0	NS	NS	NS	Young adult
Sex	NS	NS	Either	NS	Either	NS	NS	NS	NS
No. of animals/group	9	6	4 (min.)	3 (min.)	3 (prelim. test)[d] 6	6–18	6	6	At least 6
Test agent vol. and method of instillation									
Liquids	0.1 ml on the eye	Same as Draize	Liquids and solid; two or more different doses within the probable range of human exposure[c]	Same as Draize	Same as Draize	Same as Draize	Same as FHSA	Same as FHSA	Same as OECD
Solids	0.1 g	100 mg or 0.1 ml equivalent when this vol. weighs less than 100 mg; direct instillation into conjunctival sac	Manner of application should reflect probable route of accidental exposure	Same as FHSA	Same as FHSA	Same as FHSA	Same as FHSA	Same as FHSA	Same as OECD
Aerosols[j]	NS	NS	Short burst of distance approximating self-induced eye exposure	1-sec burst sprayed at 10 cm	1-sec burst sprayed at approx. 4 in.	NS	As OECD	As OECD	As OECD
Irrigation schedule	At 1 sec (3 animals) and at 4 sec (3 animals) following instillation of test agent (3 animals remain nonirrigated)	Eyes may be washed after 24-hr reading	May be conducted with separate experimental groups	Same as FHSA; in addition to substances found to be irritating; wash at 4 sec (3 animals) and at 30 sec (3 animals)	Same as FHSA	Same as FHSA	As FHSA	As FHSA	Similar to OECD; if irritation does not disappear at 72 hr after dose the effects of washing should be tested

	20 ml tap water (body temp.)	Sodium chloride solution (USP or equivalent)	NS	Wash with water for 5 min using vol. and velocity of flow which will not cause injury	Tap water or sodium chloride solution (USP or equivalent)	Same as FHSA	NS	NS	As OECD
Irrigation treatment									
Examination times (post instillation)	24 hr 48 hr 72 hr 4 Days 7 Days	24 hr 48 hr 72 hr	1 Day 3 Days 7 Days 14 Days 21 Days	1 hr 24 hr 48 hr 72 hr	24 hr[g] 48 hr 72 hr	24 hr 48 hr 72 hr	As OECD	As OECD	As OECD
Use of fluorescein	NS	May be applied after the 24-hr reading (optional)	May be used	Same as FHSA	Same as FHSA	Same as FHSA	As FHSA	As FHSA	Same as FHSA
Use of anesthetics	NS	NS	NS	May be used	May be used	NS	May be used	May be used	NS
Scoring and evaluation	Draize et al. (1944) (Table 4)	Modified Draize et al. (1944) or a slit-lamp scoring system based on CPSC (1976)	CPSC (1976)	CPSC (1976)	CPSC (1976)	CPSC (1976)	CPSC (1976)	CPSC (1976)	As FHSA

Note. FHSA, Federal Hazard Substance Act; NAS, National Academy of Sciences; OECD, Organization for Economic Cooperation and Development; IRLG, Interagency Regulatory Liason Group; CFR, Code of Federal Regulations.

[a] Office Pesticide Assessment

[b] Tests should be conducted on monkeys when confirmatory data are required.

[c] Not specified.

[d] If the substance produces corrosion, severe irritation, or no irritation in a preliminary test with three animals, no further testing is necessary. If equivocal responses occur, testing on at least three additional animals should be performed.

[e] Suggested doses are 0.1 and 0.05 ml for liquids.

[j] Currently no testing guidelines exist for gases or vapors.

[g] Eyes may also be examined at 1 hr and 7, 14, and 21 days (at the option of the investigator).

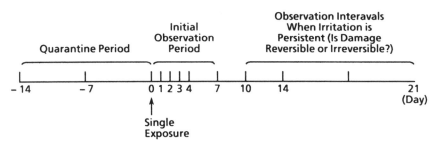

ACUTE EYE IRRITATION STUDY

Species:	Rabbit
Strain:	New Zealand White
Test Group:	9 Animals (6 Nonirrigated; 3 Irrigated)

FIGURE 8   Line chart for design and conduct of acute eye irritation study in the rabbit.

(Draize *et al.*, 1944), ocular irritation testing in rabbits has both developed and diverged. Indeed, clearly there is no longer a single test design that is used and there are different objectives that are pursued by different groups using the same test. This lack of standardization has been recognized for some time and attempts have been made to address standardization of at least the methodological aspects of the test, if not the design aspects.

One widely used study design, which begins with a screening procedure as an attempt to avoid testing severe irritants or corrosives in animals, proceeds as follows:

A. Testing article screening procedure (presented diagramatically in Fig. 9). This is mandated by OECD guidelines and recommended by other agencies.
  1. Each test substance will be screened in order to eliminate potentially corrosive or severely irritating materials from being studies for eye irritation in the rabbit.
  2. The pH of the test substance should be measured.
  3. A Primary Dermal Irritation Study will be performed prior to the study.
  4. The test substance will not be studied for eye irritation, if the test substance is a strong acid (pH is 2.0 or less) or strong alkali (pH 11.0 or greater) and/or if the test substance is a severe dermal irritant (with a Primary Dermal Irritation Index of 5–8) or causes corrosion of the skin.

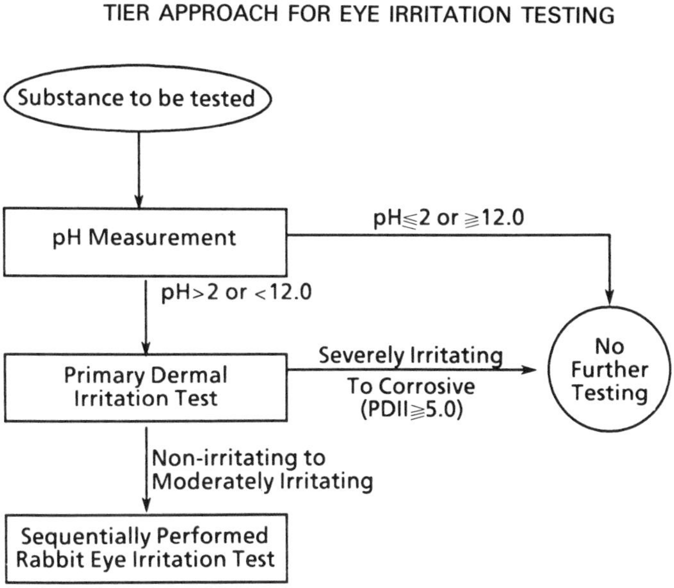

TIER APPROACH FOR EYE IRRITATION TESTING

FIGURE 9 Procedure for screening test articles prior to conduct of acute eye irritation procedure. This tier approach serves to identify corrosive and almost all strong irritants before they are tested in the rabbit eye.

5. If it is predicted that the test substance does not have the potential to be severely irritating or corrosive to the eye, continue to Section B, Rabbit Screening Procedure.

B. Rabbit screening procedure
1. A group of at least 12 New Zealand White rabbits of either sex are screened for the study. The animals are removed from their cages and placed in rabbit restraints. Care should be taken not to accidentally cause mechanical damage to the eye during this procedure.
2. All rabbits selected for the study must be in good health; any rabbit exhibiting snuffles, hair loss, loose stools, or apparent weight loss is rejected and replaced.
3. One hour prior to instillation of the test substance, both eyes of each rabbit are examined for signs of irritation and corneal defects with a hand-held slit lamp. All eyes are stained with 2.0% sodium fluorescein and examined to confirm the absence of corneal lesions.
   Fluorescein staining: Cup the lower lid of the eye to be tested and instill one drop of a 2% (in water) sodium fluorescein solution

onto the surface of the cornea. After 15 sec the eye is thoroughly rinsed with physiological saline. The eye is examined, employing a handheld long-wave ultraviolet illuminator in a darkened room. Corneal lesions, if present, appear as bright yellowish-green fluorescent areas.

4. Only 9 of the 12 animals are selected for the study. The 9 rabbits must not show any signs of eye irritation and must show either a negative or minimum fluorescein reaction (due to normal epithelial desquamation).

C. Study procedure

1. At least 1 hr after fluorescein staining, the test substance is placed on one eye of each animal by gently pulling the lower lid away from the eyeball to form a cup (conjunctival cul-de-sac) into which the test material is dropped. The upper and lower lids are then gently held together for 1 sec to prevent immediate loss of material.

2. The other eye remains untreated and serves as a control.

3. For testing liquids, 0.01 ml of the test substance is used.

4. For solids or pastes, 100 mg of the test substance is used.

5. When the test substance is in flake, granular, powder, or other particulate form, the amount that has a volume of 0.01 ml (after gently compacting the particles by tapping the measuring container in a way that will not alter their individual form) is used whenever this volume weighs less than 10 mg.

6. For aerosol products, the eye should be held open and the substance administered in a single, short burst for about 1 sec at a distance of about 4 in. directly in front of the eye. The velocity of the ejected material should not traumatize the eye. The dose should be approximated by weighing the aerosol can before and after each treatment. For other liquids propelled under pressure, such as substances delivered by pump sprays, an aliquot of 0.01 ml should be collected and instilled in the eye as for liquids.

7. The treated eyes of six rabbits are not washed following instillation of the test substance.

8. The treated eyes of the remaining three rabbits are irrigated for 1 min with room-temperature tap water, starting 20 sec after instillation.

9. In order to prevent self-inflicted trauma by the animals immediately after instillation of the test substance, the animals are not immediately returned to their cages. After the test and control eyes are examined and graded at 1 hr postexposure, the animals are returned carefully to their respective cages.

D. Observations

1. The eyes are observed for any immediate signs of discomfort after instilling the test substance. Blepharospasm and/or excessive tearing are indicative of irritating sensations caused by the test substance and the duration should be noted. Blepharospasm does not necessarily indicate that the eye will show signs of ocular irritation.

2. Grading and scoring of ocular irritation are performed in accordance with Table 8. The eyes are examined and grades of ocular reactions are recorded.

3. If signs of irritation persist at 7 days, readings are continued on Days 10 and 14 after exposure or until all signs of reversible toxicity are resolved.

4. In addition to the required observations of the cornea, iris, and conjunctiva, serious effects (such as pannus, rupture of the globe, or blistering of the conjunctivae) indicative of a corrosive action are reported.

5. Whether or not toxic effects are reversible depends on the nature, extent, and intensity of damage. Most lesions, if reversible, will heal or clear within 21 days. Therefore, if ocular irritation is present at the 14-day reading, a 21-day reading is required to determine whether the ocular damage is reversible or nonreversible.

E. Evaluation of results

The results can be evaluated by the following two methods:

1. Federal Hazardous Substances Act (FHSA) Regulations: Interpretation of data is made from the six test eyes which are not irrigated with water. Only data from Days 1, 2, and 3 are used for this evaluation; data from the 1-hr observation and Days 4, 7, 10, 14, and 21 are not used. An animal is considered as exhibiting a positive reaction if the test substance produces at any of the readings ulceration of the cornea (other than a fine stippling) (grade 1), opacity of the cornea (other than a slight dulling of the normal luster) (grade 1), inflammation of the iris (other than a slight deepening of the rugae or a slight circumcorneal injection of the blood vessels) (grade 1), or if such substance produces in the conjunctivae (excluding the cornea and iris) an obvious swelling with partial eversion of the lids (grade 2) or a diffuse crimson red color with individual vessels not easily discernible (grade 2). The test is positive if four or more of the animals in the test group exhibit a positive reaction. If no or only one animal exhibits a positive reaction, the test is considered negative. If two or three animals exhibit a positive reaction, the test is repeated using a different group of six animals. The second test

TABLE 13   Grades for Ocular Lesions

Cornea	Conjunctivae
No ulceration or opacity..................................0	Redness (refers to palpebral) and bulbar conjunctivae excluding cornea and iris)
Scattered or diffuse areas of opacity (other than slight dulling of normal luster), details of iris clearly visible .... (1)[a]	Vessels normal..
	Some vessels definitely injected.................1
Easily discernible translucent areas, details of iris slightly obscured...................................2	Diffuse, crimson red, individual vessels not easily discernible ....(2)
Nacreaous areas, no details of iris visible, size of pupil barely discernible 3	Diffuse, beefy red 3
Complete corneal opacity, iris not discernible...4	Chemosis
	No swelling 0
Iris	Any swelling above normal (includes nictitiating membrane) 1
Normal 0	Obvious swelling with partial eversion of lids ....(2)
Markedly, deepened folds, congestion swelling, moderate circumcorneal injection (any of these or combination of any thereof), iris still reacting to light (sluggish reaction is positive) ....(1)	Swelling with lids about half closed...........3
	Swelling with lids more than half closed...4
No reaction to light, hemorrhage, gross destruction (any or all of these)....................2	

[a]Numbers in parentheses indicate lowest grades considered positive under the Federal Hazardous Substances Act Regulations (CFR, 1981).

shall be considered positive if three or more of the animals exhibit a positive reaction. If only one or two animals in the second test exhibit a positive reaction, the test shall be repeated with a different group of six animals. Should a third test be needed, the substance will be regarded as an irritant if any animal exhibits a positive response. These steps are summarized in Table 13.

2. A modified Classification Scale of Ocular Responses is based on severity and persistence (derived from Green *et al.*, 1978). The most severe response seen in a group of six test animals is used for the classification. This scheme is presented in Table 9.

The U.S. EPA toxicity categories based on ocular irritation are given in Table 10.

21-DAY EYE IRRITATION STUDY IN RABBITS

This study is intended to identify the irritation potential of a test contact lens or lens disinfectant solution compared to that caused by a control lens or disinfectant solution.

Sixteen young adults (2–3.5 kg) New Zealand White rabbits are randomized into two groups.

Test and control lenses (or lenses soaked in test and control disinfectants) are inserted into the right eyes of each rabbit in the appropriate group (control or test) once daily for 21 consecutive days. The test or control contact lens will be carefully placed over the cornea of each rabbit. The lens will remain in place for 24 hr. After 24 hr, the contact lens will be removed, the eye examined, and a new lens placed on the cornea for 24 hr. This procedure will be repeated for 21 consecutive days. The treated eye of each animal is examined and scored for irritation of the cornea, iris, and conjunctiva pretest, and prior to each daily application of the contact lens and again 24 hr following the last application (study Day 22). A handheld source of illumination will be used to aid in examining the eyes. Ocular responses will be graded according to the scale in Table 8. Additional signs will be described.

ANALYSIS OF DATA

Calculations: The primary eye irritation score for each rabbit is calculated from the weighted Draize scale. The method of calculation is indicated on the scale included herein.

Interpretation: The interpretation of the scores recorded is based on the number of rabbits with positive scores. A positive score is any score for opacity of intis or a score of 2 or more for redness or chemosis.

Irritant: An irritant is a test article which under the conditions of this study causes a positive score in four to six rabbits with unwashed eyes (16 CFR 1500.3(c)(4)).

Indeterminate: If positive scores are noted in two or three animals with unwashed eyes, irritation potential of the test article is not classified.

Nonirritant: If positive scores are recorded in zero or one animal, the test article is classified as a nonirritant.

ADEQUACY OF CURRENT *IN VIVO* METHODS

To assess the adequacy of the currently employed eye irritation tests to fulfill the objectives behind their use, we must evaluate them in terms of (1) their accuracy (how well they predict the hazard to humans); (2) can comparable results be obtained by different technicians and laboratories; and (3) reproducibility and precision within any single laboratory (how well a single lab can repeat tests and accurately evaluate standard or "control" materials). We should also consider what methods and designs have been developed and are being employed as modifications to rabbit eye irritation tests to improve their performance against these criteria.

Assessing the accuracy of rabbit eye irritation tests—or indeed, of any predictive test of eye irritation—requires that the results of such tests can be compared to what happens in man. Unfortunately, the human database available in the literature or resulting from controlled tests is not large. The concerns, however, have been present almost as long as the tests have been performed (McLaughlin, 1946).

There are substantial differences between the eyes of humans and those of the rabbit and, indeed, of other species that have also been considered as test models. Beckley (1965) presented the following comparison of corneal thickness and area (as a percentage of the total area of the globe) of four species, as shown in Table 14.

The rabbit's aqueous humor also has a different pH (7.6 vs 7.1–7.3 for humans), a less effective tearing mechanism, and a nictitating membrane. Calabrese (1984) presents a comprehensive review of the anatomical and biochemical differences between the ocular systems of people and rabbits.

Some have claimed that the rabbit, in the test as it is currently performed, is more sensitive than man. Many anionic formulations, for example, are severe rabbit eye irritants but are nonirritants in humans. For other anionics, however, there is moderate human ocular irritation (such as with sodium dodecyl sulfate). However, the relative sensitivities vary from class to class of chemical. Alexander (1965) and Calabrese (1984) both have provided reviews of materials for which rabbits are more sensitive than man. MacDonald *et al.* (1983) published a review of materials that were both more or less irritating in rabbits than in humans.

TABLE 14   Corneal Thickness and Area

Species	Thickness (mm)	Area (%)
Man	0.53–0.54	7
Rabbit	0.4	25
Mouse	0.1	50
Rat	?	50

Note. In a recent publication, Berdasco *et al.* (1996) did a retrospective analysis of 118 different occular irritation tests. The results suggest that the number of rabbits could be reduced to three (current U.S. & Japanese guideline mandate six) without any change in U.S. EPA categorization. The rates of discomfort and injury were quite low with the use of an appropriate prescreening technique.

In the experience of one of the authors (SCG), reviewing more than 1000 materials, the prediction of irritancy in humans (as evaluated in medical and poison control center incidence reports) by rabbit eye test is correct about 85% of the time. Approximately 10% of the time, the rabbit test tends to overpredict irritancy, while it underpredicts it less than 5% of the time. Swanston (1985) has also published a comparative review of seven different species, including humans. For those interested in what is known about human ocular toxicity, the best source is Grant and Schuman (1993).

It should be noted, however, that rabbit eye tests do not detect ocular toxicities associated with some ocular anesthetics and eye drops (Andermann and Erhart, 1983).

The second concern, which has also been around as long as the test, is its reproducibility between laboratories. Weil and Scala (1971) published the most frequently cited study of intralaboratory reproducibility of eye and skin irritation tests. Twenty-five labs evaluated a battery of 12 materials using a common protocol. The results showed variability between laboratories, with a number of individual labs reporting consistently either more or less severe results than the other labs. A second comparative study, reported by Marzulli and Ruggles (1973), had 10 laboratories test 7 liquid materials, 2 at a time, along with a control material. The materials were selected to be intermediate-range eye irritants (5 materials) or nonirritants (2 materials). The labs utilized a common set of evaluation criteria and were found to be quite consistent in properly classifying materials as irritants or nonirritants—a somewhat less stringent comparison of reproducibility than that employed by Weil and Scala (1971). The causes and cures for such variability from lab to lab are multiple, but we have already mentioned differences in methodologies and evaluator training (to name just two major sources).

Since the Weil and Scala (1971) study, a number of authors in addition to Marzulli and Ruggles (1973), have published comparative studies which have shown a greater degree of reproducibility, though they have not involved as large or diverse a population of evaluators. Some of these are summarized in Table 15.

Behind some of these differences in evaluating the reproducibility of the rabbit eye irritation test is a fundamental disagreement as to what such tests should do (or, more precisely, what kind of data they should generate). Many believe that the tests should serve to classify materials (into two or more categories, such as nonirritants/mild irritants/moderate irritants), while others believe it to be critical that a test effectively rank materials.

Several authors have made the point that nonirritants and strong irritants are reproducibly predicted the best. For other materials, several authors have made the point that the use of concurrent reference materials (Gloxhuber, 1985) or semiannual refresher training of personnel doing scoring of results

TABLE 15   Summary of Comparative Rabbit Eye Studies

Study	Result	Reference
3 materials by 3 readers under 2 separate conditions	90% reproductibility of irritant/nonirritant classification	Bayard and Hehir (1976)
7 materials evaluated in duplicate	Test results reproducible	Williams et al. (1982)
56 materials evaluated in 3 separate protocols	Each protocol reproducible—variations between tests by different protocols	Guillot et al. (1982a,b)
29 materials (detergents) evaluated in 2 rabbits, 1 monkey, and 1 human test	Results for all nonhuman models were more severe than man, but low-volume rabbit test data were ranked comparable to human data	Freeberg et al. (1984)

vs a set of standards (McDonald et al., 1983) improves reproducibility of results and gives a set of standard results against which we can evaluate a drift in test or scoring practices.

LIMITATIONS OF THE RABBIT EYE TEST

The rabbit eye irritation test is designed to provide a range of information. First, what kinds of effects are to be expected and how severe are they? The Draize scale was never intended to provide a score such that the data are continuous and linear. That is, Draize scores are not such that a material with a score of 109 is distinguishably different than one with a score of 106. Rather, the results of scoring any one animal were intended to allow one to classify an agent as to its ability to cause or not cause irritation in that one animal.

Second, the test provides information as to rate of occurrence (or incidence) of irritation in animals. As demonstrated earlier, it is actually this information that is used to classify a material as an irritant or not.

Third, what is the time course of response, and are any or all adverse effects reversible? Earlier, the criteria for severity and reversibility were presented. Note that if a test is performed so that results (assuming there is irritation) are followed only for 72 hr as per the FHSA guidelines, the only classification of a material that is possible is either irritant or nonirritant.

If one desires to more fully characterize and classify a material in this test system (such as a severe irritant), then one must either continue observations until the responses disappear or to 21 days (at which time most lesions can be determined to be either reversible or nonreversible). In certain cases (if the responses are extreme and test animals are in continued discomfort), a judgment can be made that effects will persist to 21 days, and the animals may be humanely terminated.

Fourth, for many uses, one may wish to know if there is a sensory warning response if a chemical is splashed into the eye. For some materials, such as dimethyl sulfoxide, methyl bromide, and bis-(2-chloroethyl)sulfate, no stinging or discomfort is caused—just damage to the eye later (Ballantyne and Swanston, 1977).

Finally, will washing or irrigation of the eye (the most common first aid procedure after an accidental exposure) alleviate the effects or make them worse?

There are modifications which have been proposed and adapted for the performance of rabbit eye irritation tests themselves that should be reviewed. These modifications have been directed at the twin objectives of making the tests more accurate in predicting human responses and at reducing both the use of animals and the degree of discomfort or suffering experienced by those that are used. Some of these modifications have already been discussed:

1. *Alternative species*: Dogs, monkeys, and mice (Swanston, 1985) have all been suggested as alternatives to rabbits that would be more representative of humans. Each of these, however, also has shown differences in responses compared to those seen in humans and pose additional problems in terms of cost, handling, lack of database, etc.

2. *Use of anesthetics*: Over the years, a number of authors have proposed that topical anesthetics be administered to the eyes of rabbits prior to their use in the test. Both OECD and IRLG regulations allow such usage and the CPSC advocates their use. Numerous published (such as Falahee *et al.,* 1981) and unpublished studies have shown that such use of anesthetics can interfere with test results (usually by increasing the severity and/or duration of eye irritation findings). However, the available literature remains mixed as to the scientific validity and/or advantages of using anesthetics in these tests.

3. *Low-volume test*: An alternative which has been proposed (and which our survey showed has been adopted by a number of laboratories) is using a reduced volume/weight of test materials.

In 1980, Griffith *et al.* reported on a study in which they evaluated 21 different chemicals at volumes of 0.1, 0.03, 0.01, and 0.003 ml. These 21 chemicals were materials on which there were already human data. The volume reduction was found to not change the rank order of responses, and it was found that 0.01 ml (10 μl) gave results which best mirrored those seen in man. In 1982, Williams *et al.* reported a comparison of seven materials evaluated at 0.1 and 0.01 ml and found that the rank of results was not changed with the volume reduction, while the responses were moderated.

In 1984, Freeberg *et al.* published a study of 29 detergents (for which there were human data), each evaluated at both 0.1 and 0.01 ml test volumes in rabbits. The results of the 0.01- and 0.01-ml tests were reported to be more reflective of results in man. In 1986, Freeberg *et al.* published a further evaluation of low vs classical volume tests, in both humans and rabbits, and found that recovery times from low-volume rabbit tests gave a better correlation with results seen in humans than classical volumes.

In 1985, Walker reported an evaluation of the low-volume (0.01-ml) test which assessed its results and correlated them with those in humans and reported that 0.01 ml gave a better correlation than did 0.1 ml.

There are only two objections to the low-volume test. These are that we would lose a screen for exquisitely toxic materials (single drops of which in the eye will kill an animal, such as was reported for an organophosphonium salt by Dunn *et al.* in 1982) and that there may be some classes of chemicals for which low-volume tests may give less representative results. Neither of these is supportable. A lower volume test would still reveal exquisitely lethal materials, and no data have been produced to identify any special class of chemicals.

The American Society of Testing and Materials has published the low-volume method (Method E 1055-85) as a consensus standard procedure. It seems clear that this approach should be seriously considered by those performing *in vivo* eye irritation tests.

4. *Use of prescreens*: This modification (presented in brief earlier) may also be considered a tier approach. Its objective is to avoid testing severely irritating or corrosive materials in many (or, in some cases, any) rabbits. This approach entails a number of steps which should be considered independently.

The first step is a screen based on physicochemical properties. This usually means pH, but also should be extended to materials with high oxidation or reduction potentials (hexavalent chromium salts, for example).

Though the correlation between low pH values (acids) and eye damage in the rabbit has not been found to be excellent, all alkalis (pH 11.5 or above) tested have been reported to produce opacities and ocular damage (Murphy *et al.*, 1982). The lack of correlation between eye damage and low pH is not limited to the rabbit, but rather is an inherent property of the more complex chemical reactivities of acids. Many laboratories now use cutoffs for testing of 2.0 or lower and 11.5 or 12.0 and higher. If a material falls under the provisions of these cutoffs (or is so identified due to other physicochemical parameters), then it should be (a) not tested in the rabbit eye and assumed to be corrosive, (b) evaluated in a secondary screen such as an *in vitro* cytotoxicity test or primary dermal irritation test (Jackson and Rutty, 1985), or (c) evaluated in a single rabbit before a full-scale eye irritation test is performed. It should be kept in mind that the correlation of all the physicochemical screen parameters with acute eye test results is very concentration dependent, being good at high concentrations and marginal at lower concentrations (where various buffering systems present in the eye are meaningful).

The second commonly used type or level of prescreen is the use of primary dermal irritation (PDI) test results. In this approach, the PDI study is performed before the eye irritation study and if the score from that study (called the primary dermal irritation index or PDII and ranging from 0 to 8) is above a certain level (usually 5.0 or greater), the same options already outlined for physicochemical parameters can be exercised. There is no universal agreement on the value of this prescreen. Gilman *et al.* (1983) did not find the PDII to be a good predictor, but made this judgment based on a relatively small data set and a cutoff PDII of 3.0 or above. In 1984 and 1985, Williams reported that severe PDII scores (5.0 or greater) predicted severe eye irritation responses in 39 of 60 cases. He attributed the false positives to possible overprediction of potential human response by current PDI test procedures. On the other hand, Guillot *et al.* (1982a,b) reported good prediction of eye irritation based on skin irritation in 56 materials, and Gad *et al.* (1986) reported good prediction of severe eye irritation results based on PDIIs of 72 test materials.

5. *Staggered study starts*: Another approach, which is a form of screen, calls for starting the eye test in one or two animals, then delaying the dosing of the additional animals in the test group for 4 hr to a day. During this offset period, if a severe result is seen in the first one or two animals, the remainder of the test may be cancelled. This staggered start allows one to limit testing severe eye irritants to a few animals and yet have confidence that a moderate irritant would be detected.

6. *Use of fluorescein staining and slit lamp examination*: Two methodologies for decreasing the subjectivity of evaluations, for detection of more subtle changes in the eye, and for understanding differences are the use of fluorescein and of slit lamps for performing ocular exams.

Sodium fluorescein is a weak acid and polar molecule which is deeply colored and highly fluorescent and has a number of uses in ophthalmology in both marking damaged tissue and studying the flow of aqueous humor (Maurice, 1967). Fluorescein is frequently used for both screening eyes prior to study initiation (to ensure that only animals with healthy eyes are being included) and to evaluate recovery from grossly observed damage on the cornea.

The slit lamp biomicroscope allows for *in vivo* microscopic study of the ocular tissue (particularly the cornea). There are a range of methods for performing such exams (Sugar, 1980), all of which can be utilized by a well-trained technician.

An integrated summary of the approach presented in these design modifications is shown in Fig. 9.

TABLE 16   Rationale for Rabbit Eye Irritancy Tests

---

1. Provide whole animal and organ *in vivo* evaluation.
   The rabbit test assesses the inflammatory response of a complex organ composed of different tissues made up of numerous cell types. When a tissue or an organ becomes inflamed, the whole animal responds.
2. Either neat chemicals or whole products (complex mixtures) can be tested.
   This allows us to address the complex mixtures resulting from such processes as synthesis, augmentation, quenching, and synergism.
3. Either concentrated or diluted products can be tested.
4. Yields data on the recovery and healing processes.
5. Required screening test with the Federal Hazardous Substances Act (unless data are already available), Toxic Substances Control Act and Federal Insecticides, Fungicides and Rodenticides Act (FIFRA).
6. Quantitative and qualitative test with the Draize ocular scoring scale.
7. Amenable to modifications (irrigation, low volume, and anesthetics).
8. Extensive database and cross-reference capability.
9. The ease of handling of the rabbit.
10. The eye of the albino rabbit presents a large surface of exposed globe for observation, and the lack of pigmentation in the iris makes it easier to interpret iritis.
11. Test is conservative, providing for maximum protection by erring on the side of overprediction of irritancy in man. Because vision is our single most important sense, a greater degree of protection of these small and vulnerable organs is essential.

IN VIVO VS IN VITRO TESTS

Given the modifications that are being made to the traditional rabbit eye irritation test, what are the advantages and disadvantages of the current rabbit eye tests in providing this information? The rationale for such tests and that for seeking alternatives are presented in Tables 16 and 17. These are modifications of lists originally published by Jackson (1983).

IN VITRO TESTS

The area of ocular irritancy has been the most active grounds in toxicology for the development of true alternative (*in vitro*) tests for the past 6 years. A complete review of this effort is beyond the scope of this volume. Indeed, there is a separate book which summarizes the current status (Frazier *et al.*, 1987). However, at least a brief outline or summary of approaches being pursued is called for.

There are six major categories of approaches to alternative eye irritation tests. The first five of these aim at assessing portions of the irritation response

TABLE 17   Rationales for Seeking *in Vitro* Alternatives for Eye Irritancy Tests

Avoid whole animal and organ *in vivo* evaluation

Strict Draize scale testing in the rabbit assesses only three eye structures (conjunctiva, cornea, and iris) and traditional rabbit eye irritancy tests do not assess cataracts, pain, discomfort, or clouding of the lens.

In vivo tests assess only inflammation and immediate structural alterations produced by irritants (not sensitizers, photoirritants, or photoallergens). Note, however, that the test was (and generally is) intended to evaluate any pain or discomfort.

Technical training and monitoring are critical (particularly in view of the subjective nature of evaluation).

Rabbit eye tests do not perfectly predict results in humans if the objective is either the total exclusion of irritants or the identification of truly severe irritants on an absolute basis (that is, without false positives or negatives). Some (such as Reinhardt *et al.*, 1985) have claimed that these tests are too sensitive for such uses.

There are structural and biochemical differences between rabbit and human eyes which make extrapolation from one to the other difficult. For example, Bowman's membrane is present and well developed in man (8–12 μm thick) but not in the rabbit, possibly giving the human cornea greater protection (Prince *et al.*, 1980).

Lack of standardization.

Variable correlation with human results.

Large biological variability between experimental units.

Large, diverse, and fragmented databases which are not readily comparable.

(alterations in tissue morphology, toxicity to individual component cells, alterations in cell or tissue physiology, inflammation, or immune modulation, and alterations in repair and/or recovery processes). These methods have the limitation that they assume that one of these component parts can or will predict effects in the complete organ system. A more likely case is that, while each may serve well to predict the effects of a set of chemical structures which have that component as a determining part of the ocular irritation response, a valid assessment across a broad range of structures will require the use of a collection or battery of such tests.

The sixth category contains tests which have little or no empirical basis, such as computer-assisted structure–activity relationship models. These approaches can only be assessed in terms of how well (or poorly) they perform. Table 18 presents an overview of these categories and some of the component tests within them, as assessed by Gad (1991), along with a single reference for each test.

TABLE 18 *In Vitro* Alternatives for Eye Irritation Tests

Morphology
  Enucleated superfused rabbit eye system (Burton *et al.*, 1981)
  BALB/c 3T3 cells/morphological assays (HTD) (Borenfreund and Puerner, 1984)

Cell toxicity
  Adhesion/cell proliferation
    BHK cells/growth inhibition (Reinhardt *et al.*, 1985)
    BHK cells/colony formation efficiency (Reinhardt *et al.*, 1985)
    BHK cells/cell detachment (Reinhardt *et al.*, 1985)
    SIRC cells/colony forming assay (North-Root *et al.*, 1982)
    BALB/c 3T3 cells/total protein (Shopsis and Eng, 1985)
    BCL/D1 cells/total protein (Balls and Horner, 1985)
    Primary rabbit corneal cells/colony forming assay (Watanabe *et al.*, 1988)
  Membrane integrity
    LS cells/dual dye staining (Scaife, 1982)
    Thymocytes/dual fluorescent dye staining (Aesechbacher *et al.*, 1986)
    LS cells/dual dye staining (Kemp *et al.*, 1983)
    RCE-SIRC-P815-YAC-1/Cr release (Shadduck *et al.*, 1985)
    L929 cells/cell variability (Simons, 1981)
    Bovine red blood cell/hemolysis (Shadduck *et al.*, 1987)
    Mouse L929 fibroblasts–erythrocin C staining (Frazier, 1988)
    Rabbit corneal epithelial and endothelial cells/membrane leakage (Meyer and McCulley, 1988)
    Agarose diffusion (Barnard, 1989)
  Cell metabolism
    Rabbit corneal cell cultures/plasminogen activator (Chan, 1985)
    LS cells/ATP assay (Kemp *et al.*, 1985)
    BALB/c 3T3 cells/neutral red uptake (Borenfreund and Puerner, 1984)
    BALB/c 3T3 uridine uptake inhibition assay (Shopsis and Sathe, 1984)
    HeLa cells/metabolic inhibition test (MIT-24) (Selling and Ekwall, 1985)
    MDCK cells/dye diffusion (Tchao, 1988)

Cell and tissue physiology
  Epidermal slice/electrical conductivity (Oliver and Pemberton, 1985)
  Rabbit ileum/contraction inhibition (Muir *et al.*, 1983)
  Bovine cornea/corneal opacity (Muir, 1984)
  Proposed mouse eye/permeability test (Maurice and Singh, 1986)

Inflammation/immunity
  Chorioallantoic membrane (CAM)
    CAM (Leighton *et al.*, 1983)
    HET-CAM (Luepke, 1985)
  Bovine corneal cup model/leukocyte chemotactic factors (Elgebaly *et al.*, 1986)
  Rat peritoneal mast cells/histamine release (Jacaruso *et al.*, 1985)
  Rat peritoneal mast cells/serotonin release (Chasin *et al.*, 1979)
  Rat vaginal explant/prostaglandin relsease (Dubin *et al.*, 1984)
  Bovine eye cup/histamine (Hm) and leukotriene C4 (LtC4) release (Benassi *et al.*, 1986)

Recovery/repair
  Rabbit corneal epithelial cells–wound healing (Jumblatt and Neufeld, 1985)

Other
  EYTEX assay (Gordon and Bergman, 1986; Soto *et al.*, 1988)
  Computer-based structure–activity (Enslein, 1984; Enslein *et al.*, 1988)

REFERENCES

Aesechbacher, M., Reinhardt, C. A., and Zbinden, G. (1986). A rapid cell membrane permeability test using fluorescent dyes and flow cytometry. *Cell Biol. Toxicol.*, in press.

Alexander, P. (1965). Evaluation of the irritation potential of shampoos and conditioning rinses. *Specialties* 9, 33–37.

Andermann, G., and Erhart, M. (1983). *Meth. Find. Exp. Clin. Pharmacol.* 5, 321–333.

Ballantyne, B., and Swanston, D. W. (1977). The scope and limitations of acute eye irritation tests. In *Current Approaches in Toxicology* (B. Ballantyne, Ed.), pp. 139–157. Wright, Bristol, UK.

Balls, M., and Horner, S. A. (1985). The FRAME interlaboratory program on *in vitro* cytotoxicology. *Fd. Chem. Toxicol.* 23, 205–213.

Barnard, N. D. (1989). A Draize alternative. *Animal's Agenda* 6, 45.

Bayard, S., and Hehir, R. M. (1976). Evaluation of proposed changes in the modified Draize rabbit irritation test. Soc. Toxicol. 15th Meeting, Atlanta, GA. [Abstract 225]

Beckley, J. H. (1965). Comparative eye testing: Man vs. animal. *Toxicol. Appl. Pharmacol.* 7, 93–101.

Benassi, C. A., Angi, M. R., Salvalaio, L., and Bettero, A. (1986). Histamine and leukotriene C4 release from isolated bovine scheracharoid complex: A new *in vitro* ocular irritation test. *Chimica Agg.*

Berdasco, N. A., Gilbert, K. S., Luchar, J., and Matteson, J. L. (1996). Low rate of severe injury from dermal and ocular irritation tests and the validity of using fewer animals. *J. Am. Col. Tox.* 15, 177–193.

Borenfreund, E., and Peurner, J. A. (1984). A simple quantiitative procedure using monolayer cultures for cytotoxicity assays (HTD/NR-NE). *J. Tissue Culture Methods* 9, 7–10.

Burton, A. B. G., York, M., and Lawrence, R. S. (1981). The *in vitro* assessment of severe eye irritants. *Fd. Cosmet. Toxicol.* 19, 471–480.

Calabrese, E. J. (1984). *Principles of Animal Extrapolation*, pp. 391–402. Wiley, New York.

Chan, K. Y. (1985). An *in vitro* alternative to the Draize test. In *In Vitro Toxicology* (A. M. Goldberg, Ed.), Alternative Methods in Toxicology, Vol. 3, pp. 405–422. Liebert, New York.

Chan, P. K., and Hayes, A. W. (1985). Assessment of chemically induced ocular toxicity: A survey of methods. *Toxicology of the Eye, Ear and Other Special Senses* (A. W. Hayes, Ed.), pp. 103–143. Raven Press, New York.

Chasin, M., Scott, C., Shaw, C., and Persico, F. (1979). A new assay for the measurement of mediator release from rat peritoneal in most cells. *Int. Arch. Allergy Appl. Immun.* 58, 1–10.

Code of Federal Regulations (CFR) (1981). Revised Jan. 1, 1981, Title 16: Subchapter C—Federal Hazardous Substances Act, Part 1500.42 (test for eye irritants).

Consumer Products Safety Commission (CPSC) (1976). *Illustrated Guide for Grading Eye Irritation Caused by Hazardous Substances* (16 CFR 1500).

Draize, J. H., Woodard, G., and Calvery, H. O. (1944). Methods for the study of irritation and toxicity of substances applied topically to the skin and mucus membranes. *J. Pharmacol. Exp. Ther.* 82, 377–390.

Dubin, N. H., and De Blasi, M. C., *et al.* (1984). Development of an *in vitro* test for cytotoxicity in vaginal tissue: Effect of ethanol on prostanoid release. In *Acute Toxicity Testing: Alternative Approaches* (A. M. Goldberg, Ed.), Alternative Methods in Toxicology, Vol. 2, pp. 127–138. Liebert, New York.

Dunn, B. J., Nichols, C. W., and Gad, S. C. (1982). Acute dermal toxicity of two quarternary organophosphonium salts in the rabbit. *Toxicology* 24, 245–250.

Elgebaly, S. A., Downes, R. T., Forouhr, F., O'Rourke, J., and Kreutzer, D. L. (1986). Inflammatory mediators in alkali-burned corneas: Inhibitory effects of citric acid. Submitted for publication.

Enslein, K. (1984). Estimation of toxicology endpoints by structure–activity relationships. *Pharmacol. Rev.* 36, 131–134.

Enslein, K., Blake, V. W.,, Tuzzeo, T. M., Borgstedt, H. H., Hart, J. B., and Salem, H. (1988). Estimation of rabbit eye irritation scores by structure–activity equations. *In Vitro Toxicol.* **2**, 1–14.

Environmental Protection Agency (EPA) (1979). Acute Toxicity Testing Criteria for New Chemical Substances (EPA 560/13-9-009, 9-14).

Falahee, K. J., Rose, C. S., Olin, S. S., and Seifried, H. E. (1981). *Eye Irritation Testing: An Assessment of Methods and Guidelines for Testing Materials for Eye Irritancy.* Office of Pesticides and Toxic Substances, EPA, Washington, DC.

Food and Drug Administration (FDA) (1965). *Illustrated Guide for Grading Eye Irritation by Hazardous Substances.* FDA, Washington, DC.

Federal Hazardous Substances Act (FHSA) (1974, 1979) Chapter 2, Title 16. CFR 13009-191.12. Test for Eye Irritants.

Frazier, J. M., Gad, S. C., Goldberg, A. M., and McCulley, J. P. (1987). *A Critical Evaluation of Alternatives to Acute Ocular Irritation Testing.* Liebert, New York.

Freeberg, F. E., Griffith, J. F., Bruce, R. D., and Bay, P. H. S. (1984). Correlation of animal test methods with human experience for household products. *J. Toxicol. Cut. Ocular Toxicol.* **1**, 53–64.

Freeberg, F. E., Nixon, G. A., Reer, D. J., Weaver, J. E., Bruce, R. D., Griffiths, J. F., and Sanders, L. W. (1986). Human and rabbit eye response to chemical insult. *Fundam. Appl. Toxicol.* **7**, 626–634.

Friedenwald, J. S., Hughes, W. F., and Herrmann, H. (1944). Acid-base tolerance of the cornea. *Arch. Ophthalmol.* **31**, 279.

Gad, S. C. (1994). *In Vitro Toxicology.* Raven Press, New York.

Gad, S. C., Walsh, R. D., and Dunn, B. J. (1986). Correlation of ocular and dermal irritancy of industrial chemicals. *J. Toxicol. Cut. Ocular Toxicol.* **5**(3), 193–211.

Gilman, M. R. (1982). Skin and eye testing in animals. In *Principles and Methods of Toxicology* (A. W. Hayes, Ed.), pp. 209–222. Raven Press, New York.

Gilman, M. R., Jackson, E. M., Cerven, D. R., and Moreno, M. T. (1983). Relationship between the primary dermal irritation index and ocular irritation. *J. Toxicol. Cut. Ocular Toxicol.* **2**, 107–117.

Gloxhuber, C. H. (1985). Modification of the Draize eye test for the safety testing of cosmetics. *Fd. Chem. Toxicol.* **23**, 187–188.

Gordon, V. C., and Bergman, H. C. (1986). Eytex, an *in vitro* method for evaluation of optical irritancy. National Testing Corporation Report 26.

Grant, W. M., and Schuman, J. S. (1993). *Toxicology of the Eye,* 4th ed. Charles C Thomas, Springfield, IL.

Green, W. R., Sullivan, J. B., Hehir, R. M., Scharpf, L. F., and Dickinson, A. W. (1978). *A Systematic Comparison of Chemically Induced Eye Injury in the Albino Rabbit and the Rhesus Monkey.* The Soap and Detergent Association, New York.

Griffith, J. F., Nixon, G. A., Bruce, R. D., Reer, P. J., and Bannan, E. A. (1980). Dose–response studies with chemical irritants in the albino rabbit eye as a basis for selecting optimum testing conditions for predicting hazard to the human eye. *Toxicol. Appl. Pharmacol.* **55**, 501–513.

Guillot, J. P., Gonnet, J. F., Clement, C., Caillard, L., and Trahaut, R. (1982a). Evaluation of the cutaneous-irritation potential of 56 compounds. *Fd. Chem. Toxicol.* **201**, 563–572.

Guillot, J. P., Gonnet, J. F., Clement, C., Caillard, L., and Trahaut, R. (1982b). Evaluation of the cutaneous-irritation potential of 56 compounds. *Fd. Chem. Toxicol.* **20**, 573–582.

Interagency Regulatory Liaison Group (IRIG) (January 1981). Testing Standards and Guidelines Work Group. Recommended Guidelines.

Jacaruso, R. B., Barlett, M. A., Carson, S., and Trombetta, L. D. (1985). Release of histamine from rat peritoneal cells in vitro as an index of irritational potential. *J. Toxicol. Cut. Ocular Toxicol.* **4**, 39–48.

Jackson, E. M. (1983). Industrial practices in safety testing. In *Product Safety Evaluation* (A. M. Goldberg, Ed.), Alternative Methods in Toxicology, Vol. 1, pp. 51–65. Liebert, New York.

Jackson, J., and Rutty, D. A. (1985). Ocular tolerance assessment-integrated tier policy. *Fd. Chem. Toxicol.* **23**, 309–310.

Jumblatt, M. M., and Neufeld, A. H. (1985). A tissue culture model of the human corneal epithelium. In *In Vitro Toxicology* (A. M. Golberg, Ed.), Alternative Methods in Toxicology, Vol. 3, pp. 391–404. Liebert, New York.

Kemp, R. V., Meredith, R. W. J., Gamble, S., and Frost, M. (1983). A rapid cell culture technique for assaying to toxicity of detergent based products in vitro as a possible screen for high irritants in vivo. *Cytobios.* **36**, 153–159.

Kemp, R. V., Meredith, R. W. J., and Gamble, S. (1985). Toxicity of commercial products on cells in suspension: A possible screen for the Draize eye irritation test. *Fd. Chem. Toxicol.* **23**, 267–270.

Latven, A. R., and Molitor, H. (1939). Comparison of the toxic, hypnotic and irritating properties of 8 organic solvents. *J. Pharm. Exp. Ther.* **65**, 89–94.

Leighton, J., Nassauer, J., Tchao, R., and Verdone, J. (1983). Development of a procedure using the chick egg as an alternative to the Draize rabbit test. In *Product Safety Evaluation* (A. M. Goldberg, Ed.), Alternative Methods in Toxicology, Vol. 1, pp. 165–177, Liebert, New York.

Luepke, N. P. (1985). Hen's egg chorioallantoic membrane test for irritation potential. *Fd. Chem. Toxicol.* **23**, 287–291.

Mann, I., and Pullinger, B. D. (1942). A study of mustard gas lesions of the eyes of rabbits and men. *Proc. R. Soc. Med.* **35**, 229–244.

Marzulli, F. N., and Ruggles, D. I. (1973). Rabbit eye irritation test: Collaborative study. *J. Assoc. Off. Anal. Chem.* **56**, 905–914.

Maurice, D. M. (1967). The use of fluorescein in ophthalmological research. *Invest. Ophthalmol.* **6**, 465–477.

Maurice, D., and Singh, T. (1986). A permeability test for acute corneal toxicity. *Toxicol. Lett.* **31**, 125–130.

McCally, A. W., Farmer, A. G., and Loomis, E. C. (1933). Corneal ulceration following use of lash lure. *JAMA* **101**, 1560–1561.

McDonald, T. O., Seabaugh, V., Shadduck, J. A., and Edelhauser, H. F. (1983). Eye irritation. In *Dermatotoxicology* (F. N. Marzulli and H. I. Maibach, Eds.), pp. 555–610. Hemisphere, New York.

McLaughlin, R. S. (1946). Chemical burns of the human cornea. *Am. J. Ophthalmol.* **29**, 1355–1362.

Meyer, D. R., and McCulley, J. P. (1988). Acute and protracted injury to cornea epithelium as an indication of the biocompatability of various pharmaceutical vehicles. In *Progress in in Vitro Toxicology* (A. M. Goldberg, Ed.), pp. 215–235. Liebert, New York.

Muir, C. K. (1984). A simple method to assess surfactant-induced bovine corneal opacity in vitro: Preliminary findings. *Toxicol. Lett.* **23**, 199–203.

Muir, C. K., Flower, C., and Van Abbe, N. J. (1983). A novel approach to the search for in vitro alternatives to in vivo eye irritancy testing. *Toxicol. Lett.* **18**, 1–5.

Murphy, J. C., Osterberg, R. E., Seabaugh, V. M., and Bierbower (1982). Ocular irritancy response to various pHs of acids and bases with and without irrigation. *Toxicology* **23**, 281–291.

NAS (1977). *Principles and Procedures for Evaluating the Toxicity of Household Substances.* NAS Publication 1138, pp. 41–59.

North-Root, H., Yackovich, Demetrulias, F. J., Gucula, N., and Heinze, J. E. (1982). Evaluation of an *in vitro* cell toxicity test using rabbit corneal cells to predict the eye irritation potential of surfactants. *Toxicol. Lett.* **14**, 207–212.

Oliver, G. J. A., and Pemberton, N. A. (1985). An *in vitro* epidermal slice technique for identifying chemicals with potential for severe cutaneous effects. *Fd. Chem. Toxicol.* **23**, 229–232.

Organization for Economic Cooperation and Development (OECD) (1981). *OECD Guidelines for Testing of Chemicals,* Sect. 404, Acute Dermal Irritation/Corrosion, Paris.

Reinhardt, C. A., Pelli, D. A., and Zbinden, G. (1985). Interpretation of cell toxicity data for the estimation of potential irritation. *Fd. Chem. Toxicol.* **23**, 247–252.

Scaife, M. C. (1982). An investigation of detergent action on *in vitro* and possible correlations with *in vivo* data. *Int. J. Cosmet. Sci.* **4**, 179–193.

Selling, J., and Ekwall, B. (1985). Screening for eye irritancy using cultured Hela cells. *Xenobiotica* **15**, 713–717.

Shadduck, J. A., Everitt, J., and Bay, P. (1985). Use of *in vitro* cytotoxicity to rank ocular irritation of six surfactants. In *In Vitro Toxicology* (A. M. Goldberg, Ed.), Alternative Methods in Toxicology, Vol. 3, pp. 641–649. Liebert, New York.

Shadduck, J. A., Render, J., Everitt, J., Meccoli, R. A., and Essexsorlie, D. (1987). An approach to validation: Comparison of six materials in three tests. In *In Vitro Toxicology–Approaches to Validation,* Alternative Methods in Toxicology, Vol. 5. Liebert, New York.

Shopsis, C., and Eng, B. (1985). Uridine uptake and cell growth cytotoxicity test: Comparison applications and mechanistic studies. *J. Cell Biol.* **101**, 87a.

Shopsis, C.,and Sathe, S. (1984). Uridine uptake inhibition as a cytotoxicity test: Correlation with the Draize test. *Toxicology* **29**, 195–206.

Silverman, J. (1983). Preliminary findings on the use of protozoa (*Tetrahymena thermophila*) as models for ocular irritation testing in rabbits. *Lab. Animal Sci.* **33**, 56–59.

Simons, P. J. (1981). An alternative to the Draize test. In *The Use of Alternatives in Drug Research* (A. N. Rowan and C. J. Stratmann, Eds.). MacMillan, London.

Soto, R. J., Servi, M. J., and Gordon, V. C. (1988). Evaluation of an alternative method of ocular irritation. In *Progress in in Vitro Toxicology* (A. M. Goldberg, Ed.), pp. 289–296. Liebert, New York.

Sugar, J. (1980). Corneal examination. In *Principles and Practice of Ophthalmology, Vol. 1* (G. A. Peyman, D. R. Sanders, and M. F. Goldberg, Eds.), pp. 393–395. Saunders, Philadelphia.

Swanston, D. W. (1985). Assessment of the validity of animal techniques in eye irritation testing. *Fd. Chem. Toxicol.* **23**, 169–173.

Tchao, R. (1988). Trans-epithelial permeability of fluorescein *in vitro* as an assay to determine eye irritants. In *Progress in in Vitro Toxicology* (A. M. Goldberg, Ed.), pp. 271–284. Liebert, New York.

Walker, A. P. (1985). A more realistic animal technique for predicting human eye responses. *Fd. Chem. Toxicol.* **23**, 175–178.

Watanabe, M., Watanabe, K., Suzuki, K., Nikaido, O., Sugarhara, T., Ishii, I., and Konishi, H. (1988). *In vitro* cytotoxicity test using primary cells derived from rabbit eye is useful as an alternative for Draize testing. In *Progress in in Vitro Toxicology* (A. M. Goldberg, Ed.), pp. 285–290. Liebert, New York.

Weil, C. S., and Scala, R. A. (1971). Study of intra- and interlaboratory variability in the results of rabbit eye and skin irritation test. *Toxicol. Appl. Pharmacol.* **19**, 276–360.

Williams, S. J. (1984). Prediction of ocular irritancy potential from dermal irritation test result. *Fd. Chem. Toxicol.* **2**, 157–161.

Williams, S. J. (1985). Changing concepts of ocular irritation evaluation: Pitfalls and progress. *Fd. Chem. Toxicol.* **23**, 189–193.

Williams, S. J., Graepel, G. J., and Kennedy, G. L. (1982). Evaluation of ocular irritancy potential: Intralaboratory variability and effect of dosage volume. *Toxicol. Lett.* **12**, 235–241.

CHAPTER 5

Dermal Sensitization

Assessing materials to determine if they can act as delayed contact dermal sensitizers in humans is different on a number of grounds from the other tests we have looked at so far and, indeed, from most of the other test systems presented later in this book. These differences all stem from how the immune system, which is the mechanistic basis for this set of adverse responses, functions.

Bringing about this Coombs type IV hypersensitivity response (which we will call "sensitization," for short) requires more than a single exposure to the causative material, both in humans and in test animals. Unlike irritation responses, sensitization occurs in individuals in an extremely variable manner. A portion of the human population is considerably more liable to be sensitized while others are infrequently affected. And the response, once sensitization is achieved, becomes progressively more severe with each additional exposure. All three of these characteristics are due to the underlying mechanism for the response and influence the manner in which we conduct tests. These factors mean that *in vivo* test systems require multiple exposures of animals (unlike all of the other systems in this volume, except for photosensitization, which is related to sensitization) and tend to underpredict the potential for an adverse response in those individuals who are most susceptible to sensitization. But because the response to repeated exposures of even minimal amounts of material in these susceptible individuals can lead to such striking adverse responses, we must be concerned about them.

MECHANISMS

Our understanding of the mechanism underlying sensitization has increased greatly in recent years but still includes several alternative "models" for portions of the whole. These are best guesses as to what occurs on a molecular or cellular basis.

The outward signs of both irritation and sensitization are often similar (erythema, edema, heat, etc.) but the mechanisms leading to these two inflammatory responses are very different (Jackson, 1984). Dermal sensitization and photosensitization are delayed cellular immune responses mediated by T lymphocytes. A chemical hapten or incomplete allergen first must pass into the dermis, and then complexes with dermis protein to form a hapten–protein complex. The Langerhans' cells in the area interact with this antigen (allergen) as if it is a completely foreign protein. These Langerhans' cells then migrate to the thymus gland to "educate" the naive T cells about the allergen. The now educated T cells proliferate and leave the thymus as "sensitized cells"—that is, cells which will act as "defenders" against the foreign protein. With the proper stimulus, they can initiate the inflammatory process through the release of lymphokines, followed by an influx of granulocytes and macrophages. The role of different cytokines (such as TNF-α) in sensitization has been well explored in the past decade (Kimber, 1993). This knowledge will not only lead to different, more sophisticated assays but has already provided explanations as to why some chemicals are pulmonary sensitizors and others are contact sensitizers (Dearman and Kimber, 1991).

A number of factors influence the potential for a chemical to be a sensitizer in humans and, in turn, also influence the performance of test systems. These are summarized in Table 19. Various test systems manipulate these in different ways.

There are a number of references which explore and discuss the underlying immune system mechanisms and operation in greater detail. Particularly recommended is Gibson et al. (1983).

OBJECTIVES AND GENERAL FEATURES

Given the considerations of mechanism, degree of concern about protecting people, and practicality, the desired characteristics of a sensitization test include the following:

TABLE 19   Factors Influencing Delayed Type Sensitization Responses

1. Percutaneous absorption of agent

2. Genetic status of host

3. Immunological status of host

4. Host nutrition

5. Chemical and physical nature of potential sensitizing agent

6. Number, frequency, and degree of exposures of immune system to potential antigen

7. Concurrent immunological stimuli (such as adjuvants, innoculations, and infections). System can be "up modulated" by mild stimuli or overburdened by excessive stimulation

8. Age, sex, and pregnancy (by influencing factors 1, 3, and 4 above)

1. Be reproducible.
2. Involve fairly low technical skills so that it may be performed as a general laboratory test.
3. Not involve the use of exotic animals or equipment.
4. Use relatively small amounts of test material.
5. Be capable of evaluating almost any material of interest.
6. Be sensitize enough to detect weak sensitizers (that is, those which would require extensive exposure to sensitize other than the most sensitive individuals).
7. Predict the relative potency of sensitizing agents accurately.

Several of these desired characteristics are mutually contradictory; as with most other test systems, the methods for detecting dermal sensitization each incorporate a set of compromises.

All the *in vivo* tests have some common features, however. The most striking is that they involve at least three (and frequently four) different phases. These are, in order, the irritation/toxicity screen, the induction phase, the challenge phase, and (often) the rechallenge phase.

Irritation/toxicity screen: All assays require knowledge of the dermal irritancy and systemic toxicity of the test material(s) to be used in the induction, challenge, and rechallenge. These properties are defined in this pretest phase. Most tests desire (or will allow) mild irritation in the induction phase but no systemic toxicity. Generally, a nonirritating concentration is required for the challenge and for any rechallenge because having irritation present either confounds the results or precludes having a valid test. As will be discussed in the sections on the individual tests, even a carefully designed screen does not necessarily provide the desired guidance in selecting usable concentrations. During this phase, solvent systems are also selected.

Induction phase: This requires exposing the test animals to the test material several times over a period of days or weeks. A number of events must be accomplished during this phase if a sensitization response is to be elicited. The test material must penetrate through the epidermis and into the dermis. There, it must interact with dermis protein. The protein–test material complex must be perceived by the immune system as an allergen. Finally, the production of sensitized T cells must be accomplished. Some assays enhance the sensitivity of the induction phase by compromising the natural ability of the epidermis to act as a barrier. These enhancement techniques include irritation of the induction site, intradermal injection, tape stripping, and occlusive dressings. In contrast, events such as the development of a scab over the induction site may reduce percutaneous absorption. The attention of the immune system can be drawn to the induction site by the intradermal injection of oil-coated bacteria (Freund's complete adjuvant, which serves as a mild immunological stimulant).

Challenge phase: This consists of exposing the animals to a concentration of the test material which would normally not be expected to cause a response (usually an erythema-type response). The responses in the test animals and of the control animals are then scored or measured.

Rechallenge phase: This is a repeat of the challenge phase and can be a very valuable tool if used properly. Sensitized animals can be rechallenged with the same test material at the same concentration used in the challenge in order to assist in confirming sensitization. Sensitized animals can be rechallenged with different concentrations of the allergen to evaluate dose–response relationships. Animals sensitized to an ingredient can be challenged to a formulation containing the ingredient to evaluate the potential of the formulated product to elicit a sensitization response under adverse conditions. Conversely, animals which responded (sometimes unexpectedly) to a final formulation can be challenged with formulation without the suspected sensitizer or to the ingredient which is suspected to be the allergen. Cross-reactivity can be evaluated; that is, the ability of one test material to elicit a sensitization response following exposure in the induction phase to a different test material. A well-designed rechallenge is important and should be considered at the same time that the sensitization evaluation is being designed because the rechallenge must be run within 1 or 2 weeks after the primary challenge. Unless plans have been made for a possible rechallenge, one may have to reformulate a test material or obtain additional pure ingredient and perhaps run additional irritation/toxicity screens before the rechallenge can be run. The ability of the sensitized animals to respond at a rechallenge can fade with time; thus the reason for the rechallenge being run shortly after the challenge. In addition, some assays use sham-treated controls and these must be procured while the induction phase is in progress. One additional piece of information must be kept in mind when evaluating a rechallenge. The animal does not differentiate between an induction exposure and a challenge exposure. If one is using an assay which involves three induction exposures and one challenge exposure, then, at the rechallenge, the animal has received four induction exposures. This "extra" induction may serve to strengthen a sensitization response.

After the study is done, one must evaluate the data and decide how to translate them to the human conditions. We will look at this problem toward the end of this chapter.

HISTORY

Koch's initial observation of tuberculin reactivity was made in humans and guinea pigs. Though the rabbit and guinea pig have both been considered the animals of choice for evaluating adverse skin reactions of chemicals, from the beginning guinea pigs have been the animals of choice for predictive tests. Though it is widely believed that this is due to a relatively higher degree of susceptibility to dermal sensitization, the preference was actually based on availability, ease of handling, and the fact that the albino animal has a clear pale skin which is easily denuded of hair and on which an erythema response is easy to distinguish. Recently developed protocols have relied on the mouse as the experimental model, as will be discussed below.

Landsteiner and Jacobs (1935) first proposed a formalized predictive test in guinea pigs. Later, he and Chase (1942) used low-molecular-weight chemicals to sensitize guinea pigs and developed the theory of complete antigen formations being due to hapten–protein interactions.

The basis of many predictive tests is that devised by Landsteiner and Draize in 1944. It consists of 10 intradermal injections of the test compound into the skin of albino guinea pigs during the 3-week induction period and a single intracutaneous challenge application 14 days after the last induction injection. A standardized 0.1% test concentration is used for induction and challenge. This method was widely used and recommended until the end of the 1960s. Its disadvantage is that only strong allergens are detected, while well-known moderate allergens fail to sensitize the animals at all.

Starting in 1964, however, a wide variety of new test designs started to be proposed. Buehler (1964) proposed what is now considered the first modern test (described in detail in this chapter), which used an occlusive patch to increase test sensitivity. The Buehler test is the primary example of the so-called "epidermal" methods, which have been criticized for giving false negative results for moderate to weak sensitizers such as nickel.

A new generation of tests was established by using Freund's complete adjuvant (FCA) during the induction process to stimulate the immune system, independent of the type of hapten and independent of the method or application; that is, whether or not the substance is incorporated in the adjuvant mixture. It is claimed that this family of tests displays the same level of susceptibility to sensitization in guinea pigs as is normally observed in humans (Cronin and Agrup, 1970). The adjuvant tests include the guinea pig maximization test (GPMT; Magnusson and Kligman, 1969), optimization test (Maurer et al., 1975, 1980), split adjuvant test (Maguire and Chase, 1967), and the epicutaneous maximization test (EMT; Guillot and Gonnet, 1985).

Finally, during the past few years, two test systems which use mice instead of guinea pigs—the mouse ear swelling test (MEST; Gad et al., 1985a) and the local lymph nude assay (Kimber et al., 1986, 1994; Basketter et al., 1992a,b)— have been proposed as an alternatives. Both assays are gaining provision acceptance by most regulatory agencies as a preliminary screen. Negative results must be confirmed with a guinea pig assay.

This chain of development should be expected to continue and the overall quality and utility of tests should improve. Five tests will be presented and compared in this volume because they have features and operating characteristics which make them altercative in particular circumstances and also cause them to be representative of other available tests. These are the Buehler, guinea pig maximization, split adjuvant, mouse ear swelling, and local lymph node tests.

MODIFIED BUEHLER PROCEDURE

This is a closed patch procedure for evaluating test substances for potential delayed contact dermal sensitization in guinea pigs. The procedure, based on that described by Buehler (1965), is practical for test substances that cannot be evaluated by the traditional intradermal injection procedure of Landsteiner and Jacobs (1935) or by the GPMT for skin sensitization testing. The closed patch procedure is performed when a test substance either is highly irritating to the skin by the intradermal injection route of exposure or cannot be dissolved or suspended in a form allowing injection. It is also the method of choice for some companies. This procedure, which is one version of the Buehler test, complies with the test standards set forth in the Toxic Substances Control Act (TSCA) and other regulatory test rules and is presented diagramatically in Fig. 10. There are other versions which also comply.

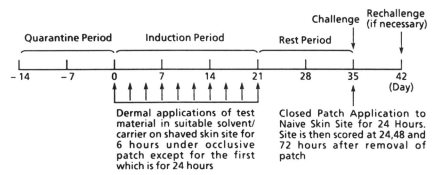

MODIFIED BUEHLER TEST DESIGN

Species: Guinea Pig
Strain: Hartley
Test Group: 15 Animals
Control Group: 6 Animals

FIGURE 10 Line chart for modified Buehler test for delayed contact dermal sensitization in the guinea pig.

Animals

1. Young albino female guinea pigs, weighing between 300 and 400 g, are used.

2. Although several proposed test rules suggest the use of male guinea pigs, the female sex is preferred because the aggressive social behavior of males may result in considerable skin damage that might interfere with the interpretation of challenge reactions. This concern occurs because animals are group housed (Marzulli and Maibach, 1983).

3. Animals that show poor growth or are ill in any way are not used because illness markedly decreases the response. Animals with skin marked or scarred from fighting are avoided. The guinea pigs are observed for at least 2 weeks to detect any illness before starting a study.

4. The guinea pigs are identified by a cage card and marking pen or any other suitable method. There is no regulatory requirement, however, for the identification of individual animals.

5. The guinea pigs are randomly assigned to test and negative control groups consisting of at least 15 and at least 6 animals each, respectively. If a pretest group is necessary, as many animals as needed for that group are randomized also.

Pretest screen
1. If practical, the dermal irritation threshold concentration should
   be established for the test substance prior to the first induction application. A concentration of the test substance that produces minimal or no irritation (erythema and/or edema formation) is determined. The highest concentration that produces no irritation is
   preferred for the dermal sensitization study challenge dose.
2. Those animals randomly assigned to the pretest group are used.
3. Each animal is prepared by clipping a 1-in. square area of hair
   from the left upper flank using a small animal clipper with a size
   No. 40 blade.
4. The test substance is diluted, emulsified, or suspended in a suitable vehicle. Vehicles are selected on the basis of their solubilizing
   capacity for the test substance and on their ability to penetrate the
   skin.
5. Different concentrations of the test substance are tested on the pretest group of guinea pigs; a few animals are used for each concentration tested.
6. A volume of 0.5 ml is applied to a patch consisting of a cotton
   pad (2.5 × 2.5 cm) occluded with impermeable surgical tape or
   placed in a Hilltop style occlusive "chamber."
7. The patch is applied to the shaved left flank of a guinea pig. The
   patch is held firmly in place for 24 hr by wrapping the trunk of
   the animal with a 3-in.-wide elastic bandage. A 2-in.-wide strip of
   tape is used to line the center adhesive side of the bandage in order to prevent skin damage from the adhesive.
8. After 24 hr of exposure, the wrappings and patches are removed.
9. Observations of skin reactions (erythema and/or edema formation)
   are recorded 48 hr after application.
10. A judgment is made as to which concentration will be used for
    the dermal sensitization study, based on the dermal irritation data
    which have been collected. The highest concentration that pro-
    duces minimal or no dermal irritation is selected.

Induction phase
1. Test group and control group guinea pigs are weighed at the beginning of the study and weekly thereafter.
2. Test control group guinea pigs are clipped as described earlier in
   this procedure.
3. If the test substance is a liquid (solution, suspension, or emulsion),
   a volume of 0.5 ml of the highest concentration found to be nonirritating in a suitable vehicle (as determined in the pretest portion of

this procedure) is applied to a patch consisting of a cotton pad (1 × 1 in.) occluded with impermeable surgical tape. If the test substance is a solid or semisolid, 0.5 g is applied. (When the test substance is in flake, granule, powder, or other particulate form, the weight of the test substance that has a volume of 0.5 ml (after compacting as much as possible without crushing or altering the individual particles, such as by tapping the measuring container) is used whenever this volume weighs less than 0.5 g.) If the test substance is a fabric, a 1-in. square is moistened with 0.5 ml of physiological saline before application.

4. The first induction patch is applied to the clipped left flank of each test group guinea pig. The patch is held firmly in place for 24 hr by wrapping the trunk of each animal with a 3-in.-wide elastic bandage. A 5-cm-wide strip of tape is used to line the center adhesive side of the bandage in order to prevent skin damage from the adhesive. A 5-cm length of athletic adhesive tape is placed over the bandage wrap as a precautionary measure to prevent unraveling.

5. After 24 hr of exposure, the wrappings and patches are removed and disposed of in a plastic bag.

6. Each dermal reaction, if any, is scored on the basis of the designated values for erythema and edema formation presented in Table 20. Observations are made 48 hr after initiation of the first induction application. Resulting dermal irritation scores are recorded.

7. After the initial induction application, subsequent induction applica-

TABLE 20 Evaluation of Skin Reactions

Skin reaction	Value
Erythema and eschar formation	
No erythema	0
Very slight erythema (barely perceptible)	1
Well-defined erythema	2
Moderate to severe erythema	3
Severe erythema (beet redness) to slight eschar formation (injuries in-depth)	4
Necrosis (death of tissue)	+N
Eschar (sloughing)	+E
Edema formation	
No edema	0
Very slight edema (barely perceptible)	1
Slight edema (edges of area well defined by definite raising)	2
Moderate edema (raised approximately 1 mm)	3
Severe edema (raised more than 1 mm and extending beyond the area of exposure)	4

Note. These scores are illustrated in the photographs in Fig. 5A. From Draize (1959).

tions (2–10) are made on alternate days (three times weekly) until a total of 10 treatments are administered. Each of these patches is removed after 6 hr of exposure. It should be noted that some use a modification which calls for one application per week for 3 weeks.

8. Observations are made 24 and 48 hr after initiation of each subsequent induction application. Dermal scores of the remaining nine induction applications are needed.

9. Clipping the hair from the left flank induction sites of test group animals and corresponding sites on negative control group animals is performed just prior to each subsequent induction application. Only the test group guinea pigs receive the induction applications.

Challenge phase

1. Fourteen days after the tenth induction application, all 10 test group, and 3 of 6 control group guinea pigs are prepared for challenge application by clipping a 1-in. square area of hair from the right side, the side opposite that which was clipped during the induction phase.

2. A challenge dose, using freshly prepared test substance (solution, suspension, emulsion, semisolid, solid, or fabric), is applied topically to the right side (which had remained untreated during the induction application) of test group animals. The left side, which had previously received induction applications, is not challenge dosed.

3. The concentration of the challenge dose is the same as that used for the first induction application. (It must be a concentration that does not produce dermal irritation after one 24-hr. application.)

4. Each of three negative control group guinea pigs is challenge dosed on the right flank at approximately the same time that the test group guinea pigs are challenge dosed.

5. All patches are held in contact with the skin for 24 hr before removal.

6. The skin sites are evaluated using the scoring system for erythema and edema formation presented in Table 20. Observations are made 48, 72, and 96 hr after initiation of the challenge application. Skin reactions are recorded.

Rechallenge phase

1. If the test substance is judged a nonsensitizing agent after the first challenge application, or causes dermal sensitization in only a few animals or causes dermal reactions that are weak or questionable, then a second and final challenge application will be performed on each test animal 7 days after the initiation of the first challenge dose.

2. Controls from the first challenge application are not rechallenged because they have been exposed to the test substance and are not longer true negative controls. The three remaining naive control group animals (not used for the first challenge) are challenged for comparison to the test group animals.

3. The product used for the first challenge application will be used for the second challenge application (including reclipping, patching method, and duration of exposure). Either the same concentration or a new concentration (higher or lower) of test substance may be used, depending on the results of the first challenge. Observations are made 48, 72, and 96 hr after initiation of the rechallenge application and skin reactions are recorded.

4. When a rechallenge application is performed, the data from both challenges are compared. If neither challenge produces a positive dermal reaction, the classification of the test substance is based on both challenge applications. If one challenge application (whether it is the first or second) produces a greater number of positive dermal reactions than the other, the classification of the test substance is based on the challenge with the most positive responses.

5. Two or more unequivocally positive responses in a group of 15 animals should be considered significant. A negative, equivocal, or single response probably ensures that a substance is not a strong sensitizer, although this is best confirmed by further testing with human subjects (NAS, 1977).

Interpretation of results

1. Judgment concerning the presence or absence of sensitization is made for each animal. The judgment is made by comparing the test animal's challenge responses to its first induction treatment response, as well as to those challenge responses of negative control animals.

2. Challenge reactions to the test substance that are stronger than challenge reactions to negative controls or to those seen after the initial induction application should be suspected as results of sensitization (NAS, 1977). A reaction that occurs at 48 hr, but resolves by 72 or 96 hr, should be considered a positive response as long as it is stronger than that which is displayed by controls at the same time interval.

Strengths and weaknesses: There are a number of both advantages and disadvantages to the Buehler methodology, which has been in use for 20 years. The relative importance and merits of each depend on the intended use of the material. The three advantages are

1. Virtually no false positives, compared to human experience, are generated by this test.
2. The techniques involved are easy to learn and very reproducible.
3. The Buehler style test does not overpredict the potency of sensitizers. That is, materials which are identified as sensitizers are truly classified as very strong, weak, or in between—not all (or nearly all) as very strong.
4. There is a large database in existence for the Buehler style test. Unfortunately, the vast majority is not in the published literature.

Likewise, there are three disadvantages associated with the Buehler style test.

1. The test gives a high rate of false negatives for weak sensitizers and a detectable rate of false negatives for moderate sensitizers. That is, the method is somewhat insensitive—particularly if techniques for occlusive wrapping are inadequate.
2. The test takes a long time to complete. If animals are on hand when started, the test is 5 or 6 weeks long. Because few laboratories keep a "pool" of guinea pigs on hand (especially because they are the most expensive of the common lab species), the usual case is that 8–10 weeks is the minimum time required to get an answer from this test.
3. The test uses a relatively large amount of test material. In the normal acute "battery," the guinea pig test systems use more material than any other test systems unless an acute inhalation study is included. With 10 induction applications, this is particularly true for the Buehler style test.

GUINEA PIG MAXIMIZATION TEST

The guinea pig maximization test was developed by Magnusson and Kligman (1969, 1970; Magnusson, 1975) and is considered a highly sensitive procedure for evaluating test substances for potential dermal sensitization. The procedure presented here is illustrated diagramatically in Figs. 11 and 12 and is one common version of the test.

Animals
1. Young adult female guinea pigs, weighing between 250 and 350 g at the initiation of the study, are used.
2. Although several proposed test rules suggest the use of male guinea pigs, the female sex is preferred because the aggressive social behavior of males may result in considerable skin damage that might interfere with the interpretation of challenge reactions.

GUINEA PIG MAXIMIZATION TEST (GPMT) DESIGN

Species: Guinea Pig
Strain: Hartley
Test Group: 15 Animals
Control Group: 6 Animals

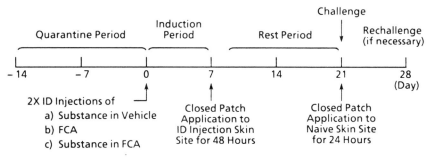

FIGURE 11   Line chart for guinea pig maximization test for dermal sensitization.

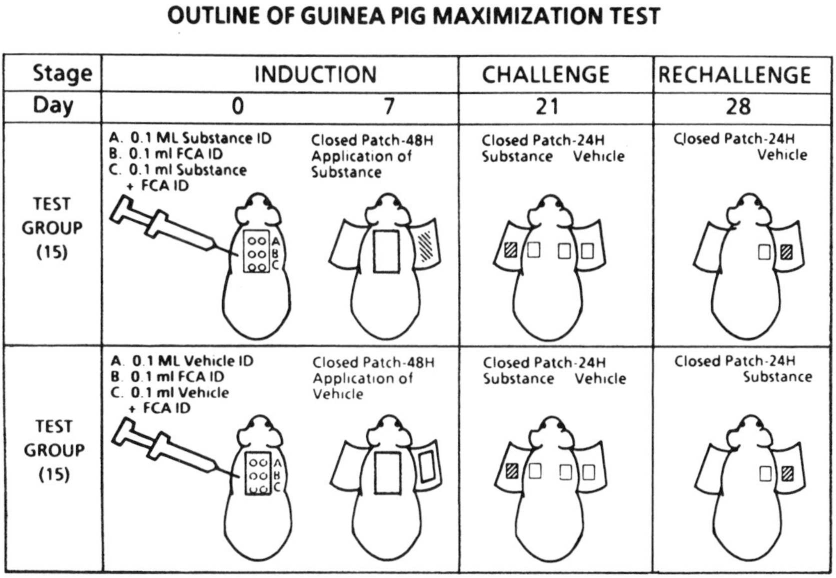

OUTLINE OF GUINEA PIG MAXIMIZATION TEST

Stage	INDUCTION		CHALLENGE	RECHALLENGE
Day	0	7	21	28
TEST GROUP (15)	A. 0.1 ML Substance ID B. 0.1 ml FCA ID C. 0.1 ml Substance + FCA ID	Closed Patch-48H Application of Substance	Closed Patch-24H Substance Vehicle	Closed Patch-24H Vehicle
TEST GROUP (15)	A. 0.1 ML Vehicle ID B. 0.1 ml FCA ID C. 0.1 ml Vehicle + FCA ID	Closed Patch-48H Application of Vehicle	Closed Patch-24H Substance Vehicle	Closed Patch-24H Substance

FIGURE 12   Illustrative figures for injection and patching of animals in GPMT.

3. Animals that show poor growth or are ill in any way are not used because illness markedly decreases the response. Animals with skin marked or scarred from fighting are avoided. The guinea pigs are observed for at least 2 weeks to detect any illness before starting a study.

4. The guinea pigs are randomly assigned to two groups: (1) a test group consisting of 15 animals, and (2) a control group consisting of 6 animals. If a pretest group is necessary, as many animals as needed for that group are randomized also.

5. Test and control group guinea pigs are weighed 1 week prior to dosing (Day −7), on the day of dosing (Day 0), and weekly thereafter.

Pretest

1. Several animals are used to pretest the test substance and vehicles to determine the topical dermal irritation threshold concentration.

2. These animals are shaved on the left flank, to which is applied a 2 × 2-cm filter paper patch which contains 0.1 ml of the test concentration.

3. The trunks of the animals are wrapped for 24 hr with a 3-in.-wide elastic bandage to hold the patch in contact with the skin.

4. Wrappings are removed after the 24 hr exposure and, based on skin reactions at 48 hr, a concentration of the test substance to be used on test is determined. Dermal irritation values are recorded for future reference.

5. In addition, several guinea pigs are utilized to determine a concentration (generally, between 1 and 5%) of test substance in vehicle and in FCA emulsion that can be injected id without eliciting a strong local or systemic toxic reaction.

6. The hair is clipped in an area of approximately 4 × 6 cm from the upper shoulder region of these animals.

7. Several concentrations of the test substance (ranging between 1 and 5%) can be injected in the same animal to compare local dermal reactions produced by the different concentrations.

8. However, if systemic toxicity is suspected, then each concentration should be tested in separate animals to determine local and systemic effects.

9. The dermal reactions (erythema, edema, and diameter) are recorded 24 hr after the id injections.

Induction stage 1 (Day 0)

1. The hair in an area of 4 × 6 cm is clipped from the shoulder region of each test and control group guinea pig on Day 0.

2. Three pairs of id injections are made with a glass 1-ml tuberculin

syringe with a 26-gauge needle, each pair flanking the dorsal midline.

3. The three pairs of id injections for test group animals are as follows:
   1. 0.1 ml test substance in appropriate vehicle
   2. 0.1 ml FCA emulsion alone
   3. 0.1 ml test substance in FCA emulsion
4. The three pairs of id injections for control group animals are as follows:
   1. 0.1 ml vehicle alone
   2. 0.1 FCA emulsion alone
   3. 0.1 ml vehicle in FCA emulsion
5. Injections 1 and 2 in the above two steps are given close to each other and nearest the head; injection 3 is given most posteriorly.
6. The date, time, and initials of those individuals performing the id injections are recorded.
7. Immediately before injection, an emulsion is prepared by blending commercial FCA with an equal volume of house distilled water or other solvent as appropriate.

   Water-soluble test materials are dissolved in the water phase prior to emulsification.

   Oil-soluble or water-insoluble materials are dissolved or suspended in FCA prior to adding water.

   Paraffin oil, peanut oil, or propylene glycol can be used for dissolving or suspending water-insoluble materials.

   A homogenizer is used to emulsify the FCA alone and the test substance in either FCA or vehicle prior to the id injections

   The concentration of the test substance for id injections is adjusted to the highest level that can be well tolerated locally and generally.
8. The adjuvant injection infiltration sometimes causes ulceration, especially when it is superficial, which lasts several weeks. These lesions are undesirable but do not invalidate the test results except for lowering the threshold level for skin irritation.

Induction stage 2 (Day 7)
1. Test substance preparation
   a. The concentration of the test substance is adjusted to the highest level that can be well tolerated.
   b. If the test substance is an irritant, a concentration is chosen that causes a weak to moderate inflammation (as determined by the pretest).

     c. Solids are micronized or reduced to a fine powder and then suspended in a vehicle, such as petrolatum or propylene glycol.

     d. Water- and oil-soluble test substances are dissolved in an appropriate vehicle.

     e. Liquid materials are applied as such, or diluted if necessary.

2. The same area over the shoulder region that received id injections on Day 0 is again shaved on both test and control guinea pigs.

3. A volume of 0.3 ml of a mildly irritating concentration (if possible) of the test substance (determined by the pretest) is spread over a 1 × 2-in. filter paper patch in a thick, even layer.

4. The patch is occluded with surgical tape and then is secured to test group animals with elastic bandage, which is wrapped around the torso of each test group animal.

5. The control group animals are exposed to 0.3 ml of 100% vehicle using the same procedure.

6. The date, time, and initials of those individuals performing the second induction are recorded.

7. The dressings of both groups are left in place for 48 hr before removal.

Challenge stage (Day 21)

1. An area of hair (1.5 × 1.5 in.) on both flanks of the guinea pigs (15 test and 3 controls) is shaved.

2. A 1 × 1-in. patch with a nonirritating concentration of test substance in vehicle (as determined by the pretest) is applied to the left flank and a 1 × 1-in. patch with 100% vehicle is applied to the right flank.

3. The torso of each guinea pig is wrapped with an elastic bandage to secure the patches for 24 hr.

4. The date, time, and initials of those individuals performing the challenge dose are recorded.

5. The patches are removed 24 hr after application.

Rechallenge (Day 28)

1. If the first challenge application of test substance does not cause dermal sensitization, causes dermal sensitization in only a few animals, or causes dermal reactions that are weak or questionable, then a second challenge application of test substance to the 15 test group guinea pigs will be conducted on Day 28 (1 week after the first challenge). The three remaining naive control group animals (not used for the first challenge) are challenged for comparison to the test group animals.

2. The three negative control group animals used on Day 21 will not be rechallenged. These animals will be terminated because they were exposed to the test substance during the first challenge and are no longer negative controls.
3. A 1 × 1-in. patch with a nonirritating concentration of test substance in vehicle is applied to the right flank of test and control group animals. The left flanks are not dosed.
4. The date, time, and initials of those individuals performing the rechallenge dose are recorded.
5. Steps 3 and 5 are followed as for Challenge stage (Day 21).

Observations—Challenge and/or rechallenge readings
1. Twenty-one hours after removing the patch, the challenge area on each flank is cleaned and clipped, if necessary.
2. Twenty-four hours after removing the patch, the first reading of dermal reactions is taken.
3. The dermal reactions are scored on a 4-point scale (as below):
   0, No reaction
   1, Scattered mild redness
   2, Moderate and diffuse redness
   3, Intense redness and swelling
4. Forty-eight hours after removing the patch, the second reading is taken and the scores are recorded.

Interpretation of results
1. Both the intensity and the duration of the test responses to the test substance and the vehicle are evaluated.
2. The important statistic in the GPMT is the frequency of sensitization and not the intensity of challenge responses. A value of 1 is considered just as positive as a value of 3 (as long as the values for controls are zero).
3. The test agent is a sensitizer if the challenge reactions in the test group clearly outweigh those in the control group. A reaction that occurs at 24 hr, but resolves by 48 hr after removal of patches, should be considered a positive response, as long as it is stronger than that which is displayed by controls. The sensitization rate (% of positive responders) is based on the greatest number of animals showing a positive response, whether it is from the 24-hr data or the 48-hr data after removal of patches.
4. When a second challenge application is performed, the data from both challenges are compared. If neither challenge produces a positive dermal reaction, the classification of the test substance is based on both challenge applications. If one challenge application

(whether it is the first or second) produces a greater number of positive dermal reactions than the other, the classification of the test substance is based on the challenge with the most positive responses.

5. Under the classification scheme of Kligman (1966, shown in Table 21), the test substance is assigned to one of five classes, according to the percentage of animals sensitized, ranging from a week grade I to an extreme grade V.

The advantages and disadvantages of the GPMT can be summarized as follows. First, the advantages:

1. The test system is sensitive and effectively detects weak sensitizers. It has a low false negative rate.
2. If properly conducted, there are no false positives—that is, materials which are identified as potential sensitizers will act as such at some incidence level in humans.
3. There is a large database available on the evaluation of compounds in this test system, and many people are familiar with the test system.

The disadvantages, meanwhile are the following:

1. The test system is sensitive; it overpredicts potency for many sensitizers. There is no real differentiation between weak, moderate, and strong sensitizers; virtually all positive test results identify a material as strong.
2. The techniques involved (particularly the intradermal injections) are not easy. Some regulatory officials have estimated that as many as 35% of the laboratories which try cannot master the system to get it to work reproducibly.
3. The test, though not as long as the Buehler, still takes a minimum of 4 weeks to produce an answer.

TABLE 21   Sensitization Severity Grading Based on Incidence of Positive Responses[a]

Sensitization rate %	Grade	Classification
0– 8	I	Weak
9– 28	II	Mild
29– 64	III	Moderate
65– 80	IV	Strong
81–100	V	Extreme

[a]From Kligman (1966).

4. The test uses a significant amount of test material.
5. One cannot evaluate fibers or other materials which cannot be injected (such as solids which cannot be finely ground and/or suspended or which are highly irritating or toxic by the iv route).
6. The irritation pretest is critical. Failure to detect irritation in this small group of animals does not guarantee against irritation in test animals at challenge.

GUINEA PIG SPLIT ADJUVANT TEST

The guinea pig split adjuvant dermal sensitization procedure for detecting contact allergenicity is based on that developed by Maguire (1973a,b, 1975) and Maguire and Chase (1967, 1972), is sensitive and effective for detection of substances and products with weak allergic potential, and will serve as a useful alternative for testing materials that cannot be injected intradermally (e.g., fabrics, nonsoluble solids, and extremely irritating or toxic materials). A concise outline of the split adjuvant technique has been documented (Klecak, 1983). This procedure is shown diagramatically in Fig. 13.)

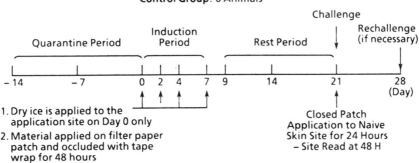

FIGURE 13 Line chart for design and conduct of split adjuvent procedure for dermal sensitization testing in guinea pigs.

Animals

1. Young adult female guinea pigs, weighing between 250 and 350 g at the initiation of the study, are used.
2. The female sex is preferred because the aggressive social behavior of males may result in considerable skin damage that might interfere with the interpretation of challenge reactions.
3. Animals that show poor growth or are ill in any way are not used because illness markedly decreases the response. Animals with skin marked or scarred from fighting are avoided. The guinea pigs are observed for at least 2 weeks to detect any illness before starting a study.
4. The guinea pigs are randomly assigned to two groups: (1) a test group consisting of 10 animals and (2) a control group consisting of 6 animals. If a pretest group is necessary, as many animals as needed for that group are randomized also.
5. Test and control group guinea pigs are weighed and the weights are recorded 1 week prior to dosing (Day -7), on the day of dosing (Day 0), and weekly thereafter.

Pretest

1. Several animals are used to pretest the test substance and vehicles to determine the dermal irritation threshold concentration.
2. These animals are clipped on the left flank (2 × 2 cm).
3. Then 0.2 ml of ointment (semisolid) or 0.1 ml of liquid is spread onto a 1.5 × 1.5-cm Whatman No. 3 filter paper patch, which is occluded on the opposite side with surgical tape.
   a. Solid test substances are micronized or reduced to a fine powder and then suspended in a vehicle, such as petrolatum or propylene glycol.
   b. Water- and oil-soluble test substances are dissolved in an appropriate vehicle.
   c. Liquid test substances are applied as such (100%), or diluted if necessary.
4. The pretest patch is then applied to the left flank. The trunk of each animal is wrapped for 24 hr with a 3-in.-wide elastic bandage to hold the patch in contact with the skin.
5. Wrappings are removed after 24 hr of exposure. Based on skin reactions at 48 hr, a concentration of the test substance to be used on test is determined. Dermal irritation values are recorded for later reference.

Induction stage
The date, time, and initials of those individuals performing the induction applications are recorded.

Day 0
1. The hair in an area of 2×2 cm is clipped behind the shoulder girdle of each test and control group guinea pig.
2. Dry ice is applied for 5 sec to the skin site of each test and control animal. Dry ice is used only for the Day 0 induction application.
3. Then 0.2 ml of ointment (semisolid) or 0.1 ml of liquid is spread onto a 1.5×1.5-cm Whatman No. 3 filter paper patch, which is occluded on the opposite side with surgical tape.
   a. The test substance is tested at a concentration that is minimally irritating (if possible), as determined by the pretest.
   b. If the substance is mixed in petrolatum or ointment, 0.2 ml is dispensed onto the patch.
   c. In the case of liquids, 0.1 ml is used.
   d. If a fabric is to be tested, a 1.5×1.5-cm sample is cut, moistened with 0.2 ml of physiological saline, and then applied under a filter paper patch.
4. Control group animals are dosed with vehicle only, not test substance.
5. The trunk of each animal is wrapped for 48 hr with a 3-in.-wide elastic bandage to hold the patch in contact with the skin.

Day 2
1. The wrapping and patch are removed from each test and control group animal 48 hr after the initial induction application.
2. A fresh patch is applied to the same site using the same procedure as described for induction Day 0 (without dry ice). Test group animals receive test substance in vehicle, and control group animals receive vehicle alone for a 48-hr period.

Day 4
1. The wrapping and patch are removed from each test and control group animal 48 hr after the application of the Day 2 induction patch.
2. An emulsion of FCA is prepared by blending commercial FCA with an equal volume of house distilled water.
3. Two volumes, each of 0.1 ml of FCA emulsion, are injected id into the induction site of each test and each control group animal with a glass 1-ml tuberculin syringe and a 26-gauge needle. These two injections flank the dorsal midline.

4. A fresh patch is applied to the same site using the same procedure as described on induction Day 2. Test group animals receive test substance in vehicle, and control group animals receive vehicle alone for a 48-hr period.

Day 6
1. The wrapping and patch are removed from each test and control group animal 48 hr after the application of the Day 4 incubation patch.

Day 7
1. A fresh patch is applied to the induction site using the same procedure as described on induction Day 2. Test group animals receive test substance in vehicle, and control group animals receive vehicle alone for a 48-hr period.

Day 9
1. The wrapping and patch are removed from each test and control group animal 48 hr after the application of the Day 7 induction patch.

Challenge stage (Day 21)
1. An area of hair (3 × 3 cm) on both flanks of the guinea pigs (10 test and 3 controls) is clipped.
2. A 1.5 × 1.5-cm filter paper patch with the highest nonirritating concentration of test substance in vehicle (as determined by the pretest) is applied to the left flank and 1.5 × 1.5-cm patch with 100% vehicle is applied to the right flank.
    a. If the test substance is liquid, 0.1 ml is applied to the patch.
    b. If the test substance is mixed in petrolatum or ointment, 0.2 ml is dispensed onto the patch.
    c. If the test substance is a fabric, a 1.5 × 1.5-cm sample is cut, moistened with physiological saline, and then applied under a patch.
3. The torso of each guinea pig is wrapped with an Elastoplast elastic bandage to secure the patches for 24 hr.
4. The date, time, and initials of those individuals performing the challenge dose are recorded.
5. The patches are removed on Day 22 and the challenge area on each flank is cleaned and clipped atraumatically.

Challenge readings
1. On Day 23, 24 hr after removing the patch, the first reading of dermal reactions is taken and results are recorded.

2. Readings of the challenge site are taken again 48 hr after removing the patch and results are recorded.
3. The intensity of the skin reaction is classified according to the following rating scale used by Maguire (1973b):

> 0 = Normal skin
> ± = Very faint, nonconfluent pink
> + = Faint pink
> + + = Pale pink to pink, slight edema
> + + + = Pink, moderate edema
> + + + + = Pink and thickened
> + + + + + = Bright pink, markedly thickened

Interpretation of results
1. The frequency, intensity, and duration of the test responses to the test substance and the vehicle are evaluated.
2. The test substance is a sensitizer if the challenge reactions in the test group clearly outweigh those in the control group.
3. Two or more unequivocally positive responses (at least a + on the rating scale) in a group of 10 animals should be considered significant. A negative, equivocal, or single response probably ensures that a substance is not a strong sensitizer, although this is best confirmed by further testing with human subjects (NAS, 1977).

Rechallenge (Day 28)
1. If the first challenge application does not cause dermal sensitization, then a second challenge application of the 10 test group guinea pigs will be conducted on Day 28 (1 week after the first challenge). The remaining naive control group animals (not used for the first challenge) are challenged for comparison to the test group animals.
2. The three negative control group animals used on Day 21 will not be rechallenged. These animals will be terminated because they were exposed to the test article during the first challenge and are no longer negative controls.
3. A 1.5 × 1.5-cm patch with the highest nonirritating concentration of test substance in vehicle is applied to the right flank of test and control group animals. The left flanks are not dosed.
4. The date, time, and initials of those individuals performing the rechallenge dose are recorded.
5. Steps 3 and 5 of the challenge procedure are repeated here.

Strengths and weaknesses: The advantages and disadvantages of the split adjuvant test can be summarized as follows. The advantages are the following:

1. The test system has a lower false negative rate for moderate and weak sensitizers than does the Buehler design.
2. If properly conducted, there are no false positives.
3. Fibers and other materials which cannot be injected intradermally can be evaluated here.

As elsewhere, there is also a list of disadvantages. These include the following:

1. The techniques involve (particularly the intradermal injection) are not easy ones.
2. The sensitivity of the test system is "bought" at the expense of making relative hazard predictions not necessarily accurate. The test system tends to overpredict potency.
3. The test still both takes a relatively long time to complete and uses a significant amount of test material.
4. There is a limited published database on test system performance, and relatively few people have experience with it.

MOUSE EAR SWELLING TEST

Several of the disadvantages associated with the previous three test systems, both stated and unstated, are reflections of limitations of the guinea pig as a model and the methodology of evaluating response in terms of observing and subjectively "grading" skin erythema.

Since Crowle (1959a,b) formally proved that passive transfer of delayed-type contact hypersensitivity exists in the mouse in 1959, research immunologists have generated a wealth of information in attempts to understand the delayed-type hypersensitivity (DTH) response in this species (Asherson and Ptak, 1968).

In particular, they have demonstrated that thymus-derived cells are necessary for inducing a DTH response (DeSousa and Parrott, 1969). Also, the mouse has been used to investigate immunosuppressive properties of certain drugs, such as fluorinated steroids and corticosteroids. All of these have led to the development of a formalized test procedure, the MEST.

The MEST is a procedure based on that which is described by Gad et al. (1985b, 1986a) for evaluating test substances for their potential to cause dermal sensitization in mice. This procedure evaluates contact sensitization by quantitatively measuring mouse ear thickness. This method is shown diagramatically in Figs. 14–16.

Animals

1. CF-1 or BALB/c female mice, 6–8 weeks old, are used. The mice are observed for at least 1 week to detect any signs of illness before

MOUSE EAR SWELLING TEST
OPTIMAL STUDY DESIGN

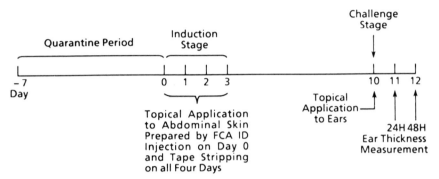

FIGURE 14   Line chart for optimal study design and conduct of MEST for dermal sensitization.

DETAILS OF MEST INDUCTION STAGE PROCEDURE

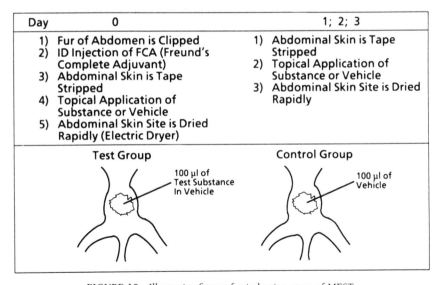

Day	0	1; 2; 3
	1) Fur of Abdomen is Clipped 2) ID Injection of FCA (Freund's Complete Adjuvant) 3) Abdominal Skin is Tape Stripped 4) Topical Application of Substance or Vehicle 5) Abdominal Skin Site is Dried Rapidly (Electric Dryer)	1) Abdominal Skin is Tape Stripped 2) Topical Application of Substance or Vehicle 3) Abdominal Skin Site is Dried Rapidly

Test Group — 100 μl of Test Substance In Vehicle

Control Group — 100 μl of Vehicle

FIGURE 15   Illustrative figures for induction stage of MEST.

DETAILS OF MEST CHALLENGE STAGE PROCEDURE

Day 10	11 & 12
1) Topical Application of Test Substance to One Ear 2) Topical Application of Vehicle to Contralateral Ear 3) Both Ears Are Dried Rapidly	Ear Thickness Measurement of Test and Control Ears is Made With Micrometer 24 & 48 Hours After Exposure

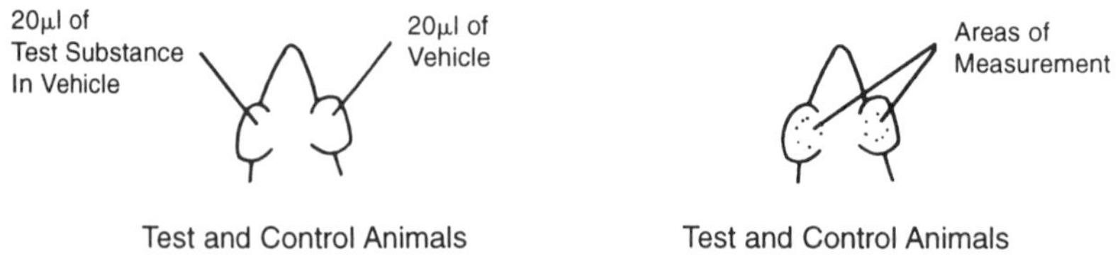

20μl of
Test Substance
In Vehicle   20μl of
                              Vehicle   Areas of
                                                                        Measurement

        Test and Control Animals   Test and Control Animals

FIGURE 16   Illustrative figures for challenge stage of MEST.

starting a study. Mice that show poor growth or signs of illness are excluded from use on a test.

2. Any mouse displaying redness of either ear prior to the start of a test should be replaced.

3. Mice, which have been randomly placed in cages upon arrival, are assigned to groups (a maximum of 5/cage) by labeling cage cards. For each test substance investigated, a pretest group of at least 8 mice, a test group of at least 15 mice, and a control group of at least 10 mice are utilized. For 2 weeks prior to initiation of testing (starting on arrival), animals are given diet supplemented with vitamin A (Thorne, 1991a,b) as shown in Fig. 17.

4. Because animals are not individually marked, they will always be handled one at a time when each phase of this procedure is performed. The following procedure is conducted to prevent mixing animals during each phase (e.g., shaving, id injections, tape-stripping, and dosing). All mice are removed from their original cage and placed in an empty cage for holding. One mouse is removed from the holding cage at a time, the phase activity is performed, and then the mouse is returned to its original cage. This step will be repeated for each of the remaining mice in the holding cage.

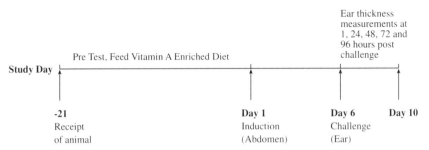

FIGURE 17   Thorne modification of the mouse ear swelling test.

Pretest

1. A dermal (abdomen and ear) irritation and toxicity probe study is conducted 1 week prior to the actual MEST in order to establish the maximum concentration of test substance that produced minimal irritation to the abdomen (belly) region after a single topical application on each of 4 days (if the substance does have potential to irritate skin) and to establish a concentration of test substance that is nonirritating to the ear after a single topical application. Also, dose levels of the test substance that produce systemic toxicity can be established during the pretest.

2. The test substance is diluted, emulsified, or suspended in a suitable vehicle. A vehicle (such as acetone, 70% ethanol, 25% ethanol, or methyl ethyl ketone) is selected which should be able to solubilize the test substance and be volatile.

3. Two mice from the pretest group are used to test each concentration of test substance. As many as four concentrations can be evaluated. The same mice used for belly irritation are also used for ear irritation testing.

4. On Day 0, the first day of the pretest, each animal is prepared by clipping the hair from the belly region using a small animal clipper with a size No. 40 blade.

5. After clipping the belly, the outer layers of epidermis (stratum corneum) of each mouse are removed from the shaved belly region with a tacky transparent tape (1-in. wide). This procedure is referred to as "tape-stripping." On Day 0, the belly skin of each mouse is tape-stripped until the application region appears shiny. While an assistant supports the dorsal portion of the mouse, the tape is pressed firmly over the clipped belly region and quickly removed; this procedure is repeated as many times as needed.

6. After tape-stripping the belly, a volume of 100 μl of test substance is applied to the belly region using a microliter pipette. At the same time, test substance is applied to the ventral surface (10 μl) and dorsal surface (10 μl) of the left ear of the mouse using a microliter pipette.

7. On Day 1, 24 hr after dosing the ears, the thickness of all probe animal ears is measured using an Oditest Model D-1000 thickness gauge.

   a. Ether is used to anesthetize the mice in a fume hood while the ears are measured.

   b. When a mouse reaches the "surgical anesthesia" stage, it is removed from the jar and gently placed on the countertop of the fume hood, which is prepared with a protective lining.

   c. While supporting the mouse with one hand, the other hand is used to press the finger lever on the Oditest gauge in order to open the flat measurement contacts. One ear of the mouse is then inserted between the contacts until it is positioned with approximately 1 or 2 mm of the outer edge of the ear showing. After positioning the ear, the finger lever is released to allow the contacts to clamp onto the ear. The measurement is read from the gage after the indicator needle is stabilized. If desired, one or two more measurements can be rapidly made to be certain of a reproducible reading.

   d. Once a reading is obtained, the other (contralateral) ear is measured in the same manner. The animal's body is turned over in order to position the other ear for measurement.

   e. Measurements are recorded.

8. On subsequent Days 1, 2, and 3, the belly region is first tape-stripped five times and then a volume of 100 μl of test substance is applied topically to the belly region using a microliter pipette.

9. On day 4, 24 hr after the last topical application, the belly skin of all animals is observed for dermal irritation. A description of the results is recorded.

10. If any signs of systemic toxicity are observed on any of the pretest days, then they should be noted.

11. Based on the results of the pretest data, a judgment is made as to which concentration will be used for topical induction applications to the belly and for topical challenge application to the ear. A minimal or mildly irritating concentration is preferable for induction, and the highest nonirritating concentration possible is used for challenge application.

Induction stage
1. Day 0
   a. The belly of each test and control group mouse is clipped free of hair.
   b. Immediately after clipping, two id injections of FCA emulsion are made at separate sites in the skin of the shaved belly (each site flanks the ventral midline). Approximately 20 μl of FCA emulsion is injected with a glass tuberculin syringe with a 30-gauge needle attached. Injections are performed in test and control mice.
   c. Following the id injections, the belly skin of test and control group animals is taped-stripped until the site gives a shiny appearance.
   d. After tape-stripping the belly, a volume of 100 μl of test substance (at a concentration determined by pretest) is topically applied to the belly skin of test group animals with a microliter pipette. Control animals receive a dose of 100 μl of vehicle.
2. Days 1, 2, and 3
   a. The skin of the belly of test and control group animals is tape-stripped five times.
   b. After tape-stripping, a volume of 100 μl of test substance is topically applied to the belly skin of test group animals and a volume of 100 μl of vehicle/solvent is topically applied to control group animals.

Challenge stage
1. Day 10
   Each test group mouse and each of 5 control group mice is dosed with 10 μl of a concentration of test substance (determined by the pretest data) on the ventral side of the left ear and 10 μl on the dorsal side of the left ear. The contralateral right ear is dosed with 10 μl of 100% vehicle on the ventral side and 10 μl on the dorsal side.
2. Day 11
   Ear thickness measurements are made 24 hr after challenge dosing. The procedure described in Section 7a–d of this standard operating procedure (SOP) is used.
3. Day 12
   Each thickness measurement is made again 48 hr after challenge dosing.

Rechallenge

1. If the test substance is judged a nonsensitizing agent after the first challenge application, causes dermal sensitization in only a few animals, or causes ear swelling that is weak or questionable, then a second and final challenge application will be performed on each test animal on Day 17.

2. The five control group mice from the first challenge are not rechallenged because they have been exposed to the test substance and are no longer true negative controls. The five remaining naive control group animals (not used for the first challenge) are challenged for comparison to the test group animals.

3. The procedure used for the first challenge application will be used for the rechallenge application. Either the same concentration or a new concentration (higher or lower) of test substance may be used, depending on the results of the first challenge.

4. Measurement of both ears is performed on Days 18 and 19 (24 and 48 hr after rechallenging, respectively). Each thickness measurement is recorded.

Interpretation of results

1. Judgment concerning the presence or absence of sensitization is made for each animal. The judgment is based on the percentage difference (% ∇) between test and control ears. A "positive" sensitization response is considered to have occurred if the test ear of an animal is at least 20% thicker than the control ear.

2. The percentage of animals in a test group that is considered "positive" is then calculated and recorded as percentage responders.

3. The negative control group ear thickness measurements are used to identify any possible dermal irritation reactions, which would be interpreted as false positive dermal sensitization responses.

4. In addition, percentage ear swelling is calculated for the test group. The left (A) and right (B) ear thickness measurements are added. Percentage ear swelling equals the sum of A (test ear thicknesses) divided by the sum of B (control ear thicknesses), multiplied by 100:

$$\% \text{ Ear swelling} = \frac{A}{B} \times 100$$

5. When a second challenge application is performed, the data from both challenges are compared. If neither challenge procedure produces a positive sensitization reaction, the classification of the test substance is based on both challenge applications. If one challenge

application (whether it is the first or second) produces a greater number of positive dermal reactions than the other, the classification of the test substance is based on the challenge with the most positive responses.

6. Two or more unequivocally positive responses in a group of 15 animals should be considered significant. A negative, equivocal, or single response probably ensures that a substance is not a strong sensitizer, although this is best confirmed by further testing with human subjects (NAS, 1977).

Strengths and Weaknesses: The MEST offers distinct advantages compared to the guinea pig dermal sensitization procedures:

1. The mouse is markedly less expensive.
2. Less vivarium space is required.
3. The duration of the test is shorter.
4. Less test substance is utilized.
5. Overall cost of the test is significantly less.
6. The test is objective, rather than subjective.
7. Materials which stain the skin may be easily evaluated. Several of the materials evaluated were colored and very difficult to evaluate by existing methods.
8. The test has a low false negative rate and no false positive rate, if properly performed.
9. The test seems to do a more accurate job of predicting relative hazard to humans.
10. The test is now regulatorily recognized under OECD and ISO standards.

Disadvantages include the following:

1. The database, though now not small, is not as extensive as that for the GPMT or Buehler tests.
2. Fewer people have experience with the test system.

A modified form of the mouse ear swelling assay has been developed by Thorne and colleagues (1991a,b). The differences between the Thorne method and the Gad method are that (in the former):

The animals are fed a vitamin A (225 IU/g feed, stored refrigerated, and offered fresh daily) for 21 days prior to induction.

The animals are receive only one induction dose (as opposed to three over 3 consecutive days).

The animals are challenged 5 days rather than 7 days after the induction dose.

Although the vitamin A pretreatment would appear to add considerable calendar time to the conduct of this test (additional 14 days of pretest), it in fact does not have that much impact—the "in-study" time is shorter. The vitamin a treatment greatly enhances the sensitivity of the assay. This is a good assay for detecting weak sensitizers. For example, in animals sensitized to cinnamaldehyde (20%), the mean ETI was 0.022 (40% of animals positive) for animals on regular feed versus an ETI of 0.063 (100% of the animals responding) for animals fed the vitamin A-enriched diet (Thorne et al., 1991b). One could easily envision a two-tiered approach in which equivocal findings in the regular MEST could be confirmed with this modification.

LOCAL LYMPH NODE ASSAY

This method has developed out of the work of Ian Kimber and associates (Kimber et al., 1986, 1994; Kimber and Weisenberger, 1989). It has the advantage over the other methods discussed in this chapter in that it provides an objective and quantifiable endpoint. The method is based on the fact that dermal sensitization requires the elicitation of an immune response. This immune response requires proliferation of a lymphocyte subpopulation. The local lymph node assay (LLNA) relies on the detection of increase DNA synthesis via tritiated thymidine incorporation. Sensitization is measured as a function of lymph node cell proliferative responses induced in a draining lymph node following repeated topical exposure of the test animal to the test article. Unlike the other tests discussed in this chapter, this assay looks only at induction because as there is no challenge phase.

The typical test (illustrated in Fig. 18) is performed using mice—normally female CBA mice 6–10 weeks of age. Female BALB/c and ICR mice have also been used. After animal receipt, they are typically acclimated to standard laboratory husbandry conditions for 7–14 days. The usual protocol will consist of at least two groups (vehicle control and test article treated) of five mice each. They are treated on the dorsal surface of both ears with 25 μl (on each

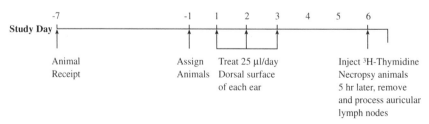

FIGURE 18   The mouse local lymph node assay.

ear) of test article solution for 3 consecutive days. Twenty-four to forty-eight hours after the last test article exposure, the animals are given a bolus (0.25 ml) dose of [^{3}H]thymidine (20 μCi with a specific activity of 5.0–7.0 Ci/mmol) in phosphate-buffered saline via a tail vein. Five hours after the injection, the animals are euthanized by CO_2 asphyxiation and the auricular lymph nodes removed.

After removal, the lymph nodes can either be pooled by group or processed individually. Single cell suspensions are prepared by gentle mechanical disaggregation through a nylon (100 μm) mesh. Cells are washed twice by centrifugation in an excess of PBS. After the final supernatant wash is removed, the cells are precipitated with cold 5% trichloroacetic acid (TCA) and kept at 4°C for 12–18 hr. The precipitate is then pelleted by centrifugation and resuspended in 1 ml 5% TCA, and the amount of radioactivity is determined by liquid scintillation counting, using established techniques for tritium.

The data are reduced to the stimulation index (SI):

$$SI = \frac{H \text{ (dpm) treated group}}{H \text{ (dpm) control group}}$$

An SI of 3 or greater is considered a positive response, i.e., the data support the hypothesis that the test material is a sensitizer.

The test article concentration is normally the highest nonirritating concentration. Several concentrations could be tested at the same time should one wish to establish a dose–response curve for induction. The test is easiest to perform if the vehicle is a standard nonirritating organic, such as acetone, ethanol, or dimethylformamide, or a solvent–olive oil blend. Until a laboratory develops its own historical control base, it is also preferable to include a positive control group. Either 0.25% dinitrochlorobenzene or 0.05% oxazalone are recommended for positive controls. If the vehicle for the positive control is different than the vehicle for the test material, then two vehicle control groups may be necessary.

This method has been extensively validated in two international laboratory exercises (Basketter et al., 1991; Loveless et al., 1996). In the earlier work (Basketter et al., 1991), there was good correlation between the results obtained with guinea pig tests and those obtained with the LLNA. In the recent report, for example, five laboratories correctly identified dinitrochlorobenzene and oxazalone as sensitizers and the fact that p-aminobenzoic acid was not (Loveless et al., 1996). Robinson and Cruze (1996) demonstrated that the sensitivity of the assay could be increased by slight abrasion (light draging of a 26-ga needle) to the ear. Arts and colleagues (1996) demonstrated that rats could be used as well as mice. Interestingly, they validated their assay (for both rats and mice) using BrDU uptake and immunohistochemical staining (rather than [^{3}H]thymidine) to quantitate lymph node cell proliferation.

This method is relatively quick and inexpensive because it uses relatively few mice (which are much less expensive than guinea pigs) and takes considerably less time than traditional guinea pig assays. It has an advantage over other methods in that it does not depend on a somewhat subjective scoring system and produces an objective and quantifiable endpoint. It does require a radiochemistry laboratory. Unless one already has an appropriately equipped laboratory used for other purposes (most likely metabolism studies), setting one up for the sole purpose of running the LLNA does not make economic sense.

TEST SYSTEM MANIPULATION (FOR ALL *IN VIVO* TEST SYSTEMS)

Increasing percutaneous absorption will increase test sensitivity. Factors which will increase absorption (and techniques for achieving them) include the following:

1. Increase surface area of solids.
2. Hydrate region of skin exposed to chemical. This can be done by wetting solids and using very occlusive wrapping of application.
3. Irritate application site.
4. Abrade application site.
5. Injection of test material (if possible).
6. Proper selection of solvent or suspending system. [See Christensen *et al.* (1984) for a discussion of the effect of vehicle in the case of even a strong sensitizer.]
7. Remove part of all of the "barrier layer" (stratum corneum) by tape-stripping the application site.
8. Increase the number of induction applications.

Though it is not a factor which increases percutaneous absorption, mildly stimulating the immune system of test animals (by such means as injecting FCA (or some other adjuvant) alone or FCA blended with the test material also increases responsiveness of the test system.

Also, it is generally believed that using the highest possible test material concentrations (mildly irritating for induction and just below irritating for challenge) will guarantee the greatest possible sensitization response and will therefore also serve to universally increase sensitivity. There are reports, however (Gad *et al.*, 1985a, for croton oil; Thorne *et al.*, 1987, for isocyanates), that this is not true for all compounds and that a multiple dose (i.e., two or more concentrations) study design would increase sensitivity. Such designs, however, would also significantly increase cost.

Concurrent or frequent positive and negative controls are essential to guard against test system failure. Any of these test systems should show 0.05% dinitrochlorobenzene (DNCB) in 70% ethanol to be a strong sensitizer.

CURRENT TEST SYSTEMS: PRACTICAL PROBLEMS AND SOLUTIONS

Virtually all the general problems associated with the use of the current test systems can be thought of as being an aspect of "What do the results mean in terms of hazard to people?" These problems arise for a number of reasons, but the major two can be traced back to two facts: First, as a population, humans will exhibit greater variability in sensitivity than an animal test system. In trying to reduce this gap, current test systems do not give a true prediction of relative hazard (i.e., what portion of the human population will be sensitized, and how easily?) in people.

Second, what is evaluated in these models may be a mixture (such as a cosmetic). At the same time, if a chemical is found to be a sensitizer, we may be concerned about structurally related compounds evoking a response in those already sensitized to the compound we have tested—that is, that there may be cross-sensitization.

Interpretation: Once we have animal sensitization test data, we must elate these to potential hazards in humans. On one end of the scale, a negative finding does not guarantee that a material will not be a sensitizer in humans, though most investigators would agree that it is unlikely that such a material would be other than a weak or mild sensitizer.

On the other end, however, it is not nearly as clear what a finding of a material being a strong or extreme sensitizer means in each of these assays. The GPMT and split adjuvant test, plus other related maximization style tests, tend to overpredict potency, and what action a manufacturer of a material may, and should, take will definitely be a reflection of both how the material is to be used and how much of a risk it will present to humans.

Accordingly, one is left with two options. First, human patch style tests can be performed, and with large enough (100–200 people) test groups of a representative nature (that is, a variety of ages, skin types, and such that resemble that of the population that will be exposed), the results will give one an understanding of what to expect in humans. This approach, however, is expensive and has both ethical and liability concerns of its own.

The second approach is to use a methodology which allows us to evaluate potency in a human model. As Gad et al. (1985b, 1986b), Gad (1987, 1988), and Thorn et al. (1987) have pointed out, such potency evaluations require dose–response testing and a number of considerations should be taken into account.

POTENCY

Starting with several assumptions, data from four different animal test systems have been used to evaluate one possible procedure for ranking the potency of known sensitizers. These assumptions were the following:

1. Because absolute (100%) responses do not give actual data points (rather, they define a portion of an unlimited response region), only partial (1–99%) response data from animal tests can be used to predict potency.

2. Because the profit transformation has already been shown to linearize sensitization dose–response data, probit values can be used to adjust different partial dose–response values to a comparable basis. This transformation is most stable in the central region (16–84%) of the response range, so partial responses in this range are most desirable.

3. Because individual molecules of material evoke the response being both measured and predicted, doses (or exposures) should be expressed on a molecular basis. Accordingly, data should be adjusted for molecular weight.

A method for calculating a potency index should have at least six characteristics.

A. It should be relatively easy to perform, requiring little more than the data and a calculator.

B. It should incorporate data as to test concentration used, incidence of response achieved, and molecular weight of the test material.

C. The resulting potency index numbers should cover a compact scale—for example, from 0 to 10—and not include negative numbers nor cover more than one order of magnitude.

D. There should be a positive correlation between potency and the index number (i.e., more potent compounds should have higher index numbers).

E. The results should serve to separate materials into clear clumps or clusters lending themselves to classification of materials into categories.

F. Data from various test systems should produce similar classification results for compounds and should predict human results which are not contrary to fact.

An earlier attempt at such an index calculating method (Gad et al., 1986a, 1987) produced results which were promising, but clearly did not fit desired characteristics C and D. This has been modified as follows:

Potency index (PI) =

$$
\text{Log}\left[\left(\frac{\text{Probit of response incidence}}{(\text{Test concentration (As a decimal fraction)}) (\text{Molecular weight})}\right) \times 1000\right]
$$

This produced results which, as shown below, generally fulfilled the desired design characteristics. A classification scheme based on the resulting index was devised, with the scale as follows:

Class I: PI > 4.0, "Severe"
Class II: 4.0 > PI ≥ 3.0, "Strong"
Class III: 3.0 > PI ≥ 2.0, "Moderate"
Class IV: 2.0 > PI ≥ 1.0, "Mild"
Class V: 1.0 > PI ≥ 0, "Weak or Questionable"

Values from this classification scheme are also assigned below.

CROSS-SENSITIZATION

A frequent situation is that one member of a structural series of compounds is tested and found to be a sensitizer. If other members of the structural series will evoke a positive response in those that have been sensitized, we call this broader response "cross-sensitization." This occurs because the structures of these materials complexed with a protein are not distinguished as different by the "educated" surveillance lymphocytes.

Any of the animal tests described here can be modified to see if cross-sensitization occurs among members of a series. The test is conducted with multiple groups of animals. Those animals which are successfully sensitized are then rechallenged with other members of the class.

MIXTURES

Mixtures become a particular problem in sensitization testing because, frequently, we are called upon first to evaluate a complex mixture in an animal test system; then, if it is found to be a sensitizer, we are called upon to determine which component is the cause of the positive response. If such a component can be identified, it is frequently possible to reformulate the mixture to serve the desired need without the problem component.

Such components can be identified by continued testing in a set of animals previously sensitized to the mixture as a whole. Groups of positively sensitized animals are rechallenged with separate samples of different suspect components to identify that which evokes a positive response. The guinea pig methods offer some advantage here, in that multiple components may be simultaneously evaluated on different sites of the same animal.

In Vitro Methods

There are actually several approaches available to *in vitro* evaluation of materials for sensitizing potential. These use cultured cells from various sources and, as endpoints, look at either biochemical factors [such as production of migration inhibition factor (MIF)] or cellular events (such as cell migration or cell "transformation").

Milner (1970) reported that lymphocytes from guinea pigs sensitized to dinitrofluorobenzene (DNFB) would transform in culture, as measured by the incorporation of tritiated thymidine, when exposed to epidermal proteins conjugated with DNFB. This work was later extended to guinea pigs sensitized to *p*-phenylenediamine. He later (1971) reported that his method was capable of detecting allergic contact hypersensitivity to DNFB in humans when he used human lymphocytes from sensitized donors and human epidermal etracts conjugated with DNFB.

Miller and Levis (1973) reported the *in vitro* detection of allergic contact hypersensitivity to DNCB conjugated to leukocyte and erythrocyte cellular membranes. This indicated that the reaction was not specifically directed toward epidermal cell conjugates.

Thulin and Zacharian (1972) extended earlier work on MIF-induced migration of human peripheral blood lymphocytes to a test for delayed contact hypersensitivity.

None of these approaches has yet been developed as an *in vitro* predictive test, but work is progressing. Milner (1983) has published a review of the history and state of this field.

Any alternative (*in vitro* or *in vivo*) test for sensitization will need to be evaluated against a battery of "known" compounds The Consumer Product Safety Commission in 1977 proposed such a battery, which is shown in Table 22.

TABLE 22   Requested Reference Compounds for Skin Sensitization Studies (U.S. Consumer Product Safety Commission)

Tribromophylophosphate	Formalin
Ditallow dimethyl ammonium methyl sulfate	Turpentine
Hydroxylamine sulfate	Potassium dichromate
Ethyl amino benzoate	Penicillin G
Iodochlorohydroxy quinoline	*p*-Phenylenediamine
(Clioquinol, Chinoform)	Epoxy systems (ethylenediamine, diethylene-
Nickel sulfate	triamine, and diglycidyl ethers)
Monomethyl methacrylate	Toleune 2,4-diisocyanate
Mercaptobenzothiazole	Oil of Bergamot

Gad *et al.* (1986a) have published comparative data on multiple animal and human test system data for some 52 materials. Such a database should be broadened and developed for other test systems.

REFERENCES

Arts, J. H. E., Droge, S. C. M., Bloksma, N., and Kuper, C. F. (1996). Local lymph node activation in rats after application of the sensitizers 2,4-dinitrochlorobenzene and trimellic anhydride. *Fd. Chem. Toxicol.* **34**, 55–62.

Asherson, G. L., and Ptak, W. (1968). Contact and delayed hypersensitivity in the mouse. I. Active sensitization and passive transfer. *Immunology* **15**, 405–416.

Basketter, D. A., Scholes, E. W., Kimber, I., Botham, P. A., Hilton, J., Miller, K., Robbins, M. C., Harrison, P. T. C., and Waite, S. J. (1991). Interlaboratory evaluation of the local lymph node assay with 25 chemicals and comparison with guinea pig test data. *Toxicol. Methods* **1**, 30–43.

Basketter, D. A., Roberts, D. W., Cronin, M., and Scholes, E. W. (1992b). The value of the local lymph node assay in quantitative structure–activity investigations. *Contact Dermatitis* **27**, 137–142.

Buehler, E. V. (1964). A new method for detecting potential sensitizers using the guinea pig. *Toxicol. Appl. Pharmacol.* **6**, 341.

Buehler, E. V. (1965). Delayed contact hypersensitivity in the guinea pig. *Arch. Dermatol.* **91**, 171–177.

Christensen, O. B., Christensen, M. B., and Maibach, H. I. (1984). Effect of vehicle on elicitation of DNCB contact allergy in the guinea pig. *Contact Dermatitis* **10**, 166–169.

Cronin, E., and Agrup, G. (1970). Contact Dermatitis X. *Br. J. Dermatol.* **82**, 428–433.

Crowle, A. J. (1959a). Delayed hypersensitivity in mice: Its detection by skin tests and its passive transfer. *Science* **130**, 159.

Crowle, A. J. (1959b). Delayed hypersensitivity in several strains of mice studied with six different tests. *J. Allergy* **30**, 442–459.

Dearman, R. J., and Kimber, I. (1991). Differential stimulation of immune function by respiratory and contact chemical allergens. *Immunology* **72**, 563–570.

DeSousa, M. A. B., and Parrott, D. M. V. (1969). Induction and recall in contact sensitivity, changes in skin and draining lymph nodes of intact and thymectomized mice. *J. Exp. Med.* **130**, 671–686.

Draize, J. H. (1959). *The Appraisal of Chemicals in Foods, Drugs and Cosmetics*, pp. 36–45. Association of Food and Drug Officials of the U.S., Austin, TX.

Draize, J. H., Woodard, G., and Calvery, H. O. (1944). Methods for the study of irritation and toxicity of substances applied topically to the skin and mucus membranes. *J. Pharmacol. Exp. Ther.* **82**, 377–390.

Gad, S. C. (1987). Scheme for the ranking and prediction of relative potencies of dermal sensitizers, based on data from several test systems. *Toxicologist*, A343.

Gad, S. C. (1988). A scheme for the ranking and prediction of relative potencies of dermal sensitizers based on data from several test systems. *J. Appl. Toxicol.* **8**, 301–312.

Gad, S. C., Dobbs, D. W., Dunn, B. J., Reilly, C., and Walsh, R. D. (1985a). Elucidation of the delayed contact sensitization response to Croton Oil. Paper presented at the American College of Toxicology in Washington, DC., Noevmber.

Gad, S. C., Dunn, B. J., and Dobb, D. W. (1985b). Development of alternative dermal sensitization test: Mouse Ear Swelling Test (MEST). *In Vitro Toxicology, Proceedings of 1984 Johns Hopkins Symposium* (A. M. Goldberg, Ed.), p. 539–551.

Gad, S. C., Darr, R. W., Dobbs, D. W., Dunn, B. J., Reilly, C., and Walsh, R. D. (1986a). Comparison of the potency of 52 dermal sensitizers in the Mouse Ear Swelling Test (MEST). Paper presented at SOT Meetings, March.

Gad, S. C., Dunn, B. J., Dobbs, D. W., and Walsh, R. D. (1986b). Development and validation of an alternative dermal sensitization test: The Mouse Ear Swelling Test (MST). *Toxicol. Appl. Pharmacol.* **84**, 93–114.

Gad, S. C., Dobbs, D. W., Dunn, B. J., Reilly, C., and Walsh, R. W. (1987). Development, validation and transfer of a new test system technology in toxicology. In *New Test Systems in Toxicology* (A. M. Goldberg, Ed.), Vol. 5, pp. 275–292. Liebert, New York.

Gibson, C. C., Hubbard, R., and Parke, D. V. (1983). *Immunotoxicology.* Academic Press, New York.

Griffith, J. F., and Buehler, E. V. (1977). Prediction of skin irritancy and sensitizing potential by testing with animals and man. In *Cutaneous Toxicity* (V. A. Drill and P. Lazar, Eds.), pp. 155–174. Academic Press, New York.

Guillot, J. P., and Gonnet, J. F. (1985). The Epicutaneous Maximization Test. *Curr. Probl. Dermatol.* **14**, 220–247.

Jackson, E. M. (1984). Cellular and molecular events of inflammation. *J. Toxicol. Cut. Ocular Toxicol.* **3**, 347.

Kimber, I. (1989). Aspects of the immune response to contact allergens: Opportunities for the development and modification of predictive test methods. *Fd. Chem. Toxicol.* **27**, 755–762.

Kimber, I. (1993). Epidermal cytokines in contact hypersensitivity: Immunological roles and practical applications. *Toxicol. In Vitro* **7**, 295–298.

Kimber, I., and Weisenberger, C. (1989). A murine local lymph node assay for the identification of contact allergens: Assay development and results of an initial validation study. *Arch. Toxicol.* **63**, 274–282.

Kimber, I., Mitchell, J. A., and Griffin, A. C. (1986). Development of a murine local lymph node assay for the determination of sensitizing potential. *Fd. Chem. Toxicol.* **24**, 585–586.

Kimber, I., Dearman, R. J., Scholes, E. W., and Basketter, D. A. (1994). The local lymph node assay: Developments and applications. *Toxicology* **93**, 13–31.

Klecak, G. (1983). Chapter 9. Identification of contact allergens: Predictive tests in animals. In *Dermatotoxicology* (F. N. Marzulli and H. I. Maibach, Eds.), 2nd ed. Hemisphere, Washington, DC.

Kligman, A. M. (1966). The identification of contact allergens by human assay. III. The maximization test. A procedure for screening and rating contact sensitizers. *J. Invest. Dermatol.* **47**, 393–409.

Landsteiner, K., and Chase, M. W. (1942). Experiments on transfer of cutaneous sensitivity to simple chemical compounds. *Proc. Soc. Exp. Biol. Med.* **49**, 288–390.

Landsteiner, K., and Jacobs, J. (1935). Studies on sensitization of animals with simple chemical compounds. *J. Exp. Med.* **61**, 643–656.

Loveless, S. E., Ladics, G. S., Greberick, G. F., Ryan, C. A., Basketter, D. A., Scholes, E. W., House, R. V., Hilton, J., Dearman, R. J., and Kimber, I. (1996). Further evaluation of the local lymph node assay in the final phase of the international collaborative trial. *Toxicology* **108**, 141–152.

Magnusson, B. (1975). The relevence of results obtained with the guinea pig maximization test. In *Animal Models in Dermatology* (H. Maibach, Ed.), pp. 76–83. Churchill Livingstone, Edinburgh, UK.

Magnusson, B., and Kligman, A. M. (1969). The identification of contact allergens by animal assay. The guinea pig maximization test. *J. Invest. Dermatol.* **52**, 268–276.

Magnusson, B., and Kligman, A. M. (1970). *Allergic Contact Dermatitis in the Guinea Pig: Identification of Contact Allergens.* Charles C. Thomas, Springfield, IL.

Maguire, H. C. (1973a). Mechanism of intensification by Freund's complete adjuvant of the acquisition of delayed hypersensitivity in the guinea pig. *Immunol. Commun.,* 1, 239–246.

Maguire, H. C. (1973b). The bioassay of contact allergens in the guinea pig. *J. Soc. Cosmet. Chem.* 24, 151–162.

Maguire, H. C. (1975). Estimation of the allergenicity of prospective human contact sensitizers in the guinea pig. In *Animal Models in Dermatology* (H. Maibach, Ed.), pp. 67–75. Churchill Livingstone, Edinburgh, UK.

Maguire, H. C., and Chase, M. W. (1967). Exaggerated delayed-type hypersensitivity to simple chemical allergens in the guinea pig. *J. Invest. Dermatol.* 49, 460–468.

Maguire, H. C., and Chase, M. W. (1972). Studies on the sensitization of animals with simple chemical compounds. XIII. Sensitization of guinea pigs with picric acid. *J. Exp. Med.* 135, 357–374.

Marzulli, F. N., and Maibach, H. L. (1983). *Dermatotoxicology,* 2nd ed. Hemisphere, Washington, DC.

Maurer, T. (1983). *Contact and Photo-Contact Allegens.* Dekker, New York.

Maurer, T., Thomann, P., Weirich, E. G., and Hess, R. (1975). The optimization test in the guinea pig. *Agents Actions* 5, 174–179.

Maurer, T., Weirich, E. G., and Hess, R. (1980). The optimization test in the guinea pig in relation to other predictive sensitization methods. *Toxicology* 15, 163–171.

McAuliffe, D. J., Hasan, T., Parrish, J. A., and Kochevar, I. E. (1986). Determination of photosensitivity by an *in vitro* assay as an alternative to animal testing. In *Alternative Methods in Toxicology* (A. M. Goldberg, Ed.), Vol. 3, pp. 31–41. Liebert, New York.

Miller, A. E., Jr., and Levis, W. R. (1973). Studies on the contact sensitization of man with simple chemicals, I. Specific lymphocyte transformation in response to dinitrochlorobenzene sensitization. *J. Invest. Dermatol.* 61, 261–269.

Milner, J. E. (1970). *In vitro* lymphocyte responses in contact hypersensitivity. *J. Invest. Dermatol.* 55, 34–38.

Milner, J. E. (1971). *In vitro* lymphocyte responses in contact hypersensitivity II. *J. Invest. Dermatol.* 56, 349–352.

Milner, J .E. (1983). *In vitro* tests for delayed skin hypersensitivity: Lymphokine production in allergic contact dermatitis. In *Dermatotoxicology* (F. N. Marzulli and H. D. Maibach, Eds.), pp. 185–192. Hemisphere, New York.

National Academy of Sciences (NAS) (1977). *Principles and Procedures for Evaluating the Toxicity of Household Substances,* Publication 1138, pp. 36–39. Prepared for the Consumer Product Safety Commission, National Academy of Sciences, Washington, DC.

Robinson, M. K., and Cruze, C. A. (1996). Preclinical skin sensitization testing of antihistamines: Guinea pig and local lymph node assay responses. *Fd. Chem. Toxicol.* 34, 495–506.

TCSA (1979). Part IV, proposed EPA Test Standards for Toxic Substances Control Act Test Rules, Part 772.112-26. *Fed. Reg.* 44(145).

Thorne, P. S. Hillebrand, J. A., Lewis, G. R., and Karol, M. H. (1987). Contact sensitivity by diisocyanates: Potencies and cross-reactivities. *Toxicol. Appl. Pharmacol.* 87, 155–165.

Thorne, P. S., Hawk, C., Kaliszewski, S. D., and Guiney, P. D. (1991a). The noninvasive mouse ear swelling assay. I. Refinements for detecting weak contact sensitizers. *Fundam. Appl. Toxicol.* 17, 790–806.

Thorne, P. S., Hawk, C., Kaliszewski, S. D., and Guiney, P. D. (1991b). The noninvasive mouse ear swelling assay. II. Testing the contact sensitizing potency of fragrances. *Fundam. Appl. Toxicol.* 17, 807–820.

Thulin, H., and Zacharian, H. (1972). The leukocyte migration test in chromium hypersensitivity. *J. Invest. Dermatol.* 58, 55–58.

CHAPTER 6

Photosensitization and Phototoxicity

Over the past 60 years, it has become clear that sunlight may interact with chemicals to adversely affect human health. Though writings from the ancient civilizations of India and Egypt clearly describe contact photosensitization due to 8-methoxysoralen in plants, it was not until this century that the phenomena has become well understood or the causative agent identified.

In 1916, Freund clearly described a photodermatitis associated with exposure to oil of bergamot (a fragrance extracted from orange rind and containing 5-methoxypsoralen). A very similar photodermatitis among sunbathers was described by Oppenheim in 1932 but was attributed to components other than the psoralens in grass and meadows. Only in 1970 did Marzulli and Maibach define in detail the phototoxicity involved.

In 1939, Epstein, in studying photosensitization due to sulfonamides, clearly differentiated the two separate conditions of photosensitization and phototoxicity. This differentiation is demonstrate in Table 23.

Schwartz and Speck (1957) extensively studied the mechanisms involved in the photosensitization (also known as photoallergy) reaction of sulfonamides (which, unlike the psoralens, produced photosensitization when they were

TABLE 23   Comparison of Phototoxicity and Photosensitization Reactions

Reaction	Phototoxic	Photosensitization
Reaction possible on first exposure	Yes	No
Delay period necessary after first exposure	No	Yes
Chemical alteration	No	Yes
Covalent binding	No	Yes
Clinical changes	Usually like sunburn	Varied morphology
Flares at distant previously involved sites possible	No	Yes
Persistent light reaction can develop	No	Yes
Cross-reactions to structurally related agents	Infrequent	Frequent
Broadening of cross reactions following repeated photopatch testing	No	Possible
Amount of drug necessary for reaction	High	Low
Incidence	Usually relatively high (theoretically 100%)	Usually very low (but theoretically could reach 100%)
Action spectrum	Usually similar to absorption	Usually higher wavelength than absorption spectrum
Passive transfer	No	Possible
Lymphocyte stimulation test	No	Possible
Macrophage migration inhibition test	No	Possible

taken orally) and greatly increased our understanding of these chemicals. Recently, the phototoxicity and photoallergic properties of the quinolone antibiotics have been an issue (Horio *et al.*, 1995).

Phototoxicity and photosensitization both require that a chemical or one of its metabolites absorb light energy to be activated. From that point on, however, they are quite different, because photosensitization is immunologically mediated but phototoxicity is not. The reader is referred to a review of the subject by Lambert *et al.* (1996) for a more detailed review.

THEORY AND MECHANISMS

The portion of the solar spectrum containing the biologically most active region is from 290 to 700 nm.

The ultraviolet (UV) part of the spectrum includes wavelengths from 200 to 400 nm. Portions of the UV spectrum have distinctive features from both the physical and biological points of view. The accepted designations for the biologically important parts of the UV spectrum are UVA, 400–315 nm; UVB, 315–280 nm; and UVC, 280–220 nm. Wavelengths less than 290 nm (UVC) do not occur at the earth's surface because they are absorbed, predominantly by ozone in the stratosphere. The most thoroughly studied photobiological reactions that occur in skin are induced by UVB. The quinolones, for example, absorb light strongly in the 300- to 400- nm wavelength range. Although UVB wavelengths represent only approximately 1.5% of the solar energy received at the earth's surface, they elicit most of the known chemical phototoxic and photoallergic reactions. The visible portion of the spectrum, representing about 50% of the sun's energy received at sea level, includes wavelengths from 400 to 700 nm. Visible light is necessary for such biological events as photosynthesis, the regulation circadian cycles, vision, and pigment darkening. Furthermore, visible light in conjunction with certain chromophores (e.g., dyes, drugs, and endogenous compounds which absorb light and therefore "give" color) and molecular oxygen induces photodynamic effects.

Understanding the toxic effects of light impinging on the skin requires knowledge of both the nature of sunlight and the skin's optical properties. Skin may be viewed as an optically heterogeneous medium, composed of three layers that have distinct refractive indices, chromophore distributions, and light-scattering properties. Light entering the outermost layer, the stratum corneum, is in part reflected—4–7% for wavelengths between 250 and 3000 nm (Anderson and Parrish, 1981)—due to the difference in refractive index between air and the stratum corneum. Absorption by urocanic acid (a deamination product of histidine), melanin, and proteins containing the aromatic amino acids tryptophan and tyrosine in the stratum corneum produces further attenuation of light, particularly at shorter UV wavelengths. Approximately 40% of UVB is transmitted through the stratum corneum to the viable epidermis. The light entering the epidermis is attenuated by scattering and, predominantly, absorption. Epidermal chromophores consist of proteins, urocanic acid, nucleic acids, and melanin. Passage through the epidermis results in appreciable attenuation of UVA and UVB radiation. The transmission properties of the dermis are largely due to scattering, with significant absorption of visible light by melanin, β-carotene, and the blood-borne pigments bilirubin, hemoglobin, and oxyhemoglobin. Lightly traversing these layers of the skin is extensively attenuated, most drastically for wavelengths less than 400 nm. Longer wavelengths are more penetrating. It has been noted that there is an "optical window"—that is, greater transmission—for light at wavelengths of 600–1300 nm, which may have important biological consequences.

Normal variations in the skin's optical properties frequently occur. The degree of pigmentation may produce variations in the attenuation of light, particularly between 300 and 400 nm, by as much as 1.5 times more in blacks than in Caucasians (Pathak, 1967). Alterations in the amount or distribution of other natural chromophores account for further variations in skin optical properties. Urocanic acid, deposited on the skin's surface during perspiration (Anderson and Parrish, 1981), and UV-absorbing lipids, excreted in sebum, may significantly reduce UV transmission through the skin. Epidermal thickness, which varies over regions of the body and increases after exposure to UVB radiation, may significantly modify UV transmission.

Certain disease states also produce alterations in the skin's optical properties. Alterations of the skin's surface, such as by psoriatic plaques, decrease transmitted light. This effect may be lessened by application of oils whose refractive index is similar to that of skin (Anderson and Parrish, 1981). Disorders such as hyperbilirubinemia, porphyrias, and blue skin nevi result in increased absorption of visible light due to accumulation or altered distribution of endogenous chromophoric compounds.

The penetration of light into and through dermal tissues has important consequences. This penetration is demonstrated in Fig. 19. Skin, as the primary organ responsible for thermal regulation, is overperfused relative to its metabolic requirements (Anderson and Parrish, 1981). It is estimated that the

SCHEMATIC REPRESENTATION OF LIGHT PENETRATION INTO SKIN.

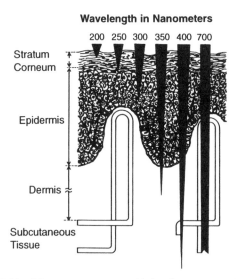

FIGURE 19   Schematic penetration of light of varying wavelengths into the skin.

average cutaneous blood flow is 20–30 times that necessary to support the skin's metabolic needs. The papillary boundaries between epidermis and dermis allow capillary vessels to lie close to the skin's surface, permitting the blood and important components of the immune system to be exposed to light. The equivalent of the entire blood volume of an adult may pass through the skin, and potentially be irradiated, in 20 min. This corresponds to the time required to receive 1 or 2 MEDs (the MED is defined as the minimal dose of UV irradiation that produces definite, but minimally perceptible, redness 24 hr after exposure). The accessibility of incidence radiation to blood has been exploited in such regimens as phototherapy of hyperbilirubinemia in neonates, where light is used as a therapeutic agent. However, in general, there is a potential for light-induced toxicity due to irradiation of blood-borne drugs and metabolites.

FACTORS INFLUENCING PHOTOTOXICITY/PHOTOSENSITIZATION

There are a number of factors which can influence an agent acting either as a phototoxin or a photoallergen. In addition to all those factors previously reviewed in chapter 5, there are also the following:

1. The quantity and location of photoactive material present in or on the skin.
2. The capacity of the photoactive material to penetrate into normal skin by percutaneous absorption as well as into skin altered by trauma, such as maceration, irritation, and sunburn.
3. The pH, enzyme presence, and solubility conditions at the site of exposure.
4. The quantity of activating radiation to which the skin is exposed.
5. The capacity of the spectral range to activate the materials on or within the skin.
6. The ambient temperature and humidity.
7. The thickness of the horny layer.
8. The degree of melanin pigmentation of the skin.
9. The inherent "photoactivity" of the chemical; does it weakly or strongly absorb light?

Basically, any material that has both the potential to absorb ultraviolet light (in the UVA or UVB regions) and the possibility of dermal exposure or distribution into the dermal region should be subject to some degree of suspi-

TABLE 24   Known Phototoxic Agents

In humans		In animals	
Compound	Route	Compound	Route
Aminobenzoic acid derivatives	Topical	Acradine	Topical
		Amiodarone	Oral
Amyldimethylamino benzoate, mixed *ortho* and *para* isomers	Topical	Anthracine	Topical
		Bergapten (5-methoxypsolaren)	Topical
Anthracene acridine	Topical	Bithionol	Topical
Bergapten (5-methoxypsoralen)	Topical	Chlorodiazepoxide	ip
Cadmium sulfide	Tattoo	Chlorothiazide	ip
Chlorothiazides	Oral	Chlorpromazine	Topical
Coar tar (multicomponent)	Topical	Demeclocycline	ip
Dacarbazine	Infusion	Griseofulvin	ip
Disperse blue 35 (anthaquinone-base dye)	Topical	Kynuremic acid	Oral
Nalidixic acid	Oral	Nalidixic acid	Oral
Padimate A or Escalol 506 (amyl-*p*-dimethylamino benzoate)	Topical	Prochlorperazine	ip
		Quinokine methanol	ip
		Quinolone (antibacterial)	Oral
Psoralens	Oral, topical	Tetracyclines	ip, topical
Quinolone (antibacterial)	Oral	Xanthotoxin (8-methoxypsoralen)	Oral, ip, im
Sulfanilamide	id		
Tetracyclines	Oral		
Xanthotoxin (8-methoxypsoralen)	Topical, oral		

cion as to potential phototoxicity. As shown in Table 24, a large number of agents have been identified as phototoxic or photoallergenic agents. Of these, tetrachlorosalicylanilide (TCSA) is most commonly used as a positive control in animal studies.

PREDICTIVE TESTS FOR PHOTOTOXICITY

Before we start on our description of the different methods, we will first cover some basics on light dosimetry. The intensity of the irradiation used in phototoxicity testing is determined with a light meter, which provides output as watts per m^2. The shelves on which the animals rest during the exposure periods are normally adjustable in order to control the dose of light to the exposure area. The irradiation from fluorescent lights will vary somewhat from day to day, depending on temperature, variations in line current, etc. The dose the animals receive is generally represented as joules/cm^2. A joule is equal to 1 watt/sec. Therefore, the dose of light is dependent on the time of exposure. For example, in their review, Lambert *et al.* (1996) discuss dosages of UVA light of 9 or 10 J/cm^2 in the UVA spectral region. If the irradiation from the light is found to be 20 W/m^2 at the exposure site, then the time of exposure required to obtain the target dose of light (in J) is calculated as

$$(\text{time of exposure}) = \frac{\text{Wsec}}{J} \frac{9J}{cm^2} \frac{m^2}{20\,W} \frac{10^4\,cm^2}{m^2} \frac{min}{60\,sec} = 75\,min$$

If, with the same set of lights, 2 weeks later the irradiation is determined to be 19 W/m^2, then the exposure period would have to be 79 min.

There are three recommended protocols for assessing topical phototoxicity potential—rabbit, guinea pig, and mouse. The first described here is that for the rabbit. The traditional methodology for a predictive test for phototoxicity has been an intact rabbit test (Marzulli and Maibach, 1970). This test is conducted as follows (and illustrated diagrammatically in Fig. 20):

A. Animals and animal husbandry
    1. Strain/species: Female New Zealand White rabbits
    2. Number: 6 rabbits per test; 2 rabbits for positive control

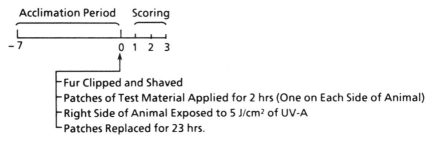

PHOTOTOXICITY ASSAY

Species:	New Zealand white Rabbits
Test Group:	6 Rabbits
Positive Control:	2 Rabbits

Acclimation Period Scoring

−7   0 1 2 3

   Fur Clipped and Shaved
   Patches of Test Material Applied for 2 hrs (One on Each Side of Animal)
   Right Side of Animal Exposed to 5 J/cm² of UV-A
   Patches Replaced for 23 hrs.

FIGURE 20　Line chart for the design and conduct of phototoxicity assay using rabbits.

    3. Age: Young adult

    4. Acclimation period: At least 7 days prior to study

    5. Food and water: Commercial laboratory feed and water are freely available.

B. Test article

    1. A dose of 0.5 ml of liquid or 500 mg of a solid or semisolid will be applied to each test site.

    2. Liquid substances will be used undiluted.

    3. For solids, the test article will be moistened with water (500 mg test article/0.5 ml water or another suitable vehicle) to ensure good contact with the skin.

    4. The positive control material will be a lotion containing 1% 8-methoxypsoralen.

C. Experimental procedures

    1. Animals will be weighed on the first day of dosing.

    2. On the day prior to dosing, the fur of the test animals will be clipped from the dorsal area of the trunk using a small animal clipper, then shaved clean with a finer bladed clipper.

    3. On the day of dosing, the animals will be placed in restraints.

    4. One pair of patches (approximately 2.5 × 2.5 cm) per test article will be applied to the skin of the back, with one patch on each side of the backbone.

    5. A maximum of two pairs of patches may be applied to each animal and the patches must be at least 2 in. apart.

    6. The patches will be held in contact with the skin by means of an occlusive dressing for the 2-hr exposure period.

    7. After the 2-hr exposure period, the occlusive dressing, as well as the patches on the right side of the animal, will be removed (aluminum foil).

    8. The left side of the animal will be covered with opaque material.

    9. The animal will then be exposed to approximately 5 J/cm^2 of UVA (320–400 nm).

    10. After exposure to the UVA light, the patches on the right side of the animal, as well as the occlusive dressing, will be replaced.

    11. The dressing will again be removed approximately 23 hr after the initial application of the test article. Residual test article will be carefully removed, where applicable, using water (or another suitable vehicle).

    12. Animals will be examined for signs of erythema and edema and the responses scored at 24, 48, and 72 hr after the initial test article application according to the Draize reaction grading system previously presented in this volume.

13. Any unusual observation and mortality will be recorded.

D. Analysis of data: The data from the irradiated and nonirradiated sites are evaluated separately. The scores from erythema and eschar formation, and edema at 24, 48, and 72 hr, are added for each animal (six values). The six values are then divided by 3, yielding six individual scores. The mean of the six individual animal irritation scores represents the mean primary irritation score (maximum score = 8, as in the primary dermal irritation study). This method was developed after a human model had been developed.

GUINEA PIG

Recently, a standardized protocol for using the guinea pig for phototoxicity testing has been proposed (Nilsson *et al.,* 1993), which has been the subject of an international validation exercise. This is detailed below and in Fig. 21A.

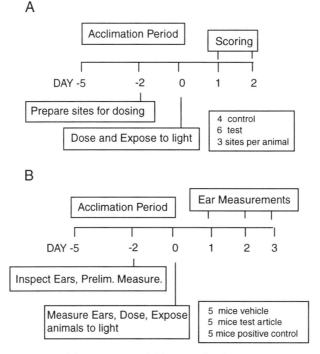

FIGURE 21 (A) Guinea pig and (B) mouse for phototoxicity testing.

A. Animals and animal husbandry
   1. Strain/species: Males Hartley guinea pig
   2. Number: At least 10 (two groups)
        Irradiation controls: 4 animals
        Test material treated: 6 animals
   3. Age: Young adult, 300–500 g
   4. Acclimation period: At least 5 days
   5. Feed/water: *Ad libitum*
B. Test material
   1. Vehicle: Test assumes that material will be in solution. Use the most volatile, nonirritating organic solvent possible, e.g., ethanol, acetone, dimethylacetamide, or some combination.
   2. Treatment: There can be up to four sites per animal, each measuring 1.5×1.5 cm (2.25 cm^2). In general, one side should be for a vehicle control, and another for a positive control [8-methoxypsoralen (8-MOP), 0.005% in ethanol].
   3. Dosage: A dose of 0.025–0.050 ml is applied using a micropipetor to each site.
C. Experimental procedure
   1. Animals will be weighed on the first day of dosing.
   2. Preparation: Approximately 48 hr prior to treatment, removed the hair from a 6×8-cm area on the back with a fine clipper. On the day of dosing, animals are dosed as described previously. Tests are situated as to prevent mixing of test solutions after application. No patches or wraps are used.
   3. Immediately after dose application, the animals are placed in a restraint while keeping the test sites uncovered. Prior to irradiation the heads are covered to prevent ocular damage from the light exposure.
   4. Thirty minutes after dosing, animals are exposed to a nonerythmogenic dose of light in the UVA band (should have peak intensity between 335 and 365 nm). The dose of light should be 9 or 10 J/cm^2 for UVA and 0.1–0.3 J/cm^2 for UVB.
   5. Immediately after light exposure, the animals are wiped clean if necessary and returned to their home cages.
   6. Animals are inspected and scored at 24 and 48 hr postexposure according to the following:
        0, No reaction
        1, Slight erythema
        2, Moderate erythema
        3, Severe erythema, with or without edema
   The reader should note that this scoring scheme is the same one

used for dermal sensitization scoring, whereas the scoring method for the rabbit model discussed previously is that used for dermal irritation studies.

7. Any unusual clinical signs noted during exposure should be noted. The following descriptive parameters can be calculated from the data.

Phototoxic irritation Index (PTII)

$$= \frac{(\text{number of positive sites}) \times 100}{(\text{number of exposure sites})}$$

$$\text{Phototoxicity severity index (PSI)} = \frac{(\text{total of scores})}{(\text{total of observations})}$$

Lovell and Sanders (1992) had previously proposed a similar model for assessing topical phototoxicity potential in the guinea pig. Their model differed from that proposed by Nilson et al. (1993) with regard to the following:

Only one test site per animal was used

Test sites were smaller (about 1.6 cm²)

Amounts applied were less (about 10 μl)

Light intensity was set at 15 J/cm².

Their paper made no reference to the use of a restrainer.

Assessments were conducted at 4, 24, 48, and 72 hr.

The scoring system was as follows

0, Normal

2, Faint/trace erythema

4, Slight erythema

6, Definite erythema

8, Well-developed erythema

(intermediate scores were indicated by odd numbers.)

They recommend the use of acridine (weak phototoxin) or anthracene (strong phototoxin) for positive controls.

MOUSE EAR SWELLING MODEL

Gerberick and Ryan (1989) proposed a method for using the mouse in topical phototoxicity testing. This is detailed below and in Fig. 21B.

A. Animals and animal husbandry
   1. Strain/species: Female BALB/c mice
   2. Number: At least 10 (two groups, three groups if positive control is included)

Solvent/irradiation controls: 5 animals
Test material treated: 5 animals
Positive control (8-MOP): 5 animals

3. Age: Juvenile, weighing 20–25 g
4. Acclimation period: At least 5 days
5. Feed/water: *Ad libitum*

B. Test material

1. Vehicle: Test assumes that material will be in solution. Use the most volatile, nonirritating organic solvent possible, e.g., ethanol, acetone, dimethylacetamide, or some combination.
2. Treatment: Each ear on each mouse in a group is treated with the same solution. For example, the test article treated group is treated only with test article solution.
3. Dosage: 8 μl per each side of each ear applied using a micropipette.

C. Experimental procedure

1. Animals will be weighed on the first day of dosing.
2. Preparation: Approximately 48 hr prior to treatment, the ears are inspected and animals assigned to treatment groups. Animals with swollen or damaged ears are excluded from test. Preliminary ear thickness measurements are taken.
3. On the day of dosing, animals are placed in specially designed restrainers, ear thickness measurements are taken, and the animals are dosed as described previously. No patches or wraps are used.
4. Thirty to 60 min after dose application, the animals (while still in restrainers) are exposed to a nonerythmogenic dose of light in the UVA band (150 W short-arc UV solar simulator with internal 1-mm UG-11 and WG320 filters with peak intensity between 290 and 410 nm). Irradiation in W/cm^2 should be determined using a radiometer with an appropriate UVA or UVB detector. Light should be between 5 and 7 J/cm^2 for UVA and 0.2–0.4 J/cm^2 for UVB.
5. Only the right ear is exposed. The left ear is protected from light by the researchers hand. Immediately after light exposure, the animals are wiped clean if necessary and returned to their home cages.
6. Ear thickness measurements are taken at 24, 48, and 72 hr postdosing, using a handheld dial micrometer. The ear is positioned so that the contact plates of the micrometer could be placed toward the outer edge of the ear. The spring-loaded lever of the micrometer is slowly released until the plates come into contact with the surface of the ear as judged visually. Care is taken so that the plates do not close too quickly or tightly on the ear, causing compression of any edema that might be present. Two measurements are taken

at adjacent sites on each ear and the average ear thickness is determined.

7. Changes in ear thickness from the pretreatment baseline are calculated and expressed as mm $\times 10^{-2}$. A statistically significant (paired t test) increase in ear thickness in the irradiated ears vs the nonirradiated ears within the test article treated groups is considered sufficient evidence for phototoxicity, providing that there was not a statistically significant change in the control group.

This method has obvious advantages over the guinea pig and rabbit models described previously. The animals are less expensive to obtain and maintain. Once one learns the appropriate measurement techniques, the method is very objective and reliable. Examples of known photosensitizers are shown in Table 24.

ALTERNATIVE DESIGNS: *IN VIVO* SYSTEMS

There are at least three *in vivo* alternatives to this traditional test. The first uses just the ear of the rabbit. The rabbit ear provides a site which is of sufficient size with uniform, thin skin without a thick, hairy coat—thus, offering advantages over the whole body rabbit and mouse models. The external surface of the pinna is shaved with clippers and radiation is delivered using a xenon arc solar simulator with multiple liquid light guides (Solar Light Co., Philadelphia, PA) adjusted to provide intensity steps varying by 40%. Depending on the test situation, exposures range from 0.5 to 12 min. In the absence of phototoxic agents or sunscreens, a 1-min exposure will generally produce detectable erythema from the midrange light guides. The intensity of the erythema is graded and corresponds with the radiation flux. In phototoxicity testing, the flux is decreased by 50% or more. Exposure of the rabbit ear treated with 8-MOP at these flux levels results in erythema and edema. The developers of this test system (Marks *et al.*, 1986) report it to give comparable results to the traditional test system.

The second *in vivo* alternative uses the hairless mouse, in which one can measure the dorsal skin thickness using vernier skinfold calipers. In this way, the degree of dermal edema induced by phototoxic agents is measured readily and is not subject to the problems of visual assessment of erythema in rodent skin. These latter studies examined the ability of psoralens and UVA to induce the enzyme ornithine decarboxylase (ODC). ODC is the rate-limiting enzyme in the biosynthesis of polyamines. The polyamines appear to be important precursors of cellular hyperplasia, while ODC in itself appears to be a useful marker of cellular damage. Noteworthy here is that psoralens that were phototoxic, i.e., 8-MOP and 5-methoxypsoralen (5-MOP), and UVA significantly induced ODC and edema in the hairless mouse, but a nonphototoxic psoralen, i.e., 3-carbethoxypsoralen (3-CP) and UVA have failed to induce either. These studies also examined the ability of the different psoralens and of UVA to inhibit the rate of thymidine incorporation into the epidermis. 8-MOP and 5-MOP produced a profound suppression of thymidine incorporation 4 hr following psoralen and UVA irradiation. However, 3-CP produced no significant change in DNA synthesis. Thus, it would seem that for those phototoxic substances that have an effect on cellular DNA, the thymidine incorporation assays *in vivo* are useful (Lowe, 1986).

ADVANTAGES AND DISADVANTAGES

The classic and alternative tests share common advantages and disadvantages. On the plus side, they

Have no appreciable false negative rate.
Are relatively easy to perform.
Are relatively inexpensive.

The disadvantages are limited to the following:

Photometers must be carefully calibrated to control UV exposure.
Results are subjective rather than objective.
Significant amounts of test material are used.

PREDICTIVE TESTS FOR PHOTOSENSITIZATION

There are at least five *in vivo* photosensitization test methods. Only two of these (the Armstrong assay and Harber and Shalita method) will be presented here. The other three (the Vinson and Borselli method, Guillot *et al.* method, and a method using mice) are not generally considered mainstream methods, but are mentioned because they could be of interest.

Though the pattern of evolution of predictive animal tests is not as clear as that of dermal sensitization tests, the two methods presented here each represent a distinct phase of that development.

Harber and Shalita Method

This method is the older of the two and uses dermal exposure without any adjuvent to increase the response. This method was originally published by Harber and Shalita in 1975, and is presented diagrammatically in Fig. 22.

HAUBER AND SHALITA PHOTOSENTIZATION TEST

Species: Guinea Pig (Hartley Strain)
Test Group: 10 Animals
Vehicle Control Group: 6 Animals (Positive Control
Group Optional)

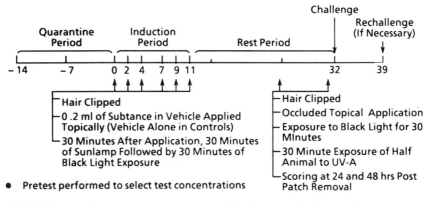

FIGURE 22   Line chart for the design and conduct of the Hauber and Shalita assay for photosensitization.

A. Animals
   1. Young adult female Hartley strain guinea pigs, weighing between 300 and 400 g at the start of the study, are used. The female sex is preferred because the aggressive social behavior of males may result in considerable skin damage that might interfere with the interpretation of challenge reactions.
   2. Animals that show poor growth or are ill in any way are not used because illness markedly decreases the response. Animals with skin marked or scarred from fighting are avoided. The guinea pigs are quarantined and observed for at least 2 weeks to detect any illness before starting a study.
   3. The guinea pigs are randomly assigned to a test group of 10 animals and negative control group of 6 animals. If a pretest group is necessary, as many animals as needed for that group are randomized also.
   4. Test and control group guinea pigs are weighed 1 week prior to dosing (Day −7), on the day of dosing (Day 0), and weekly thereafter.
B. Pretest (if necessary)
   1. Several animals are used to pretest different concentrations of test substance in vehicle (usually acetone) to determine the topical

dermal irritation threshold concentration on skin that is exposed to UVB and UVA irradiation sequentially and on skin that is exposed to UVA irradiation alone.

2. The hair of these animals is clipped over the whole dorsal region.

3. A volume of 0.2 ml of each test concentration is applied twice to each guinea pig (1) to the nuchal region and (2) to the dorsal lumbar region.

4. Thirty minutes after application, the treated nuchal sites are irradiated with sunlamp (fluorescent "sunlamp" tubes (UVB irradiation): type of tubes, Westinghouse FS40; skin distance, 15 cm; dose, measured and calculated at time of exposure; exposure time, 30 min; emission, 285–350 nm) emissions (UVB for 30 min while the lumbar sites are shielded with elastoplast tape.

5. After the UVB exposure, the tape is removed from the lumbar region, and both the treated nuchal sites and lumbar sites are irradiated with black light [fluorescent "black light" tubes (UVA irradiation): type of tubes, GE F40 BL; skin distance, 10 cm; dose, measured and calculated at time of exposure; exposure time, 30 min; emission, 320–450 nm; a pane of window glass (3-mm thick) is used to eliminate passage of radiation of lower than 320 nm] emissions (UVA) for 30 min.

6. The animals are returned to their respective cages after the UVA exposure.

7. Twenty-four hours after the initial exposure to the test substance, the nuchal and lumbar skin sites are scored for erythema formation.

8. A concentration is chosen for induction applications that causes a mild or weak erythema response at the nuchal sites. If the test substance does not cause an erythema response, then the highest concentration level that is practical should be used for induction.

9. The highest concentration of the test substance that is nonirritating to the lumbar sites is used for challenge application. Two lower concentrations of the test substance, prepared by serial dilution from the highest concentration, are also used for the challenge application.

C. Induction stage—Days 0, 2, 4, 7, 9, and 11

1. The hair in an area of approximately 3 × 3 cm is clipped from the nuchal region of each test and control group guinea pig.

2. A volume of 0.2 ml of a relatively high concentration of the test substance in either acetone or ethanol is applied to the shaved nuchal region of each test group guinea pig. The concentration will be the highest level that can be well tolerated locally and generally by the guinea pig, as determined by a pretest for dermal irritation.

3. A volume of 0.2 ml of solvent (acetone or ethanol) is applied to the shaved nuchal region of each control group guinea pig.

4. Thirty minutes after application, the treated nuchal sites of test and control guinea pigs are irradiated with sunlamp emissions for 30 min and black light emissions for 30 min, successively. The lumbar region of the back is shielded from the light sources during the irradiation procedures with elastic bandage which is wrapped around the torso of each animal.

5. The clipping, topical exposure to test substance, and irradiation procedures are repeated six times during a 12-day period (typical study days are 0, 2, 4, 7, 9, and 11).

D. Challenge stage—Day 32

1. Elicitation of contact photosensitivity is performed 21 days from the last sensitizing (induction) exposure.

2. The hair of the dorsal lumbar region of each of 10 test group and 3 of 6 control group guinea pigs is clipped for the first time.

3. Three different concentrations of test substance using the solvent used for induction, as determined from the pretest, are applied topically to this region; test and control animals are treated alike. Each concentration is applied to the right and left side of the dorsal midline, as depicted in Fig. 23.

4. The torso of each test and control guinea pig is wrapped in Saran Wrap (1 layer thick) after the test chemical is applied. The Saran Wrap is held in place at the ends with athletic adhesive tape. The same tape is used to shield the left side of each animal from the UVA light source.

EXPOSURE AND UV-ILLUMINATION PATTERN FOR PHOTOSENSITIZATION TESTS

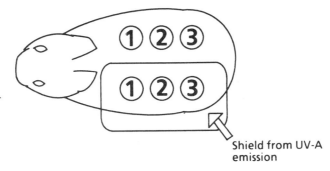

Shield from UV-A emission

FIGURE 23   Illustrative figure for dermal exposure and UV irradiation of guinea pigs for photosensitization test.

5. Thirty minutes after application, the right side of each animal is exposed to nonerythrogenic (>320 nm) UVA emissions for 30 min. The radiation is passed through a pane of window glass 3 mm thick in order to eliminate passage of radiation lower than 320 nm.

6. After the black light exposure, all animals are unwrapped, returned to their respective cages, and placed in a darkened room for 24 hr.

E. Challenge readings

1. If the test substance leaves a colored residue, the excess test material is removed by washing with a suitable solvent at 24 hr so that the area of challenge skin can be evaluated accurately.

2. All test sites, both irradiated and nonirradiated, are scored and interpreted 24 and 48 hr after the initial test substance application and subsequent exposure to black light irradiation.

3. Erythema is scored as follows:

   0, No erythema
   1, Minimal, but definite erythema
   2, Moderate erythema
   3, Considerable erythema
   4, Maximal erythema

4. Erythema scores are recorded.

F. Rechallenge

1. If the test substance is judged a nonphotosensitizing agent after the first challenge application, a second and final challenge application will be performed on each test group animal 7 days after the initiation of the first challenge dose.

2. Controls from the first challenge application are not rechallenged because they have been exposed to the test substance and are no longer true negative (naive) controls. The three remaining naive control group animals (not used for the first challenge) are challenged for comparison to the rechallenge of test group animals.

3. The procedure used for the first challenge application will be used for the second challenge application. Either the same procedure will be used or new concentrations of test substance, including reshaving, the same patching method, and the same duration of exposure will be used. Observations are again made 24 and 48 hr after the second challenge application and skin reactions are recorded.

G. Interpretation of results

1. The negative control group of animals, having received no previous photosensitive (induction) exposures, serves to identify any phototoxic or primary irritant (nonphototoxic) substances.

2. An erythema score of 1 or more is considered a positive response.
3. Interpretation of data is based on the dermal score for erythema, as in Table 25.

Armstrong Assay

This method, originally published by Ichikawa *et al.* (1981), introduced the use of adjuvents in a photosensitization test system.

This assay has been recommended by the Cosmetic, Toiletries and Fragrances Association. It is of interest that the EPA has not made public a concern about photoallergens because several pesticides have similar structures to fra-

TABLE 25   Dermal Erythema Interpretation in Photosensitization

Test group		Control group		
Irradiated	Nonirradiated	Irradiated	Nonirradiated	Interpretation
0	0	0	0	No contact photosensitization No contact sensitization No phototoxicity No primary dermal irritation
1–4	0	0	0	Contact photosensitization No contact sensitization No phototoxicity No primary dermal irritation
1–4	1–4	0	0	No contact photosensitization (unless sum of scores exceeds 2× of nonirradiated scores) Contact sensitization (non-photo) No phototoxicity No primary dermal irritation
1–4	0	1–4	0	Contact photosensitization[a] No contact sensitization Phototoxicity No primary dermal irritation
1–4	1–4	1–4	1–4	No contact photosensitization No contact sensitization No phototoxicity Primary dermal irritation

[a] Contact photosensitization only if the incidence and degree of positive responses of the test group are judged to clearly exceed those of the control group.

ARMSTRONG PHOTOSENSITIZATION TEST

Species: Guinea Pig (Hartley Strain)
Test Group: 20 Animals
Vehicle Control Group: 10 Animals (Positive Control
                            Group Optional)

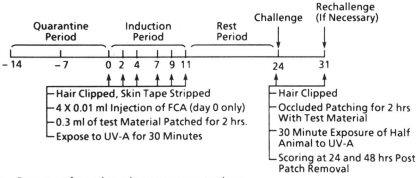

- Pretest performed to select test concentrations

FIGURE 24   Line chart for the design and conduct of the Armstrong assay for photosensitization.

grances and numerous pesticides are known to form reactive species in the presence of UV light. This test is illustrated in Fig. 24.

Lights—The Armstrong assay uses UVA light (320–400 nm) in the induction and challenge phase. The UVA lights are commonly known as "black lights" and can be purchased as "BLB" fluorescence-type bulbs from major light manufacturers. However, the selection of the light source is critical because the range of wavelengths emitted by the bulb is controlled by the phosphor coating and different manufacturers use different phosphors to produce BLB lights. There may even be different phosphors used by the same manufacturer and there is no code on the bulbs to indicate which phosphor is being used. Cole *et al.* (1984) reported an excellent study of this problem. The General Electric BLB emits effective energy only at wavelengths longer than 350 nm, whereas the entire spectrum between 315 and 400 nm is covered by the Sylvania BLB bulb. Less than 2% of the total energy emitted by the General Electric BLB light is between 250 and 350 nm, whereas 42% of the energy from the Sylvania BLB light falls in this range. There are known photoallergens which require the energy contained in the spectrum below 345 nm for activation and thus give a false negative if the incorrect light source is used. The best precaution is to determine the emission spectrum of the lights which are to be used in the assay.

It is necessary to determine the total energy being emitted by the lights in order to calculate the proper J/cm^2 exposure. An International Light Model 700 provides a relatively inexpensive means of measuring the light energy when fitted with a cosine-corrected UVA detector (W150s quartz diffuser, UVA-pass filter SEE015 detector). The device has a peak sensitivity of 360 nm and width of 50 nm. A bank of eight bulbs is readily prepared by bolting together two industrial four-bulb (48-in. long) reflectors. Two sets of these will allow 40 animals to be treated at one time. The lights are allowed to warm 30 min before use. They are turned off just before the animals are placed under them and then turned back on. The light intensity is measured at several locations at the level of the top of the backs of the animals and the correct exposure time is then calculated. The lights are adjusted to be between 4 and 6 in. above the back and 10 J/cm^2 is the proper exposure.

Patching—The Hill Top Chamber (see Buehler assay) provides a good patching system in this assay. A volume of 0.3 ml is used. The animal restrainers described in the Buehler assay work well for holding the animals during the patching and the exposure to the light as well as in providing excellent occlusion.

Induction site preparation—The majority of hair is removed from the intended patching site with a small animal clipper fitted with a No. 40 blade. The assay has a frequent requirement for the complete removal of hair using a depilatory (Whitehall Laboratories, New York) which is applied and left in contact with the skin for no more than 15 min. It must be washed away completely with a stream of warm running water. The animals are dried with a towel and the inside of the cages wiped clean of any depilatory before returning the guinea pigs.

When required, the epidermis is partially removed by tape-stripping. The skin must be completely dry or the stripping will be ineffective. A length of tape approximately 8 in. long is used. Starting at one end of the tape, it is placed against the skin and rubbed with the finger a few times to cause good adhersion. It is then pealed away, taking with it some dry epidermis cells. A new section of the tape is then applied to the skin and the procedure repeated four or five times. The skin will have a shiny appearance due to the leakage of moisture from the dermis. The tape should not be jerked away from the skin because this can cause the rupture of dermal capillaries.

The potential of the animal to respond to a sensitizer is enhanced by the injection of Freund's complete adjuvant (Calbio-chem-Behring, San Diego, CA, or Difco, Detroit, MI). The adjuvant is diluted 1:1 with sterile water before using. The injections must be intradermal. In the Armstrong assay, a pattern of four 0.1-ml injections is given just prior to the first induction patching in the nuchal area. All four injections should fit under the edge of the area to be covered by the Hill Top Chamber. It is advisable to perform the skin-stripping operation before the injections because adjuvant can leak onto the skin and prevent effective removal of the epidermis.

The occlusion of the patches is done in the same manner as described in the Buehler assay (Chapter 5). The test site(s) is exposed to the UVA light after 2 hr of occlusion. The animal is left in the restrainer and the dental dam above the test site to be exposed is cut and the patch is removed. Sites not to be exposed are left patched. Excess material is wiped from the site to be exposed and the remaining parts of the animal are covered with aluminum foil. All patches are removed after the light-exposure step, the patched areas wiped free of excess material, and the animal returned to the cage.

Grading—The grading is the same as used in the Buehler assay.

Vehicles—With the exception of water, it is desirable to use a vehicle for the inductions which is different from the one used at the challenge (see Buehler assay). Because the control animals in the Armstrong assay are sham treated (including any vehicle), one can patch the test and control animals with vehicle at the challenge if the same vehicle must be used for both the induction and the challenge. It is advantageous to use a vehicle which dissolves the test material, though suspensions may not be avoided in all cases.

Irritation screens—The irritation screen is used to determine acceptable concentrations for the induction phase (i.e., one which does not produce eschar with repeated exposure or systemic toxicity) and the challenge phase (no more than slightly irritating). Each concentration must be tested with and without exposure to UVA light, as both conditions are used in the challenge. Thus, to evaluate four concentrations requires that eight animals be used. Each animal receives a pair of patches with each pair being a different concentration (i.e., each concentration is patched on four animals). One of each pair of patches is placed on the left side and the corresponding concentration on the remaining patch is placed on the right side. The hair is removed by depilation on the day of patching. The patches on the right side are removed after 2 hr of occlusion, the remaining parts of the animal are covered with foil, and the right side is exposed to 10 J/cm^2 of UVA light. Animals are returned to their cages after the exposure. If different solvents are being used in the induction and challenge phase, then two separate screens need to be run.

Conducting the Armstrong assay—Combining the discussed techniques in a specific regimen yields the assay as follows:

1. Irritation/toxicity pretest (8 animals)

    Day 0: Remove the hair from the lumbar region by clipping and depilitation. Apply two concentrations on each animal on adjacent left-side/right-side locations for a total of four dose concentrations. Occlude the patches for 2 hr (± 15 min). Expose the right side to

10 J/cm² of UVA light after removing the patches on the right side. Remove the remaining patches and excess material after the exposure to light.

Day 1: Grade all test sites 24 hr (±1 hr) after removal of all patches (24-hr grade).

Day 2: Repeat the grading 48 hr (+2 hr) after removing the patches (48-hr grade)

2. Induction (20 tests + 10 sham controls + any rechallenge controls)

Day 0: Weigh all test and control animals. Remove the hair from the nuchal area with clippers and depilatory. Remove the epidermis by stripping four or five times with tape. Make four 0.1-ml id injections of a 1:1 dilution of Freund's complete adjuvant in an area to be covered by the patch. Cover this area on the test animals with a Hill Top Chamber which has 0.3 ml of test material preparation. Patch the sham controls with water or solvent on the patch. Occlude with dental dam and restrain in a holder for 2 hr (±15 min). Remove the patches, cover the nonpatched areas with foil, and expose to 10 J/cm² of UVA light for 30 min.

Days 2, 4, 7, 9, 11: Repeat the activities of Day 0, with the following exceptions: Do not weigh animals and do not inject adjuvant. Move the patch back when the original induction site becomes too damaged but keep it in the nuchal area. Dipilation may not be needed at each induction.

3. Challenge (20 tests + 10 sham control animals 9–13 days after last induction exposure)

Day 0: Weigh all animals, clip the lumbar region free of hair, and dipilate. Do not strip the skin. Patch each animal with a pair of adjacent patches (one on the left side and one on the right side) containing 0.3 ml of a nonirritating concentration of test material on a Hill Top Chamber. Occlude the patches and restrain the animal for 2 hr (±15 min). Remove the patches from the right side and cover the remaining animal with foil. Expose the right side to 10 J/cm² of UVA light. Remove the remaining patch and any excess material.

Day 1: Grade all challenge sites, keeping separate the grades of the sites exposed to light and those not exposed to light 24 hr (±1 hr) after removal of the patches (24-hr grade).

Day 2; Repeat the grading 48 hr (±2 hr) after removal of the patches (48-hr grade).

4. Rechallenge

All or selected animals may be rechallenged with the same or a different test material 7–12 days after the challenge. Use 10 new sham-treated controls and naive test sites on all animals following the same procedure as used in the challenge.

5. Interpretation of results

Determine the number of positive responders (number of animals with a score >1 at either the 24- or 48-hr grading or with a score 1 unit higher than the highest score in the control). Determine the average score at 24 and at 48 hr for the test and control groups using face values. Keep the data for the sites exposed to light separate from the data from sites not exposed to light.

Strengths and weaknesses: The Armstrong assay was found to give responses in the guinea pig which were consistent with what has been observed in humans: positive responses for 6-methyl coumarin and musk ambrette. One major disadvantage is that the procedure is time-consuming with six induction exposures; additional work might demonstrate that fewer exposures will yield the same results. The procedure is very stressful on the animals because of the injection of adjuvant and the multiple skin strippings and depilations. As with any assay involving the intradermal injection of adjuvant, there is often a problem with using the results of the irritation screen in naive animals to accurately predict the results that will be seen in the sham controls at the challenge. If the material being tested is a nonirritant or if one selects a concentration of an irritant which is far below the irritating concentration, then the screen does an adequate job of predicting the background irritation level in the challenge controls. However, if a slightly irritating concentration of an irritant is used, then the screen often underpredicts the irritation response and a high background level of irritation is observed at the challenge in the sham controls. The interpretation of the results of the challenge becomes difficult. The use of animals in the irritation screen which have had a prior injection of adjuvant might provide a viable alternative and reduce the number of times that rechallenges must be run because of high background levels of irritation. The Armstrong assay was designed to evaluate materials for their photoactivated sensitization potential and not their potential to be nonphotoactivated dermal sensitizers. At this time, there is no background data which will allow for properly positioning results of the Armstrong assay with regard to human risk if the assay indicates that a test material is a sensitizer or that a material is both a sensitizer and a photoallergen. Thus, it is highly recommended that a "standard" sensitization assay which can be related to humans be run before or in conjunction with the photosensitization assay. The use of a subjective grading system can be a source of significant verification.

Positive control—The recommended positive control is musk ambrett. TCSA will also give positive results, but this material has been reported to be an allergen without UV light activation. Animals are induced with a 10% w/v solution of musk ambrett in acetone and sham controls are patched with acetone alone. The Hill Top Chamber is used for all patchings. The challenge is also done in acetone. A note of warning: Both types of UVA lights yield the same results. Typical results are as follows:

Group	Challenge level	Incidence[a]	Severity 24 hr	Severity 48 hr	Maximum score 24 hr	Maximum score 48 hr
Test						
No UV light	0.01%	0 of 20	0.0	0.0	0	0
UV light		17 of 20	2.0	1.8	3	3
No UV light	0.01%	0 of 20	0.0	0.0	0	0
UV light		17 of 20	0.6	0.4	2	1
Control						
No UV light	0.01%	0 of 10	0.0	0.0	0	0
UV light		0 of 10	0.0	0.0	0	0
No UV light	0.01%	0 of 10	0.1	0.0	±	0
UV light		0 of 10	0.1	0.0	±	0

IN VITRO TEST SYSTEMS

There are *in vitro* assays for both phototoxicity and photosensitization.

The Daniels test for phototoxicity utilizes the yeast *Candida albicans* as a test species and has been in use for more than 20 years (Daniels, 1965). The measured endpoint is simply cell death. The test is simple to perform and cheap but does not reliably predict the phototoxicity of all classes of compounds (for example, sulfanilamide). Test systems utilizing bacteria have been suggested as alternatives over the past 10 years (Harter *et al.*, 1976; Ashwood-Smith *et al.*, 1980) for use in predicting the same endpoint. Recently, ICI has conducted studies on an *in vitro* phototoxicity assay which involves using three cultured cell lines: the A431 human epidermal cell line, a derived epidermal carcinoma, normal human epidermal keratinocytes, a primary cell line derived from cosmetic surgery, and the 3T3 Swiss mouse fibroblast cell line.

The protocol of this assay involves subculturing the particular cell type into microtiter tissue culture grade plates and incubating over a period of 24 hr. Following incubation, the cultures are exposed to the test compound at a concentration which has been predetermined as nontoxic. After a 4-hr exposure to the compound, the cell cultures are exposed to either UV A (320–400 nm) or UV AB (280–400 nm) radiation for varying lengths of time. The degree of enhanced toxicity effected by either UV A or UV AB radiation in the presence of the test compound relative to the control is assessed using the MTT assay.

MTT, abbreviated from 3-(4,5-dimethylthiazol-2-yl)2,5-diphenyltetrazolium bromide, undergoes a reduction reaction which is specific to mitochondrial dehydrogenases in viable cells. Work on validation of this test using 30 compounds of known phototoxic potential has shown a high degree of correlation between *in vitro* and *in vivo* results.

The area of development of *in vitro* photosensitization assays has been a very active one, as the review of McAuliffe *et al.* (1986) illustrates. Such tests have focused on being able to predict the photosensitizing potential of a compound and variously employ cultured mammalian cell lines, red blood cells, microorganisms, and biochemical reactions. McAuliffe's group has developed and proposed a test that measures the incorporation of tritiated thymidine into human peripheral blood mononuclear cells as a predictive test (Morison *et al.*, 1982). They claim to have internally validated the test using a battery of known photosensitizers. Bockstahler *et al.* (1982) have developed and proposed another *in vitro* test system which uses the responses of two *in vitro* mammalian virus–host cell systems to the photosensitizing chemicals proflavine sulfate and 8-MOP in the presence of light as a predictive system. They found that infectious simian virus 40 (SV40) could be induced from SV40–transformed hamster cells by treatment with proflavine plus visible light or 8-MOP plus near-UV radiation. The same photosensitizing treatments inactivated the capacity of monkey cells to support the growth of herpes simplex virus. SV40 induction and inactivation of host cell capacity for herpesvirus growth might be useful as screening systems for testing the photosensitizing potential of chemicals. Advantages and disadvantages were found to be associated with both of these test systems.

REFERENCES

Anderson, R. R., and Parrish, J. A. (1981). The optics of skin. *J. Invest. Dermatol.* 77, 13–19.

Ashwood-Smith, M. J., Poulton, G. A., Barker, M., and Midenberger, M. (1980). 5-Methoxypsoralen, an ingredient in several suntan preparations, has lethal mutagenic and clastogenic properties. *Nature (London)* 285, 407–409.

Bockstahler, L. E., Coohill, T. P., Lytle, C. D., Moore, S. P., Cantwell, J. M., and Schmidt, B. J. (1982). Tumor virus induction and host cell capacity inactivation: Possible *in vitro* test for photosensitizing chemicals. *JNCI* 69, 183–187.

Cole, C. A., Forbes, P. D., and Davis, R. E. (1984). Different biological effectiveness of blacklight fluorescent lamps available for therapy with psoralens plus ultraviolet A. *J. Am. Acad. Dermatol.* 11, 599.

Daniel, F. (1965). A simple microbiological method for demonstrating phototoxic compounds. *J. Invest. Dermatol.* 44, 259–263.

Epstein, S. (1939). Photoallergy and primary photosensitization to sulfanilamide. *J. Invest. Dermatol.* 2, 43–51.

Freund, E. (1916). Uber bisher noch nicht beschriebene kunstliche Hantvertarbungen. *Dermatol. Wochenscher.* 63, 931–936.

Gerberick, G. F., and Ryan, C. A. (1989). A predictive mouse ear swelling model for investigating topical phototoxicity. *Fd. Chem. Toxicol.* **12**, 813–819.

Harber, L. C., and Baer, R. L. (1972). Pathogenic mechanisms of drug-induced photosensitivity. *J. Invest. Dermatol.* **58**, 327.

Harber, L. C., and Shalita, A. R. (1975). The guinea pig as an effective model for the demonstration of immunologically-mediated contact photosensitivity. In *Animal Models in Dermatology* (H. Maibach, Ed.), pp. 90–102. Churchill Livingstone, Edinburgh, UK.

Harter, M. L., Felkner, I. C., and Song, P. S. (1976). Near-UV effects of 5,7-dimethoxycoumarin in *Bacillus subtilis. Photochem. Photobiol.* **24**, 491–493.

Horio, T., Kohachi, K., Ogawa, A., Inoue, T., and Ishihara, M. (1995). Evaluation of photosensitizing ability of quinolones in guinea pigs. *Drugs* **49**(Suppl. 2), 283–285.

Ichikawa, H., Armstrong, R. B., and Harber, L. C. (1981). Photoallergic contact dermatitis in guinea pigs: Improve induction technique using Freund's complete adjuvant. *J. Invest. Dermatol.* **76**, 498–501.

Lambert, L., Warmer, W., and Kornhauser, A. (1996). Animal models for phototoxicity testing. *Toxicol. Methods* **2**, 99–114.

Lovell, W. W., and Sanders, D. J. (1992). Phototoxicity testing in guinea pigs. *Fd. Chem. Toxicol.* **30**, 155–160.

Lowe, N. J. (1986). Cutaneous phototoxicity reactions. *Br. J. Dermatol.* **115**(Suppl. 31), 86–92.

Marks, R., Gabriel, K. L., Hershman, R. J., and Affrime, A. (1986). The rabbit ear as an animal model for phototoxicity and photobiology studies. *J. Am. College Toxicol.* **5**(6), 606.

Marzulli, F. M., and Maibach, H. I. (1970). Perfume phototoxicity. *J. Soc. Cosmet. Chem.* **21**, 685–715.

McAuliffe, D. J., Hasan, T., Parrish, J. A., and Kochevar, I. E. (1986). Determination of photosensitivity by an *in vitro* assay as an alternative to animal testing. In *In Vitro Toxicology* (A. M. Goldberg, Ed.), pp. 30–41. Liebert, New York.

Morison, W. L., McAuliffe, D. J., Parrish, J. A., and Bloch, K. J. (1982). *In vitro* assay for phototoxic chemicals. *J. Invest. Dermatol.* **78**, 460–463.

Nilsson, R., Maurer, T., and Redmond, N. (1993). A standard protocol for phototoxicity testing: Results from an interlaboratory study. *Contact Dermatitis* **28**, 285–290.

Oppenheim, M. (1932). Dermatite bullense striee consective aux fains de soleil les pues (dermatitis bullosa striata pratensis). *Ann. Dermatol. Syph.* **3**, 1–7.

Pathak, M. A. (1967). Photobiology of melanogenesis: Biophysical aspects. In *Advances in Biology of Skin, Vol. 8, The Pigmentary System* (W. Montagna and F. Hu, Eds.), pp. 400–419. Pergamon, New York.

Schwartz, K., and Speck, M. (1957). Experimentalle Untersuchungen zur Frage der Photoallergie der Sulfonamide. *Dermatologica* **114**, 232–243.

CHAPTER 7

Lethality Testing

Lethality tests are designed to determine the dosages that cause death in the model species of choice. It is acute toxicity testing with death as the single endpoint, and no other variables are examined or other data collected. This practice of using such narrowly defined protocols has come under criticism as being wasteful of resources, from a practical point of view, and immoral, from an animal rights point of view. These issues have been extensively examined in a variety of different forums and need not be revisited here (Rowan, 1981; Zbinden and Flury-Roversi, 1981; Zbinden, 1986; Sperling, 1976). We agree that there is considerably more to defining an acute toxicity profile than determining the median lethal dosage (LD_{50}) and that there are only uncommon situations in which solely an LD_{50} is of scientific value. Even in these situations, a so-called "precise" LD_{50} is not warranted. There are two general situations in which lethality is of prime concern; in dose range-finding studies and in studies performed primarily for regulatory hazard classification. There are occasions, however, when lethality data are needed for narrowly defined regulatory or labeling purposes. Substances may be legally classified as poisons on the basis of acute lethality data (Table 26). As of this writing, the Environmental

TABLE 26 Classification of Chemical Hazards[a]

| Commonly used term | Single oral dose, rats LD_{50} | Routes of administration | | Probable lethal dose for man |
		Inhalation 4 hr vapor exposure mortality 2/6–4/6 rats (ppm)	Single application to skin of rabbits LD_{50}	
Extremely toxic	1 mg or less/kg	10	5 mg or less/kg	A taste, a drop, 1 grain
Highly toxic	1–50 mg/kg[b]	10–100	5–43 mg/kg	1 teaspoonful (4 ml)
Moderately toxic	50–500 mg/kg	100–1000	44–340 mg/kg	1 ounce (30 gm)
Slightly toxic	0.5–5 g/kg	1,000–10,000	0.35–2.81 g/kg	1 pint (250 gm)
Practically g/kg quart or non-toxic	5–15 g/kg	10,000–100,000	22.6 or more g/kg	>1 quart or >1 liter

[a]From Deichemann and Gerarde (1966).
[b]By law, those materials with oral LD_{50}'s of 50 mg/kg or less in rats are classified as class B poisons and must be labeled "Poison." Class A poisons are defined not by testing, but rather by inclusion on a regulatorily mandated list (CFR 173, Section 173.326):

S 173.326 Poison A.

(a) For the purpose of Parts 170–189 of this subchapter extremely dangerous poison. Class A are poisonous gases or liquids of such nature that a very small amount of the gas, or vapor of the liquid, mixed with air is dangerous to life. This class includes the following:

(1) Bromactone.
(2) Cyanogen.
(3) Cyanogen chloride containing less than 0.9 percent water.
(4) Diphosgene.
(5) Ethyldichlorarsine.
(6) Hydrocyanic acid (see Note 1 of this paragraph).
(7) [Reserved]
(8) Methyldichlorarsine.
(9) [Reserved]
(10) Nitrogen peroxide (tetroxide).
(11) [Reserved]
(12) Phosgene (diphosgene).
(13) Nitrogen tetroxide–nitric oxide mixtures containing up to 33.2 percent weight nitric oxide.

NOTE 1: Diluted solutions of hydrocyanic acid of not exceeding 5 percent strength are classed as poisonous articles. Class B (see S 173–343).

(b) Poisonous gases or liquids, Class A as defined in paragraph (a) of this section, except as provided in S 173.331, must not be offered for transportation by rail express. (29 FR 18753, Dec. 29, 1964. Redesignated at 32 FR 5606, Apr. 5, 1967, and amended by Amdt. 173–94, 41 FR 16081, Apr. 15, 1976; Amdt. 173–94A, 41 FR 40883, Sept. 20, 1976).

TABLE 27   EPA Hazard Classification

Study	Toxicity categories[a]			
	Category I	Category II	Category III	Category IV
Acute oral	Up to and including 50 mg/kg	>50–500 mg/kg	>500–5000 mg/kg	>5000 mg/kg
Acute dermal	Up to and including 200 mg/kg	>200–2000 mg/kg	>2000–5000 mg/kg	>5000 mg/kg
Acute inhalation	Up to and including 0.05 mg/liter	>0.05–0.5 mg/liter	>0.5–2 mg/liter	>2 mg/liter

[a]Based on median lethal dose (LD_{50}). Each acute toxicity study is assigned a toxicity category (I–IV) for precautionary labeling.

Protection Agency (EPA) is in the process of harmonizing the guideline for the Office of Prevention, Pesticides and Toxic Substances (EPA, 1996) so that one set of guidelines will be applicable to both TUSCA and FIFRA. While this background document discusses ways to minimize animal usage, it is clear that lethality is still the primary endpoint for hazard categorization (see Table 27). Clearly, the dosages which cause death are legitimate regulatory concerns for chemicals in commerce. In other cases, preliminary lethality data are required to plan a more extensive definitive study. Protocol designs which gather more of the extensive data necessary for profiling acute systemic toxicity are similar in design to lethality tests and are considered in detail in Chapter 9.

HISTORICAL PERSPECTIVE

In general, toxicological research can be divided into two broad areas: descriptive and mechanistic. Descriptive research is that which is conducted to empirically describe or characterize the properties of a chemical. Toxicity testing is a descriptive exercise and may be defined as the formalized process of exposing animals to a hitherto unknown or uncharacterized chemical for the purposes of characterizing the potentially harmful effects of that chemical. Such a definition must encompass lethality testing of some sort. Like all toxicity testing, it is assumed that the findings in animals will have some predictive value in determining the possible responses of human beings. The issue of interspecies extrapolation is discussed in detail in Chapter 12.

The history of lethality testing is as old as the history of toxicology. As reviewed by Decker (1987) and Bruce and Doull (1986), the history of toxicology prior to the modern era was essentially the history of the art of poisoning. The early practitioners of this art were not interested in safety issues. Their primary concern was to find substances, preferably with no taste or smell, that would cause acute death. In that less enlightened period of human history, slaves and peasant children, rather than animals, were often the experimental models of choice. In Western civilization, the use of experimental animals in biological research started during the 18th century. Clearly, because of the work of Pasteur, Ehrlich, and others, the practice was well entrenched by the beginning of the 20th century. In a more narrow sense, it is less clear when animals were first used for toxicity testing, in general, or lethality testing, in particular. An early example of toxicity testing occurred in 1774 when Priestely exposed a mouse in a bell jar to newly discovered oxygen. Little did the good reverend suspect that he was helping to pioneer two modern lines of inquiry—first, the use of animals in defining biological activity, and, second, the study of oxygen toxicity. Orfilia, considered by some to be the father of modern toxicology, published experimental lethality data on cats in the early 1800s. By the middle of that century, Magendie and Bernard characterized the neuromuscular effects of cuarie. The work of these early toxicologists was largely mechanistic in that it was dedicated, for example, to determining why cuarie is lethal. Little thought was given in that period to formalized, descriptive protocols for assessing toxicity or safety in animals. Interestingly, both Orfilia and Magendie were criticized for using animals in their research (Decker, 1987). Hence, the debate over the use of animals in toxicologic research is hardly a new one.

In the early debates in the U.S. Congress on the Pure Food and Drug Act (passed in 1906), there was little mention of experimental animals. When Harvey Wiley, chief of the Bureau of Chemistry, Department of Agriculture, and driving force in the enactment of this early law, did his pioneering work (started in 1904) on the effects of various food preservatives on health, he did so using only human subjects and with no prior experiments in animals (Anderson, 1958). Hence, in one of those strange ironies of history, work that led to the establishment of the (U.S.) Food and Drug Administration (FDA) would probably not have been permitted under the current guidelines of the agency. Wiley's studies were not double-blinded, so it is also doubtful that his conclusions would have been accepted by the present agency or the modern scientific community.

When did modern Western society become concerned with lethality testing? For what reasons were protocols developed for describing lethality in animals in quantitative terms for the purposes of making scientific, regulatory, or marketing decisions? Interestingly, in this age of genetic engineering, few people realize that biologically derived materials were the subject of regulations well before the passage of the Pure Food and Drug Act in 1906. In 1901, a diphtheria epidemic broke out in St. Louis because of improperly manufactured antidiptheria toxin. In response to the resulting public outcry, Congress passed the Virus Act of 1902 (Pendergrast, 1984). It regulated all viruses, serums, toxins, antitoxins, and other such products sold for the prevention or cure of disease in man. Among other things, the bill eventually established consistent potency criteria. In fact, by World War II the FDA was requiring batch-to-batch certification and release for biologicals, a policy that remains in effect for certain drugs. Hence, the earliest lethality testing was for the purpose of establishing consistent potencies of biologicals, such as diptheria toxin, and not for evaluating synthetic chemicals.

One of the earliest publications discussing lethality testing (Sudmersen and Glenny, 1910) was an investigation into the lethality of diptheria toxin in guinea pigs. The Sudmersen and Glenny paper describes lethality empirically in terms of percentage of dead animals at each dosage because methods for calculating lethality curves and the median lethal dosage had not yet been developed. The authors reported that lethal response to a given dosage of toxin varied with time of the year. Hence, years before the term LD_{50} came into parlance, supposedly as an exact indicator of toxicity, data had been published attesting to the volatility and imprecision of this calculated parameter.

Because the first use of lethality testing was in describing potency of biologicals, it only makes sense that the same methods were soon applied to extracted botanicals. [Note: There is no doubt that both the Germans and English tested in animals the various poison gases employed during World War I. Little of this work, however, appears to have been published in the open scientific literature, though portions of it have recently been made public (see Harris and Paxman, 1982, for example).] In 1926, deLind van Wijngaarden published on the lethality of digitalis extracts. Interestingly, he did not plot his data as mortality vs dose. He delivered his extracts intravenously and titrated the dosage until he achieved complete heart stoppage. He was thus able to determine the precise lethal dosage for each animal, and noted that these followed a bell-shaped or Gaussian distribution. His experiments took 5 years and used more than 500 cats, an effort that would have been excessive and expensive by today's standards. However, he did conclude that no more than 9 cats would normally be required to "calibrate" an extract of digitalis. Trevan (1927), in a pivotal paper, described the lethality of stropanthin, cocaine, and insulin. Modern reviews have focused a great deal of attention on the large number of frogs used by Trevan. Most of the data he discussed, however, were derived from experiments in mice using cocaine or insulin. We suspect that so little attention was given to this aspect of Trevan's paper, even though it comprised the major portions of his work (which ran 31 pages and contained 11 figures and six tables of data), because it has never been replicated. For some of the lethality curves reported by Trevan, well over 900 mice were dosed. Again, such efforts would be excessive and expensive by today's standards but were necessitated, in part, by the less rigorous method of deriving lethality curves and calculating the median lethal dosage (LD_{50}). Modern methods of data transformation and statistical analysis were, at that time, still in their infancy. He also recognized that it was not necessary to describe an entire dosage–response curve in order to calculate an LD_{50}. He, in fact, recommended that lethality determinations start with small groups of 2 or 3 animals each and that larger groups be used for confirmatory purposes.

Behrens (1929) confirmed the observations of both deLind van Wijngaarden and Trevan. It is clear, from his article, that the use of animals for standardizing digitalis extracts was accepted to the point of being incorporated into the German and Dutch pharmacopoeias. The objective of his paper was to compare the cat and frog methods and develop a basis for using fewer animals. He concluded that the frog method was superior and that no more than 44 frogs needed to be used, which was considerably less than the 100–200 frogs prescribed in the German pharmacopoeia of that period. Interestingly, these early papers are often criticized with regard to the numbers of animals used, but the objectives and conclusions are often ignored.

Both Trevan and Behrens noted that when the percentage of animals that died at specific dosages was plotted against the logarithm of the dosage, the resulting curve (the lethal dosage curve) had a sigmoidal shape slope and range that was "characteristic" for the species and the test substance. Shackell (1925) first pointed out that such curves are integrated or cumulative frequency curves (or ogives) and coined the term "dose respond ogive" (curve). Trevan noted that these curves owe their shape to the fact that different individual animals require different quantities of poison for death to occur. It was also Trevan who identified the midpoint on this curve as being the dosage that would kill 50% of the animals exposed. He designated that point as the median lethal dose, or LD_{50}, and, thus, is widely credited with having developed the classical LD_{50}. Trevan and Behrans essentially read the LD_{50} directly from their mortality dose–response curves.

Lethality testing of biologicals and botanicals was essentially a response to governmental regulation. It was only natural that similar methods would be applied to synthetic chemicals. Major chemical companies started establishing toxicity or industrial health laboratories during the 1930s; the lethality testing of synthetic chemicals was established by the 1930s. However, there were no regulatory requirements for such tests. In fact, there was no premarketing toxicity testing of synthetic chemicals required at all. In 1937, an elixir of sulfanilamide dissolved in ethylene glycol was introduced into the marketplace. More than 100 people died as a result of ethylene glycol toxicity. The public response to this tragedy helped prompt Congress to pass the Federal Food, Drug, and Cosmetic Act of 1938 (Pendergrast, 1984). It was this law that mandated the premarket testing of drugs for safety in experimental animals. By the mid-1940s, most chemical and pharmaceutical companies were routinely testing new chemicals for lethality (at G. D. Searle, records for lethality testing extend back to 1942). In fact, until the 1960s, preclinical or premarketing toxicity data packages normally consisted of little more than acute lethality data. New laws, increased scientific sophistication, and greater societal concern over sublethal chronic toxicity have led to more extensive and expensive preclinical or premarketing toxicity testing packages, where acute lethality is a small, but still real, concern.

The protocols used to assess lethality have changed considerably since the 1920s. While the principles originally described by Trevan have never been questioned, the methods for calculating the LD_{50} have become more sophisticated and the need for the high degree of precision has been questioned. The practical result is that in using modern protocols, relatively few animals are required to obtain sufficient lethality data to meet most purposes.

PROTOCOL DESIGNS

General Considerations

Whatever type of experimental protocol one chooses to use in a lethality test, there are certain principles and criteria that should be universally applied. These principles are especially relevant in studies in which small numbers of animals will be used.

First, a wide variety of intrinsic and extrinsic factors can influence the outcome of a lethality test. These included species, strain or substrain, age, weight, and sex of the animals, husbandry practices (i.e., type of bedding, cage population, etc.), environmental conditions, feed and water quality, nutritional state, volume and vehicles of test substance delivery, etc. These have been discussed ad nauseum by a variety of authors (Morrison *et al.*, 1968; Balazs, 1976; Auletta, 1988) and are discussed in Chapters 11 and 12. The point to be made here is that the criteria for all these factors should be specified in detail in the protocol and strict adherence to the protocol observed. Otherwise, intrastudy comparisons are invalid. Small differences in protocols can cause large differences in the LD_{50} and are probably the major causes of the considerable laboratory-to-laboratory variation in the LD_{50}'s (Lorke, 1983).

Second, because the animals will generally receive a single exposure, great care must be given to the preparation and delivery of the test articles. In a chronic study, occasional miscalculations or misdelivery of the dosage will not generally greatly effect study outcome, but will clearly have a greater effect on the conclusions of a lethality screen. One should always include appropriate safeguards. We routinely triple check dosage calculations, do up-front homogeneity and concentration validation of the mixing procedures, and mix only in calibrated and precise glassware (i.e., volumetric rather than Erlenmeyer flasks).

Third, one must make sure that all animals are successfully dosed, and that accidental deaths are identified as such. In acute rodent studies, we routinely assign spare animals to a dosing group. Permanent numbers are not assigned until we are certain that the dose has been successfully delivered (i.e., "Was the supposedly ip dose accidentally delivered iv?," "Was there reflux from the site?," etc.). Spare animals not dosed are returned to the pool of animals available for the study. Animals found dead should be examined for evidence of accidental trauma. For example, it is not uncommon for a rat to suddenly move while being gavaged. This may result in a torn esophagus that may take a day or two to become evident. Depending on administration route, one must pay close attention to dosing techniques and the volume limitations imposed by these techniques. For example, 20 ml/kg is the maximum volume that should be given po to a rodent. These considerations be covered in detail in Chapter 10. Deaths that are clearly accidental should not be considered in the final conclusions.

Fourth, lethality protocols, by the nature of the question they address, do not specify all dosages. This can sometimes result in a study in which absurdly high dosages are administered. Hence, all protocols should clearly state what the ceiling or limit dosage will be and the reasons for selection.

CLASSICAL (TRADITIONAL) DESIGNS

The classical or traditional methods of determining the lethality of a substance have been established since the 1920s. In discussing this type of study design, it is assumed that what is desired is an LD_{50} and the slope of the lethality curve. In general, these are only necessary for meeting specific regulatory guidelines. If less precise information will suffice (which is generally the case), other protocols can be used and these are described in sections which follow. Briefly, this type of protocol species that animals (of the same species/strain, sex, and age) be divided into groups. All the animals in a specified group receive the same dosage. Different groups are treated at different dosages. All animals are treated by the same route. The animals are then held and observed for a set and consistent period of time—usually 14 days. Different regulatory agencies have somewhat different protocol requirements; these are summarized in Tables 28A, 28B, 29A, and 29B.

Mortality in each group is calculated on the basis of the number of animals that die during the observation period and is normally presented in percentage terms: (number dead/number dosed) $\times$ 100. If mortality at each dosage is plotted against dosages, a sigmoidal dose–response curve is obtained. The LD_{50}

TABLE 28A Summary of Regulatory Testing Guidelines—Acute Dermal Toxicity Tests

	FHSA	DOT	TSCA	FIFRA
	Test animals			
Species	Rabbit	Rabbit	Rat, rabbit, or guinea pig[a]	Rat, rabbit, or guinea pig[a]
Age	NS	NS	Young adult	Adult
Weight				
Rat	NA	NA	200–300 g	200–300 g
Rabbit	2.3–3 kg	NS	2–3 kg	2–3 kg
Guinea pig	NA	NA	350–450 g	350–450 g
	Limit test			
Amount (mg/kg)	2000[b]	200[c]	2000	At least 200
Acceptable mortality	Less than half	None	None	None
Exposure period[d]	24 hr	24 hr	24 hr	24 hr
	LD_{50} determination			
Minimum no. animals per group	10	10	10[e]	10[e]
No. of groups	NA	NA	3	At least 3
Vehicle control	NR	NR	Yes[f]	No[g]
	Observations			
Observation period	14 Days	48 hr	14 Days[h]	14 Days[h]
Body weight	NS	NS	Weekly[i]	Weekly[i]
Necropsy	NR	NR	Yes	Optional[j]
Histopathology	NR	NR	Optional[k,l]	NS

Note: NS, not specified; NR, not required; NA, not applicable.
[a]Rabbit is preferred.
[b]To be considered not "toxic."
[c]To define class B pioson. Class A poisons defined by inclusion on list (see Table 26).
[d]In general, all guidelines for acute dermal toxicity require 24-hr exposure under occluded conditions.
[e]5 males and 5 females.
[f]Required unless historical data are available to determine acute toxicity of vehicle.
[g]The toxic characteristics of the vehicle should be known.
[h]14 days in minimum duration; study may be extended if delayed death (e.g., more than 24 hr postdosing) occurs.
[i]Body weights pretest, weekly, and at death.
[j]Should be considered where indicated.
[k]Should be considered for animals surviving more than 24 hr.
[l]Clinical chemistry studies should also be considered.

is simply the dosage, either observed or calculated, that yields 50% mortality. Seldom are such curves reported as such because the LD_{50} is difficult to read off a curvilinear plot and the small number of dosages normally used make drawing an accurate lethal dosage curve difficult. It is most common to probit transform the data to obtain a rectilinear plot.

TABLE 28B Summary of Regulatory Testing Guidelines—Acute Dermal Toxicity Tests

	OECD/EC	J MAFF	FDA[a]	IRLG
		Test animals		
Species	Rat, rabbit, or guinea pig	One mammalian species, (rat, rabbit, guinea pig, etc.)	Two species by using the clinical formulation, plus 24-hr exposure by dermal route in one species	Rat, rabbit, or guinea pig[b]
Age	Adult	Adult	NS	Young adult
Weight				
Rat	200–300 g	200–300 g	NS	200–300 g
Rabbit	2–3 kg	2–3 kg	NS	2–3 kg
Guinea kpig	350–450 g	350–450 g	NS	350–450 g
Exposure period	24 hr	24 hr	24 hr	24 hr
		Limit test		
Amount (mg/kg)	2000	2000	NA	$\geq$2000 or $\geq$2 ml/kg
Acceptable mortality	None	None	NA	None
		LD_{50} determination		
Minimum no. animals per group	10[c,d]	10[c]	NS	10[c,d]
No. or group	At least 3	At least 3	NS	At least 3
Vehicle control	No[e]	No[e]	NS	NS[e]
		Observation		
Observation period	14 Days[f]	14 Days[f]	Dermal, 14 days	14 Days[f]
Body weight	Weekly[g]	Weekly[g]	NS	Weekly[g]
Necropsy	Optional[h]	Optional[h]	NS	Yes—animals that die; others optional
Histopathology	Optional[i]	Optional[i]	NS	Optional for gross lesions

Note. NS, not specified; NA, not applicable.

[a]When an NDA is filed it should include acute toxicity data by the intended route of administration and also by the oral route. This is to provide information on the situation in which overdose or accidental ingestion has occurred.

[b]Rabbit is preferred.

[c]5 males and 5 females.

[d]Smaller numbers may be used, especially in the case of the rabbit.

[e]The toxic characteristics of the vehicle should be known.

[f]14 Days is minimum duration; study may be extended if delayed death (e.g., more than 24-hr postdosing) occurs.

[g]Body weights pretest, weekly, and at death.

[h]Should be considered where indicated.

[i]Should be considered for animals surviving for more than 24 hr.

TABLE 29A   Summary of Regulatory Testing Guidelines—Acute Oral Toxicity Tests

	FHSA	DOT	TSCA	FIFRA
Test animals				
Species	Rat	Rat	Rat/mouse[a]	Rat
Age	NS	NS	Young	Young adult
Weight	200–300 g	200–300 g	NS[b]	NS[b]
Limit test				
Amount (mg/kg)	5000[c]	50[c,d]	5000	5000
Acceptable mortality	Less than half	Less than half	None	None
LD_{50} determination				
Minimum no. animals per group	10	10	10[e]	10[e]
No. of groups	NA	NA	3	At least 3
Vehicle control	NR	NR	Yes[f]	No[g]
Observations				
Observation period	14 Days	48 hr	14 Days[h]	14 Days[h]
Body weight	NS	NS	Weekly[i]	Weekly[i]
Necropsy	NR	NR	Yes	Optional[j]
Histopathology	NR	NR	Optional[k,l]	NS

Note. NS, not specified; NR, not required; NA, not applicable.
[a] Preferred species (several mammalian species acceptable).
[b] Weight not specified, but weight variation not to exceed ± 20% of the mean weight for each sex.
[c] See Table 26.
[d] To define class B poison. Class A poisons are defined by inclusion on list.
[e] Smaller numbers may be used, especially in the case of the rabbit.
[f] Required unless historical data are available to determine acute toxicity of vehicle.
[g] The toxic characteristics of the vehicle should be known.
[h] 14 days is minimum duration; study may be extended if delayed lethality (e.g., death more than 24 hr postdosing) occurs.
[i] Body weights pretest, weekly, and at death.
[j] Should be considered where indicated.
[k] Should be considered for animals surviving more than 24 hr.
[l] Clinical chemistry studies should also be considered.

Traditionally, because of FDA and foreign regulatory guidelines, protocols have frequently been designed as batteries, including both sexes of two species (generally rats and mice) and two routes of administration. At least one route must be the intended or the most probable human exposure route. Hence, such protocols generally result in the generation of eight lethal dosage curves (1/route/sex/species). In the drug industry (where this approach is common), the two routes are generally oral and ip for an oral drug and oral and iv for intravenous. While such extensive data packages may still be required for regulatory purposes, scientifically they are of little value. First, there is no reason to assume that either the rat or the mouse is the better predictor for

TABLE 29B Summary of Regulatory Testing Guidelines—Acute Oral Toxicity Tests

	OECD/EC	J MAFF	FDA	IRLG
		Test animals		
Species	Rat/mouse[a]	Rat plus one other	3 (at least 1 a nonrodent)	Rat[a]
Age	Young adult	Young adult	NS	NS
Weight	NS[b]	NS	NS	Mean ± 20%
		Limit test		
Amount (mg/kg)	5000	5000	NA	≧5000
Acceptable mortality	None	None	NA	None
		LD$_{50}$ determination		
Minimum no. animals per group	10[c]	10[c]	NS[d]	10[c]
No. of group	At least 3	5	NS	At least 3, prefer 4
Vehicle control	No[e]	NS[a]	NS	NR
		Dosing solution		
Volume	Constant	NS	NS	Constant if possible. Aqueous solutions ≦20; others ≦10 m/kg
Concentration	Variable	NS	NS	Variable
		Observations		
Observation period	14 Days[f]	14 Days[f]	≧14 Days	14 Days[f]
Body weight	Weekly[g]	Weekly[g]	NS	Weekly
Necropsy	Optional[h]	Optional[h]	Nonrodents that die	Yes—animals that die; others optional
Hispathology	Optional[i]	Optional[i]	NS	Optional for gross lesions

Note. NS, not specified; NR, not required; NA, not applicable.
[a]Rat is preferred.
[b]Weight not specified, but weight variation not to exceed ≧20% of the mean weight for each sex.
[c]5 males and 5 females.
[d]No longer required (FDA, 1996).
[e]The toxic characteristics of the vehicle should be known.
[f]14 days is minimum duration; study may be extended if delayed lethality (e.g., death more than 24 hr postdosing) occurs.
[g]Body weights pretest, weekly, and at death.
[h]Should be considered where indicated.
[i]Should be considered for animals surviving more than 24 hr.

man than the other—or for each other (see Table 30). The only general correlation between the rat and mouse LD$_{50}$ is that when one is high, so is the other. It has been our experience that having the lethality data from two different rodents, rather than single species, does not generally change one's conclusions nor improve one's understanding of the toxicity of a drug or chemical or the potential hazard to man. We recommend that a simple prelimi-

TABLE 30   Sample Data Set: Comparison of Lethality of
Various Drugs in Rats vs Mice

Drug	LD_{50} (mg/kg) Rat	Mouse	LD_{50} ratio (rat/mouse)
SC–37407	310	72	4.31
SC–36602	3200	980	3.26
SC–27166	569	247	2.30
SC–31828	880	450	1.96
SC–32840	4700	2900	1.62
SC–29169	890	650	1.37
SC–35135	420	440	0.95
SC–38394	2200	4700	0.47

Note. Drugs were given orally by gavage to adult animals, same sex for each comparison. The results are from previously unpublished studies on unmarketed drugs of G. D. Searle & Co.

nary screen be performed to pick out the most sensitive species, and a rigorous protocol applied only to that species. The two-route requirement was developed primarily in order to gain information about the bioavailability of the test substance for pharmaceuticals. Certainly more sophisticated and scientific methods of using animals now exist to gather such information. In fact, some investigators often divide the oral LD_{50} by the parenteral LD_{50} to calculate the potency index (for example, see Table 31). The utility of this number in making safety considerations is in doubt. Basically, it simply formalizes what is commonly known and accepted—that route changes toxicity. As a gross rule of thumb, the iv LD_{50} will be 10% of that of the oral, and the ip will be roughly 30% of oral. The reasons for these differences are discussed in Chapter 10. Lethality assessment should generally be limited to the intended or most likely route (or routes, when appropriate) of human exposure.

Number and Size of Dosage Groups

As amply discussed, the precision with which the curves are described will depend on the number of groups (hence, dosages) and the number of animals in each group. Between 1940 and 1980, the standard was to use from four to six dosages with 10 animals per dosage. Some regulatory guidelines even called for achieving 95% confidence limits within ±10% of the calculated value. The current emphasis is on limiting the number of animals used for lethality testing, particularly with recognition of the limited value of such "precise" data. Hence, the number and size of dosage groups will depend, to an extent, on the methods

TABLE 31   Sample Data Set: Differences in Lethality Due to
Route of Administration

Drug	LD$_{50}$ (mg/kg)		Potency ratio
	Oral	ip	po/ip
SC–27166	300	110	2.7
SC–32840	4700	1600	2.9
SC–38394	2200	1000	2.2
SC–25469	1200[a]	880	1.4[a]
SC–36250	5000[a]	1100	4.5[a]
	Oral	iv	po/iv
SC–31828	880	20	44
SC–35135	420	25	17
SC–37407	310	21	15
SC–34871	2400[a]	67	36
SC–36602	3200	79	41

[a]Adult male rats, where indicated (>), higher dosages were not
given because of the physical characteristics of the drug or because
a limit dosage had been achieved.

of statistical analysis. The classic statistical methods for analyzing lethality data (or, indeed, any quantal dosage response data) were published between 1930 and 1960 and have been extensively reviewed by Armitage and Allen (1950) and Morrison et al. (1968). These will be discussed in greater detail in Chapter 11, but are mentioned here with regard to the demands these methods make on protocol design, i.e., specifically, the number of dosage groups, the spacing of the dosages, and the number of animals per dosage group. The probit and moving average methods are the most commonly used today. In general, all methods of calculation and computation are more precise if the designs are symmetrical (i.e., the dosages are evenly spaced and the group sizes are equal). The probit method first developed by Bliss (1935, 1937) and later refined by Finney (1971, 1985) is considered to be the most precise but requires at least two groups of partial responses (i.e., mortality greater than 0% but less than 100%). This may require dosing more than three groups until this criteria is met. It also does not deal effectively with groups that had either 0 or 100% lethality. (The most common correction for these is to substitute 0.1 for 0% and 99.7 for 100%.) The moving average method, first described by Thompson and Weil (1952), does not require partial responses and deals effectively with complete responses and, therefore, can produce an acceptable estimate of an LD$_{50}$ with as few as three groups of 3–5 animals each. This method requires that the dosages be separated by a constant geometric factors (e.g., 2, 4, and 8 mg/kg) and that groups be of equal size. Weil

(1952), and later Gad and Weil (1982, 1986), have published tables that allow for the easy calculation of the LD_{50} with $K = 3$ (four dosage groups). The LD_{50} for $K < 3$ can be easily calculated without the aid of tables. In addition, methods for estimating the confidence limits of this calculated LD_{50} have also been published (Gad and Weil, 1986). Traditionally, the moving average method has not been more extensively used because, while it yielded an estimate of the LD_{50}, it did not give the slope of the (probit transformed) lethality curve. However, Weil (1985) published a method for calculating a slope from the same data. Hence, an estimate of the LD_{50} and slope can be obtained from as few as three groups and 5 animals per group, providing at least one group shows a response less than 50% and another shows a response greater than 50%.

The Litchfield–Wilcoxon (Litchfield and Wilcoxon, 1949) method was once commonly used. It is certainly a valid method and poses no additional restrictions on study design than those imposed by the probit method. Modern handheld calculators and the ready availability of simple computer programs have made other methods more convenient to run. The Litchfield–Wilcoxon method has become a victim of technology. However, at least one software company has adopted the Litchfield for its acute toxicity protocol package.

The normit χ^2 developed by Berkson (1955), is also sometimes used. Like the probit method, the normit χ^2 does not absolutely require equally spaced dosages or equal group sizes, but does require at least one partial response. Hence, using the normit χ^2 method, fewer dosage groups may be needed than with the probit method. According to Waud (1972), the correction for including complete responses is better than that used for probit analysis but is still "tainted." His method supposedly deals adequately with complete responses but is extremely complex and, probably for this reason, is rarely used.

Karber (1931) published a simple method, which has been often described but rarely cited, for calculating an LD_{50}. It does not require that dosages be equally spaced, but widely divergent dosages will lead to a biased result. The method was originally described for groups of equal size, but groups of slightly different size can be used, providing that they do not differ by more than a few animals each. In this case, mean group size can be inserted into Karber's formula with little change in accuracy. The formula is very simple and one can calculate an acceptable estimate of the LD_{50} quickly with only a few arithmetic computations. This method, unlike those mentioned previously, does not allow for calculating the confidence limit or slope of the probit response curve. Hence, if these calculated parameters are not sought, this method allows one a bit more freedom in picking dosages.

While much has been written about the influence of gender on acute lethality, most authors now agree that there is seldom any substantial difference in the LD_{50} due to sex (DePass *et al.*, 1984). In those instances in which there is a sex-related difference, females tend to be more sensitive than males (see Chapter 12). If one is willing to accept this amount of uncertainty, only one sex needs to be tested. Alternatively, as few as two or three animals per sex per dosage can be used. Schutz and Fuchs (1982) have demonstrated that, by pooling sexes, there is seldom any substantial difference in the LD_{50} calculations with five per sex vs three per sex groups. If there are no substantial differences between sexes (i.e., 0% mortality for males and 100% for females at a dosage), the results from the sexes can provide a pooled LD_{50}. For most safety considerations, an LD_{50} derived on this basis will be acceptable and will result in the use of fewer animals.

Selection of Dosages

In setting the dosages, a few common-sense rules have to be applied. First, the intrinsic biological and chemical activity of the chemical must be considered. Zbinden and Flury-Roviers (1981) have documented several cases in which lethality was of no biological relevance. The oral lethality of tartaric acid, for example, was due to the caustic action of a high concentration of acid in the GI tract. In these instances, limit tests (discussed below) are more appropriate. Additionally, it is uncommon that a completely unknown chemical is tested. Factors such as known pharmacological profile, chemical or physical characteristics including molecular weight, particient coefficient, etc., and the toxicity of related chemicals should be considered. For example, it is likely that a polymeric, poorly soluble molecule will not be bioavailable and an initial dosage of 100 mg/kg is too low. A little homework will permit one to pick dosages with more confidence, and thereby save both time and resources.

Second, no method will yield a reliable LD_{50} if all dosages given caused 100% lethality. Therefore, one is best advised to pick widely spaced, rather than closely spaced, dosages. In general, the best dosage regimen includes one that will definitely produce close to 100% lethality, another that will produce marginal lethality, and one in between. If this pattern is obtained, adding more groups does not generally change the results. This point is illustrated by the data in Table 32. For two drugs, an LD_{50} of 300 mg/kg was obtained using six groups of 10 mice each. Essentially the same result is obtained if the second, fourth, and sixth groups are eliminated and not used in the calculations. Behrens (1929) noted this phenomenon almost 60 years ago.

Widely spaced dosages also decrease the likelihood of nonmonotonic data, where mortality does not necessarily increase with dosage (see Table 33). This can frequently occur when the test chemical has a shallow does–response curve and the group size is small (three or four animals.) While it is possible to calculate an LD_{50} from such data, the slope and confidence limits will not be very accurate. Nonmonotonic data can also occur if the lethality is indeed

TABLE 32   Sample Data Sets: LD_{50} Calculations Using Fewer Dosages[a]

SC–27166		Theophylline	
Dosage (mg/kg)	Mortality	Dosage (mg/kg)	Mortality
100	0/10	280	0/10
180	0/10	320	3/10
240	4/10	370	5/10
320	7/10	430	9/10
560	9/10	500	10/10
1000	10/10	670	10/10
$LD_{50} = 300$		$LD_{50} = 300$	
Using every other dosage			
100	0/10	280	0/10
240	4/10	370	5/10
560	9/10	500	10/10
$LD_{50} = 290$		$LD_{50} = 290$	

[a]Adult male mice; drugs given by gavage.

biphasic and there are a few documented occurrences of such cases. If one suspects that this is occurring, additional dosages should be examined. For safety considerations, only the first part of the curve, the lowest LD_{50}, is of importance.

Timing

The greatest precision in any lethality curve is obtained when the number of experimental variables is kept to a minimum. Hence, it is best if all the animals

TABLE 33   Sample Data Sets: Homogeneous versus Heterogeneous Data

Homogeneous (normotonic)		Heterogeneous (nonnormotonic)	
SC–31828 (adult rats, both sexes)		SC–38394 (adult male rats)	
Dosage (mg/kg)	Mortality	Dosage (mg/kg)	Mortality
300	0/20	620	0/10
600	1/20	1600	2/10
800	10/20	2100	8/10
1000	17/20	2800	5/10
		3700	8/10
		5000	8/10

used for determining a specific curve are dosed on the same day and, if possible, at the same time of day. This limits age-related and diurnal effects. If only a total of 15 animals are being dosed, this is not an impossible task for a single well-trained technician. However, if the test substance is of unknown lethality, it is not prudent to deliver all doses on the same day. Hence, it is not unusual for a single dosage group to be treated on the first day of an experiment and the dosages for the second and third groups to be adjusted up or down pending the results of the first group (see Fig. 25). Generally most acute deaths will occur within 24 hr of dosing. Delayed deaths (those occurring more than 24 hr after dosing) are relatively rare and generally restricted to the 72-hr period following dosing (Gad *et al.*, 1984; Bruce, 1985). Hence, generally, waiting for 24 hr between doses will yield sufficient data to choose the next dosage. For example, if all but one of the animals dosed in the first group die, there is no doubt that the next dosage should be adjusted downward considerably, whether or not the final animal eventually dies. All the dosing for a single curve can be completed in 3 days. If a day or chemical are being tested in traditional protocols with two species by two routes and separate sexes (eight curves), the two initial groups by a route can be treated on the first day of the dosing period and the second route initiated on the next day. Subsequent dosages can be adjusted on alternate days. This is a matter of individual

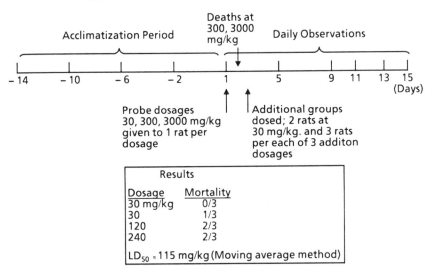

FIGURE 25   Line chart for the design and conduct of a typical dosage probe for lethality.

preference. Little real impact on the eventual result will occur if there is as much as 2 or 3 days between dosing sets. After that, however, the changing age of the animals may result in a change in sensitivity. As reviewed by Balazs (1976), for example, the ratios of the LD_{50}'s obtained in adult animals to those in neonates vary from 0.002 to 160. This is further illustrated by the sample data in Table 34. One can use longer observation periods between dosing days if separate animal orders are timed for delivery to ensure that all animals dosed are the "same" age. As a rule of thumb, the animals should not differ in age by more than 15%; hence, the younger the animals, the smaller the age window.

Summary

The classical lethality testing protocol calls for the definition of a lethality curve and the midpoint on this curve, the LD_{50}. The curve is defined by plotting the mortality against the logarithm of suitably spaced dosages. The number and size of the dosage groups dictate the precision of the curve and the LD_{50}. The probit method is considered the standard and is, in fact, dictated by certain regulations. In general, the method of calculation and analysis will impose certain restraints on the number of dosages studied. At least three are required. Three animals per dosage are the minimum required for acceptable results. The slope of the probit plot is considered by some to be an important parameter of toxicity. The moving average method will yield nearly an identical LD_{50}, can also yield an estimate of the slope of the probit curve, and can deal with complete responses and nonmonotonic data better than the probit method. Depending on the specific objectives of the study, there is generally no need to treat sexes separately or study more than one species.

DOSE PROBES

Dose probing protocols (see Fig. 25) are of value when one needs the information supplied by a traditional protocol but has no preliminary data

TABLE 34   Sample Data Set: Age-Related Changes in Lethality of SC–27166 in Rats

	Age	LD_{50} (95% fiducial limit)
Neonatal	1 Day	24 (18– 33)
Juvenile	21 Days	140 (120–160)
Adult	63–70 Days	260 (220–300)

Note. SC–27166 was given orally by gavage. The neonatal and juvenile rats were studied due to a specific regulatory concern about the potential use of this drug in neonates and children.

on which to choose dosages. In this protocol, one animal per dosage is dosed at each of three widely spaced dosages, where the top dosage is generally the maximum deliverable. The method works best if the dosages are separated by constant multiples, e.g., 3000, 300, and 30 mg/kg (a logarithmic progression). Subsequent dosages are selected on the basis of the results of these probe animals. If none of the animals die, the protocol defaults to a limit test (described below) and two more animals are dosed at the top dosage to confirm the limit.

If 1 or 2 animals die, then two additional dosages between the lethal and nonlethal dosages are chosen and 3 animals treated per dosage. Selection of these dosages is a matter of personal judgment. If, for example, one wishes to apply the moving average method of calculation, these subsequent dosages can be either even fractions of the top dosage or even multiples of low dosage. In either case, 2 or 3 animals are dosed at the initial dose and 3 or 4 animals at each of the two or three new dosages. The result should be three or four groups of 3 or 4 animals each, which should probably provide sufficient data for calculating the LD_{50} and the slope of the curve. The results from the two initial high dosages are not included in the calculations. In most cases, this design yields sufficient information and uses only up to 18 animals.

In a few instances, all the animals may die following the first-day probe. In that case, the probe activity continues on Day 2 with two more animals dosed at two more widely spaced lower dosages, i.e., 3 and 0.3 mg/kg. This could continue daily until a nonlethal dosage was identified. Unless one has grossly misestimated the toxicity of the test substance, it is unlikely that the probing process could take more than 3 days. Carrying our example into 3 days of dosing would have resulted in probing the 3 μg/kg to the 3 g/kg range and it is a rare chemical that is lethal at less than 3 μg/kg. Once a nonlethal dosage is identified, additional animals and/or dosages can be added, as discussed previously.

There are two disadvantages to dose probing studies. First, as with the up-and-down method, delayed deaths pose difficulties. Hence, all animals should be observed for at least 7 days after dosing. Second, if the follow-up dosages do not yield at least one partial response, the next decision point is ill-defined. Should more animals be dosed at some different dosage? The resulting data sets may be cumbersome and difficult to analyze by the moving average method. One should also have a backup method of analysis described in the protocol. Alternatively (and this is true regardless of protocol design), if no partial response dosage is identified, one can simply conclude that the LD_{50} is between two dosages, but the data do not permit the calculation of confidence limits of the LD_{50} or the slope of the curve. This can happen if the dosage response is fairly steep. If one absolutely needs a single number in order, for example, to fill out a DOT shipping document, then we recommend taking the conservative approach and using the highest identifiable dosage at which no lethality is observed.

Lorke (1983) has developed a similar protocol design. His probe (or dose ranging) experiment consists of 3 animals per dosage at 10, 100, and 1000 mg/kg. The results of the experiment dictate the dosages for the second round of dosing as shown in Table 34A. Animals were observed for 14 days postdosing. Lorke (1983) compared the results obtained when 1–5 animals were used per dosage group for the second test. He concluded that using only 1 animal per group gave unreliable results in only 7% of chemicals tested. Hence, the Lorke design can produce a reasonable estimate of the LD_{50} using 14 animals. Schutz and Fuchs (1982) have proposed a dose probing type of protocol that adequately deals with delayed deaths (Fig. 26). All animals are observed for 7 days before subsequent dosages are given. Dosing is initiated at two widely delivered dosages with 1 rat each. A third probe dosage is determined pending the outcome of the first two probes. A fourth may also be used. After that, groups of 3 or 4 animals are used at subsequent dosages, which will also include a repeat of a probe dose. The process generally requires four to six dosing periods and will result in a minimal data set for calculating an LD_{50}, three or four groups of 4 animals each with at least two groups having mortality greater than 0 but less than 100%.

The Schutz and Fuchs protocol will greatly reduce animal usage. It does require between 6 and 7 weeks to complete the test, as opposed to the 2–4 weeks needed to complete a conventional test. It would require that one order

TABLE 34A   Dosage Selection for the Lorke (1983) Dose Probing Protocol Design

10	100	1000	Dosages chosen for the second test			
0/3[a]	0/3	0/3		1600	2900	5000
0/3	0/3	1/3	600	1000[b]	1600	2900
0/3	0/3	2/3	200	400	800	1600
0/3	0/3	3/3	140	225	370	600
0/3	1/3	3/3	50	100[b]	200	400
0/3	2/3	3/3	20	40	80	160
0/3	3/3	3/3	15	25	40	60
1/3	3/3	3/3	5	10[b]	20	40
2/3	3/3	3/3	2	4	8	16
3/3	3/3	3/3	1	2	4	8

Doses (mg/kg): Result of the probe experiment — 10, 100, 1000.

[a]Number of animals which died/number of animals used.
[b]The result from the probe is inserted for these doses.

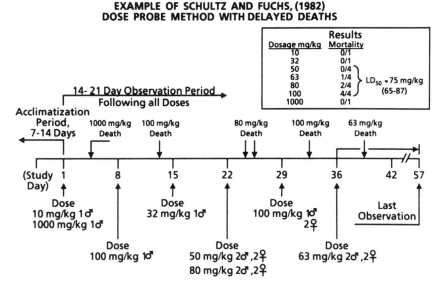

FIGURE 26   Line chart for the design and conduct of a Schultz and Fuchs (1982) style dose probe for lethality.

several small shipments of animals. However, because this method is not very labor-intensive, these problems can be overcome by running several tests in parallel.

THE UP-AND-DOWN METHOD

Using classical or traditional protocols, 15–30 animals per set may be required to calculate a single LD_{50}. This is because the method relies on the analysis of group responses. There are protocols which can provide for the estimation of the LD_{50} by analyzing the responses of individual animals. Deichemann and LeBlanc (1943) published an early method which provided an estimate of an LD_{50} using no more than 6 animals. All animals were dosed at the same time. The dosage range was defined as 1.5 × a multiplication factor (e.g., 1.0, 1.5, 2.2, 3.4, and 5.1 ml/kg). The approximate lethal dose (ALD), as they defined it, was the highest dose that did not kill the recipient animal. The resultant ALD differed from the LD_{50} (as calculated by the probit method from more complete data sets) by from −22 to 33%.

The Deichemann method was a little too approximate. Later, Dixon and

Wood (1948), followed by Brownlee *et al.* (1953), developed the method in which single animals were exposed per dosage, but subsequent dosages were adjusted up or down by some constant factor depending on the outcome of the previous dosage. The method (Fig. 27) has been developed more extensively by Bruce (1985). In this method, individual animals are dosed at different dosages on successive days. If an animal dies, the dosage for the next animal is decreased by a factor of 1.3. Conversely, if an animal lives, the next dosage is increased by a factor of 1.3. The process is continued until five animals have been dosed after reversal of the first observation. For example, if the first treated animal lives, an additional five animals are dosed, counting from the first death. The data are analyzed with the maximum likelihood methods SAS procedure NLIN (Bruce, 1985). Alternatively, one can use the tables developed by Dixon (1965). In general, only six to nine animals are required—unless, of course, the initial dosages are grossly high or low. When compared to the LD_{50} obtained by more classical protocols, excellent agreement is obtained with the up/down method (Bruce, 1985). As with classical protocols, sexes should be tested separately. However, as mentioned, a further reduction in animals can be effected if one is willing to accept that females are of the same or increased sensitivity as males.

There are three main disadvantages to using the up/down method. The first is regulatory, the second is procedural, and the third is scientific. First, many regulatory guidelines imply a requirement for the use of traditional protocols. Some also specify the method of calculation. Second, the sequential dosing

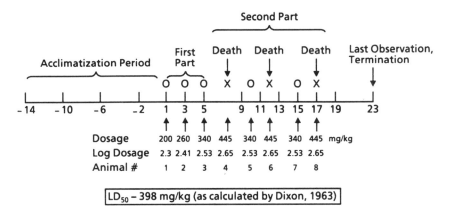

FIGURE 27 Line chart for the design and conduct of an up-and-down style lethality estimating test.

design is inappropriate for substances that cause delayed deaths. As reported by various authors (Gad et al., 1984; Bruce, 1985), such deaths (beyond 2 days' postdosing) are rare but not unknown. They are most prevalent when animals are dosed by the intraperitoneal route with a chemical that causes peritonitis. Death secondary to severe liver or gastrointestinal damage may also take more than 2 days to occur. To guard against possible spurious results, all animals should be maintained and observed for at least 7 days after dosing. If delayed deaths occur, the original data set must be corrected and the LD_{50} recalculated. A substantial number of delayed deaths could result in a data set from which an LD_{50} cannot be calculated, in which case the test should be rerun with longer observations between doses. Third, the up/down method produces a number, not a curve. Hence, it cannot be used in experiments in which changes in curve slope or shape are of importance.

PYRAMIDING STUDIES

Using this type of design (Fig. 28), one can obtain information about lethality with the minimum expenditure of animals. A minimum of two animals are

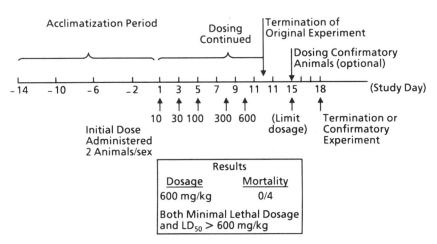

FIGURE 28 Line chart for the design and conduct of a pyramiding style systemic toxicity test (used for larger nonrodent species).

dosed throughout the study, usually on alternate days (e.g., Monday, Wednesday, and Friday) but the dosage increases at each session may be 1, 3, 10, 30, 100, 300, and 1000, and 3000 mg/kg, or 10, 20, 40, 80, 160, 320, 640, and 1280 mg/kg. One is literally stepping or pyramiding up the lethality–dosage curve. Dosing continues in this fashion until one or both animals die or until some practical upward limit is reached. For drugs, there is seldom any need to go higher than 1000 mg/kg for nonrodents and 3000 mg/kg for rodents. Because this design uses so few animals, it is commonly used for assessing lethality in nonrodent species. An exploratory study typically uses an animal of each sex. A study intended to support a regulatory submission will typically use two animals per sex.

There are three conclusions that can be reached on the basis of data from a pyramiding dosage study. First, if none of the animals die, then both the threshold, or minimum lethal dosage (MLD), and the LD_{50} are greater than the top or limit dosage. Second, if all the animals die at the same dosage, then both the MLD and the LD_{50} are reported as being between the last two dosages given. This is not uncommon and is an indication that the lethality curve has a steep slope. Third, one animal may die at one dosage, and remaining deaths may occur at a subsequent dosage. In this case, the MLD is reported as being between the lowest nonlethal dosage and the dosage at which the first death occurred, while the LD_{50} is reported as being between this latter dosage and the dosage at which the last animal dies. For nonrodents, this type of data is sufficient to support almost all regulatory submissions.

There are some disadvantages to the pyramiding dose protocol. First, it cannot produce a lethality curve or provide for the calculation of an LD_{50}. Second, this method cannot identify delayed deaths. If an animal, for example, dies 1 hr after the second dosage, one has no way of determining whether it was actually the second dosage or a delayed effect of the first. For this reason it is of little value to observe the animals for any more than a few days after the last dosage. Third, if the test article has an unusually long half-life, bioaccumulation can lead to an underestimation of the acute lethal dosage. On the other hand, pharmacological accommodation can lead to a spuriously high estimate of lethality. Depending on the importance of the finding, one may wish to confirm that the highest dosage administered was nonlethal by dosing two naive animals at the same dosage. Fortunately, the minimum 48-hr period between dosing sessions will minimize such effects. Because of this design feature, it may take as long as 3 weeks to complete the dosing sequence. However, because there is generally no need for a 1- or 2-week postdosing holding period, the actual study does not take any more calendar time than a traditional test.

For nonrodents (especially monkeys), if none of the animals die during the dosing period, there may be no reason to sacrifice such animals. They can be saved and used, following a reasonable "washout" period, to assess the toxicity of a different chemical.

Limit Tests

There are inocuous substances that are simply not very lethal, and little useful information is to be gained by forcing increasing amounts of chemicals into experimental animals. In a review of propylene carbonate (Elder, 1987), a frequently used cosmetic ingredient (i.e., intended human exposure by the dermal route), an oral LD_{50} of 29.1 g/kg was cited. The maximum concentration in any one product is 25%. Hence, a 55-kg person would have to consume 640 g (1.4 lb) to approach 1/10 of the oral LD_{50}. Eating a few pounds of lipstick or eyeliner is not a common form of accidental or intentional intoxication. For evaluating the lethality of such substances, the limit test (Fig. 29) is the most appropriate protocol. The limit test is also appropriate for the testing of chemicals not intended for consumer exposure but for which there is a regulatory need for lethality data. The DOT classifies shipping hazards on the basis of lethality in rodents. As such, lack of lethality of statutorily set dosages (i.e., limit) ends any further testing needs. In the limit test, a single dosage of the test article is given to one group, generally of five animals. The limit dosage should be set on the basis of the chemical or physical properties of the test article and/or on the basis of an upward safety margin. If the substance is

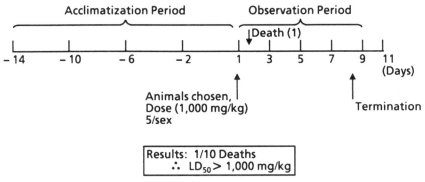

FIGURE 29 Line chart for the design and conduct of a typical limit test protocol for evaluating lethality.

acidic, a sufficiently large dosage ip will cause considerable peritoneal damage but will yield no useful toxicological information. Alternatively, if the anticipated acute human dosage of a drug is 0.3 mg/kg, there is probably no reason to test dosages in excess of 100 mg/kg (300-fold the human dose). In general, there is never any reason to test at dosages higher than 5 g/kg and rarely any reason to exceed 3 g/kg. In the case of propylene carbonate, the authors also cite limit dosage studies in which the limit was set at 5 g/kg. There were no deaths. Clearly, the safety conclusion based on this information is no different than that based on the LD_{50} of 29.1 g/kg.

There are three possible outcomes to a limit test. If none of the animals die, then the conclusion is that the minimum lethal dosage is greater than the limit dosage. If fewer than 50% of the animals die, then the conclusion is that the LD_{50} is greater than the limit dosage. If more than 50% of the animals die, then one has a problem. Depending on the reasons for performing the test, one could reset the limit and repeat the study or one could assess lethality by a different protocol. Alternatively, the change in the limit could reflect a change in the chemical or biological properties of the test substance that should be evaluated further.

FIXED DOSE PROCEDURE

The fixed dose design (Fig. 30) was proposed by the British Toxicology Society (1984). It is designed to supply the data needed for classification or labeling purposes. It is essentially a three-step limit test.

Five rats per sex are given 50 mg/kg. If survival is less than 90%, a second group of animals is given 5 mg/kg. If survival is again less than 90%, the substance is classified as "very toxic"; otherwise, it is classified as "toxic."

If, after the 50 mg/kg dose, survival is 90% but there is evident toxicity, no further dosages are given and the substance is classified as "harmful." If, on the other hand, there is no evident toxicity at 50 mg/kg, another group of rats is given 500 mg/kg. If there is again 90% survival and no evident toxicity, the substance is "unclassified" or is "slightly toxic."

This procedure was the successful subject of an international validation study (van den Heuvel, 1990). It may result in a decrease in animal usage. More important, it uses not only lethality, but also "evident toxicity." For hazard classification, in all likelihood, this refers to obvious signs of CNS effect, such as seizures or prostation. Some results are shown in Table 35. These have led to acceptance by European regulator authorities (van den Heuvel *et al.,* 1990).

This protocol was evaluated in an international validation effort involving 33 different laboratories (van den Heuvel, 1990). The acute oral toxicity of

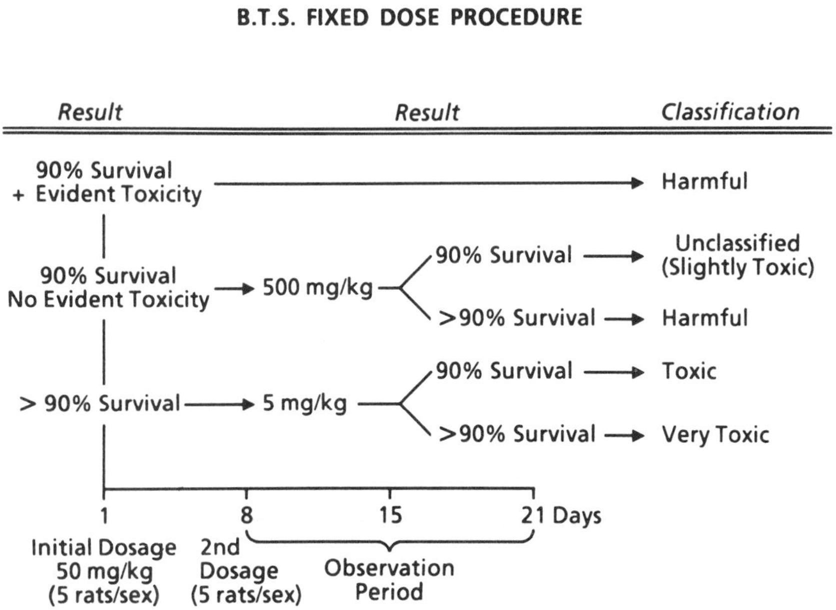

B.T.S. FIXED DOSE PROCEDURE

FIGURE 30   Line chart for the design and conduct of the British Toxicology Society (BTS) fixed dose protocol for evaluating acute systemic toxicity.

20 preparations was evaluated using a fixed dose procedure in the vat and the results compared with those obtained using classical lethality data. The results are summarized in Table 35. The data indicate that the fixed dose procedure produces consistent results with little interlaboratory variations and that this procedure enables preparations to be ranked according to the EEC classification system based on acute oral toxicity. The procedure uses fewer animals, relies on endpoints other than lethality, and the toxicity rankings are compatible with the rankings based on classical (LD_{50}) lethality testing.

QUALITY CONTROL SCREENS

Lethality testing was first used for standardization of biological and/or botanical drug preparations. This is, in fact, a practice that continues to this day. The FDA mandates that certain preparations be released on a batch basis and expects to see the LD_{50} as part of the release documentation. Drug companies may do final lethality screens on wholly synthetic finished preparations prior to release for either clinical trials or wholesale distribution. Finished food

TABLE 35   A Comparison of Classification of Selected Chemicals by the LD_{50} and Fixed-Dose Tests

Compound	LD_{50} test classification	Fixed-dose tests: Number of laboratories classifying compound as			
		Very toxic	Toxic	Harmful	Unclassified
Nicotine	Toxic	—	23	3	—
Sodium pentachlorophenate	Harmful	—	1	25	—
Ferrocene	Harmful/unclassified	—	—	3	23
2-Chloroethyl alcohol	Toxic	—	19	7	—
Sodium arsenite	Toxic	—	25	1	—
Phenyl mercury acetate	Toxic	2	24	—	—
p-Dichlorobenzene	Unclassified	—	—	—	26
Fentin hydroxide	Toxic	—	8	17	1
Acetanilide	Harmful	—	—	4	22
Quercetin diydrate	Unclassified	—	—	—	26
Tetrachlorvinphos	Unclassified	—	—	1	25
Piperidine	Harmful	—	2	24	—
Mercuric chloride	Toxic	—	−25	1	—
1-Phenyl-2-thiourea	Toxic/harmful	12	12	2	—
4-Aminophenol	Harmful	—	—	17	9
Naphthalene	Unclassified	—	—	—	26
Acetonitrile	Harmful	—	—	4	22
Aldicarb (10%)	Very toxic	22	—	—	—
Resorcinol	Harmful	—	—	25	1
Dimethyl formamide	Unclassified	—	—	—	26

From van den Heuvel et al. (1990) with permission.

products are often also batch tested prior to distribution. Quality control screens are simple in that they are conducted to help assure the quality of a specific product lot prior to human exposure. They do not provide data to make general conclusions about the safety of a properly prepared product. The protocols contain predefined expectations as to what constitutes a "Pass" or "Fail." Quality assurance screens fall roughly into two different categories. The first is composed of those conducted to standardized biologically derived materials for potency. The second consists of those tests for gross contamination or adulteration, i.e., "a cyanide test." Another way of looking at these two different tests is that the first is a two-sided question: Is the test batch of a vaccine, for example, of greater or lesser potency (and, in this case, the endpoint is death) than a known standard? In the second, the question is single sided: Is the material of unexpectedly high lethal potency?

For questions of the first kind, greatest precision and surety of result will be obtained when complete lethal dosage curves are defined for both the test batch and the standard. Such tests can be expensive and time-consuming. Resources can be saved by not including the standard in every test and relying on historical data, providing that one's historic database is broad and consisting. Slight shifts (especially upward shifts) in the LD_{50} are of little consequence. Alternatively, we recommend that, for each test, one group be dosed with the standard and another with the same batch. Such quality control (QC) tests should be conducted with two groups of 5–10 animals dosed at the expected LD_{50}. If mortality falls within the expected range of 40–60%, then no further action may be necessary.

For questions of the second kind, cyanide tests are appropriately conducted as limit tests where slight shifts (especially upward shifts) in the LD_{50} are of little consequence. Only five animals are tested at a set limit dose. Depending on how many times material is screened, an occasional animal may die because the MLD is usually in the range of the LD_{01}. Hence, if an animal dies, the test should be repeated before proceeding. If the result is the same or if more than one animal dies during the initial limit test, then there is cause for concern and the material should not be released until the cause for enhanced lethality is understood. It must be stressed that in no way are these tests a substitute for chemical analysis. One cannot, and should not, come to any conclusions concerning the amounts or concentrations of the active ingredients in a preparation solely on the basis of lethality data.

It may still be common practice in some laboratories to use traditional lethality protocols to conduct QC tests of both types. As mentioned, such tests are often unnecessary. Considerable savings in resources can be realized by the adoption of limit test protocols, where appropriate. Until 1984, a substantial number of the mice ordered by the Department of Toxicology of G.D. Searle R&D were for quality assurance testing. In 1984, we adopted limit test protocols for QC testing, with the result that the number of mice ordered was cut roughly by 34%, while the number of QC tests increased by 30%. Incidentally, because of cost, quality assurance limit tests are almost exclusively conducted on mice. Other species should be used only when there is a compelling scientific reason.

The authors have little practical experience in using lethality data for the standardization of biological materials. We, therefore, restrict our comments on the problems of quality assurance testing to protocols designed to detect gross contamination or adulteration. Traditional protocols can sometimes provide data that are unnecessarily complicated for the purposes of QC testing. For example, changes in the dosage form changed the LD_{50} of a well-studied drug, theophylline (Table 36). One dosage form consistently yielded an LD_{50} higher than expected on the basis of comparison to neat chemical. As it turned out, the formulation was one designed for controlled release and the increased LD_{50} (hence, decrease in lethality) could be explained by the decrease in immediate absorption. If this test had been conducted as a limit test at 200 mg/kg, the time and effort necessary to reconcile this finding with the protocol

TABLE 36 Sample Data: Theophylline Quality Assurance Data

Dosage (mg/kg)	Mortality	
	Neat chemical	CR–24 dosage form
280	0/10	0/10
370	3/10	0/10
500	8/10	2/10
670	10/10	10/10
	LD_{50} = 420 mg/kg	LD_{50} = 30 mg/kg

Note. In both cases, unfasted CD–1 male mice 5 or 6 weeks of age from the same supplier were used.

specification would have been saved because a decrease in lethality was not of any consequence.

Even with the limit test protocol, false positives (i.e., enhanced lethality not due to gross contamination or adulteration) can be obtained. In the overwhelming majority of cases, this will be due to increased bioavailability. If a positive limit response is obtained, changes in bioavailability should always be investigated (providing, of course, that the test article was administered by the oral route). The data summarized in Table 37 provide an example of a "false positive" due to enhanced bioavailability. Two lots of drug preparation were tested at the same limit dosage of 1400 mg/kg. The limit had been set on the basis of previous results with the drug formulated 2 : 1 with microcrystalline cellulose. In the two tests in question, all variables were controlled (vehicle, time of day, age, sex, strain of mice, and even the technician doing the dosing). The only difference was that the drug in lot D454 was formulated 2 : 1 with polyvinylprovidone (PVP), while that in D259 was formulated 2 : 1 with microcrystalline cellulose. Further investigation demonstrated that this one simple change was sufficient to more than double the peak plasma concentrations and the areas under the curves.

TABLE 37 Quality Assurance Testing of SC–33643 in Adult Male Mice

Dosage(s) (mg/kg)	Lot No. D 259 (avicel formulation)	Lot No. D 454 (PVP formulation)
1400	0/10[a]	8/10[a]
720	—	4/10[b]

[a]Mortality: number dead/number dose.
[b]The original limit dose was 1400 mg/kg. Subsequent experimentation indicated that a lower limit (720 mg/kg) was justified because of enhanced bioavailability of the PVP formulation.

The other leading cause of false positives is the use of unhealthy animals. Mice should be purchased only from approved vendors (those that produce animals that consistently meet your institutional criteria of quality) and acclimated to laboratory conditions for several days before the start of the study. Young, recently weaned mice may have a difficult time learning to drink from an automatic watering system. Even under the best of circumstances, it is not unusual for a few mice to die of no apparent cause during the acclimation period. Hence, a limit test conducted prior to appropriate acclimization could yield a false positive. Mice should be held for at least a week before the start of a study.

While we have a good deal of experience with false positives, we have no concrete examples of a false negative. Given the moral and legal implications of a false negative, this is good news. A false negative could lead to the release of materials that are injurious to man. A false negative could arise only in some very unusual circumstances. For example, the preparation could be grossly contaminated with a substance highly poisonous to man but innocuous to mice.

Using Lethality Data in Safety Assessment: The MLD

The LD_{50} is simply a calculated point on a lethality curve. The shape or slope of this curve is also an important characteristic of the test substance. However, unless one does a great deal of acute toxicity testing, a slope of 1.5 vs a slope of 4 has very little meaning. For safety considerations, the dosage that kills 50% of the animals is not as important as the dosage at which lethality first becomes apparent (i.e., the threshold or minimum lethal dosage). For example, if the oral LD_{50}'s of two different substances, A and B, were 0.6 and 2.0 g/kg, respectively, what would we conclude about the relative safety of these compounds? Further, let's assume these two substances are drugs, and that the estimated human dosage of drug A is 0.5 mg/kg and of drug B is 5 mg/kg. Do our conclusions concerning the relative safety of these two drugs change? In fact, the LD_{50}'s of both drugs are so high that both are considered only slightly toxic (0.5–5.0 g/kg); the same conclusion would have been reached had these been nonpharmaceuticals. One can also compute the lethality safety margin or index (LSI, equal to LD_{50}/EHD, where EHD is the estimated human dose) for these two drugs; both are so large (1200 for A and 400 for B) that there is still no toxicology relevant difference between the two drugs. Let's now assume that the lethality curve for substance A is very steep, such that 0.4 g/kg causes death in a very small percentage of animals. It is, in fact, the lowest dose administered that causes death. This is the MLD or estimated minimum lethal dosage (EMLD). Let's now assume that the lethality curve for B is very shallow, such that its MLD is also 0.4 g/kg. Does this change our safety considerations of these two drugs? One can calculate a new more conservative lethality index (MLD/EHD) of 800 for A and 80 for B. As a very general rule of thumb, an LSI of less than 100 for lethality is cause for mild concern, one less than 10 is cause for caution, and one less than 1 should be cause for extreme caution. In the case of our two hypothetical drugs, the development of drug B should be approached with more caution than drug A, despite the fact that B has a higher LD_{50}. This is demonstrated in Fig. 34. There are drugs sold over the counter, however, that have lethality safety indices of less than 10. For example, the MLD of indomethacin in rats is 3.7 mg/kg (from data reported by Schiantarelli and Cadel, 1981), while the maximum recommended human dose is 200 mg (2.9 mg/kg for a 70-kg person); hence, indomethacin has an LSI of 1.3. Such a finding is only cause for some caution, but does not in and of itself justify restricting the use or sale or a drug. Hence, because it results in a more conservative safety factor and also takes into consideration the slope of the lethality curve, we recommend the use of the MLD rather than the LD_{50} in calculating acute lethality safety indices.

A number of different safety factors and therapeutic indices (TI) have been proposed in the literature. Despite their similarity, some distinction should be made between these two. A therapeutic index applies only to drugs and is the ratio between a toxic dosage (LD or TD: the toxic end point does not always have to be death) and the pharmacologically effective (ED) dosage in the same species. The TI of Gaddum (LD_{50}/ED_{50}) is the most commonly used. A safety index can be calculated for all xenobiotics, not just drugs. A safety factor is the ratio of likely human exposure (or dosage) and the dosage that causes death or other forms of toxicity in the most sensitive experimental animal species. The most conservative (lethality) safety index (LSI) is obtained by dividing the maximum estimated human dosage or exposure by either the minimum lethal dosage or the maximum nonlethal dosage.

MLD PROTOCOLS

Stating that the MLD preferable to the LD_{50} for safety considerations in one thing; trying to determine what a specific MLD may or could be is another. There are no commonly used experimental designs that have the MLD as an endpoint. Assuming a log-dose response, the MLD may become a function of group size. Theoretically, if enough animals are dosed, at least one animal could die at any dosage of any chemical. Because there are neither an infinite number of animals in the world nor the technicians to dose them, there are practical considerations that can and should be applied to determining an

MLD. As a practical rule of thumb, we recommend that the estimated LD_{01}, the dose that would be expected to kill 1% of the experimental animals so exposed, be used as an estimate of the MLD. If one already has sufficient data to describe a lethality curve, an LD_{01} can be calculated as easily as the LD_{50}. This is often the case with acute toxicity data obtained to support regulatory submission. In such a case, both numbers (the LD_{01} and the LD_{50}) should be calculated and included in regulatory submission.

How is the MLD found if one does not choose to do a complete lethality curve using classical or traditional protocols? Clearly, the up-and-down method is inappropriate. A modified pyramiding dosage design may be the most appropriate. With this design, groups of animals are treated with stepwise increases in dosage until death occurs or a limit dosage is attained. If one has no idea as to what the initial dosage should be or how to graduate the dosages, a dose probing experiment can be conducted. If the dose probing experiment produces no deaths, two or three more animals can be dosed at the limit dose to confirm the results, and the lethality determination is now complete. If the probe experiment does produce death, then the additional dosages can be graduated between the lowest lethal and the highest nonlethal dosages. A typical progression may preceed as follows (Fig. 31): On Day 1 of the study, three probe animals are dosed at 10, 100, and 1000 mg/kg. The animal at 1000 mg/kg dies within a few hours of dosing. The two remaining animals are dosed at 300 mg/kg on Day 3. Neither die. They are then dosed at 500 mg/kg on Day 5. One dies. Three additional animals should be dosed on Day 7 or 8 at a dosage between the previous two, i.e., 400 mg/kg. If none dies, then 500

EXAMPLE OF MLD PYRAMIDING DOSAGE PROTOCOL

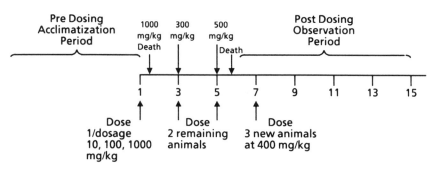

FIGURE 31 Line chart for the design and conduct of a pyramiding style protocol with the objective of determining a MLD.

mg/kg is a good estimate of the MLD and 400 mg/kg is a good estimate of the maximum nonlethal dosage (MNLD). While different by definition, there is usually not a great deal of distance between these two points, as this example illustrates. In fact, even for a comparatively well-defined lethality curve, the confidence limits about the LD_{01} will be quite broad and encompass both these points, the MLD and MNLD. Because this design permits the reuse of animals, acceptable estimates of the lethality limits of a chemical can be obtained using as low as six animals.

Malfors (1983) has proposed a similar method for determining what he terms the MNLD. Rather than initiating the study with probe animals, his design calls for three consecutive pyramiding type studies with the steps becoming increasingly small. For example, 2 animals will be sequentially dosed at 2, 200, and 2000 mg/kg. If death occurs at 2000 mg/kg, a new pair of animals is initiated at 200 mg/kg, and sequential dosages are increased by a factor of 1.8 until death occurs. Then another pair of animals is initiated at the highest nonlethal dosage, and successive dosages are increased by a factor of 1.15. The result of this exercise will be two dosages, one apparently nonlethal and the other lethal, separated by a factor of 1.15. Six animals are dosed at each dosage. If none die at the lower dosage and 1 dies at the higher dose, then the lower dose is considered to be the MNLD. He recommends at least 24 hr between dosing sessions. While this method may have some utility, there are some disadvantages. First, the recommended limiting dosage of 6.5 g/kg is too high. Second, 24 hr between doses may be too short to allow for recovery. Third, even with only 24 hr between doses, this is a time-consuming procedure and may take up to 2 weeks to complete the dosing. Third, it does not save on the use of animals because it may use 18–20 animals. One would almost be better off dividing these animals into four groups and obtaining a traditional lethality curve and calculating both the LD_{01} and the LD_{50}.

For nonrodents, dose probing is generally not used. The initiating dosage is normally in the range of 1 to 5 times projected human exposure. The limit is generally in the area of 1 g/kg or 100–200 × the human dosage. The normal study will include two animals of each sex treated with the test article. For lethality studies (in general), there is seldom any need to include control animals. If the projected human exposure is 4 mg/kg, the initial dosage will be 20 mg/kg and succeeding dosages increased stepwise at half-log intervals; thus, 20, 60, 200, and 600 mg/kg doses are separated by at least 48 hr. The MLD is reported as simply being between the highest observable nonlethal and the lowest lethal dosage, or at greater than the limit dosage—in this case, 600 mg/kg. Rarely are such studies done with nonrodents solely for determining lethality. To do so would be a waste of time and animals. We generally included extensive physical examinations, including ECGs and rectal temperatures, careful observations of behavior and activity, and extensive clinical laboratory workups after each dose. These will be discussed in more detail in Chapter 9.

The pyramiding dose study is not without disadvantages. The small number of animals used can cause simple random variation resulting in misestimation of lethality. It is a well-accepted statistical maxim that the smaller the sample size, the greater the impact of any random variation from the population characteristic. This may be especially true for a nonrodent species that is drawn from an outbread population. Second, the pyramiding dose regimen can permit the development of tolerance. For example, we conducted pyramiding dosage studies to range-find dosages for the 2-week study on 1,4-benzodiazepine. Lethality was observed at 600 mg/kg in the pyramiding study. For the subsequent 2-week study, top dose was set at 300 mg/kg and both dogs died of CNS depression on the first day of dosing.

ALTERNATIVES TO LETHALITY TESTING

To a significant extent, the bulk of this chapter has been an attempt to present and explain the *in vivo* alternatives to the traditional LD_{50} test (as illustrated in Fig. 32).

EXAMPLE OF TYPICAL TRADITIONAL ACUTE LETHALITY PROTOCOL

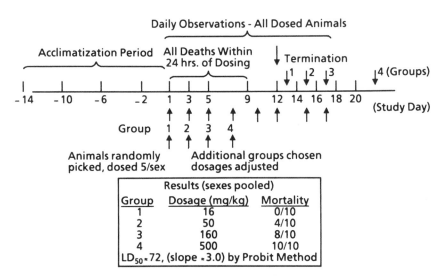

FIGURE 32   Line chart for the design and conduct of a traditional acute lethality (LD_{50}) study.

Such alternatives seek to both reduce the amount of suffering and the number of animals involved in lethality testing and to make the testing process as scientifically valid and economically efficient as possible. There are also, however, "*in vitro*" alternatives which use lower forms of life (invertebrates or bacteria), no intact organisms (cultured cells such as hepatocytes), or no living materials at all [the structure–activity relationship (SAR) methodologies]. Each of these three approaches represents an additional large difference between the objective of such testing (predicting lethality in humans) and the model being used to achieve the objective.

Some researchers have shown a good correlation between the lethality of chemicals to *Daphnia magna* (the LC_{50} of the material dissolved in water) and the oral LD_{50} of the same chemicals in rats. This correlation is nonlinear, but still suggestive that more toxic materials could be at least initially identified and classified in some form of screening system based on *Daphnia*. A broader range of chemical structures will need to be evaluated, however, and some additional laboratories will need to confirm the finding. It must also be kept in mind that the metabolic systems (and many of the other factors involved in species differences, as presented in Chapter 12) and other factors which contribute to a nonlinear correlation may also make the confidence in prediction of human effects in cases in which accuracy is critical (such as a pharmaceutical with a narrow therapeutic index but high potential patient benefit) unacceptable.

TABLE 38   Sample Data Set: Variability of Cytotoxicity of MNNG and 3MC in the $TK^{+/-}$ Mouse Lymphoma Cell Line

Study No.	MNNG (0.04 μg/mg)	3MC (5 μg/ml)
SA 1944	46%	42%
SA 1954	90%	75%
SA 1960	70%	75%
SA 1961	58%	78%
SA 1962	69%	46%
SA 2004	57%	98%
SA 2005	80%	72%
	67 ± 15%	57 ± 26%

Note. The results are as percentage of relative suppression of cell growth with comparison to concurrent (vehicle treated) control cultures. Studies were conducted over an 18-month period from 1982 to 1984. Cultures were derived from a common seed lot and all materials and methods between studies uniform. MNNG, n-methyl-n'-nitrosoguanadine; 3MC, 3-methylcholanthrene. With 3MC, rat liver S9 metabolic activation system was included.

LACK OF CORRELATION BETWEEN THE LD$_{50}$s IN MICE AND THE LC$_{50}$s IN THE TK$^{+/-}$ MOUSE LYMPYOMA CELL LINE FOR A DIVERSE GROUP OF DRUGS

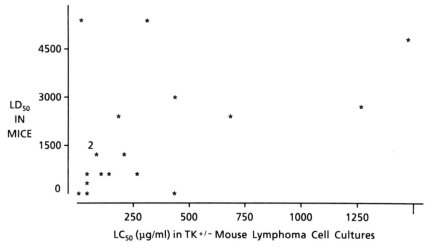

FIGURE 33   Graph showing a comparison of the lethalities of a group of 18 drugs of diverse structure in *in vivo* (mouse) and *in vitro* (cultured mouse lymphoma cells) test systems. Correlation of these LD$_{50}$/LC$_{50}$ values is very poor, though extreme high and low scale values seem to be more closely associated in the two systems.

Others (Kurach *et al.*, 1986) have developed and suggested a system based on cultured mammalian hepatocytes. The system does metabolize materials in a manner similar to that of mammalian target species and has shown promise in a limited battery of chemicals. But such cell culture and bacteria (as some have suggested) screening systems have significant weaknesses for assessing the lethality of many classes of chemicals. They lack any of the integrative functions of a larger organism and, thus, would miss all agents which act by disrupting such functions (such as the organophosphate pesticides and most other neurologically mediated lethal agents).

Finally, there are systems which do not directly use any living organisms, but rather seek to predict the lethality (in particular, the LD$_{50}$) of a chemical based on what is known about structurally related chemicals. Such SAR systems have improved markedly over the past 10 years (Enslein *et al.*, 1983; Lander *et al.*, 1984) but are still limited. Accurate predictions are usually possible only for those classes of structures in which data have previously been generated on several members of the classes. For new structural classes, the value of such predictions is minimal. Phillips *et al.*

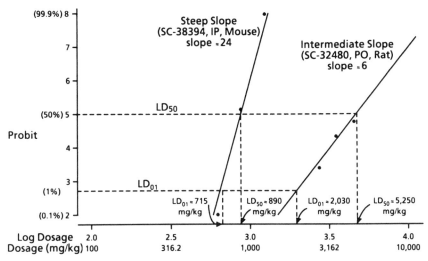

FIGURE 34   Graph illustrating differences in slopes of lethality–response curves of two different compounds.

(1990) extensively reviewed the literature on SAR and *in vitro* methods. They confirmed that SAR methods have been very imprecise in LD_{50} predictions. Best success has been obtained with chemicals that are closely related chemicals with common physical properties. They concluded that the LD_{50} is a toxic endpoint that may not be predictable when applied to unrelated chemicals because different mechanisms of toxic action are involved. The successful application of SAR to predict the LD_{50} based strictly on structural considerations may not be possible until biological mechanisms can somehow be worked into the computer modeling systems. Likewise, very few studies have found good correlations between *in vitro* and *in vivo* tests. Phillips *et al.* (1990) proposed that the luck of correlation may be because cytotoxicity is surely an important determinant in acute systemic toxicity. They also point out that such tests ignore the importance of pharmacokinetic behavior and metabolic transformation. Good correlations have been obtained, however, where the *in vitro* system involves the same toxic mechanisms as the *in vivo* lethality. For example, the LD_{50} of neurotoxins can be best predicted with *in vivo* neural cell systems. Hence, for both SAR and *in vitro* cell culture system, the blanket application of technology has not been successful in replacing lethality testing and probably will not be successful until a greater level of sophistication, i.e., involvement of specific mechanistic considerations, is obtained.

However, QC testing may be an area that is very amenable to alternative methods, given the narrow focus of the question(s) asked and the high throughput and fast turnaround times required. Cytotoxicity, for example, in a defined cell line is as valid a biological endpoint as lethality in a group of mice. Such tests should always include known standards or "positive controls" because, as illustrated by the data in Table 38, even the most rigorously defined *in vitro* system will have considerable test-to-test variation.

A key difference in QC testing vs acute toxicity testing is that in the former comparisons are made to known standards or results, whereas in the latter, the emphasis is on describing the unknown. Recently, "alternative" (*in vitro*) methods in acute toxicity testing have gained increasing attention. *In vitro* methods, however, may not be generally reliable with regard to predicting lethality. For example, the LD_{50} in mice vs the LC_{50} in mouse lymphoma cell culture (Clive *et al.*, 1979) for a wide assortment of chemicals are compared in Table 38. There was no general correlation between the LC_{50} and LD_{50} (Fig. 33) in this case. Given the imprecision of some LD_{50} values due to the steep slope of the lethality curve (as illustrated in Fig. 34) this should not be a surprise.

REFERENCES

Anderson, O. (1958). *The Health of a Nation: Harvey W. Wiley and the Fight for Pure Food.* University of Chicago Press, Chicago.

Armitage, P., and Allen, I. (1950). Methods of estimating the LD50 in quantal response data. *J. Hygiene* **48**, 398–422.

Aulette, C. (1988). Acute systemic toxicity testing. In *Handbook of Product Safety Assessment* (S. Gad, Ed.). Dekker, New York.

Balazs, T. (1976). Assessment of the value of systemic toxicity studies in experimental animals. In *Advances in Modern Toxicology Vol. 1, Part 1, New Concepts in Safety Evaluation* (M. Mehlman, R. Shapiro, and H. Blumenthal, Eds.), pp. 141–153. Hemisphere, Washington, DC.

Behrens, B. (1929). Evaluation of digitalis leaves in the frog experiments. *Arch. Exp. Pathol. Pharmacol.* **140**, 236–256.

Berkson, J. (1955). Estimate of the integrated normal curve by minimum normit chi-square with particular reference to bioassay. *J. Am. Stat. Assoc.* **50**, 529–549.

Bliss, C. (1935). The calculation of the dosage mortality curve. *Anal. Appl. Biol.* **22**, 134–167.

Bliss, C. (1957). Some principles of bioassay. *Am. Scientist* **45**, 449–466.

British Toxicology Society (1984). A new approach to the classification of substances and preparations on the basis of their acute toxicity. A report by the British Toxicology Society Working Party on Toxicity. *Hum. Toxicol.* **3**, 85–92.

Brownlee, K., Hodges, J., and Rosenblatt (1953). The Up-and-Down Method with small samples. *J. Am. Stat. Assoc.* **48**, 262–277.

Bruce, M., and Doull, J. (1986). Origin and scope of toxicology. In *Casarett and Doull's Toxicology* (C. Klaassen, M. Amdur, and J. Doull, Eds.), 3rd ed., pp. 3–10. Macmillan, New York.

Bruce, R. (1985). An up-and-down procedure for acute toxicity testing. *Fundam. Appl. Toxicol.* **5**, 151–157.

Clive, D., Johnson, K., Spector, J., Batson, A., and Brown, M. (1979). Validation and characterization of the L5178Y/TK mouse lymphoma mutagen assay system. *Mutat. Res.* **59**, 61–108.

Decker, W. (1987). Introduction and history. In *Handbook of Toxicology* (J. Haley and W. Berndt, Eds.), pp. 1–19. Hemisphere, Washington, DC.

Deichemann, W., and Gerarde, H. (1969). *Toxicology of Drugs and Chemicals.* Academic Press, New York.

deLind van Wijngaarden, C. (1926). Investigations on the activity of digitalis preparations, Part II: On the accuracy of digitalis calibration on cats. *Arch. Exp. Pathol. Pharmacol.* **113**, 40–58.

DePass, L. R., Myers, R. C., Weaver, E. V., and Weil, C. S. (1984). An assessment of the importance of number of dosage levels, number of animals per dosage level, sex and method of LD_{50} and slope calculations in acute toxicity studies. In *Alternate Methods in Toxicology, Vol. 2: Acute Toxicity Testing: Alternate Approaches* (A. M. Goldberg, Ed.), pp. 139–154. Liebert, New York.

Dixon, W. J., and Wood, A. M. (1948). A method for obtaining and analyzing sensitivity data. *J. Am. Stat. Assoc.* **43**, 109–126.

Elder, L. (Ed.) (1987). Final report on the safety assessment of propylene carbonate in safety assessment of cosmetic ingredients. *J. Am. Coll. Toxicol.* **6**, 1–22.

Enslein, K., Lander, T. R., Tomb, M. E., and Craig, P. N. (1983). *A Predictive Model for Estimating Rate Oral LD50 Values.* Princeton Scientific, Princeton, NJ.

Environmental Protection Agency (EPA) (1996). Health Effects Test Guidelines. OPPTS 870.1000 Acute Toxicity Testing—Background. EPA 712-C-96-189. EPA, Washington, DC.

Finney, D. J. (1971). *Probit Analysis,* 3rd ed. Cambridge University Press, New York.

Finney, D. (1985). The median lethal dose and its estimation. *Arch. Toxicol.* **56**, 215–218.

Food and Drug Administration (FDA) (1996). Single dose acute toxicity testing for pharmaceuticals; Revised guidance *Fed. Reg.* August 26, 61(166) 43934-43935.

Gad, S., and Weil, C. (1982). Statistics for toxicologists. In *Principles and Methods of Toxicology* (A. Hayes, Ed.), pp. 273–320. Raven Press, New York.

Gad, S., and Weil, C. (1986). *Statistics and Experimental Design for Toxicologists.* Telford Press, Caldwell, NJ.

Gad, S., Smith, A., Cramp, A., Gavigan, F., and Derelanko, M. (1984). Innovative designs and practices for acute systemic toxicity studies. *Drug Chem. Toxicol.* **7**, 423–434.

Harris, R., and Paxman, J. (1982). *A Higher Form of Killing.* Hill and Wang, New York.

Karber, G. (1931). Contribution to the collective treatment of pharmacological serial experiments. *Arch. Exp. Pathol. Pharmacol.* **162**, 480–483.

Kurach, G., Vossen, P., Deboyser, D., Goethals, F., and Roberfubid, M. (1986). An *in vitro* model for acute toxicity screening using hepatocyes freshly isolated from adult mammals. In *In Vitro Toxicology* (A. Goldberg, Ed.). Liebert, New York.

Lander, T., Enslein, K., Craig, P., and Tomb, N. (1984). Validation of a structure–activity model of rat oral LD50. In *Acute Toxicity Testing: Alternative Approaches* (A. Goldberg, Ed.). Liebert, New York.

Litchfield, J., and Wilcoxon, F. (1949). A simplified method of evaluating dose–effect experiments. *J. Pharmacol. Exp. Ther.* **96**, 99–113.

Lorke, D. (1983). A new approach to practical acute toxicity testing. *Arch. Toxicol.* **54**, 275–287.

Malmfors, T., and Teiling, A. (1983). LD_{50}—Its value for the pharmaceutical industry in safety evaluation of drugs. *Acta Pharmacol. Toxicol.* **52**(suppl. 2), 229–246.

Morrison, J., Quiton, R., and Reinert, H. (1968). The purpose and value of LD_{50} determinations. In *Modern Trends in Toxicology, Vol. I* (E. Boyland and R. Goulding, Eds.), pp. 1–17. Appleton-Century-Crofts, London.

Muller, H., and Kley, H. (1982). Retrospective study on the reliability of an "approximate LD_{50}" determined with a small number of animals. *Arch. Toxicol.* **51**, 189–196.

Osterberg, R. E. (1983). Today's requirements in food, drug, and chemical control. *Acta Pharmacol. Toxicol.* **52**(suppl. 2), 210–228.

Pendergrast, W. (1984). Biological drug regulation. In *The Seventyfifth Anniversary Commemorative Volume of Food and Drug Law*, pp. 293–305. Food and Drug Law Institute, Washington, DC.

Phillips, J., Gibson, W., Yum, J., Alden, C., and Hurd, G. (1990). Survey of the QSAR and *in vitro* approaches for developing non-animal methods to supersede the *in vivo*. LD_{50} test. *Fd. Chem. Toxicol.* **28**, 375–394.

Rowan, A. (1981). The LD_{50} Test: A critique and suggestions for alternatives. *Pharm. Technol.* April, 65–92.

Schiantarelli, P., and Cadel, S. (1981). Piroxicam pharmacological activity and gastrointestinal damage by oral and rectal route: Comparison with oral indometacin and phenylbutazone. *Arzneim-Forsch/Drug Res.* **31**, 87–92.

Schutz, E., and Fuchs, H. (1982). A new approach to minimizing the number of animals in acute toxicity testing and optimizing the information of the test results. *Arch. Toxicol.* **51**, 197–220.

Shackell, L. (1925). The relationship of dosage to effect. *J. Pharmacol. Exp. Ther.* **31**, 275–288.

Sperling, F. (1976). Nonlethal parameters as indices of acute toxicity: Inadequacies of the acute LD_{50}. In *Advance in Modern Toxicology Vol 1, Part 1: New Concepts in Safety Evaluation* (M. Mehlman, R. Shapiro, and H. Blumenthal, Eds.), pp. 177–191. Hemisphere, Washington, DC.

Sudmersen, H., and Glenny, A. (1910). Variations in susceptibility of guinea-pigs to diphteria toxin. *J. Hygiene* **9**, 399–408.

Thompson, W., and Weil, C. (1952). On the construction of table for moving average interpolation. *Biometrics* **8**, 51–54.

Trevan, J. (1927). The error of determination of toxicity. *Proc. Roy. Soc. B* **101**, 483–514.

van den Heuvel, M., Clark, D., Fielder, R., Koundakjian, P., Oliver, G., Pelling, D., Tomlinson, N., and Walker, A. (1990). The international validation of a fixed-dose procedure as an alternative to the classical LD_{50} test. *Fd. Chem. Toxicol.* **28**, 469–482.

Waud, D. (1972). Biological assays involving quantal responses. *J. Pharmacol. Exp. Ther.* **183**, 577–607.

Weil, C. (1952). Table for convenient calculation of median effective dose (LD_{50} or ED_{50}) and instructions in their use. *Biometrics* **8**, 249–263.

Weil, C. (1983). Economical LD_{50} and slope determination. *Drug Chem. Toxicol.* **6**, 595–603.

Zbinden, G. (1986). Invited contribution: Acute toxicity testing, public responsibility and scientific challenges. *Cell Biol. Toxicol.* **2**, 325–335.

Zbinden, G., and Flury-Roversi, M. (1981). Significance of the LD_{50} test for the toxicological evaluation of chemical substances. *Arch. Toxicol.* **47**, 77–99.

CHAPTER 8

Safety Considerations for the Administration of Agents by the Parenteral Routes

There are a number of special concerns about the safety of materials which are injected (parenterally administered) into the body as a matter of course. By definition, these concerns are all associated with materials that are the products of the pharmaceutical and (in some minor cases) medical device industries. Such parenteral routes include three major ones—intravenous (iv), intramuscular (im), and subcutaneously (sc)—and a number of minor routes (such as intraarterial) which will not be considered here.

Administration by the parenteral routes raises a number of safety questions in addition to the usual systemic safety questions. These include local irritation (vascular, mucosal, muscular, or subcutaneous), pyrogenicity, blood compatibility, and sterility (Avis, 1985). The background of each of these, along with the underlying mechanisms and factors which influence the level of occurrence of such an effect, are briefly discussed below.

Irritation: Tissue irritation upon injection, and the accompanying damage and pain, is a concern which must be addressed for the final formulation which is to be either tested in humans or marketed, rather than for the active ingredient. This is because most of the factors are either due to or influenced

197

by aspects of formulation design (see Avis, 1985, for more information on parenteral preparations). These factors are not independent of which route (iv, im, or sc) will be used and, in fact (as will be discussed later), are part of the basis for selecting between the various routes.

The lack of irritation and damage at the injection site is sometimes called local tolerance. Some of the factors which affect tolerance are not fully under the control of an investigation and are also not related to the material being injected. These include body movement, temperature, and animal age. Other factors which can be controlled, but are not inherent to the active ingredient, include solubility, tonicity, and pH. Finally, the active ingredient and vehicle can have inherent irritative effects and factors such as solubility (in the physiological milleau they are being injected into), concentration, volume, molecular size, and particle size. Gray (1978) and Ballard (1968) discuss these factors and the morphological effects of their not being addressed.

Pyrogenicity: Pyrogenicity is the induction of a febrile (fever) response induced by the parenteral (usually iv or im) administration of exogenous material. Usually, pyrogenicity is associated with microbiological contamination of a final formulation, but is now of increasing concern because of the increase in interest in biosynthetically produced materials. Generally, ensuring sterility of product and process will guard against pyrogenicity.

Blood compatibility: The concern here is really that the cellular components of the blood will not be disrupted and that serum- or plasma-based responses are not triggered. Therefore, two mechanisms must be assessed regarding the blood compatibility of component materials. These include the material's effect on the cellular components causing membrane destruction and hemolysis and the activation of the clotting mechanism resulting in the formation of the thromboemboli. Many materials (such as the polyurethanes) are found to be relatively nonthrombogenic. The conditioning of materials contacting blood may employ the adhesion of heparin molecules to improve surface compatibility. For some materials, surface conditioning is accomplished by the adsorption of benzalkonium chloride prior to heparin treatment. Test procedures to assess these blood interaction mechanisms have included both *in vivo* and *in vitro* procedures for the determination of hemolysis and formation of thromboemboli.

Many of the nonactive, ingredient—related physicochemical factors which influence irritation (tonicity, pH, and particle size, for example) also act to determine blood compatibility. But the chemical features of a drug entity itself—its molecular size and reactivity—can also be of primary importance.

Sterility: This is largely a concern to be answered in the process of preparing a final clinical formulation and will not be addressed in detail in this chapter. However, it should be clear that it is essential to ensure that no viable microorganisms are present in any material to be parenterally administered (except for vaccines).

PARENTERAL ROUTES AND RATES

There are at least 13 different routes which do not involve oral administration and require injection or placing of a material under the skin or in a body compartment (other than the digestive tract). Therefore, these qualify as parenteral routes. These are:

1. Intravenous (iv)	8. Epidural
2. Subcutaneous (sc)	9. Intrathecal
3. Intramuscular (im)	10. Intracisternal
4. Vaginal	11. Intracardiac
5. Intraarterial	12. Intraventricular
6. Intradermal	13. Intraocular
7. Intralesional	14. Intraperitoneal (ip)

Only the first four are discussed in detail here. The intention of many of these routes of administration is to place the drug into the systemic circulation. There are a number of these routes, however, by which the drug exerts a local effect, and most of the drug does not enter the systemic circulation (e.g., intrathecal, intraventricular, intraocular, and intracisternal). Certain routes of administration may exert both local and systemic effects depending on the characteristics of the drug and excipients (e.g., subcutaneous).

The choice of a particular parenteral route will depend on the required time of onset of action, the required site of action, and the characteristics of the fluid to be injected, among other factors.

The need for a rapid onset of action usually requires that an iv route be used, although at a certain stage of cardiopulmonary resuscitation (for example), the need for a rapid effect may require the use of an intracardiac injection. The required site of action may influence the choice of route of administration (e.g., certain radiopaque dyes are given intraarterially near the site being evaluated; streptokinase is sometimes injected experimentally into the coronary arteries close to coronary vessel occlusion during a myocardial infarction to cause lysis of the thrombus and therefore reestablish coronary blood flow).

The characteristics of the fluid to be injected will also influence which parenteral routes of administration are possible to consider. The compatibility of the fluid used must be evaluated with other fluids (e.g., saline, dextrose, of Ringer's lactate) that the drug may be combined with for administration to the patient, as well as with the components of the blood itself.

There are certain clinical situations in which a parenteral route of administration is preferred to other possible routes. These include the following:

A. When the amount of drug given to a subject must be precisely controlled (e.g., in many pharmacokinetic studies), it is preferable to use a parenteral (usually iv) route of administration.

B. When the "first-pass effect" of a drug going through the liver must be avoided, a parenteral route of administration is usually chosen, although a sublingual route or dermal patch will also avoid the firstpass effect.

C. When one requires complete assurance that an uncooperative subject has actually received the drug and has not rejected it (e.g., via forced emesis).

D. When subjects are in a stupor, coma, or otherwise unable to take a drug orally.

E. When large volumes (i.e., more than 1 liter) of fluid are injected (such as in peritoneal dialysis, hyperalimentation, fluid replacement, and other conditions). Drugs given in large volumes require special consideration of fluid balance in the patients receiving the large volumes and careful consideration of the systemic effects of injection fluid components (for example, amino acids and their nephorotoxicity).

Each of the three routes we are concerned with here has a specific set of either advantages and disadvantages or specific considerations which must be kept in mind.

INTRAVENOUS

The iv route is the most common method of introducing a drug directly into the systemic circulation. It has the following advantages:

1. Rapid onset of effect.
2. Usefulness in situations of poor gastrointestinal absorption.
3. Avoidance of tissue irritation if present with im or other routes (e.g., nitrogen mustard).
4. More precise control of levels of drug than with other routes, especially to toxic drugs, where the levels must be kept within narrow limits.
5. Ability to administer large volumes over time by a slow infusion.
6. Ability to administer drugs at a constant rate over a long period of time.

It also suffers from disadvantages:

1. Higher incidence of anaphylactic reactions than with many other routes.
2. Possibility of infection or phlebitis at site of injection.
3. Greater pain to patients than with many other routes.

4. Possibility that embolic phenomena may occur—either air embolism or vascular clot—as a result of damage to the vascular wall.
5. Impossibility of removing or lavaging drug after it is given except by dialysis.
6. Inconvenience in many situations.
7. Possibility that rapid injection rates may cause severe adverse reactions.
8. Patient dislike of, and psychological discomfort with, the injection procedure.

For best results, intravenous fluids should possess the following characteristics:

1. Must be an aqueous solution. Administration of particulates can have unwanted sequalae.
2. Should be isoosmotic; otherwise, hemolysis and local irritation can occur (more critical in repeated dose studies than in acute studies).
3. Should be neutral in pH. The further from neutrality the pH, the greater the likelihood of localized irritation and other sequalae. Solution of pH less than 4 or greater than 9 will be frankly toxic (depending on volume and rate).
4. Should be sterile.
5. Should be room temperature or warmer when being administered to small animals.

When it comes to iv injection or infusion, the standard questions are how much and how fast? For bolus injection (administered in 2 min or less with the syringe held in hand), most species tolerate up to 10 ml/kg. For infusion, the volumes can be increased dramatically. For adult rats, the 40×2 relationship is a handy rule of thumb; that is, they can generally tolerate 40 ml/kg administered at a rate of 2 ml/min or less. As the volume goes up, the rate must come down proportionally. For example, a volume of 80 ml/kg must be administered at 1 ml/min or less. For mice, the similar proportional rule of thumb is 50×1. With dogs, because of their size, rate of administration is more limiting than total volume. The rule of thumb in this case is that just about any volume can be administered but at a rate no faster than 0.5 ml/min/kg.

For iv fluids, it must be determined how the dose will be given (i.e., by bolus or slow injection, intermittent or constant infusion, or by constant drip) and whether special equipment will be used to control and monitor the flow. Drugs with short half-lives are usually given by a constant drip or infusion technique. All iv fluids given immediately subsequent to an iv drug must be evaluated for their compatibility with the study drug. Suspensions are generally not given iv because of the possibility of blocking the capillaries.

SUBCUTANEOUS

Drugs given by the sc route are forced into spaces between connective tissues, as with im injections. Vasoconstrictors and drugs that cause local irritation should not be given sc in usual circumstances because inflammation, abscess formation, or even tissue necrosis may result. When daily or even more frequent sc injections are made, the sites of injection should be continuously changed to prevent local complications. Fluids given sc must have an appropriate tonicity to prevent pain. Care must be taken to prevent injection of the drug directly into veins.

The absorption of drugs from a sc route is influenced by blood flow to the area, as with im injections. The rate of absorption may be retarded by cooling the local area to cause vasoconstriction, adding epinephrine to the solution for the same purpose (e.g., with local anesthetics), decreasing blood flow with a tourniquet, or immobilizing the area. The opposite effect may be achieved with the enzyme hyaluronidase, which breaks down mucopolysaccharides of the connective tissue matrix and allows the injected solution to spread over a larger area and thus increase its rate of absorption or by warming the injection region.

In addition to fluids, solid forms of drugs may be given sc. This has been done with compressed pellets of testosterone placed under the skin, which are absorbed at a relatively constant rate over a long period.

INTRAMUSCULAR

The im route is frequently used for drugs dissolved in oily vehicles or for those in a microcrystalline formulation that are poorly soluble in water (e.g., procaine or penicillin G). Advantages include rapid absorption in many cases, often in under 30 min. Other advantages of the im route include the opportunity to inject a relatively large amount of solution and a reduction in pain and local irritation compared with sc injections. Potential complications include infections and nerve damage. The latter usually results from the choice of an incorrect site for injection.

Although the time to peak drug concentration is often on the order of 1 or 2 hr, depot preparations given im are absorbed extremely slowly. Numerous physical–chemical properties of the material given im will affect the rate of absorption from the site within the muscle (e.g., ionization of the drug, lipid solubility, osmolality of the solution, and volume given). The primary sites used for im injections are the gluteal (buttocks), deltoid (upper arm), and vastus lateralis (lateral thigh) muscles. The rate of drug absorption and the peak drug levels obtained will often differ between sites used for im injections.

This is related to differences in blood flow among muscle groups. The site chosen for an im injection in humans and some animals may be a critical factor in whether or not the drug exhibits an effect (Schwartz *et al.,* 1974).

BOLUS VS INFUSION

Technically, for all the parenteral routes (but in practice only for the iv route), there are two options for how a material may be introduced into the body. These options (bolus and infusion) are defined on the single basis of rate of injection but differ on a wide range of grounds.

The most commonly exercised option is the bolus or "push" injection in which the injection device (syringe or catheter) is appropriately entered into the vein and a defined volume of material is introduced through the device. The device is then removed. In this operation, it is relatively easy to restrain an experimental animal and the stress on the animal is limited. Though the person doing the injection must be skilled, it takes only a small amount of time to do so. Also, the one variable to be controlled in determining dosage is the total volume injected (assuming dosing solutions have been properly prepared).

There are also limitations and disadvantages for the bolus approach. Only a limited volume may be so injected, which may disallow use of the route when volumes to be introduced (due to either low active compound solubility or a host of other reasons) are high. Only two devices (syringe and catheter) are available for use in the bolus approach. Also, if a multiple-day course of treatment is desired (e.g., every day for 15 days), separate injections must be made at discrete entry sites.

The infusion approach involves establishing a fixed entry point into the vein, then slowly passing the desired test material through that point over a period of time (30 min is about minimum while continuous around-the-clock treatment is at least therapeutically possible). There are a number of devices available for establishing this entry point; catheter, vascular port (Garramone, 1986), or osmotic pump (Theeuwes and Yum, 1976). Each of these must, in turn, be coupled with some device to deliver the dosing solution at a desired rate. The osmatic pump, which is implanted, is also its own delivery device. Other options are gravity-driven "drips," syringes by hand (not practical or accurate over any substantial period of time), or syringe pumps. Very large volumes can be introduced by infusion over a protracted period of time, and only a single site need be fitted with an entry device.

However, infusion also has its limitations. Skilled labor is required, and the setup must be monitored over the entire period of infusion. Larger animals must be restrained, while there are special devices which avoid this requirement for smaller animals. The restraint and protracted manipulation are more stressful on animals. Over a period of time, one must regularly demonstrate patency of a device—that is, that entry into the vascular system continues to exist. Finally, one is also faced with having to control two variables in controlling dose—both total volume and rate.

When are the two approaches (bolus and infusion) interchangeable? Why select one over the other? The reasons for selecting infusion are usually limited to two: (1) when a larger volume must be introduced than is practical in a bolus injection or (2) tolerance is not sufficient if the dose is given all at once (i.e., an infusion will "clear" a higher daily dose than will single injection). When, for safety studies, a bolus can be used to clear a human infusion dosing is a matter of judgment. If the planned clinical infusion is less than half an hour, practicality dictates that the animal studies be accomplished by bolus. In other situations, pharmacokinetics (in particular, the half-life of the drug entity) should be considered in making the decision.

TEST SYSTEMS FOR PARENTERAL IRRITATION

There are no regulatory guidelines or suggested test methods for evaluating agents for muscular/vascular irritation. Because such guidelines are lacking, but the evaluation is necessary, those responsible for such evaluations have tried to develop and employ the most scientifically valid procedures.

Hagan (1959) first suggested a method for assessing im irritation, but this approach did not include a grading system for evaluation of the irritation. The method also used the sacrospinalis muscles, which are somewhat difficult to dissect or repeatedly inject.

Shintani et al. (1967) developed and proposed the methodology which currently seems to be more utilized. It uses the vastus lateralis muscle and includes a methodology for evaluation, scoring, and grading of the irritation. Additionally, Shintani et al. investigated the effects of several factors such as pH of the solution, drug concentration, volume of injection, the effect of repeated injections, and the time to maximum tissue response. In a previously unpublished study, this laboratory evaluated the Shintani method. The results of this study generally agreed with those of Shintani. Differences in irritation scores were most often found for those agents (10% urethane and 1% calcium chloride) that caused slight, mild, or moderate irritation. Differences between the results of the studies may be due to the small number of animals used in the trust (one animal/agent/time point). The inherent variability of scoring (especially mild irritation) suggests group size should be sufficiently large.

Additionally, concurrent control solutions should be given because the Shintani method requires that an animal's irritation score be deleted if the control score is 3 or greater.

The actual test procedure is described below.

ACUTE INTRAMUSCULAR IRRITATION IN THE MALE RABBIT

1. Overview of study design
   Each rabbit is injected as follows:

Site (M. vastus lateralis)	Treatment (1.0 ml/site)
Left	(test article)
Right	(vehicle)

   Day 1: Injection of all treatment groups (9 rabbits)
   Day 2: Sacrifice and evaluation—24-hr posttreatment group (3 rabbits)
   Day 3: Sacrifice and evaluation—48-hr posttreatment group (3 rabbits)
   Day 4: Sacrifice and evaluation—72-hr posttreatment group (3 rabbits)
   No. of animals: 9

2. Administration
   Route: The test article is injected into the M. vastus lateralis of each rabbit.
   Dose: The dose selected is chosen to evaluate the severity of irritation and represents a concentration that might be used clinically. This volume has been widely used in irritation testing.
   Frequency: Once only.
   Duration: 1 day.
   Volume: 1.0 ml/site.

3. Test system
   Species, age, and weight range: Male New Zealand White rabbits, weighing 2–5 kg, are used. The New Zealand White rabbit has been widely used in muscle irritation research for many years and is a reasonably sized, even-tempered animal which is well adapted to the laboratory environment.
   Selection: Animals to be used in the study are selected on the basis of acceptable findings from physical examinations and body weights.
   Randomization: Animals are ranked by body weight and assigned a number between 1 and 3. The order of numbers assigned (e.g., 1–3–2) is chosen from a table of random numbers. Animals assigned number 1 are

in the 24-hr posttreatment group, those assigned number 2 are in the 48-hr posttreatment group, and those assigned number 3 are in the 72-hr posttreatment group.

4. In-life observations

Daily observations: Once daily following dosing.

Physical examinations: Once within the 2 weeks before the first dosing day.

Body weight: Should be determined once before the start of the study.

Additional examinations may be done by the study director to elucidate any observed clinical signs.

5. Postmortem procedures

Irritation is evaluated as follows: Three rabbits are sacrificed by a lethal dose of barbiturate at approximately 24, 48, or 72 hr after dosing. The left and right vastus lateralis muscles of each rabbit are excised. The lesions resulting from injections are scored for muscle irritation on a numerical scale of 0–5 as follows:

Scoring of intramuscular irritation (Shintani *et al.*, 1967)

Reaction criteria	Score
No discernible gross reaction.	0
Slight hyperemia and discoloration.	1
Moderate hyperemia and discoloration.	2
Distinct discoloration in comparison with the color of the surrounding area.	3
Brown degeneration with small necrosis.	4
Widespread necrosis with an appearance of "cooked meat" and occasionally an abscess involving the major portions of the muscle.	5

Average score	Grade
0.0–0.4	None
0.5–1.4	Slight
1.5–2.4	Mild
2.5–3.4	Moderate
3.5–4.4	Marked
4.5 or greater	Severe

SHINTANI METHOD (SHINTANI ET AL., 1967)

1. Overview of study design

Rabbits will be injected as follows:

Group	No. of animals	Treatment site	Treatment	Evaluation
1	2	M. vastus lateralis (left) and cervicodorsal subcutis (left)	_____	24 hr
		M. vastus lateralis (right) and cervicodorsal subcutis	_____	24 hr
2	2	M. vastus lateralis (left) and cervicodorsal subcutis (left)	_____	72 hr
		M. vastus lateralis (right) and cervicodorsal subcutis (right)	_____	72 hr
3	2	Auricular vein (left)	_____	24- and 72-hr evaluations
		Auricular vein (right)	_____	

Day 1: Injection of all groups (6 rabbits)

Day 2: Evaluation of group 3 (2 rabbits); sacrifice and evaluation of group 1 (2 rabbits)

Day 4: Evaluation of group 3 (2 rabbits); sacrifice and evaluation of group 2 (2 rabbits)

2. Administration

Intramuscular: M. vastus lateralis.

Subcutaneous: cervicodorsal subcutis.

Intravenous: auricular vein.

Dose: The doses and concentration selected are chosen to evaluate the severity of irritation. The dose volumes have been widely used in irritation testing.

Frequency: Once only.

Duration: 1 day.

Volume: M. vastus lateralis and cervicodorsal subcutis, 1.0 ml/site; auricular vein; 0.5 ml/site.

3. Test system

Species, age, and weight range: Male New Zealand White rabbits, weighing 2–5 kilograms, are used.

Selection: Animals to be used in the study are selected on the basis of acceptable findings from physical examinations.

Randomization

Assignment to treatment groups: Animals are ranked by body weight and assigned a number between 1 and 3. The order of numbers assigned (e.g., 1–3–2) is chosen from a table of random numbers. Animals assigned number 1 are in group 1, those assigned number 2 are in group 2, and those assigned number 3 are in group 3.

4. In-life observations

Daily observations: Once daily following dosing.

Physical examinations: Once within the 2 weeks before the first dosing day.

Body weight: Determined once before the start of the study.

Additional examinations may be done by the study director to elucidate any observed clinical signs.

5. Postmortem procedures

Intramuscular irritation is evaluated as follows: Rabbits are sacrificed by a lethal dose of barbiturate approximately 24 and 72 hr after dosing. The left and right vastus lateralis muscles of each rabbit are excised. The reaction resulting from injection is scored for muscle irritation on a scale of 0–5 as follows:

Scoring of intramuscular irritation (Shintani *et al.*, 1967)

Reaction criteria	Score
No discernible gross reaction.	0
Slight hyperemia and discoloration.	1
Moderate hyperemia and discoloration.	2
Distinct discoloration in comparison with the color of the surrounding area.	3
Brown degeneration with small necrosis.	4
Widespread necrosis with an appearance of "cooked meat" and occasionally an abscess involving the major portions of the muscle.	5

Subcutaneous irritation is evaluated as follows: Rabbits are sacrificed by a lethal dose of barbiturate approximately 24 and 72 hr after dosing. The subcutaneous injection sites are exposed by dissection, and the reaction is scored for irritation on a scale of 0–5 as follows:

Scoring of subcutaneous irritation

Reaction criteria	Score
No discernible gross reaction.	0
Slight hyperemia and discoloration.	1
Moderate hyperemia and discoloration.	2
Distinct discoloration in comparison with the surrounding area.	3
Small areas of necrosis.	4
Widespread necrosis, possibly involving the underlying muscle.	5

Average score	Grade
0.0–0.4	None
0.5–1.4	Slight
1.5–2.4	Mild
2.5–3.4	Moderate
3.5–4.4	Marked
4.5 or greater	Severe

Intravenous irritation is evaluated as follows: Rabbits are sacrificed by a lethal dose of barbiturate following the 72-hr irritation evaluation. The injection site and surrounding tissue are grossly evaluated approximately 24 and 72 hr after dosing on a scale of 0–3 as follows:

Scoring of intravenous irritation

Reaction criteria	Score
No discernible gross reaction.	0
Slight erythema at injection site.	1
Moderate erythema and swelling with some discoloration of the vein and surrounding tissue.	2
Severe discoloration and swelling of the vein and surrounding tissue with partial or total occlusion of the vein.	3

Average score	Grade
0.0–0.4	None
0.5–1.4	Slight
1.5–2.4	Moderate
2.5 or greater	Severe

Additional examinations may be done by the study director to elucidate the nature of any observed tissue change.

ALTERNATIVES

The Shintani method is an acceptable and established procedure for routine evaluation of im irritation. However, the scoring is entirely a subjective evaluation and there is unavoidable discomfort for the test animals. It would be desirable to supplement the Shintani evaluation with another more objective index of muscle damage. Review of the literature in this area indicates that serum creatinine phosphokinase (CPK) analysis might serve the purpose of providing a more objective endpoint. The literature on CPK is summarized below.

Serum CPK is not a totally specific indicator of muscle damage. The CPK isoenzyme from skeletal muscle (MM), however, can be differentiated from those isoenzymes in heart (MB) and brain (BB).

Only MM CPK is elevated after im injection (Klein et al., 1973). Therefore, it may not be necessary to separate isoenzymes. However, if there is any possibility of myocardial or brain damage from the agent used, isoenzyme determination should be employed.

Although serum MM CPK is a good marker for muscle damage, it may reflect other factors. Exercise and stress are examples of some of the factors that may cause CPK elevation. Thus, handling of the animal may cause significant CPK elevation. Many investigators train their animals (i.e., acclimate the animals to handling) prior to use.

A method has been described that avoids nonspecific CPK elevation (Svendsen et al., 1979). The injection site is dissected and homogenized, and the CPK remaining in the muscle is determined and compared to the CPK activity in normal muscle. This procedure is advantageous because it is not necessary to train the animals. However, this procedure would be more labor-intensive because the injection site must be dissected and homogenized prior to CPK determination. This procedure would also prohibit evaluations of the irritation at 24 and 48 hr because muscle CPK depletion is only calculated 72 hr after dosing.

The time course of CPK elevation varies with species and the irritating agent (Steiness et al., 1978). In rabbits, serum CPK reaches a peak approximately 6 hr after the im injection and returns to normal between 48 and 72 hr after injection. Scoring of in vivo tests could thus be done by measuring evolved CPK levels.

Based on the information available on muscle CPK as a damage marker and on recent developments in tissue culture, three alternative models have been developed and proposed. The first of these uses chicken pectoral muscle as a model (Hem et al., 1975), with the actual end point still being a subjective grading of observed tissue irritation. This model is reported to give results comparable to those of the rabbit model.

The second alternative utilizes the paw of the rat as an alternative model and uses a measurement of the paw-licking response of the animal as an evaluation criteria (Celozzi et al., 1980). This method is reported to give results comparable to those from the rabbit model and is not terminal to the animal (Comereski et al., 1986).

The last current alternative is a truly in vitro one, utilizing a cultured rat skeletal muscle cell line (the L6) as a model and measuring creatine kinase levels in media afterwards as an evaluation endpoint. It is reported to give results which are positively rank correlated with those of the in vivo model for antibiotics (Williams et al., 1987).

PYROGENICITY

The United States Pharmacopeia describes a pyrogen test using rabbits as a model. This test is the standard for limiting risks of a febrile reaction to an acceptable level and involves measuring the rise in body temperature in a group of three rabbits for 3 hr after injection of 10 ml of test solution.

APPARATUS AND DILUENTS

Render the syringes, needles, and glassware free from pyrogens by heating at 250°F for not less than 30 min or by any other suitable method. Treat all diluents and solutions for washing and rinsing of devices or parenteral injection assemblies in a manner that will ensure that they are sterile and pyrogen-free. Periodically perform control pyrogen tests on representative portions of the diluents and solutions for washing or rinsing of the apparatus.

TEMPERATURE RECORDING

Use an accurate temperature-sensing device, such as a clinical thermometer, or thermistor probes or similar probes that have been calibrated to ensure an accuracy of $\pm 0.1°C$ and have been tested to determine that a maximum reading is reached in less than 5 min. Insert the temperature-sensing probe into the rectum of the test rabbit to a depth of not less than 7.5 cm and, after a period of time, not less than that previously determined as sufficient, record the rabbit's temperature.

TEST ANIMALS

Use healthy, mature rabbits. House the rabbits individually in an area of uniform temperature between 20 and 23°C and free from disturbances likely to excite them. The temperature should vary no more than $\pm 3°C$ from the selected temperature. Before using a rabbit for the first time in a pyrogen test, condition it not more than 7 days before use by a sham test that includes all of the steps as directed under Procedure, except injection. Do not use a rabbit for pyrogen testing more frequently than once every 48 hr, prior to 2 weeks following a maximum rise of its temperature of 0.6°C or more while being subjected to the pyrogen test, or following its having been given a test specimen that was adjusted to be pyrogenic.

Procedure

Perform the test in a separate area designated solely for pyrogen testing and under environmental conditions similar to those under which the animals are housed and free from disturbances likely to excite them. Withhold all food from the rabbits used during the period of the test. Access to water is allowed at all times but may be restricted during the test. If rectal temperature measuring probes remain inserted throughout the testing period, restrain the rabbits with light-fitting Elizabethan collars that allow the rabbits to assume a natural resting posture. Not more than 30 min prior to the injection of the test dose, determine the "control temperature" of each rabbit; this is the base for the determination of any temperature increase resulting from the injection of a test solution. In any one group of test rabbits, use only those rabbits whose control temperatures do not vary by more than 1°C from each other, and do not use any rabbit having a temperature exceeding 39.8°C.

Unless otherwise specified in the individual protocol, inject into an ear vein of each of three rabbits 10 ml of the test solution per kilogram of body weight, completing each injection within 10 min after the start of administration. The test solution is either the product, constituted if necessary as directed in the labeling, or the material under test. For pyrogen testing of devices or injection assemblies, use washings or rinsings of the surfaces that come in contact with the parenterally administered material or with the injection site or internal tissues of the patient. Ensure that all test solutions are protected from contamination. Perform the injection after warming the test solution to a temperature of 37 ± 2°C. Record the temperature at 1, 2, and 3 hr subsequent to the injection.

Test Interpretation and Continuation

Consider any temperature decreases as zero rise. If no rabbit shows an individual rise in temperature of 0.6°C or more above its respective control temperature, and if the sum of the three individual maximum temperature rises does not exceed 1.4°C, the product meets the requirements for the absence of pyrogens. If any rabbit shows an individual temperature rise of 0.6°C or more, or if the sum of the three individual maximum temperature rises exceeds 1.4°C, continue the test using five other rabbits. If not more than three of the eight rabbits show individual rises in temperature of 0.6°C or more, and if the sum of the eight individual maximum temperature rises does not exceed 3.7°C, the material under examination meets the requirements for the absence of pyrogens.

An alternative for pyrogen testing has recently been accepted not only for in-process control for pharmaceutical products but also for release testing of such products and for devices. It is an *in vitro* test based on the gelling or color development of a pyrogenic preparation in the presence of the lysate of the amebocytes of the horseshoe crab (*Limulus polyphemus*). The Limulus test, as it is called, is simpler, more rapid, and of greater sensitivity than the rabbit test (Cooper, 1975). Although it detects only the endotoxic pyrogens of gram-negative bacteria, this probably will not significantly limit its use because most environmental contaminants gaining entrance to sterile products are gram negative.

BLOOD COMPATIBILITY

The standard test (and its major modifications) currently used for this purpose is technically an *in vitro* one, but it requires a sample of fresh blood from a dog or other large donor animal. The test was originally developed by The National Cancer Institute for use in evaluating cancer chemotherapeutic agents (Prieur *et al.*, 1973) and is rather crude, though definitive.

The variation described here is one commonly utilized. It uses human blood from volunteers, eliminating the need to keep a donor colony of dogs. This test procedure is described below.

1. Test system: Human blood. Collect 30 ml heparinized blood for whole blood and plasma (3 tubes) and 30 ml clotted blood for serum (2 tubes) from each of 6 donors.

2. Precipitation potential

For each donor, set up and label 8 tubes: 1–8.

Add 1 ml serum to tubes 1–4.

Add 1 ml plasma to tubes 5–8.

Add 1 ml formulation to tubes 1 and 5.

Add 1 ml vehicle to tubes 2 and 6.

Add 1 ml physiological saline to tubes 3 and 7 (negative control).

Add 1 ml 2% nitric acid to tubes 4 and 8 (positive control).

Observe tubes 1–8 for qualitative reactions (e.g., precipitation or clotting) before and after mixing.

If a reaction is observed in the formulation tubes (tubes 1 and/or 5), dilute the formulation in an equal amount of physiological saline ($\frac{1}{2}$ dilution) and test 1 ml of the dilution with an equal amount of plasma and/or serum. If a reaction still occurs, make serial dilutions of the formulation in saline (i.e., $\frac{1}{4}$, $\frac{1}{8}$, etc.).

If a reaction occurs in the vehicle tubes (tubes 2 and/or 6), repeat in a manner similar to (2).

3. Hemolytic potential

For each donor, set up and label 8 tubes: 1–8.

Add 1 ml whole blood to each tube.

Add 1 ml formulation to tube 1.

Add 1 ml vehicle to tube 2.

Add 1 ml of $\frac{1}{2}$ dilution of formulation in saline to tube 3.

Add 1 ml of $\frac{1}{2}$ dilution of vehicle in saline to tube 4.

Add 1 ml of $\frac{1}{4}$ dilution of formulation in saline to tube 5.

Add 1 ml of $\frac{1}{4}$ dilution of vehicle in saline to tube 6.

Add 1 ml physiological saline to tube 7 (negative control).

Add 1 ml distilled water to tube 8 (positive control).

Mix by gently inverting each tube three times.

Incubate tubes for 45 min 37°C.

Centrifuge 5 min 1000g.

Separate the supernate from the sediment.

Determine hemoglobin concentrations to the nearest 0.1 g/dl on the supernate (plasma).

If hemoglobin concentrations of the above dilutions are 0.2 g/dl (or more) greater than the saline control, repeat the procedure, adding 1 ml of further serial dilutions ($\frac{1}{8}$, $\frac{1}{16}$, etc.) of formulation or vehicle to 1 ml of blood until the hemoglobin level is within 0.2 g/dl of the saline control.

There are two proposed, true *in vitro* alternatives to this procedure (Mason *et al.*, 1974; Kambic *et al.*, 1976), but neither has been either widely evaluated or accepted.

VAGINAL IRRITATION

Few, if any, products are administered via the vagina that are intended for systemic absorption. Thus, this route has not been as widely studied and characterized as others. On the other hand, large numbers of different products (douches, spermicides, antiyeast agents, etc.) have been developed that require introduction into the vagina in order to assert their localized effects. Increased research into different birth control and antiviral prophylaxis will result in more vaginal products in the future. All these must be assessed for vaginal irritation potential.

Considerable research (Eckstein *et al.*, 1969; Auletta, 1994) has indicated that the rabbit is the best species for assessing vaginal irritation. There are those investigators, however, who consider the rabbit too sensitive and recommend the use of ovariectomized rats. Ovariectomy results in a uniformly thin, uncornified epithelium which is more responsive to localized effects. This model is used when the results from a study with rabbits are questionable

(Auletta, 1994). The routine progression of studies consists of first doing an acute primary vaginal irritation study, then a 10-day repeated dose study in rabbits, followed (if necessary) by a repeated dose study in rats. These protocols are summarized below. Longer-term vaginal studies have been conducted in order to assess systemic toxicity of the active agents, when administered by these routes (while the intended effects may be local, one cannot assume that there will be no systemic exposure).

ACUTE PRIMARY VAGINAL IRRITATION STUDY IN THE FEMALE RABBIT

1. Overview of study design: One group of six adult rabbits received a single vaginal exposure and observed for 3 days with periodic examination (1, 24, 48, and 72 hr postdosing) of the genitalia. Animals are then euthanized and the vagina is examined macroscopically.

2. Administration
   Route: The material is generally introduced directly into the vagina using a lubricated 18 French rubber catheter attached to a syringe for quantification and delivery of the test material. Gentle placement of the catheter is important because one needs to ensure complete delivery of the dose without mechanical trauma. For rabbits, the depth of insertion is about 7.5 cm, and the catheter should be marked to about that depth. After delivery is completed, the tube is slowly withdrawn. No attempt is made to close or seal the vaginal orifice. Alternative methods may be used to administer more viscous materials. The most common is to backload a lubricated 1-ml tuberculine syringe, then warm the material to close to body temperature. The syringe is then inserted into the vagina and the dose administered by depressing the syringe plunger.
   Dosage: The test material should be one (concentration, vehicle, etc.) that is intended for human application.
   Frequency: once.
   Duration: 1 day.
   Volume: 1 ml per rabbit.

3. Test system
   Species, age, and weight range: Sexually mature New Zealand White rabbits are generally used, weighing between 2 and 5 kg. The weight is not as important as the fact that the animals need to be sexually mature.
   Selection: Animals should be nuliparous and nonpregnant. Animals should be healthy and free of external genital lesions.
   Randomization: Because there is only one group of animals, randomization is not a critical issue.

TABLE A   Scoring Criteria for Vaginal Irritation

Value	
	Erythema
0	No erythema
1	Very slight erythema (barely perceptible)
2	Slight erythema (pale red in color)
3	Moderate to severe erythema (definite red in color)
4	Severe erythema (beet or crimson red)
	Edema
0	No edema
1	Very slight edema (barely perceptible)
2	Slight edema (edges of area well defined by definite raising)
3	Moderate edema (raised approximately 1 mm)
4	Severe edema (raised more than 1 mm and extending beyond area of exposure)
	Discharge
0	No discharge
1	Very slight discharge
2	Slight discharge
3	Moderate discharge
4	Severe discharge (moistening of considerable area around vagina)

4. In-life observations

Daily observations: At least once daily for clinical signs.

Detailed Physical Examination: Once during the week prior to dosing.

Body weight: Day of dosing.

Vaginal irritation: Scored at 1, 24, 48, and 72 hr postdosing. Scoring criteria are shown in Table A.

5. Postmortem procedures: Rabbits are euthanized by lethal dose of a barbiturate soon after the last vaginal irritation scores are collected. The vagina is opened by longitudinal section and examined for evidence of mucosal damage such as erosion, localized hemorrhage, etc. No other tissues are examined. No tissues are collected. After the macroscopic description of the vagina is recorded, the animal is discarded.

Repeated Dose Vaginal Irritation in the Female Rabbit

1. Overview of Study Design: Four groups of five adult rabbits each receive a single vaginal exposure daily for 10 days. The genitalia are examined daily. Animals are then euthanized and the vagina is examined macroscopically and microscopically.

2. Administration

Route: The test materials are introduced directly into the vagina using a lubricated 18 French rubber catheter, using the techniques described previously for acute studies.

Dosage: The test material should be one (concentration, vehicle, etc.) that is intended for human application. There will also be a sham-negative control (catheter in place but nothing administered), a vehicle control, and a positive control (generally 2% nonoxynol-9).

Frequency: once daily.

Duration: 10 days.

Volume: 1 ml per rabbit for each material.

3. Test system

Species, age, and weight range: Sexually mature New Zealand White rabbits are generally used, weighing between 2 and 5 kg. The weight is not as important as the fact that the animals need to be sexually mature.

Selection: Animals should be nuliparous and nonpregnant. Animals should be healthy and free of external genital lesions.

Randomization: At least 24 animals should be on pretest. Randomization to treatment groups is best done using a computerized blocking by body weight method or a random number generation method.

4. In-life observations

Daily observations: At least once daily for clinical signs.

Detailed physical examination: Once during the week prior to dosing and immediately prior to necropsy.

Body weight: First, fifth, and last day of dosing.

Vaginal irritation: Scored once daily. Scoring criteria shown in Table A.

5. Postmortem procedures: Rabbits are euthanized by lethal dose of a barbiturate soon after the last vaginal irritation scores are collected. The vagina is isolated using standard prosection techniques and then opened by longitudinal section and examined for evidence of mucosal damage such as erosion, localized hemorrhage, etc. No other tissues are examined. The vagina and cervix are collected and fixed in 10% neutral buffered formalin. Standard hematoxylin/eosin stained, paraffin-embedded histologic glass slides are prepared by routine methods. Three levels of the vagina (low, mid, and upper) are examined and graded using the scoring system shown in Table B. Each level is scored separately and an average is calculated. Irritation is rated as follows:

Score	Rating
0	Nonirritating
1–4	Minimal irritation
5–8	Mild irritation
9–11	Moderate irritation
12–16	Marked irritation

TABLE B   Microscopic Scoring Procedure for Vaginal Sections[a]

	Value
Epithelium	
Intact–normal	0
Cell degeneration or flattening of the epithelium	1
Metaplasia	2
Focal erosion	3
Erosion or ulceration, generalized	4
Leukocytes	
Minimal—<25 per high-power field	1
Mild—25–50 per high-power field	2
Moderate—50–100 per high-power field	3
Marked—>100 per high-power field	4
Injection	
Absent	0
Minimal	1
Mild	2
Moderate	3
Marked with disruption of vessels	4
Edema	
Absent	0
Minimal	1
Mild	2
Moderate	3
Marked	4

[a]From Eckstein et al. (1969).

The score for each rabbit is then averaged and acceptability ratings are given as follows:

Average score	Acceptability ratings
0–8	Acceptable
9–10	Marginal
11 or greater	Unacceptable

REPEATED DOSE VAGINAL IRRITATION IN THE OVARIECTOMIZED RATS

This study is very similar in design to that described previously for rabbits, with the following (sometimes obvious) exceptions. Mature ovariectomized female rats can be obtained from a commercial breeder. A 15% surplus should be obtained. Ten animals per group should be used (40 total for the study).

The vaginal catheter is placed to a depth of approximately 2.5 cm and the treatment volume should be 0.2 ml.

REFERENCES

Auletta, C. (1994). Vaginal and rectal administration. *J. Am. Col. Toxicol.* **13**, 48–63.

Avis, K. E. (1985). Parenteral preparations. In *Remington's Pharmaceutical Sciences* (A. R. Gennaro, Ed.), pp. 1518–1541, Mack, Easton, PA.

Ballard, B. E. (1968). Biopharmaceutical considerations in subcutaneous and intramuscular drug administration. *J. Pharm. Sci.* **57**, 357–378.

Celozzi, E., Lotti, V. J., Stapley, E. O., and Miller, A. K. (1980). An animal model for assessing pain-on-injection of antibiotics. *J. Pharm. Methods* **4**, 285–289.

Comereski, C. R., William, P. D., Bregman, C. L., and Hottendorf, G. H. (1986). Pain on injection and muscle irritation: A comparison of animal models for assessing parenteral antibiotics. *Fundam. Appl. Toxicol.* **6**, 335–338.

Cooper, J. F. (1975). *Bull. Parenteral Drug Assoc.* **29**, 122.

Eckstein, P., Jackson, M., Millman, N., and Sobero, A. (1969). Comparison of vaginal tolerance tests of spermical preparations in rabbits and monkeys. *J. Reprod. Fertil.* **20**, 85–93.

Garramone, J. P. (1986). *Vascular Access Port Model SLA Users Manual.* Norfolk Medical Products, Skokie, IL.

Gray, J. E. (1978). Pathological evaluation of injection injury. In *Sustained and Controlled Release Drug Delivery System* (J. Robinson, Ed.), pp. 351–405. Dekker, New York.

Hagan, E. C. (1959). *Appraisal of the Safety of Chemicals in Foods, Drugs and Cosmetics,* p. 19. Association of Food and Drug Officials of the United States, Austin, TX.

Hem, S. L., Bright, D. R., Banker, G. S., and Pogue, J. P. (1975). Tissue irritation evaluation of potential parenteral vehicles. *Drug Dev. Commun.* **1**, 471–477.

Kambic, H. E., Kiraly, R. J., and Yukihiko, N. (1976). A simple *in vitro* screening test for blood compatibility of materials. *J. Biomed. Mat. Res. Symp.* **7**, 561–570.

Klein, M. S., Shell, W. E., and Sobel, B. E. (1973). Serum creatine phosphokinase (CPK) isoenzymes after intramuscular injections, surgery, and myocardial infarction. Experimental and clinical studies. *Card. Res.* **7**, 412–418.

Mason, R. G., Shermer, R. W., Zucker, W. H., Elston, R. C., and Blackwelder, W. C. (1974). An *in vitro* test system for estimation of blood compatibility of biomaterials. *J. Biomed. Mat. Res.* **8**, 341–356.

Prieur, D. J., Young, D. M., Davis, R. D., Cooney, D. A., Homan, E. R., Dixon, R. L., and Guarino, A. M. (1973). Procedures for preclinical toxicologic evaluation of cancer chemotherapeutic agents: Protocols of the laboratory of toxicology. *Cancer Chemother. Rep. Part 3* **4**, 1–30.

Schwartz, M. L., Meyer, M. B., Covino, B. G., and Narang, R. M. (1974). Antiarrhythmic effectiveness of intramuscular lidocaine: Influence of different injection sites. *J. Clin. Pharmacol.* **14**, 77–83.

Shintani, S., Yamazaki, M., Nakamura, M., and Nakayama, I. (1967). A new method to determine the irritation of drugs after intramuscular injection in rabbits. *Toxicol. Appl. Pharmacol.* **11**, 293–301.

Steiness, E., Rasmussen, F., Svendsen, O., and Nielsen, P. (1978). A comparative study of serum creatine phosphokinase (CPK) activity in rabbits, pigs and humans after intramuscular injection of local damaging drugs. *Acta Pharmacol. Toxicol.* **42**, 357–364.

Svendsen, O., Rasmussen, F., Nielsen, P., and Steiness, E. (1979). The loss of creatine phosphokinase (CPK) from intramuscular injection sites in rabbits. A predictive tool for local toxicity. *Acta Pharmacol. Toxicol.* **44**, 324–328.

Theeuwes, F., and Yum, S. I. (1976). Principles of the design and operation of generic osmotic pumps for the delivery of semisolid or liquid drug formulations. *Ann. Biomed. Eng.* **4**, 343–353.

United States Pharmacopeia (USP) (1995). *The United States Pharmacopeia,* pp. 1718–1719. U.S. Pharmacopeial Convention, Rockville, MD.

Williams, P. D., Masters, B. C. Evans, L. D., Laska, D. A., and Hottendorf, G. H. (1987). An *in vitro* model for assessing muscle irritation due to parenteral antibiotics. *Fundam. Appl. Toxicol.* **9**, 10–17.

CHAPTER 9

Systemic Acute Toxicity Testing

It is unfortunate that the terms acute lethality testing and acute toxicity have become synonomous. There is indeed a difference that we would like to stress in this book. As described by Zbinden and Flury-Roversi (1981) and Zbinden (1986) the classical LD_{50} test has several shortcomings, not the least of which is that there is no good correlation between mortality and morbidity. In fact, the Food and Drug Administration (FDA) expects to see more than lethality data in acute toxicity studies (FDA, 1984) and no longer expects or desires to see pure lethality (LD_{50}) data. The Pharmaceutical Manufacturers Association has taken a similar position (LeBeau, 1983) in that acute toxicity testing should encompass more than LD_{50} determinations. The regulatory requirements for acute toxicity data, including lethality, are included in Tables 28A, 28B, 29A, and 29B in Chapter 7 and were also reviewed by Auletta (1988).

In concise terms, lethality testing is single-endpoint testing with death as the single endpoint. Acute testing is generally multi-endpoint testing and has as its objective the more complete characterization of the acute biological effects of a chemical free of chronicity and/or test article accumulation considerations. The Organization for Economic Cooperation and Development

(OECD) guidelines define acute toxicity as the adverse effects occurring within a short time of administration of a single dose of a substance or multiple doses given within 24 hr (OECD, 1981; Chan *et al.*, 1982). Such effects include not only lethality but also accompanying clinical signs and target organs. These data are probably of greater value in making safety decisions than the LD_{50} because, although lethal dosages will vary considerably between species, target organs are fairly uniform between species (Zbinden, 1983). Defining target organs may include not only gross and microscopic examinations but also specialized function testing such as behavioral tests. Because such testing requires that the test article enters the general systemic circulation, this type of testing is logically called acute systemic toxicity testing. In Chapter 7, the methodologies available for lethality testing were described. Here the additions and modifications to these protocols are described that permit more broad scope ("shotgun") toxicity testing. Special features of acute studies performed by the inhalation route are discussed in Chapter 13.

Acute systemic toxicity testing is largely descriptive in nature. There are occasions when more mechanistic data are required, and these types of studies are discussed in the last section of this chapter. Various needs exist for acute toxicity data. First, they are needed to support marketing registration. The regulatory uses of acute toxicity are discussed in detail by LaFlamme (1983) and Osterberg (1983). Second, acute toxicity testing also provides the information for describing a chemical's acute toxic syndrome so that intoxicated patients can be diagnosed and treated. Other health professionals, such as environmental toxicologists and industrial hygienists, also require acute toxicity data. For example, acute toxicity data are required for the completion of material safety data sheets. Third, acute toxicity data provide a basis for planning repeated dose studies, although they are rarely done for this reason alone because there are often large differences between acute and chronic toxic dosages (Brown, 1983). Fourth, for small-volume, nonpharmaceutical chemicals, an extensive acute toxicity test may be the only work done to define systemic toxicity, or any biological activity for that matter. These, and other uses of acute toxicity data, are detailed in Table 39.

Acute toxicity tests generally are performed with a definite sequence. First, a family of closely related chemicals will be exposed to a battery of screens to choose a candidate with the most desirable properties. Screens may be toxicological or pharmacological in nature. Once a candidate is identified for development, more extensive toxicity tests will be performed and a definitive acute toxicity test will be among the first done. Finally, specific mechanistic studies will be done to better define toxicity or to examine a specific safety question, such as the effects of combined drug treatment. These different protocols are discussed in the sections that follow.

The FDA generally requires acute toxicity data to be included in a new

TABLE 39   Purpose of Acute Systemic Toxicity Testing

Biological
Standardization of potent, biological drugs
Information on general poisonous potential of chemicals
Determination of therapeutic index of new drugs
Dosage range for Longer Duration Toxicity Test
Specific biological characterization, e.g., Tachyphylaxis
Information on bioavailability
Identification of potential target organs
Screens for selection of chemicals for development
Safety
Prediction of lethal dose in human beings
Prediction of symptomatology, reversibility, and possible treatment of human intoxication
Predict hazards of drug combinations
Hazard assessment for specific patient classes, e.g., neonates
Setting exposure limits for chemicals in the work place
Government regulations
Integral part of registration documents
Basic information for classification poisons
Completion of material safety data sheets
Other
Models for exploration of basic biological phenomena
Models for interaction studies between environmental factors and chemical toxins
Describe mechanisms of toxicity identified postmarketing in human beings

Note. In part, from Zbinden (1984).

drug application. The acute studies should be done with the intended clinical or market formulation. Generally, the routes of administration should include both PO and the intended clinical route (if not PO). The agency's intent is to ensure the availability of information to describe an overdose and/or accidental exposure situation. In general, data in at least one rodent (generally the rat) and one nonrodent (dog or nonhuman primate) will be expected.

There has been some recent discussion on whether or not single-dose (i.e., acute) toxicity studies should be used to support single-dose bioavailability and tolerance studies in human subjects (Monro and Mehta, 1966; Choudary et al., 1996). Currently, 2-week repeated-dose toxicity studies are generally the minimum expected to support initial clinical trial. Altering this guideline would represent a major change, especially given the success of the current system in protecting human subjects in initial clinical trials. As of this writing, the status and progress of this proposal is not known.

Imaging agents represent a special case in which single-dose studies are currently accepted to support single-dose clinical trials. Given their intended use, it is rare that imaging or contrast agents would be given repeatedly over long periods of time. Well-conducted complete acute studies in two species (generally the rat and rabbit) will be sufficient to support the general toxicology requirement for an Investigational New Drug Application.

The FDA has published revised guidelines for Acute Toxicity testing [*Fed. Reg.* 61 (166), 43 934 26 Aug. 1996]. Studies in animals should ordinarily be conducted using two routes of administration: the intended human clinical route and the intravenous route, if feasible. Studies should be conducted in two species—rodent and nonrodent. The recommended protocols for rodents are best described as supplemented acute protocols.

SCREENS

Screens are not safety studies in the regulatory sense. They are the studies done, as the name implies, to examine several chemicals in order to select those with the most desirable properties for development or eliminate those that have undesirable properties. There is nothing novel about screening; the process has been an integral part of pharmaceutical research for decades (Irwin, 1962). In a pioneering paper, Smyth and Carpenter (1944) described a screening process for gathering preliminary data on the oral, dermal, and inhalation toxicity of a chemical. In their discussion they clearly state the underlying rationale for toxicity screening,

> Opinions upon the toxicity, hazards of manufacture, and fields for safe use must be expressed regarding many chemicals which will never be produced in quantity. Large expenditures of time and money upon securing these basic conclusions is nost justified. Later, when a few of the new compounds are obviously going to be made commercially, more detailed studies can be undertaken (pp. 270).

Screens are designed for speed, simplicity, and minimal resource expenditure. They are designed to answer positive, single-sided questions. Whatever the outcome, it will be confirmed or invalidated by future studies. For example, lack of effect in an initial screen does not mean that toxicity will not be manifested with a different formulation or in a different species. It is for this reason that screens should not, as stated by Zbinden *et al.* (1984), be seen as replacements for thorough safety testing. An acute toxicity screen is normally the first leg in a decision tree or tier testing process for selecting a chemical or drug candidate for development. An example of this process is given in Fig. 35.

GENERAL TOXICITY

There are three types of toxicity screens. The first is the general toxicity screen. In this type of study, animals (often, for economic reasons, mice) are exposed

**EXAMPLE OF USE OF SCREENS IN SELECTING
DRUG CANDIDATES FOR DEVELOPMENT**

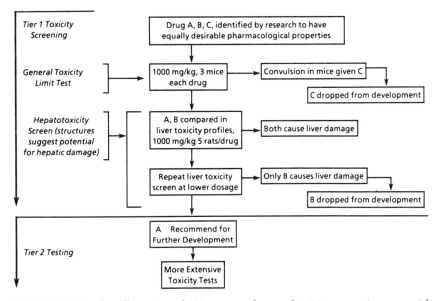

FIGURE 35   Flowchart illustrating a decision tree to the use of toxicity screens in commercial compound development.

to two or three predefined dosages of chemical. No more than three mice per dosage are necessary and no control group is required. An example of this type of protocol is shown in Fig. 36. It obviously resembles the traditional acute lethality test. The animals are carefully observed for death and obvious signs of toxicity, such as convulsions. No attempt should be made to quantify the severity of a response. There is seldom any need to have an observation period of more than 4 or 5 days. Because of the quantal nature of the data, interpretation is straightforward. There are four possible outcomes: (1) No death or signs of toxicity seen at dosages up to _____; (2) there were no deaths, but evident signs of toxicity seen at _____; (3) there were evident signs of toxicity at _____ and deaths at _____; and (4) deaths and evident signs of toxicity both occurred at _____ . These types of tests may also provide the preliminary information for picking the dosages for more definitive actue studies.

Using these data, there are two ways to determine how to proceed with the development of a drug or chemical. On a relative basis, the drugs or chemicals under consideration can be ranked according to screen results and the one

EXAMPLE OF GENERAL TOXICITY SCREEN

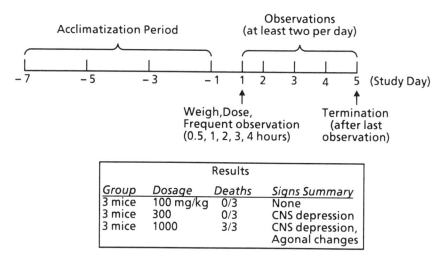

FIGURE 36   Line chart for the design and conduct of a general toxicity screen.

that appears to be the least toxic can be chosen for future development. Alternatively, decisions can be made on an absolute basis. All candidates that are positive below a certain dosage are dropped, and all those that are negative at or above that dosage will continue to the next tier of testing. If absolute criteria are used, the screen need be done only at the critical dosage. If only one dosage is examined, the test is a limit test. A limit test of this kind is the simplest form of toxicity screen and, depending on the nature of subsequent testing, it is highly recommended.

Fowler and colleagues (1979) have described a rat toxicity screen (illustrated in Fig. 37) which is more extensive and detailed than the one previously described. It includes two rounds of dosing. In the first round, up to 12 rats are (singly) exposed to six different dosages by two different routes for the purpose of defining the maximally tolerated dose (MTD). In the second round of dosing, 16 rats are dosed at (0.60) MTD and sacrificed on a serially timed basis for blood sample collections for test article concentration determinations and clinical laboratory tests. In our opinion, these features make this design too complicated, time-consuming, and expensive to run as an initial screen. This type of test is better suited to second-tier screening. We recommend that one use the data from the first screen to design the more extensive follow-up study to include fewer dosages and interim sacrifice points. Fowler *et al.*

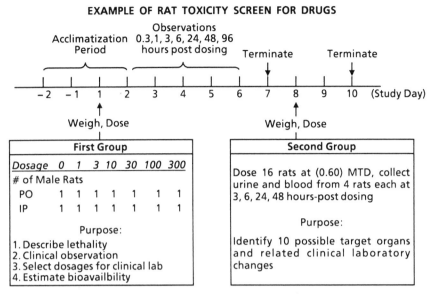

FIGURE 37   Line chart for the design and conduct of Fowler's style screen for acute toxicity screen for drugs (from Fowler *et al.*, 1979).

do conclude that their screen disclosed most toxicity uncovered by more conventional studies. This screen was most successful in defining acute CNS, liver, or kidney toxicity (Fowler *et al.*, 1979). Lesions that require long-term exposure, such as those generally involving the eyes, will not be detected in this type of screen.

Up-and-down or pyramiding designs can be used for these types of studies but generally are not because of the time involved. In addition, if several chemicals are being compared, an up-and-down study in which death occurs at different dosages can be complicated to run. It is much easier to test several chemicals at the same time using a limit test design. Because only individual animals are dosed, these designs can be used when there is a very limited amount of test article available and there is little prior data on which to base an unexpected toxic dosage.

Hazelette and colleagues (1987) described a rather novel pyramiding dosage screen that they term the rising dose tolerance (RDT) study (Fig. 38). The study uses a paraacute rather than an acute dosing regimen. The rats are exposed for 4 days to the initial dosage followed by 3 days of recovery before the next 4-day dosing period at the next highest dosage. This process is repeated for the three dosing cycles. Plasma and urine samples are collected for clinical

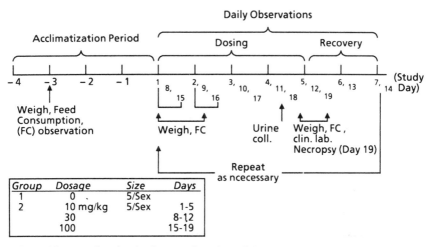

FIGURE 38   Line chart for the design and conduct of the Hazelette style rising dose tolerance study for acute systemic toxicity study.

chemistry and urinalysis as well as test article determinations. Necropsies and microscopic examinations are performed. While this study design is novel, it appears to provide considerable acute data. It is also possible that this design could generate sufficient data to plan a pivotal subchronic study and, therefore, replace a traditional 2-week study, resulting in considerable savings of time and animals. This is not a simple study and, therefore, not appropriate as an initial screen, but it would appear to be appropriate for a second tier-type test.

Specific Toxicity Screening

The second type of acute toxicity screen is the specific toxicity test. These are done when one has a specific toxicological concern. These types of test are done, for example, when one has a priori structure–activity data suggesting that a family of chemicals can be hepatotoxic. A screen to select the chemical with the least hepatotoxic potential is then in order. These tests are also done, as described by Zbinden (1983), to examine for a specific toxicological effect that may be easily overlooked in a routine safety study. He gives, as an example, screens that are designed to detect specific lesions to the hemostatic process. As pointed out by Irwin (1962) over two decades ago, such tests have their

three groups will be required. If more than one chemical is included in the study, then a single dosage (limit) group per chemical is the best design.

Strictly speaking, an acute toxicity study is conducted to examine the effect of a single dose of a single compound. In designing specific toxicity screens, however, deviation from this principle is permissible if it increases screen sensitivity. For example, the sensitivity of mice to most hepatotoxins will be enhanced by prior treatment with phenobarbital. Hence, the sensitivity of a hepatotoxicity screen will be enhanced if the mice are pretreated with pheno-barbital. Alternatively, some lesions require more than one exposure to the toxin to become fully manifested. For example, the authors discovered that the cardiotoxicity of a drug in development was not apparent after a single dose but would become well developed after three repeated high dosages. Screens to examine possible backup or replacement candidates were designed to include a 3-day dosage regimen. Hence, the use of response enhancers and/ or para-acute dosing regimens can be integral parts of an acute toxicity screen. The term subacute was originally used to refer to studies using dosages less than those used in acute studies. Currently, however, the term is frequently used to describe treatment periods of a few days. In fact, the terms subacute and subchronic have almost become synonomous: a state of affairs that lacks a certain amount of logic. We recommend that subacute be reserved for its original intention, that para-acute be used to describe dosing periods of a week or less, and that subchronic be used to described studies of 4–13 weeks of duration.)

While screens are designed for simplicity, the details of the protocol still have to be established and rigorously maintained. For example, the test animals should always be of the same species, age, and sex, and purchased from the same supplier. (Species other than the mouse are used when one has reason to believe that a different species substantially increases screen sensitivity.) The nutritional state of the animals (fed vs fasted) should always be the same. Incidently, it has often been stated that fasting of a few hours is sufficient for mice. We have critically assessed this assertion by comparing the stomach contents of mice denied feed versus those permitted to feed *ad libitum* during normal working hours. There were no differences. Evidently, because mice are nocturnal animals, they simply stop feeding when the room lights come on (most animals quarters are maintained on 12-hr light/dark cycles).

The screen should be validated for consistency of response with both positive and negative control articles. A positive control article is one which is known to reliably produce the toxic syndrome the screen is designed to detect. Concurrent control groups are not required. Rather, control groups should be evaluated on some regular basis to ensure that screen performance is stable (see Chapter 12). Because a screen does rely on a biological system, it is not a bad idea to test the control "benchmarks," particularly the positive, on a routine periodic basis. Not only does that give one increased confidence in the screen but it also provides an historical base against which to compare the results of new test articles. Zbinden and colleagues refer to positive control as the reference compound, and they have discussed some of the general criteria to be applied in the selection of reference compounds (Zbinden et al., 1984). Any changes to the protocol should trigger revalidation. Any analytical methods should be subjected to precision, accuracy, sensitivity, and selectivity validation.

Interpretation of specific toxicity screen data is not as straightforward as that of a general toxicity screen. This is because the data will often be continuous, following a Gaussian or normal distribution. This has two ramifications. First, for results around the threshold, it may be very difficult to differentiate between positive and negative responses. Second, for any one parameter, there is a real chance of false statistical significance (type I erorrs), especially if small numbers of animals are used. This is one of the reasons that specific toxicity screens should include more than one variable because it is unlikely for three false positives to occur in the same group of animals. An undetected false positive could lead to dropping a promising candidate in error. False negatives, on the other hand, may not be as critical (other than the time lost and the resources spent) because the more extensive subsequent tests should eventually lead to the discovery of the test article's toxic properties.

The problems described in the preceding paragraph assume that the screen will include a traditional ("negative" or vehicle) control group, and that the data from the test article treated groups will be compared to those of the control group by standard methods. These problems will be minimized if no control group and, therefore, no traditional statistical comparisons are included. In addition, the decrease in the number of animals used simplifies the study and decreases the number of animals required. Data can be interpreted by comparison to a historical control database as described by Zbinden (1984). The threshold, or test criterion, X_c, is calculated according to the following formula:

$$X_c = m + (z)s$$

where m is the population mean, s is the standard deviation, and z is an arbitrary constant. This is illustrated in Fig. 40. This is essentially a method of converting continuous data to quantal data: It is used to determine if individual animals are over the test threshold, not if the group mean is over the threshold. Analysis of screening data by comparison to experience (i.e., historical control data) and an activity criterion are discussed in greater detail in Chapter 12 and by Gad (1988). The higher the z value, the lower the probability of a false positive, but the lower the sensitivity of the screen. Again, including multiple parameters in the screen helps alleviate this problem. Zbinden has proposed a ranking procedure in which various levels of suspicion

SETTING THRESHOLDS USING HISTORICAL CONTROL DATA

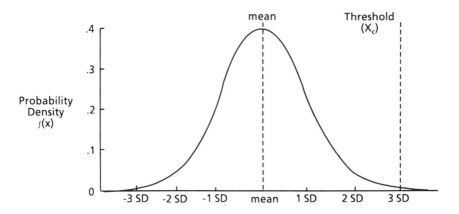

FIGURE 40   Graph illustrating use of historical control data to set screen activity criteria. Gaussian ("normal") distribution of screen parameter. 99.7% of the observations in the population are within three standard deviations (SD) of the historic mean. Here the threshold, i.e., the point at which a datum is outside of normal was set X_c = mean + 3 SD.

or a level of certainty are assigned to the result of a toxicity screen. This is simply a formalized fashion of stating that the more animals that respond and the greater the severity of the response, the more certainty one has in making a conclusion. If relative comparisons are being made, this system provides a framework for ranking test articles and selecting those to continue to the next tier of testing. On an absolute basis, however, such a ranking system is of limited usefulness. The test is either positive—that is, a majority of the animals at a dosage are over the threshold—or negative.

With regard to specific toxicity screening, behavioral toxicity screening is an area currently generating a great deal of interest. As reviewed by Hopper (1986), there are several reasons for this interest. First, the Toxic Substance Control Act (TSCA) of 1976 legislatively recognized behavioral measures as essential to examining chemicals for neurotoxic potential. Second the structure and function of the central nervous system are not amenable to traditional methods of examination in that profound behavioral changes can be induced in the absence of any detectable morphological lesions. This large and somewhat controversial subject is outside the scope of this chapter. Specific screening strategies are presented and critically discussed by Hopper (1986). Gad (1982) developed a neuromuscular screen that incorporates some simple behavioral assessments and has been subsequently modified and utilized [as the functional observation, battery, or (FOB)] as the fundamental neurotoxicity screen. This is discussed in greater detail in a subsequent section of this chapter.

ALTERNATIVES

Because toxicity testing can be expensive, and also because of the ethical considerations in testing in live animals, there is considerable interest in the use of alternative or *in vitro* methods of toxicity assessment. The greatest success in this area is in the use of mammalian cells or bacterial cultures in mutagenicity testing. Considerable progress, however, has also been made in the area of using mammalian cells for nongenetic toxicity testing. For example, in 1981 Stammati *et al.* published a review focusing on the literature through 1979 on the use of cell culture systems in assessing the toxic potential of chemicals; almost 400 references were cited (Stammati *et al.*, 1981).

Despite the progress made in this area, the use of *in vitro* methods for predicting toxicity or in making safety decisions is fraught with problems. First, in isolated cells, the integrative response of the intact organism in which the hormonal, hemostatic, or nervous system responses will effect toxicity is absent. Second, the role of metabolism and disposition toxicity cannot be assessed. Third, cells *in vitro* may not respond in the same fashion as those *in vivo*. The concentration of cytochrome P450 in isolated hepatocytes, for example, decreases rapidly following isolation unless special procedures are followed (Stark *et al.*, 1986).

The problems associated with using isolated cells for predicting lethality were discussed in Chapter 7. While the use of *in vitro* methods in general toxicity testing will require a great deal of additional work, these techniques can be used for identifying the potential for causing specific target organ damage. Hence, it is in the area of specific toxicity screening that alternative methods or *in vitro* investigation will probably be most useful. It is much simpler to investigate hepatotoxicity in isolated cells than in groups of rats and mice. Once a procedure or protocol is standardized, large numbers of chemicals can be screened at much less cost than would be incurred using more traditional *in vivo* methods. The reader is referred to reviews by Stark *et al.* (1986) and Greim *et al.* (1986) on this subject.

Currently, the use of *in vitro* methods for specific toxicity screening is of greatest value in ranking drugs or chemicals for specific target organ potential (as opposed to making absolute judgments about individual chemicals). Sorensen and Acosta (1985), for example, investigated and ranked several nonsteroidal anti-inflammatory drugs for hepatotoxic potential using rat hepatocyte cultures. Trypan blue exclusion, lactate dehydrogenase leakage, and urea synthesis, as well as histologic evaluation, were used to assess cytotoxicity. Excellent agreement between these different parameters was obtained. Indomethacin was the most hepatotoxic, while aspirin was "nontoxic," even though both have been reported to be clinically hepatotoxic in human subjects. Acosta and Ramos (1984) ranked four of the tricyclic antidepressants for cardiotoxic potential using cultures of myocardial cells, measuring LDH leakage, trypan blue exclusion, and beating rates. In contrast to the results obtained in the aforementioned experiments with hepatocytes and NSAIDs, all four tricyclic compounds were cardiotoxic *in vitro*, although amitriptyline was the most potent. Hence, some *in vitro* investigations have proven more successful than others. *In vitro* screens, like traditional *in vivo* screens, are designed primarily to identify potential hazards (i.e., "a single-sided question"). Additional experiments will always be required to confirm the results of an *in vitro* screen. Numerous other examples of seemingly effective *in vitro* screens of one form or another have been reported, but almost all are focused on specific target organ toxicities (where the limitations of such systems in assessing integrative effects are minimized) or on broad predictions based on cytotoxicity. Progress in producing either mathematical or cell culture models which adequately predict toxicity for novel structures in intact organisms is not likely in the immediate future.

QUALITY ASSURANCE SCREENS

These types of screens differ from those already discussed in that they are not conducted to choose chemicals for development. Rather, they are conducted to ensure the quality and potency of specific batches of finished products prior to wholesale release. This is sometimes referred to as biological standardization. The use of lethality for this purpose was discussed in Chapter 7. However, endpoints other than death are also used for quality assurance testing. In fact, many of these tests are mandated by inclusion in the pharmacopias of several Western countries. Dayan (1983) has described what he terms abnormal toxicity and pyrogenicity tests for the quality assurance testing of biologicals, antibiotics, and parentral preparations (see Chapter 8). The reader is referred to the article by Dayan (1983) for a more extensive discussion of this topic.

ACUTE SYSTEMIC TOXICITY CHARACTERIZATION

These are the studies performed to more completely define the acute toxicity of a drug or chemical. They are more extensive and time-consuming than screens and are normally the type of study done to satisfy regulatory requirements or when a material is to be a small-volume, commercial product and these studies will serve as the "definitive" toxicity study. In design, these tests resemble lethality tests but the protocols specify the collection of more data. A list of the types of data that can be obtained in well-conducted acute toxicity test is given in Table 40. Given that these studies usually include control groups, the classical or traditional design is the most common because this allows for the most straightforward statistical analyses. In addition, while staggered dosing days for different groups is still a fairly common practice, data analyses may be more sensitive if all animals are dosed on the same day.

TABLE 40 Information, Including Lethality, That Can Be Gained in Acute Toxicity Testing

Lethality/mortality
   LD_{50} with confidence limits
   Shape and slope of lethality curves
   Estimation of max nonlethal dose or minimum lethal dose (LD_{01})
   Time to death estimates

Clinical signs
   Times of onset and recovery
   Thresholds
   Agonal vs nonagonal (i.e., do signs occur only in animals that die?)
   Specific vs general responses
   Separation of dose–responses curves from lethality curves

Body weight changes
   Actual loss vs decreased consumption
   Recovery
   Accompanied by changes in feed consumption
   Changes in animals that die vs those that survive

Target organ identification
   Gross examinations
   Histological examinations
   Clinical chemical changes
   Hematological changes

Specialized function tests
   Immunocompetency
   Neuromuscular screening
   Behavioral screening

Pharmacokinetic considerations
   Different routes of administration yielding differences in toxicity
   Plasma levels of test article
   Areas under the curves, volume of distribution, half-life
   Recovery of test article
   Distribution to key organs
   Relationship between plasma levels and occurrence of clinical signs

This requires that one has preliminary screen data that permits selection of appropriate dosages. Studies of more than one species and/or more than one route should be limited to those instances when required by statute.

In general, traditionally designed acute toxicity tests can be divided into three types, which can be called the minimal acute toxicity test, the complete acute toxicity test, and the supplemented acute toxicity test. Of these, the minimal protocol is by far the most common and will be discussed first. The other two represent increasing orders of complexity by adding additional parameters of measurement to the basic minimal study.

MINIMAL ACUTE TEST

An example of a typical study is given in Fig. 41. This study resembles a traditional lethality test in terms of the number of groups and the number of animals per group. Standard protocols consist of three or four groups of test article treated animals and one group of control animals, each consisting of five animals/sex/dosage. Traditionally, the emphasis in these types of studies was on determining the LD_{50}, time to death, slope of the lethality curve, the prominent clinical signs, as illustrated by the data reported by Jenner *et al.* (1964). Recent designs specify, in addition to lethality and clinical observations, that body weights be recorded during, and gross necropsies performed at the end of, the postdosing observation period. An example is the article by Peterson *et al.*, (1987) on the acute toxicity of the alkaloid of *Lupinus anqustifolius* in

EXAMPLE OF MINIMAL ACUTE TOXICITY PROTOCOL

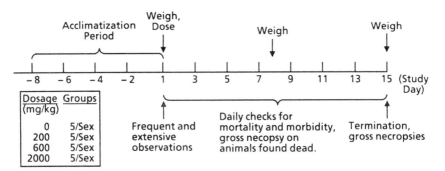

FIGURE 41   Line chart for the design and conduct of a minimal ("bare bones") acute systemic toxicity study.

which the LD_{50}'s, time to death, clinical signs, body weight effect, and gross necropsy findings were all discussed.

For nonpharmaceuticals, these studies are generally conducted on rats using the most likely routes of human exposure. While it is strictly traditional, mice are rarely used as the sole species in an acute toxicity study. For pharmaceuticals, where acute toxicity data in more than one species is often required, these studies will be done as batteries on rats and mice. In addition, because many drugs will be given by more than one route to human patients, these batteries will include groups treated by two different routes. For tests on nonrodent species, as required for pharmaceutical, a different design is used and this is discussed separately.

For lethality tests, it was mentioned that the animals should be acclimated to laboratory conditions for 7–14 days prior to dosing. For acute toxicity tests, however, this pretreatment period should be more than just a holding period. At the very least, animals should be checked daily for signs of ill health and/ or abnormal behavior. Body weights may also be determined. These data should be used to exclude abnormal animals from the test. Such data also provide an additional basis for interpreting the data gathered during the postdosing period. Finally, these activities acclimate the animals to the frequent handling that is necessarily part of an acute toxicity test.

In selecting dosages for an acute systemic toxicity study, the same general rules apply as with lethality testing: (1) There is no sense in testing dosages higher than the physical properties of the test article permit (at what point will the stomach not hold more is not a legitimate toxicological question); (2) the highest dosage should be no larger than a $100-300\times$ multiple of the anticipated human dosage; and (3) widely spaced dosages are better than narrowly spaced dosages. This is particularly cogent in an acute toxicity test because clinical signs may occur at dosages considerably less than those which cause death. Also, as discussed by Sperling (1976) and Gad (1982), the effects at the high dosages may mask the effects that would be observed at the low dosages. Because human beings are more likely to be exposed to lower dosages than experimental animals, these low-dosage effects are important parameters to define.

It is often stated that a well-conducted acute toxicity test should contain sufficient data to calculate an LD_{50}. This is not necessarily the case. Simpler, less resource-intensive protocols should be used for defining lethality (see Chapter 7). Because it is rare that an extensive acute protocol would be attempted without preliminary lethality data, the lethality objectives of acute systemic testing are not critical. Ideally, the highest dosage should elicit marked toxicity (such as lethality), but it is not required to kill off the animals dosed to satisfy the need to show due diligence in stressing the test system. If one already has sufficient preliminary data to suspect that the top dosage will be nonlethal or otherwise innocuous, the test can be conducted as a limit test, consisting of one test article treated group and one control group.

It is important to note that all the factors (husbandry, etc.) that have been shown to affect the outcome of a lethality test (see Chapter 7) will also affect the outcome of an acute toxicity test. Many investigations into the sources of variability in acute toxicity testing have been conducted and these have been reviewed by Elsberry (1986). The factors causing the greatest variation included lack of specifications for sex, strain, supplier, weight range, etc. When clearly defined, detailed protocols were used, interlaboratory variation was found to be minimal. Hence, it is equally important that the details of the protocol be well described and obeyed. It is not appropriate to draw dosage–response conclusions by comparing groups that differ substantially in age or have been fed, fasted, or otherwise manipulated differently. Guidelines for standardization of acute toxicity testing were proposed by the interagency regulatory liason group (IRLG, 1981; Elseberry, 1986). These do not differ markedly from those mandated by TSCA (see Tables 28A, 28B, 29A, and 29B, Chapter 7).

CLINICAL SIGNS

The nonlethal parameters of acute toxicity testing have been extensively reviewed by Sperling (1976) and Balazs (1970, 1976). Clinical observations or signs of toxicity are perhaps the most important aspect of a minimal acute test because they are the first indicators of drug- or chemical-related toxicity or morbidity, and they are necessary in the interpretation of other data collected. For example, body weight loss would be expected if an animal had profound CNS depression lasting several hours.

With regard to clinical signs and observations, there are some basic definitions that should be kept in mind. Symptomatology is the overall manifestation of toxicity. Signs are overt and observable (Brown, 1983). Symptoms are apparent only to the subject of intoxication (e.g., headache) and cannot be described or reported by speachless animals (Balazs, 1970). Clinical signs can be reversible or irreversible. Reversible signs are those that dissipate as the chemical is cleared from the body (Chan et al., 1982) and are generally not accompanied by permanent organ damage. Irreversible signs are those that do not dissipate and are generally accompanied by organic damage. Signs can also represent a normal biological response or reaction (Chan et al., 1982). For example, stressed animals will have higher blood glucose due to the release of adrenal glucocorticoids). These are generally reversible. They are also called nonspecific in that any number of agents or stimuli can evoke the same response and, second, because they are probably not (at least one does not have the evidence to determine otherwise) due to the direct action of the test article.

Responses can also be abnormal in that they are not due to a homeostatic process. The increases in serum urea and creatinine due to kidney damage, for example, are abnormal responses. These are often irreversible, but this is not always the case, depending on the repair capacity or functional reserve of the target organ. These may also be called primary effects because they reflect the direct action of a test article. Agonal signs are those occurring immediately prior to, or concomitantly with, death. They are obviously irreversible, but not necessarily reflective of a specific test article effect. Most animals, for example, display dyspnea prior to death. It is, therefore, important to distinguish between signs that occur in animals that die and those that do not.

In their simplest form, clinical observations are those done on an animal in its cage or, preferably, in an open plane, such as the top of a counter or laboratory cart. These are considered passive observations. One can gain even more information by active examination of the animal, such as the animal's response to stimulation. Fowler *et al.* divide their clinical evaluation of toxicity into those signs scored by simple observations (e.g., ataxia), those scored by provocation (e.g., righting reflex), those scored in the hand (e.g., mydriasis), and those scored by monitoring (e.g., rectal temperature). Cage pans should always be examined for unusually large or small amounts of excreta or excreta of abnormal color or consistency. A list of typical observations are summarized in Table 41. An even more extensive table has been prepared by Chan *et al.* (1982). Given the fact that the number of different signs displayed are not infinite and that some are simply easier to discern than others, most clinical signs are referable to the CNS (e.g., lack of activity), the GI tract (e.g., diarrhea), or the general autonomic nervous system (e.g., increased salivation or tearing). This is illustrated by the data from some past acute toxicity studies (conducted at G.D. Searle R&D) summarized in Table 42.

Other signs can be detected by a well-trained observer, but are, nonetheless, less common than those described previously. Respiratory distress can be diagnosed by examining the animals breathing motions and listening for breathing noises. Cardiovascular signs are generally limited to palor, cyanosis, and/ or hypothermia. Changes in cardiac function can be difficult to detect in small animals and generally consist of "weak" or "slow" beating. Arrhythmias can be difficult to detect because the normal heart rate in a rodent is quite rapid. ECGs are difficult to record from rodents. Therefore, the assessment of potential acute cardiovascular effect of a drug or chemical is usually restricted to a nonrodent species, usually the dog.

Given the subjective nature of recognizing clinical signs, steps must be taken to ensure uniformity (Is the animal depressed or prostrated?) of observation so that the data can be analyzed in a meaningful fashion. There are three ways of achieving this. First, signs should be restricted to a predefined list of simple descriptive terms, such as those given in Appendix D. Second, if a computerized

TABLE 41   Clinical Observation in Acute Toxicity Tests

Organ system	Observation and examination	Common signs of toxicity
CNS and somato-motor	Behavior	Unusual aggressiveness, unusual vocalization, restlessness, sedation
	Movements	Twitch, tremor, ataxia, catatoni, paralysis, convulsion
	Reactivity to various stimuli	Irritability, passivity, anesthesia, hyperesthesia
	Cerebral and spinal reflexes	Sluggishness, absence
	Muscle tone	Rigidity flaccidity
Autonomic nervous system	Pupil size	Myosis, mydriasis
Respiratory	Nostrils	Discharge (color vs uncolored)
	Character and rate	Bradypnoea, dyspnoea, Cheyne–Stokes breathing, Kussmaul breathing
Cardiovascular	Palpation of cardiac region	Thrill, bradycardia, arrhythmia, stronger or weaker beat
Gastrointestinal	Events	Diarrhea, constipation
	Abdominal shape	Flatulence, contraction
	Feces consistency and color	Unformed, black or clay colored
Genitourinary	Vulva, mammary glands	Swelling
	Penis	Prolapse
	Perineal region	Soiled
Skin and fur	Color, turgor, integrity	Reddening, flaccid skinfold, eruptions, piloerection
Mucous membranes	Conjunctiva, mouth	Discharge, congestion, hemorrhage cyanosis, jaundice
Eye	Eyelids	Ptosis
	Eyeball	Exopthalmus, nystagmus
	Transparency	Opacities
Others	Rectal or paw skin temperature	Subnormal, increased
	Injection site	Swelling
	General condition	Abnormal posture, emaciation

Note. From Balazs (1970).

data acquisition system is not available, the use of standardized forms will add uniformity to the observation and recording processes. An example of such a form is shown in Fig. 42. Third, technicians should be trained, preferably using material of known activity, so that everyone involved in such evaluations is using the same terminology to describe the same signs. Animals should be

TABLE 42 Summary of Clinical Observations from Actual Acute Toxicity Tests

Druge (route)	Indication	Acute clinical signs[a]
SC-37407 (po)	Analgesic (opiate)	Reduced motor activity, mydriasis, reduced fecal output, hunched posture, convulsions (tonic), ataxia
SC-35135 (po)	Arrhythmias	Reduced motor activity, lost righting reflex, tremors, dyspneas, ataxia, mydriasis
SC-32840 (po)	Intravascular thrombosis	Reduced motor activity, ataxia, lost righting reflex, closed eyes, red/clear tears
SC-31828 (po)	Arrhythmias	Reduced activity, dyspneas, ataxia, lost righting reflex, red/clear tears
SC-25469 (po)	Analgesic (nonopiate)	Reduced motor activity, ataxia lost righting reflex, dyspnea, convulsions (clonic)

[a]The six most frequent signs in descending order of occurrence.

GENERAL TOXICOLOGY   ACUTE OBSERVATION RECORD   SA_____

SC_____

(Days, other than Study Day 1, on which no signs are observed are recorded on the Log of Animal Observations)

Species	Sex	Route	(mg/kg) Dose Level	Animals Coded*	Date Dosed

Study Day					Page of
OBSERVATIONS: Time Date	Period After Dosing in M:Minutes or H:Hours				NOTES:
No Signs Observed					*An. Code An. ID
Reduced Motor Activity					
Ataxia					
Lost Righting Reflex					
Convulsions ( )					*Animal Code for Recording Observations
Mydriasis					
					Read and Understood
					Date
DEATH					
Observer					

FIGURE 42 An example of a form for the recording of clinical observations in acute systemic toxicity studies.

observed continuously from the time of dosing for several hours on the day of treatment. Times of observation should be recorded as well as the actual observations. After the day of dosing, observations generally need consist only of brief checks for sign remission and the development of new signs of morbidity. Data should be collected in such a way that the following could be concluded for each sign: (1) estimated times of onset and recovery, (2) the range of threshold dosages, and (3) whether signs are observed only in animals that die.

An example of clinical signs provoked by a specific drug is given in Table 43. Incidences are broken down by dosage group and sex. These data illustrate the fact that mortality can censor the occurrence of clinical signs. Reduced fecal output was a more frequent observation at the intermediate dosages because most of the animals died at the higher dosages. Therapeutic ratios (discussed in Chapter 7) are traditionally calculated using the LD_{50}. A more sensitive therapeutic ratio could be calculated using the ED_{50} for the most prominent clinical sign. However, while it may be possible to describe a dosage–response curve (which may, in fact, have a different slope than the lethality curve) for a clinical sign, and calculate the ED_{50}, in practice this is rarely done. It is more common for the approximate threshold dosages or no-observable-effect levels to be reported. A typical minimal acute toxicity study can be summarized as shown in Table 44.

TABLE 43   Example of Clinical Observations Broken Down by Dosage

	Acute toxicity study of SC–37407 signs observed in rats treated orally (No. exhibiting sign within 14 days after treatment/no. treated)									
	Dose level (mg/kg)									
	0		50		160		500		1600	
Signs observed	M	F	M	F	M	F	M	F	M	F
Reduced motor activity	—	—	—	—	—	—	5/5	5/5	4/5	4/5
Mydriasis	—	—	—	—	3/5	4/5	4/5	5/5	5/5	5/5
Reduced fecal output	—	—	5/5	5/5	3/5	5/5	—	1/5	—	—
Hunched posture	—	—	—	—	—	1/5	3/5	3/5	—	—
Convulsions (tonic)	—	—	—	—	—	—	5/5	1/5	5/5	3/5
Ataxia	—	—	—	—	—	—	5/5	4/5	2/5	1/5
Tremors	—	—	—	—	—	—	1/5	2/5	1/5	—
Death	0/5	0/5	0/5	0/5	0/5	0/5	5/5	4/5	5/5	5/5

Note. —, The sign was not observed at that dose level.

TABLE 44   Example of Acute Toxicity Summary (Acute Toxicity of SC-34871)

Species/ route	Dose (mg/kg)	Dead/ dosed	LD$_{50}$ (mg/kg)	Signs observed	Treatment to death intervals
Rat (po)	2400	0/10	>2400[a]	None	None
Rat (iv)	16	0/10	~67	Reduced motor activity at 50 mg/kg; convulsions, dyspnea, lost righting reflex at 160 mg/kg	0–2 hr
	50	2/10			
	160	10/10			
Mouse (po)	500	0/10	>2400	None	None
	1600	0/10			
	2400	0/10			
Mouse (iv)	50	1/10	120 (75–200)[b]	Reduced motor activity, ataxia at 160 mg/kg; tremors, convulsions, dyspnea at 500 mg/kg	0–2 hr
	160	6/10			
	500	10/10			

[a]Limit dosage.
[b]Fiducial limits.

COMPLETE ACUTE TESTING

An example of the next level test, the complete acute toxicity test, is given in Fig. 43. As stated by Dayan (1983), the value of doing more than the minimal test will depend on the nature of subsequent testing. Complete acute tests are more common with nonpharmaceuticals because they may be the only toxicity test conducted. In fact, it may be the only test for any biological activity. These studies are similar in design to minimal studies, but include feed consumption, more frequent body weight determinations, and more detailed and frequent clinical sign assessment. Groups will consist of at least 10 animals per group so that some animals can be sacrificed 24–48 hr postdosing for more immediate examination of any test article-induced pathological changes. Remaining animals will be sacrificed at the end of the 2-week postdosing observation period and examined for possible recovery from any pathological change. Blood will be collected at both sacrifices for clinical chemistry and/or hematology determinations. In short, the complete protocol is designed to provided for a more in-depth search for target organs than the minimal protocol. This type of study has been well described by Gad and coworkers (1984).

BODY WEIGHT CONSIDERATIONS

Body weight and feed consumption are frequently determined parameters in toxicity testing. To an extent, the ability of an animal to gain or maintain

EXAMPLE OF COMPLETE ACUTE TOXICITY PROTOCOL

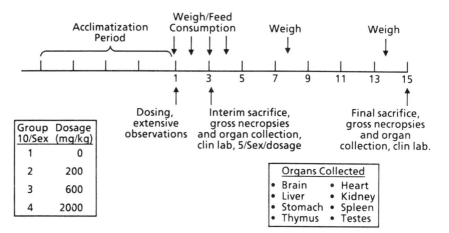

FIGURE 43 Line chart showing the design and conduct of a "complete" or full acute systemic toxicity study.

weight may be considered a sensitive, but nonspecific, indicator of health. This is certainly true in subchronic or chronic studies but is open to some question with regard to acute studies carried out at or near lethal dosages. With the minimal protocol, body weights are determined on Day 1 (prior to dosing), Day 7, and Day 14, which are the days mandated by most regulatory guidelines. One of the problems with this practice is that it is not well founded: If an animal has not died within 7 days postdosing, it has probably recovered and its body weight may not be noticeably different from normal by Day 14. The complete protocol addresses this problem by specifying more frequent body weight determinations (daily for the first 3–5 days of the observation period) so that not only can initial decreases (if they occur) be detected but also recovery can be charted. Feed consumption measurements may be made at the same times. It is difficult to determine the causes behind body weight changes in the absence of feed consumption data. Body weight loss accompanied by normal feed consumption implies something very different than body weight loss (or lack of gain) accompanied by lack of feed consumption. In the absence of feed consumption data, however, changes in body weight should still be considered indicative of a change in an animal's health status.

The more frequent body weight and, sometimes, feed consumption determinations are one of the reasons that the complete, rather than the minimal, protocol is used more frequently for nonpharmaceuticals. Drugs will almost always be subjected to at least one subchronic study. Body weight and feed consumption determinations are a standard feature of such studies. Additionally, changes in body weight and feed consumption are more likely in a subchronic than in an acute study because the animals are dosed continuously between body weight determinations.

Another reason that body weight determinations, especially the infrequent ones specified by a minimal study, are of questionable value in acute studies has to do with problems associated with the statistical analysis of the data. Deaths may substantially alter group size and complicate analysis. If two of five animals die, there is a 40% decrease in group size and a substantial diminution of the power of any statistical test. In addition, the resulting data sets are censored: Comparisons will often be between the control group, a low-dosage group in which all the animals survive, and a high-dosage group in which less than 50% of the animals survive to the end of the observation period. One has to wonder how important body weight changes are if they occur at dosages that are acutely lethal. The data in Table 45 may serve to illustrate this point. Body weight changes tended to occur only at dosages that were acutely lethal. Additionally, one would suspect that the censoring of body weights in groups where death occurs is not random. That is, the animals which die in a group are most likely those which are most sensitive, while those which survive are the most resistant or robust. This problem can be addressed by building exclusionary criteria into a protocol. For example, in our routine acute toxicity studies in rodents, we statistically analyze body weight data only in groups that had less than 50% mortality.

PATHOLOGY CONSIDERATIONS

One of the objectives of any well-conducted toxicity study is to identify target organs. There is some question, however, concerning the utility of extensive pathologic assessments as part of an acute study. Gross necropsies are generally the minimum requested by most regulatory bodies. Hence, minimal protocols will include necropsies on all animals found dead and those sacrificed following the 2-week postdosing observation period. Examples of the types of findings are given in Table 46. The gross observations seen acutely rarely predict the toxicity that will be seen when the chemical is given for longer periods of times. This is not surprising, in that most drug- or chemical-related histologic lesions are the result of chronicity. That is, discernable lesions tend to result from the cumulative effect of dosages that are acutely tolerated.

The data in Table 46 also demonstrate that substantial gross macroscopic findings are rare in minimal acute studies and seldom suggestive of a specific effect. There are several reasons for the lack of specificity. The first is the

TABLE 45   Examples of Body Weight Changes in Rats from Minimal Acute
Toxicity Studies

Drug (route)	Dosage (mg/kg)	Body wt change[a]	Mortality
SC-32561	0	45 ± 4	0/10
po	5000	39 ± 10	0/10
ip	0	43 ± 4	0/10
	500	43 ± 9	0/10
	890	44 ± 11	0/10
	1600	6 ± 14*	2/10
	2800	24 ± 20*	3/10
SC-36250	0	38 ± 10	0/10
po	5000	34 ± 10	0/10
ip	0	34 ± 6	0/10
	670	50 ± 8*	2/10
	890	46 ± 8*	3/10
	1200	45 ± 4	4/10
	1400	35[b]	9/10
SC-36602	0	38 ± 9	0/10
iv	58	38 ± 3	0/10
	67	36 ± 7	2/10
	77	49 ± 5*	3/10
	89	41 ± 7	7/10
po	0	38 ± 5	0/10
	2100	41 ± 5	3/10
	2800	38 ± 5	7/10
	3700	26 ± 6	7/10

[a]Body wt changes (in g) reflect the mean body weight changes (in g) for that group during the
  first week of the postdosing observation period.
[b]Only one surviving animal.
*Statistically different from control (0 dosage group), $p \leq 0.05$.

TABLE 46   Examples of Gross Necropsy Findings from Acute Toxicity Studies

Drug	Acute gross pathology	Subchronic target organs[a]
SC-36602	Distended stomach and intestine, bloody fluid in intestine, congested lung, pale liver	None
SC-38394	None	Liver, testes, bone marrow, thymus, kidney
SC-32840	None	Heart, stomach, kidney, bladder
SC-25469	Peritonitis (ip route only)	None
SC-36250	Peritonitis (ip route only)	Adrenal, liver, thyroid
SC-27166	None	Liver

[a]Organs which showed any evidence of test article-related changes in repeated dose studies of 2
  weeks or longer in duration.

rather limited nature of gross observations in the first place. Second, for animals found dead, it is difficult to separate the chemical-associated effects from agonal and/or autolytic changes. Finally, it is difficult to come to a conclusion about the nature of a gross lesion without histological assessment.

If there are any identifiable gross lesions, there are often differences between animals that die and those that survive to the end of the observation period. The reason for these differences are very simple. An animal that dies less than 24 hr after chemical exposure probably has not had sufficient time to develop a well-defined lesion. As mentioned in Chapter 7, most deaths occur in 24 hr. Animals that survive for the 2-week observation period have probably totally recovered and will have no apparent lesions. Hence, the best chance in identifying test article-specific lesions lies in the animals that die 24–72 hr postdosing. This is, in fact, one of the problems with acute pathology data; that is, comparing animals found dead with those sacrificed at a different time, and comparing both to controls. A complete protocol, where groups of animals are sacrificed 24–48 hours after dosing, at least partially solves this problem.

Many guidelines suggest microscopic confirmation of gross lesions "when necessary"; however, these are seldom done because of the autolytic nature of many of the lesions. On the other hand, the practice of collecting and examining only gross lesions is difficult to justify because it does not permit in-depth comparisons. Pathological examinations in general and histological assessments in particular are most meaningful when the same organs are collected and examined from all animals regardless of the circumstances of death. Elsberry (1986) recommends that the gastrointestinal tract, kidney, heart, brain, liver, and spleen be specifically examined routinely in acute studies. Given the timing issues discussed in the previous paragraph, the amount of effort may not be worth the result. In an attempt to get around these problems, Gad and co-workers (1984) have developed a complete protocol that includes groups of satellite animals that are sacrificed 24 hr after exposure and necropsied, and a standardized organ list is collected, weighed, and prepared for histological assessment. This list routinely includes the "first-line organs": brain, thyroid, liver, kidneys, heart, and adrenals. The same organs are collected from all other animals, i.e., those that die as a result of the chemical and those that are sacrificed at termination (see Fig. 43). The examination of these tissues is dictated by other findings and these criteria are discussed in detail by Gad *et al.* (1984).

Organ weights are routinely taken in most repeated-dose studies, but this is rarely done in acute studies. Some investigators believe that a single dose of a chemical will not have an effect that changes an organ weight that is not readily apparent upon gross observation, especially if organs are only collected at the end of a 2-week postdosing observation period. In reality, however, it is not unusual to find significant differences in organ weights which are not

EXAMPLE OF SUPPLEMENTED ACUTE TOXICITY PROTOCOL

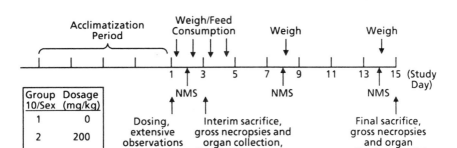

FIGURE 44 Line chart showing the design and conduct of a supplemented (or "heavy") acute systemic toxicity study. This illustrates the approach to such studies when they are to serve as the "definitive" systemic toxicity study for some period of time.

of a supplemented study is one in which additional ("satellite") groups of animals will be dosed with radiolabeled compound in order to gain information about the pharmacokinetics of the test article. Another common practice is the addition of other examinations or measurements in order to gain more information about a potential target organ. An example of this would be recording ECGs in rats, which is too complicated and time-consuming to do on a routine basis but should be done when one suspects that the heart is a potential target organ. One way of describing such a study is that it is a complete toxicity study with a specific screen "piggybacked."

An excellent example of a supplemented protocol is that described by Gad and colleagues (1984). A neuromuscular screen was developed (Gad, 1982) and incorporated into their routine acute toxicity protocol for testing nonpharmaceuticals. Doing so allows for the more systematic and quantifiable examination of effects on the CNS than reliance on simple clinical observations. The screen consists of a battery incorporating standard clinical observations plus some behavioral assessment techniques already described in the literature. These are summarized in Table 47. This screen has as an advantage that it uses noninvasive techniques and, therefore, will require the use of no additional animals. It is important to note that this screen should only be used at appropriate times. If an animal is already displaying signs of CNS depression, little useful data will be gathered by examining behavior. It is probably a better practice to use the neuromuscular screen on Days 2, 7, and 14 postdosing in an attempt to identify more subtle or lingering effects and to chart recovery

TABLE 47　Standard Clinical Observations and Some Behavioral Assessment Techniques

Observation	Nature of data generated[a]	Correlates to which neural component[b]
Locomotor activity	S/N	M/C
Righting reflex	S	C⅓M
Grip strength (forelimb)	N	M
Body temperature	N	C
Salivation	Q	P
Startle response	Q	S/C
Respiration	S	M/P/C
Urination	S	P/M
Mouth breathing	Q	S
Convulsions	S	C
Pineal response	Q	Reflex
Piloerection	Q	P/C
Diarrhea	S	GI tract/PM
Pupil size	S	P/C
Pupil response	Q	P/C
Lacrimation	Q	S/P
Impaired gait	S	M/C
Stereotypy	Q	C
Toe pinch	S	S (surface pain; spinal reflex)
Tail pinch	S	S (deep pain)
Wire maneuver	S	C/M
Hindleg splay	N	P/M
Positional passivity	S	S/C
Tremors	S	M/C
Extensor thrust	S	C/M
Positive geotropism	Q	C
Limb rotation	S	M/C

[a]Data quantal (Q), scalar (S), or interval (N). Quantal data are characterized by being of an either/or variety, such as dead–alive or present–absent. Scalar data are such that one can rank something as less than, equal to, or greater than other values but cannot exactly quantitate the difference between such rankings. Interval data are continuous data where one can assign (theoretically) an extremely accurate value to a characteristic that can be precisely related to other values in a quantitative fashion.
[b]Peripheral (P), sensory (S), muscular (M), or central (C).

from these effects. For drugs or chemicals that produce no observable CNS effect following dosing, the neuromuscular screen can be done a few hours postdosing. The more extensive and detailed nature of the data generated by the neuromuscular screen permits more confidence in the conclusion that the test article had no effect on the CNS. This is also an example of due diligence in safety testing. This neuromuscular screen, called a FOB, has become the standard initial or first-tier screen for neurotoxicity under FDA and EPA guidelines.

Any suspect target organ can be investigated in much the same fashion. Depending on the invasiveness of the supplementary techniques, satellite groups may or may not need to be added to the study. Care must be taken in this regard to prevent the study from becoming too cumbersome and too complicated to conduct. It may be better to address some questions as separate and different studies. For this reason, it is also difficult to address more than one supplementary question in any one study.

ACUTE TOXICITY TESTING WITH NONRODENT SPECIES

The designs described thus far assume that the test species being used is a rodent. Nonrodent species are also used for acute toxicity testing. The FDA, for example, requires acute toxicity testing in at least one nonrodent species. The animals most often used are dog, monkey, and ferret (although animal health agents and agricultural chemicals may have to be tested in farm stock animals, and the EPA will require tests in aquatic nonvertebrates for chemicals that may be released into the aquatic environment). While the rabbit is not technically a rodent, it is the species of choice for a variety of tests, such as dermal toxicity, in which the rabbit is treated essentially like a large rodent. This section is written with the dog and monkey in mind. Clearly, there are some profound differences between these species and rodents with regard to handling, husbandry, and dosing. These are discussed in Chapters 11. Here we will focus on the design differences in toxicity testing in large species.

For financial, procurement, and ethical reasons, acute systemic toxicity testing on nonrodents is seldom done with traditionally designed protocols. The minimal acute study requires 30–50 animals. Complete and supplemented studies will usually require more animals still. At a cost of $400 per beagle dog or $1600 per monkey, the animal costs alone are enough to make such studies with nonrodent species prohibitively expensive. Vivarium space and husbandry costs are also much higher with nonrodent species than with rodents. Nonrodents also require a much longer prestudy quarantine period than rodents: at least 6–8 weeks for dogs and 18–24 weeks for monkeys. Treatment during the quarantine period is more extensive than that given rodents. The animals should be given frequent physical examinations including complete clinical laboratory panels and appropriate tests for common illnesses. Special care must be taken with monkeys because not only can they be vectors of human disease but also they can contract human diseases, and a sick animal can compromise study outcome. All these factors dictate that these animals be used sparingly. Hence, it is most common to study acute systemic toxicity in nonrodent animals using a pyramiding dosage design using relatively few animals. The typical study will consist of two test article animals per sex and two control animals per sex for a total of eight animals. A typical protocol is shown in Fig. 45.

The use of larger animals permits more extensive observation of each individual. Hence, following each dose, animals can be given complete physical examinations that include palpations, behavioral checks, spinal reflex checks, pupillary light responses, respiration rate, ECG recording, and rectal temperature measurement. Blood samples can also be collected following each dose to determine standard clinical chemistry and hematology profiles. Hence, while fewer animals are used with the pyramiding dosage protocol, more information per animal is collected.

The small number of animals used in a pyramiding dosage study makes it difficult to do standard statistical comparisons. This can be overcome to a certain extent by taking advantage of two of the design aspects of the pyramiding protocol. First, pretreatment (i.e., Day −1) data can and should be obtained on all animals for all parameters examined or determined. In-study comparisons can be made both to pretreatment data and to concurrent control animals. Such comparisons can be made not only on the basis of absolute numbers but also on the magnitude of any changes. Second, all animals are measured repeatedly throughout the study. Hence, with a true test article-related effect,

EXAMPLE OF PYRAMIDING DOSE STUDY FOR ACUTE TOXICITY TESTING IN NONRODENT SPECIES

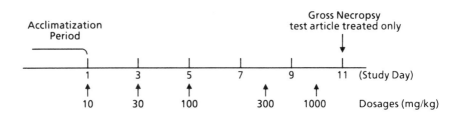

FIGURE 45   Line chart showing the design and conduct of a pyramiding style acute systemic toxicity study. Such studies are conducted when a larger nonrodent species is the test model.

the magnitude of change should increase following each dose. This is, in fact, the only way one can make any dosage–response or threshold conclusions using the pyramiding protocol.

Seldom are nonrodent animals studied by routes other than the intended or likely routes of human exposure. Hence, the most common routes in these types of protocols are oral, intravenous, and respiratory. Rarely is the test article delivered to nonrodent species by the intraperitoneal route. Routes are discussed in Chapter 10, but some discussion is appropriate here because of the design considerations. Orally, test articles are normally given in capsules to dogs and by gavage to monkeys. Nonrodents have to be restrained if dosed by gavage, and this can make the process very labor intensive. This is minimized by the small number of animals specified by the pyramiding protocol. In contrast, because of the differences in size, it is much easier to deliver a test article intravenously to nonrodents than to rodents. For topical studies, the rabbit is the nonrodent of choice because it is easier to prevent a rabbit from grooming the delivery site and it takes considerably less material to deliver a comparable dose to rabbits than it does a dog. Acute dermal studies are not, however, usually done with a pyramiding study design.

The biggest problem with the pyramiding protocol is accommodation. If no toxicity is observed, one is never certain whether the chemical is innocuous or whether the animals developed tolerance during the study. The escalating dosage feature of the pyramiding protocol is an excellent vehicle for the development of tolerance. One can check this by dosing additional naive animals at the limit dosage to confirm, as it were, a negative result. Another problem, which is most peculiar to the dog, is emesis. Too much of almost anything will make a dog vomit. This is always somewhat of a surprise to toxicologists whose prior experience is primarily with rodents, which cannot vomit. One should pay close attention to dogs the first hour after capsule delivery. If the dog vomits most of the dose, the actual dosage absorbed could be grossly overestimated. This can be a particular problem if one is using the results of a pyramiding dosage study to set the dosages for a repeated dose study. Dogs can develop tolerance to the emetic effect of a set dosage. When this occurs, absorbtion and resulting blood concentrations of test article can increase dramatically, resulting in more florid toxicity than expected on the basis of the pyramiding study. Another problem is that emesis can result in secondary electrolyte changes, especially decreases in chloride, that can be taken for a direct test article effect. If emesis is a severe problem, one can study toxicity in a different nonrodent species or divide larger dosages into two or three divided dosages on the day of dosing.

As with traditionally designed rodent studies, the pathology component of pyramiding studies usually consists of gross necropsies followed by (when appropriate and necessary) histological assessment of gross lesions. Because of study design, one cannot normally determine any dosage–response relationship with regard to gross findings. In addition, the small number of animals make definitive conclusions difficult. Usually gross lesions are defined in absolute terms with few comparisons to control animals. Suspect target organs should be further investigated in subsequent subchronic studies or in rigorous and specific mechanistic studies. Because of the limited value of the pathology data generated by the pyramiding protocol, control animals should not be sacrificed but rather should be saved for reuse.

ACUTE MECHANISTIC STUDIES

Mechanistic studies are those conducted to refine one's understanding of the toxic effect of a chemical or drug. They may be broadly defined as those studies conducted to test a hypothesis rather than to gather data which describe toxicity. It should be stressed that mechanistic studies differ from specific toxicity screens because the latter are primarily descriptive in nature. An LD_{50} is descriptive. The study which determines the relationship between the oxidative metabolism and liver toxicity of a test article is mechanistic. Such studies are, of course, the mainstay of the academic toxicologist. In a safety setting, mechanistic studies are done when one needs more information in order to interpret the results of a toxicity study. In the pharmaceutical industry, they will be run to gain better understanding of an untoward effect noticed in clinical trials or postmarketing surveillance.

There are no regulatory requirements for such studies. They may need to be conducted, however, in order to gain the data necessary to support the interpretation of a controversial finding from a safety study submitted to a regulatory body. In these circumstances the data from the mechanistic study will also have to submitted, and a good faith effort to comply with the appropriate Good Laboratory Practices (GLPs) should be made. For studies submitted to the FDA, GLPs are described in (FFDCA)/21 CFR 58. For studies to be submitted to the EPA, GLPs are described in (FFDCA)/40 CFR 160 and (TSCA)/40 CFR 792. These describe standard of conduct, not design criteria (McClain, 1983).

Clearly, all the studies that may be encompassed by the definition of a mechanistic study cannot be covered here. The important point to be made is that the protocol must be tailored to the question under study. One should not try to "shoehorn" a mechanistic study into a descriptive protocol. In the pharmaceutical industry, the most glaring example of this practice is in the study of drug–drug interactions. This is also an appropriate area of discussion for this book because it is an area where lethality testing has been misused. Traditionally, possible drug–drug toxic interactions were assessed by comparing the LD$_{50}$ of each drug to that of a drug mixture. As reviewed by Zbinden (1986), this approach is completely inadequate because it ignores the mechanisms of drug action. For example, this approach failed to detect the potentiating effect cimetidine has on the action of dicoumarol anticoagulants because it employed acute death, rather than changes in promthrombin time or partial thromboplastin time, as an endpoint (Zbinden, 1986). In addition, this approach ignores the fact that multiple drugs are often given simultaneously (the well-known synergystic effect of ethanol and sedatives on the CNS does not need to be mentioned here). In the clinical situation, it is more often the case that an acute effect will be overlayed on a chronic effect. For example, many drug–drug interactions are due to altered rates of metabolism because of the metabolic-inducing or -inhibiting effects of the first drug that will exert on the second drug.

REFERENCES

Acosta, D., and Ramos, K. (1984). Cardiotoxicity of tricyclic antidepressants in primary cultures of rat myocardial cells. *J. Toxicol. Environ. Health* 14, 137–143.

Auletta, C. (1988). Acute systemic toxicity testing. In *Handbook of Product Safety Assessment* (S. Gad, Ed.), pp. 43–71. Dekker, New York.

T. Balazs, (1970). Measurement of acute toxicity. In *Methods in Toxicology* (G. Paget, Ed.), pp. 49–81. F. A. Davis. Philadelphia.

Balazs, T. (1976). Assessment of the value of systemic toxicity studies in experimental animals. In *Advances in Modern Toxicology, Vol 1, Part 1: New Concepts in Safety Evaluation* (M. Mehlman, R. Shapiro, and H. Blumenthal, Eds.), pp. 141–153. Hemisphere, Washington, DC.

Brown, V. (1983). Acute toxicity testing. In *Animals and Alternatives in Toxicity Testing* (M. Balls, R. Riddell, and A. Worden, Eds.), pp. 1–13. Academic Press, New York.

Chan, P., O'Hara, G., and Hayes, A. (1982). Principles and methods for acute and subchronic toxicity. In *Principles and Methods of Toxicology* (A. Hayes, Ed.), pp. 1–51. Raven Press, New York.

Choudary, J., Contrera, J., DeFelice, A., DeGeorge, J., Farrelly, J., Fitsgerald, G., Goheer, M., Jacobs, A., Jordon, A., Meyers, L., Osterberg, R., Resnick, C., Sun, C., and Temple, R. (1996). Response to Monro and Mehta proposal for use of single-dose toxicology studies to support single-dose studies of new drugs in humans. *Clin. Pharmacol. Ther.* 59, 265–267.

Dayan, A. (1983). Complete programme for acute toxicity testing—Not only LD$_{50}$ determination. *Acta Pharmacol. Toxicol.* 52 (Suppl. 2), 31–51.

Elsberry, D. (1986). Screening approaches for acute and subacute toxicity studies. In *Safety Evaluation of Drugs and Chemicals* (W. Lloyd, Ed.), pp. 145–151. Hemisphere, Washington DC.

Food and Drug Administration, Office of Science Coordination (1984). Final report on acute studies workshop sponsored by the U.S. Food and Drug Administration.

Fowler, J., and Rutty, D. (1983). Methodological aspects of acute toxicity testing particularly LD$_{50}$ determinations present use in development of new drugs. *Acta Pharmacol. Toxicol.* 52 (Suppl. 2), 20–30.

Fowler, J., Brown, J., and Bell, H. (1979). The rat toxicity screen. *Pharmacol. Ther.* 5, 461–466.

Gad, S. (1982). A neuromuscular screen for use in industrial toxicology. *J. Toxicol. Environ. Health* 9, 691–704.

Gad, S. (1988). An approach to the design and analysis of screening data in toxicology. *J. Am. Col. Toxicol.* 7, 127–138.

Gad, S., Smith, A., Cramp, A., Gavigan, F., and Derelanko, M. (1984). Innovative designs and practices for acute systemic toxicity studies. *Drug Chem. Toxicol.* 7, 423–434.

Greim, H., Andrae, U., Forster, U., and Schwarz, L. (1986). Application, limitations and research requirements of *in vitro* test systems in toxicology. *Arch. Toxicol.* (Suppl. 9), 225–236.

Hazelette, J., Thompson, T., Mertz, B., Vuolo-Schuessler, L., Green, J., Tripp, S., Robertson, P., and Traina, V. (1987). Rising dose tolerance (RDT) study: A novel scenario for obtaining preclinical toxicology/drug metabolism data. *Toxicologist* 7. [Abstract No. 846]

Hopper, D. (1986). Behavioral measures in toxicology screening. In *Safety Evaluation of Drugs and Chemicals* (W. Lloyd, Ed.), pp. 305–321. Hemisphere, New York.

Interagency Regulatory Liason Group (IRLG), Office of Consumer Affairs (1981). *Testing Standards and Guidelines Work Group (HFE–88)*.

Irwin, S. (1962). Drug screening and evaluative procedures. *Science* 136, 123–128.

Jenner, P., Hagan, E., Taylor, J., Cook, E., and Fitzhugh, O. (1964). Food flavorings and compounds of related structure. I. Acute oral toxicity. *Fd. Cosmet. Toxicol.* 2, 327–343.

LeBeau, J. (1983). The role of the LD_{50} determination in drug safety evaluation. *Reg. Toxicol. Pharmacol.* 3, 71–74.

McClain, R. (1983). Generating, interpreting and reporting information in toxicity studies. *Drug Info. J.* 17, 245–255.

Monro, A., and Mehta, D. (1996). Are single-dose toxicology studies in animals adequate to support single doses of a new drug in humans? *Clin. Pharmacol. Ther.* 59, 258–264.

The Organization for Economic Cooperation and Development (OECD) (1981). *OECD Guidelines for Testing of Chemicals*. OECD, Paris.

Osterberg (1983). Today's requirements in food, drug, and chemical control. *Acta Pharmacol. Toxicol.* 52 (Suppl. 2), 201–228.

Peterson, D., Ellis, Z., Harris, D., and Spadek, Z. (1987). Acute toxicity of the major alkaloids of cultivated Lupinus angustifolius seeds to rats. *J. Appl. Toxicol.* 7, 51–53.

Stammati, A., Silano, V., and Zucco, F. (1981). Toxicology investigations with cell culture systems. *Toxicologist* 20, 91–153.

Stark, D., Shopsis, C., Borenfreund, E., and Babich, H. (1986). Progress and problems in evaluating and validating alternative assays in toxicology. *Fd. Chem. Toxicol.* 24, 449–455.

Smyth, H., and Carpenter, C. (1944). The place of the range finding test in the industrial toxicology laboratory. *J. Ind. Hyg. Toxicol.* 26, 269–273.

Sorensen, E., and Acosta, D. (1985). Relative toxicities of several nonsteroidal antiinflammatory compounds in primary cultures of rat hepatocytes. *J. Toxicol. Environ. Health* 16, 425–440.

Sperling, F. (1976). Nonlethal parameters as indices of acute toxicity: Inadequacy of the acute LD_{50}. In *Advances in Modern Toxicology, Vol 1, Part 1: New Concepts in Safety Evaluation*. M. Mehlman, R. Shapiro, and H. Blumenthal, Eds.), pp. 177–191. Hemisphere, New York.

Zbinden, G., and Flury-Roversi, M. (1981). Significance for the LD_{50}-test for the toxicological evaluation of chemical substances. *Arch. Toxicol.* 47, 77–99.

Zbinden, G. (1984). Acute toxicity testing, purpose. In *Acute Toxicity Testing: Alternative Approaches* (A. Goldberg, Ed.), pp. 5–22. Liebert, New York.

Zbinden, G. (1986). Invited contribution: Acute toxicity testing, public responsibility and scientific challenges. *Cell Biol. Toxicol.* 2, 325–335.

Zbinden, G. (1983). Current trends in safety testing and toxicological research. Naturwissenschaften 69, 255–259.

Zbinden, G., Elsner, J., and Boelsterli (1984). Toxicological screening. *Reg. Toxicol. Pharmacol.* 4, 275–286.

CHAPTER 10

Routes, Formulations, and Vehicles

Among the cardinal principles of both toxicology and pharmacology is that the means by which an agent comes in contact with or enters the body (i.e., the route of exposure or administration) does much to determine the nature and magnitude of an effect. However (particularly for acute toxicology), an understanding of routes and their implications is not rigorous. Also, in the day-to-day operations of performing studies in animals, such an understanding of routes, their manipulation, means and pitfalls of achieving them, and the art and science of vehicles and formulations is essential to the sound and efficient conduct of a study.

To some extent, this volume has already addressed aspects of two sets of routes. Chapters 3 and 5 addressed most aspects of the dermal (percutaneous) routes, the major exception being vehicles and their aspects. Chapter 8 presented some aspects of the three primary parenteral routes (the intravenous, subcutaneous, and intramuscular). These aspects will not be repeated (but will be referenced) here.

As presented in Table 48, there are at least 26 potential routes of administration, of which 10 are commonly used in acute toxicology and, therefore, will be addressed here.

TABLE 48   Potential Routes of Administration

Oral routes
   Oral[a] (po)
   Inhalation[a]
   Sublingual
   Buccal

Placed into a natural orifice in the body other than the mouth
   Intranasal
   Intraauricular
   Rectal
   Intravaginal
   Intrauterine
   Intraurethral

Parentheral (injected into the body or placed under the skin)
   Intravenous[a] (iv)
   Subcutaneous[a] (sc)
   Intramuscular[a] (im)
   Intraarterial
   Intradermal[a] (id)
   Intralesional
   Epidural
   Intrathecal
   Intracisternal
   Intracardia
   Intraventricular
   Intraocular
   Intraperitoneal[a] (ip)

Topical routes
   Cutaneous[a]
   Transdermal[a] (also called percutaneous)
   Ophthalmic[a]

[a]Commonly used in toxicology.

MECHANISMS

There are three primary sets of reasons why differences in route of administration are critical in determining the effect of an agent upon a biological system. These are (1) local effects, (2) absorption and distribution, and (3) metabolism.

LOCAL EFFECTS

Local effects are those which are peculiar to the first area or region of the body that a test material gains entry to and/or contacts. For example, for the dermal route, these include irritation, corrosion, and sensitization (as previously discussed in Chapters 3 and 5). Likewise, for the parenteral routes, we have already discussed irritation, pyrogenicity, sterility, and blood compatibility. In general, the same categories of possible adverse effects (irritation, immediate immune response, local tissue/cellular compatibility, and physicochemical interactions) are the mechanisms of, or basis for, concern.

In general, no matter what the route, certain characteristics will predispose a material to have local effects (and, by definition, if not present, tend to limit the possibility of local effects). These factors include pH, redox potential, high concentration, and being solids with low flexibility and sharp edges. These characteristics will increase the potential for irritation by any route and, subsequent to irritation, other appropriate regional response (for orally administered materials, for example, emesis and diarrhea).

ABSORPTION/DISTRIBUTION

For a material to be toxic (local effects are largely not true toxicities by this definition), the first requirement is that it be absorbed into the organism (for which purpose being in the cavity of the gastrointestinal (GI) tract does not qualify).

There are characteristics which influence absorption by the different routes, and these need to be understood by any person trying to evaluate and/or predict the toxicities of different moieties. Some key characteristics and considerations are summarized below by route.

A. Oral and rectal routes (gastrointestinal tract)
  1. Lipid-soluble compounds (nonionized) are more readily absorbed than water-soluble compounds (ionized).
    a. Weak organic bases are in the nonionized, lipid-soluble form in the intestine and tend to be absorbed there.
    b. Weak organic acids are in the nonionized, lipid-soluble form in the stomach and one would suspect they would be absorbed there, but the intestine is more important because of time and area of exposure.
  2. Specialized transport systems exist for some moieties: sugars, amino acids, pyrimidines, calcium, and sodium.
  3. Almost everything is absorbed—at least to a small extent (if it has a molecular weight below 10,000).
  4. Digestive fluids may modify the structure of a chemical.
  5. Dilution increases toxicity because of more rapid absorption from the intestine, unless stomach contents bind the moiety.
  6. Physical properties are important—for example, dissolution of metallic mercury is essential to allow absorption.

7. Age—neonates have a poor intestinal barrier.
8. Effect of fasting on absorption depends on the properties of the chemical of interest.

B. Inhalation (lungs)
  1. Aerosol deposition
    a. Nasopharyngeal—5 μm or larger in man, less in common laboratory animals.
    b. Tracheobronchiolar—1–5 μm.
    c. Alveolar—1 μm.
  2. If a solid, mucociliary transport may serve to clear from lungs to GI tract.
  3. Lungs are anatomically good for absorption.
    a. Large surface area (50–100 m^2).
    b. Blood flow is high.
    c. Close to blood (10 μm between gas media and blood).
  4. Absorption of gases is dependent on solubility of the gas in blood.
    a. Chloroform, for example, has high solubility and is all absorbed; respiration rate is the limiting factor.
    b. Ethylene has low solubility and only a small percentage is absorbed—blood flow limited absorption.
    c. Parenteral routes—discussed in Chapter 8.
    d. Dermal routes—discussed in Chapter 5.

It is rare in acute toxicology for the absorption and bioavailability of a compound by any particular route to be either studied or determined. However, as a generalization, there is a pattern of relative absorption rates which extends between the different routes that are commonly employed. This order of absorption (by rate from fastest to slowest and, in a less rigorous manner, in degree of absorption from most to least) is iv > inhalation > im > ip > sc > oral > id > other dermal.

Absorption (total amount and rate), distribution, metabolism, and species similarity in response are the reasons for selecting particular routes in toxicology. In acute toxicology, however, these things are rarely known to us. So the cardinal rule for selecting routes of use in acute testing is to use those routes which mirror the principal route for human exposure. If this route of human exposure is uncertain, or if there is the potential for either a number of routes or the human absorption rate and pattern being greater, then the common practice becomes that of the most conservative approach. This approach stresses maximizing potential absorption in the animal species (within the limits of practicality) and selecting from among those routes commonly used in the laboratory that which gets the most material into the animal's system as quickly and completely as possible to evaluate the potential toxicity. Under this approach, many compounds are administered intraperitoneally in acute testing, though there is no real potential for human exposure by this route.

Assuming that a material is absorbed, distribution of a compound in an acute study is usually of limited interest. In so-called "heavy" acute studies (Gad *et al.*, 1984) in which acute systemic toxicity is intensive and evaluated to the point of identifying target organs, or in range-finder-type study results for refining the design of longer-term studies, distribution would be of interest. Some factors which can serve to alter distribution are listed in Table 49.

Likewise, metabolism is generally of only limited concern in most acute studies. There are some special cases, however, in which metabolic considera-

---

TABLE 49 Selected Factors That May Affect Chemical Distribution to Various Tissues

Factors relating to the chemical and its administration
  Degree of binding of chemical to plasma proteins (i.e., agent affinity for proteins) and tissues
  Chelation to calcium, which is deposited in growing bones and teeth (e.g., tetracyclines in young children)
  Whether the chemical distributes evenly throughout the body (one compartment model) or differentially between different compartments (two- or more compartment model).
  Ability of chemical to cross the blood–brain barrier
  Diffusion of chemical into the tissues or organs and degree of binding to receptors that are and are not responsible for the drug's beneficial effects
  Quantity of chemical given
  Route of administration/exposure
  Partition coefficients (nonpolar chemicals are distributed more readily to fat tissues than are polar chemicals)
  Interactions with other chemicals that may occupy receptors and prevent the drug from attaching to the receptor, inhibit active transport, or otherwise interfere with a drug's activity
  Molecular weight of the chemical
Factors relating to the test subject
  Body size
  Fat content (e.g., obesity affects the distribution of drugs that are highly soluble in fats)
  Permeability of membranes
  Active transport for chemicals carried across cell membranes by active processes
  Amount of proteins in blood, especially albumin
  Pathology or altered homeostasis that affects any of the other factors (e.g., cardiac failure and renal failure)
  The presence of competitive binding substances (e.g., specific receptor sites in tissues bind drugs)
  pH of blood and body tissues
  pH of urine[a]
  Blood flow to various tissues or organs (e.g., well-perfused organs usually tend to accumulate more chemical than less well-perfused organs)

---

[a]The pH of urine is usually more important than the pH of blood.

tions must be factored in seeking to understand differences between routes and the effects which may be seen.

The first special case is parenteral routes, where the systemic circulation presents a peak level of the moiety of interest to the body at one time, tempered only by the results of a single pass through the liver.

The second special case arises from inhalation exposures. Because of the arrangements of the circulatory system, inhaled compounds enter the full range of systemic circulation without any "first pass" metabolism by the liver. Keberle (1971) and O'Reilly (1972) have published reviews of absorption, distribution, and metabolism that are relevant to acute testing.

COMMON ROUTES

Each of the 10 routes most commonly used in acute toxicity studies has its own peculiarities, and for each there are practical considerations and techniques ("tricks") which should be either known or available to the practicing toxicologist.

DERMAL

For all agents of concern in acute toxicology (except for therapeutics), the major route by which the general population is most frequently exposed is the percutaneous. Brown (1980) has reviewed background incidence data on pesticides, for example, which shows such exposures to be common.

Much of what needs to be said about nonspecific factors which influence percutaneous absorption has already been presented in Chapters 3 and 5. There are portions which are more relevant for discussion here as part of the general case.

Percutaneous (or dermal route) entry into the body really is by five separate means (Marzulli, 1962; Scheuplein, 1965 and 1967):

Between the cells of the stratum corneum
Through the cells of the stratum corneum
Via the hair follicles
Via the sweat glands
Via the sebaceous glands

Certain aspects of the material of interest and of the ambient conditions of the test animals can also influence absorption (Blank and Scheuplein, 1964):

Small molecules penetrate skin better than large molecules.

Undissociated molecules penetrate skin better than do ions.

Preferential solubility of the toxicant in organic solvents indicates better penetration characteristics than preferential solubility in water.

The less viscous or the more volatile the toxicant, the greater is its penetrating ability.

The nature of the vehicle for the toxicant and the concentration of the toxicant in the vehicle both affect absorption (vehicles will be discussed later in this chapter).

The hydration (water content) of the stratum corneum affects penetrability.

The ambient temperature can influence the uptake of toxicant through the skin. The warmer it is, the greater the blood flow through the skin and, therefore, the greater is percutaneous absorption.

Molecular shape (particularly symmetry) influences absorption (Medved and Kundiev, 1964). There are at least two excellent texts on the subject (Brandau and Lippold, 1982; Bronaugh and Maibach, 1985) which go into much greater detail.

Parenteral

This group of routes has also already been discussed as the subject of Chapter 8.

In predictive toxicology (other than for therapeutic agents) parentheral routes see limited use and are primarily restricted to the ip route. This approach serves both to maximize potential hazard and to provide a means (if done in conjunction with studies via other routes) for evaluating the relative absorption and metabolic effects.

Kruger et al. (1962) demonstrated the efficiency of absorption of some chemicals injected ip, while Lukas et al. (1971) showed that compounds administered ip are absorbed primarily through the portal circulation.

A prime practical consideration in the use of the ip route for acute testing should be the utilization of aseptic techniques to preclude bacterial or viral contamination. If these are not exercised, the resulting infected and compromised animals cannot be expected to produce either valid or reproducible indications of actual chemical toxicity.

Compounds which are more lipophilic will be more quickly absorbed systemically by the ip route but not by the im or sc routes.

In the iv route, anaphalactic reactions, caused by administration of an agent to an animal previously sensitized to it or to a particularly sensitive species such as a guinea pig, may be especially severe—probably because of the sudden massive antigen–antibody reactions. When the drug is given by other routes, its access to antibody molecules is necessarily slower; moreover, its further absorption can be retarded or prevented at the first sign of a serious allergic reaction.

Embolism is another possible complication of the iv route. Particulate matter may be introduced if a drug intended for intravenous use precipitates for some reason,or if a particular suspension intended for intramuscular or subcutaneous use is inadvertently given into a vein. Hemolysis or agglutination of erythrocytes may be caused by injection of hypotonic or hypertonic solutions or by more specific mechanisms.

Agents injected into the larger muscle masses are generally absorbed rapidly.

Blood flow through muscles in a resting animal is about 0.02–0.07 ml/min per gram of tissue, and this flow rate may increase many times during exercise as additional vascular channels open. Large amounts of solution can be introduced intramuscularly, and there is usually less pain and local irritation than is encountered by the subcutaneous route. Ordinary aqueous solutions of chemicals are usually absorbed from an intramuscular site within 10–30 min, but faster or slower absorption is possible, depending on the vascularity of the site, the ionization and lipid solubility of the drug, the volume of the injection, the osmolality of the solution, animal temperature, and other variables. Small molecules are absorbed directly into the capillaries from an intramuscular site, whereas large molecules (e.g., proteins) gain access to the circulation by way of the lymphatic channels. Radiolabeled compounds of widely different molecular weights (maximum 585) and physical properties have been shown to be absorbed from rat muscle at virtually the same rate, about 16% per minute (i.e., the absorption process is limited by the blood flow).

Drugs that are insoluble at tissue pH or that are in an oily vehicle, form a depot in the muscle tissue, from which absorption proceeds very slowly.

Absorption from subcutaneous injection sites is affected by the same factors that serve to determine the rate of absorption from im sites (Schou, 1971). Blood flow through these regions is generally poorer than in muscles, so the absorption rate is generally slower.

The rate of absorption from an sc injection site may be retarded by immobilization of the limb, local cooling to cause vasoconstriction, or application of a tourniquet proximal to the injection site to block the superficial venous drainage and lymphatic flow. Adrenergic stimulants, such as epinephrine, in small amounts will serve to constrict the local blood vessels and, therefore, slow systemic absorption. Cholinergic stimulants (such as methacholine) will conversely induce very rapid systemic absorption subcutaneously. Other agents may also alter their own rate of absorption by affecting local blood supply or capillary permeability.

A prime determinant of the absorption rate from an sc injection is the total surface area over which the absorption can occur. Although the subcutaneous tissues are somewhat loose and moderate amounts of fluid can be administered, the normal connective tissue matrix prevents indefinite lateral spread of the injected solution. These barriers may be overcome by agents which break down mucopolysaccharides of the connective tissue matrix; the resulting spread of injected solution leads to a much faster absorption rate.

ORAL

The most common route for the evaluation of acute toxicity is oral. This is because of both ease of performance and it is the most readily noticed route of exposure. Also, though the dermal route may be as common, it is much easier to accurately measure and administer doses by the oral route.

Enteral routes technically include any which will put a material directly into the GI tract, but the use of those other than the oral (such as rectal) is rare in toxicology. Though there are a number of variations and peculiarities which are specific to different animal species (which will be reviewed in the next chapter), there is also a great deal of commonality across species in methods, considerations, and mechanisms.

MECHANISMS OF ABSORPTION

Ingestion is generally referred to as "oral" or "peroral" (po) exposure and includes direct intragastric exposure in experimental acute toxicology. The regions for possible agent action and absorption should be considered separately.

Because of the rich blood supply to the mucous membranes of the mouth (buccal cavity), many compounds can be absorbed through them. Absorption from the buccal cavity is limited to nonionized lipid-soluble compounds. Buccal absorption of a wide range of aromatic and aliphatic acids and basic drugs in human subjects has been found to be parabolically dependent on log P, when P is the octanol–water partition coefficient. The ideal lipophilic character (log P_o) for maximum buccal absorption has also been shown to be in the range of 4.2–5.5 (Lein et al., 1971). Compounds with large molecular weights are poorly absorbed in the buccal cavity and because absorption increases linearly with concentration and there is no discrimination between optical enantiomorphs of several compounds known to be absorbed from the mouth, it is believed that uptake is by passive diffusion rather than active transport chemical moieties.

A knowledge of the buccal absorption characteristics of a chemical can be important for the case of accidental poisoning. It is possible that although the agent taken into the mouth is voided on being found objectionable, significant absorption may already have occurred before any material has been swallowed.

Unless voided, most materials in the buccal cavity are swallowed and enter the gastrointestinal tract. No significant absorption occurs in the esophagus and the agent passes on to enter the stomach. It is common practice in acute toxicity testing to avoid the possibility of buccal absorption by intubation ("gavage") or by the administration of the agent in gelatine capsules designed to disintegrate in the gastric fluid.

Absorption of chemicals with widely different characteristics can occur at different levels in the gastrointestinal tract (Schanker, 1960). The two factors primarily influencing this regional absorption are (a) the lipid–water partition characteristics of the undissociated toxicant, and (b) the dissociation constant which determines the amount of toxicant in the dissociated form.

Therefore, weak organic acids and bases are readily absorbed as uncharged lipid-soluble molecules, whereas ionized compounds are absorbed only with difficulty and nonionized toxicants with poor lipid-solubility characteristics are absorbed slowly. Lipid-soluble acid molecules can be absorbed efficiently through the gastric mucosa but bases are not absorbed in the stomach.

In the intestines the nonionized form of the toxicant is preferentially absorbed and the rate of absorption is related to the lipid–water partition coefficient of the toxicant. The highest pK value for a base compatible with efficient gastric absorption is about 7.8 and the lowest pK_a for an acid is about 3.0, although a limited amount of absorption can occur outside these ranges. The gastric absorption and the intestinal absorption of a series of compounds with different carbon chain lengths follows two different patterns. Absorption from the stomach increases as the chain lengthens from methyl to n-hexyl, whereas intestinal absorption increases over the range methyl to n-butyl and then diminishes as the chain length further increases. Houston et al. (1974) concluded that to explain the logic of optimal partition coefficients for intestinal absorption it was necessary to postulate a two-compartment model with a hydrophilic barrier and a lipoidal membrane and that if there is an acceptable optimal partition coefficient for gastric absorption it must be at least 10 times greater than the corresponding intestinal value.

The rate and extent of absorption of biologically active agents from the GI tract are crucial to the course of an organism's response. This has major implications as to the formulation of test material dosages and also for how production (commercial) materials may be formulated so as to minimize potential accidental intoxications. Formulation will be discussed later in this chapter.

There are a number of separate mechanisms involved in absorption from the gastrointestinal tract.

PASSIVE ABSORPTION

The membrane lining of the tract has a passive role. As toxicant molecules move from the bulk water phase of the intestinal contents into the epithelial cells, they must pass through two membranes in series because one is a layer of water and the other the lipid membrane of the microvillus surface (Wilson and Dietschy, 1974). The water layer may be the absolutely rate-limiting factor for passive absorption into the intestinal mucosa, but it is not rate limiting for active absorption. The concentration gradient as well as the physicochemical properties of the toxicant and of the lining membrane are the controlling factors. Chemicals that are highly lipid soluble are capable of passive diffusion and they pass readily from the aqueous fluids of the gut lumen through the lipid barrier of the intestinal wall and into the bloodstream. The interference in the absorption process by the water layer increases with increasing absorbability of the substances in the intestine (Winne, 1978).

Aliphatic carbamates are rapidly absorbed from the colon by passive uptake (Wood *et al.*, 1978) and it is found that there is a linear relationship between log k_a and log P for absorption of these carbamates in the colon and the stomach, whereas there is a parabolic relationship between these two values for absorption in the small intestine. The factors to be considered are:

P, octanol-buffer partition coefficient

k_a, absorption rate constant

t, time

$t_{\frac{1}{2}}$, half-life $= \dfrac{\ln 2}{k_a}$

Organic acids that are extensively ionized at intestinal pHs are absorbed primarily by simple diffusion.

FACILITATED DIFFUSION

Temporary combination of the chemical with some form of "carrier" occurs in the gut wall, and the transfer of the toxicant across the membranes is facilitated. This process is also dependent on the concentration gradient across the membrane, and there is no energy utilization in making the translocation. In some intoxications, the carrier may become saturated, and this can be a rate-limiting step in the absorption process.

ACTIVE TRANSPORT

As above, the process depends on a carrier, but differs in that the carrier provides energy for translocation from regions of lower concentration to regions of higher concentration.

PINOCYTOSIS

This is the process by which particles are absorbed and can be an important factor with the ingestion of particulate formulations of chemicals (e.g., dust formulations, suspensions of wettable powders, etc.), although it must not be confused with the absorption by one of the above processes of agent that has been released from the particles.

ABSORPTION VIA LYMPHATIC CHANNELS

Some lipophilic chemicals may be absorbed through the lymphatics dissolved in lipids.

CONVECTIVE ABSORPTION

Compounds with molecular radi of less than 4 nm can pass through pores in the gut membrane. The membrane exhibits a molecular sieving effect.

Characteristically, within certain concentration limits, if a chemical is absorbed by passive diffusion, then the concentration of toxicant in the gut and the rate of absorption are linearly related. However, if absorption is mediated by active transport, the relationship between concentration and rate of absorption conforms to Michaelis–Menten kinetics and a Lineweaver–Burk plot (i.e., reciprocal of rate of absorption plotted against reciprocal of concentration) gives a straight line.

Differences in the physiological chemistry of the gastrointestinal fluids can have a significant effect on toxicity. Both physical and chemical differences in the gastrointestinal tract can lead to species differences in susceptibility to acute intoxication. The antihelminthic pyrvinium chloride has an identical LD_{50} value when administered intraperitoneally to rats and mice (approximately 4 mg/kg) but, when administered orally, the LD_{50} value in mice was found to be 15 mg/kg, whereas for the rat, the LD_{50} values were 430 mg/kg for females and 1550 mg/kg for males. It is thought that this is an absorption difference rather than a metabolic difference (Roszkowski, 1967).

As will be shown in the next section, most of any exogenous chemical absorbed from the gastrointestinal tract must pass through the liver via the hepatic–portal system (leading to the so-called "first-pass effect") and, as mixing of the venous blood with arterial blood from the liver occurs, consideration and caution are called for in estimating the amounts of chemical in both the systemic circulation and the liver itself.

Despite the gastrointestinal absorption characteristics discussed previously, it is common for absorption from the alimentary tract to be facilitated by dilution of the toxicant. Borowitz *et al.* (1971) have suggested that the concentration effects that they observed with atropine sulfate, aminopyrine, sodium salicylate, and sodium pentobarbital were due to a combination of rapid stomach emptying and the large surface area for absorption of the drugs.

Major structural or physiological differences in the alimentary tract (e.g., species differences or surgical effects) can give rise to modifications of toxicity. For example, ruminant animals may exhibit metabolism of toxicants in the gastrointestinal tract in a way that is unlikely to occur in nonruminants.

The presence of bile salts in the alimentary tract can affect absorption of potential toxicants in a variety of ways.

ABSORPTION

Test chemicals are given most commonly by mouth. This is certainly the most convenient route, and it is the only one of practical importance for self-administration. Absorption, in general, takes place along the whole length of the gastrointestinal tract, but the chemical properties of each molecule determine whether it will be absorbed in the strongly acidic stomach or in the nearly neutral intestine. Gastric absorption is favored by an empty stomach, in which the chemical, in undiluted gastric juice, will have good access to the mucosal wall. Only when a chemical would be irritating to the gastric mucosa is it rational to administer it with or after a meal. However, the antibiotic grisofulvin is an example of a substance with poor water solubility, the absorption of which is aided by a fatty meal. The large surface area of the intestinal villi, the presence of bile, and the rich blood supply all favor intestinal absorption.

The presence of food can impair the absorption of chemicals given by mouth. Suggested mechanisms include reduced mixing, complexing with substances in the food, and retarded gastric emptying. In experiments with rats, prolonged fasting has been shown to diminish the absorption of several chemicals, possibly by deleterious effects on the epithelium of intestinal villi.

Chemicals that are metabolized rapidly by the liver cannot be given for systemic effect by the enteral route because the portal circulation carries them directly to the liver. An example is lidocaine, of value in controlling cardiac arrhythmias. This drug is absorbed well from the gut but is completely inactivated in a single passage through the liver.

The principles governing the absorption of drugs from the gastrointestinal lumen are the same as those for the passage of drugs across biologic membranes elsewhere. Low degree of ionization, high lipid/water partition coefficient of the nonionized form, and small atomic or molecular radius of water-soluble substances all favor rapid absorption. Water passes readily in both directions across the wall of the gastrointestinal lumen. Sodium ion is probably transported actively from lumen into blood. Magnesium ion is very poorly absorbed and therefore acts as a cartharic, retaining an osmotic equivalent of water as it passes down the intestinal tract. Ionic iron is absorbed as an amino acid complex, at a rate usually determined by the body's need for iron. Glucose and amino acids are transported across the intestinal wall by specific carrier systems. Some compounds of high molecular weight (polysaccharides and large proteins) cannot be absorbed until they are degraded enzymatically. Other substances are not absorbed because they are destroyed by gastrointestinal enzymes; insulin, epinephrine, and histamine are examples. Substances that form insoluble precipitates in the gastrointestinal lumen or that are not soluble either in water or in lipid clearly cannot be absorbed.

Absorption of Weak Acids and Bases

Human gastric juice is very acid (about pH 1), whereas the intestinal contents are nearly neutral (actually very slightly acid). The pH difference between plasma (pH 7.4) and the lumen of the gastrointestinal tract plays a major role in determining whether a drug that is a weak electrolyte will be absorbed into plasma or whether it will be excreted from plasma into the stomach or intestine. For practical purposes, the mucosal lining of the gastrointestinal tract is impermeable to the ionized form of a weak acid or base, but the nonionized form equilibrates freely. The rate of equilibration of the nonionized molecule is directly related to its lipid solubility. If there is a pH difference across the membrane, then the fraction ionized may be considerably greater on one side than on the other. At equilibrium, the concentration of the nonionized moiety will be the same on both sides, but there will be more total drug on the side where the degree of ionization is greater. This mechanism is known as ion trapping. The energy for sustaining the unequal chemical potential of the acid or base in question is derived from whatever mechanism maintains the pH difference. In the stomach, this mechanism is the energy-dependent secretion of hydrogen ions.

Consider how a weak electrolyte distributes across the gastric mucosa between plasma (pH 7.4) and gastric fluid (pH 1.0). In each compartment, the Henderson–Hasselbach equation gives the ratio of the concentrations (base)/(acid). The negative logarithm of the acid dissociation constant is designated by the symbol pK_a rather than using the more precisely correct pK_a'.

$$pH = pK_a + \log \frac{(base)}{(acid)}$$

$$\log \frac{(\text{base})}{(\text{acid})} = \text{pH} - \text{p}K_a$$

$$\frac{(\text{base})}{(\text{acid})} = \text{antilog } (\text{pH} - \text{p}K_a)$$

The implications of the above are obvious. Weak acids are absorbed readily from the stomach. Weak bases are not absorbed well; indeed, they would tend to accumulate within the stomach at the expense of agent in the bloodstream. Naturally, in the more alkaline intestine, bases would be absorbed better and acids more poorly.

It should be realized that although the principles outlined here are correct, the system is dynamic, not static. Molecules that are absorbed across the gastric or intestinal mucosa are removed constantly by blood flow; thus, simple reversible equilibrium across the membrane does not occur until the agent is distributed throughout the body.

Absorption from the stomach, as determined by direct measurements, conforms, in general, to the principles outlined previously. Organic acids are absorbed well because they are all almost completely nonionized at the gastric pH; indeed, many of these substances are absorbed faster than ethyl alcohol, which had long been considered one of the few compounds that were absorbed well from the stomach. Strong acids whose $\text{p}K_a$ values lie below 1, which are ionized even in the acid contents of the stomach, are not absorbed well. Weak bases are absorbed only negligibly, but their absorption can be increased, as expected, by raising the pH of the gastric fluid. All this is shown in Table 50, which shows the results of experiments in which drugs were placed in the ligated stomachs of rats and the residual amounts determined after 1 hr. Of special interest is the effect of changing the stomach pH by addition of sodium bicarbonate. Acids such as salicylic and nitrosalicyclic acids, with $\text{p}K_a$'s well on the acid side of neutrality, are absorbed much more poorly when the gastric acidity had been neutralized because they were then almost completely ionized. Very weak acids, such as thiopental and phenol, were little affected by the same pH change because, even at pH 8, they remained almost wholly nonionized.

The three barbituric acid derivatives presented (Table 51; thiopental, barbital, and secobarbital) are interesting because, although they have about the same $\text{p}K_a$, the extent of their gastric absorption differed considerably. This is related to the difference in lipid–water partition coefficients of their nonionized forms. Measurements in a number of organic solvents have revealed that thiopental has the highest partition coefficient, secobarbital a considerably smaller one, and barbital the lowest of all.

As for bases, only the weakest are absorbed to any appreciable extent at normal gastric pH, but their absorption can be increased substantially by

TABLE 50 *In Situ* Intestinal Absorption of Chemicals from Solutions of Various pH Values in the Rat[a]

| | | Percentage absorbed | | | |
| | | pH of intestinal solution | | | |
	pK_a	3.6–4.3	4.7–5.0	7.2–7.1	8.0–7.8
Base					
Aniline	4.6	40 ± 7 (9)	48 ± 5 (5)	58 ± 5 (4)	61 ± 8 (0)
Aminopyrine	5.0	21 ± 1 (2)	35 ± 1 (2)	48 ± 2 (2)	52 ± 2 (2)
p-Toluidine	5.3	30 ± 3 (3)	42 ± 3 (2)	65 ± 4 (3)	64 ± 4 (2)
Quinine	8.4	9 ± 3 (3)	11 ± 2 (2)	41 ± 1 (2)	54 ± 5 (4)
Acid					
5-Nitrosaclicylic	2.3	40 ± (2)	27 ± (2)	<2 (2)	<2 (2)
Salicylic	3.0	64 ± 4 (4)	35 ± 4 (2)	30 ± 4 (2)	10 ± 3 (6)
Acetylsalicylic	3.5	41 ± 3 (2)	27 ± 1 (2)	—	—
Benzoic	4.2	62 ± 4 (2)	36 ± 3 (4)	35 ± 4 (3)	5 ± 1 (2)
p-Hydroxypro-piophenone	7.8	61 ± 5 (3)	52 ± 2 (2)	67 ± 6 (5)	60 ± 5 (2)

[a]The percentage absorbed is expressed as mean ± range; numbers in parentheses indicate number of animals (from Hogben *et al.* 1959, Table 1).

neutralizing the stomach contents. The quaternary cations, however, which are charged at all pH values, were not absorbed at either pH.

The accumulation of weak bases in the stomach by ion trapping mimics a secretory process; if the chemical is administered systemically, it accumulates in the stomach. Dogs given various drugs intravenously by continuous infusion to maintain a constant drug level in the plasma had the gastric contents sampled by means of an indwelling catheter. The results, representing concentrations after 30–60 min, are shown in Table 51. Both acids and bases behaved according to expectation. The stronger bases (pK_a >5) accumulated in stomach contents to many times their plasma concentrations; the weak bases appeared in about equal concentrations in gastric juice and in plasma. Among the acids, only the weakest appeared in detectable amounts in the stomach. It may be wondered why the strong bases, which are completely ionized in gastric juice, and whose theoretical concentration ratios (gastric juice/plasma) are very large, should nevertheless have attained only about a 40-fold excess over plasma. Direct measurements of arterial and venous blood showed that essentially all the blood flowing through the gastric mucosa was cleared of these agents; obviously, no more chemical could enter the gastric juice in a given time than was brought there by the circulation. Another limitation comes into play when the base pK_a exceeds 7.4; now, a major fraction of the circulating base is cationic and a decreasing fraction is nonionized so that the effective concentration gradient for diffusion across the stomach wall is reduced.

TABLE 51   Absorption of Organic Acids and Organic Bases from the Rat Stomach[a]

	pK_a	Percentage absorbed in 1 hr	
		0.1 M HCl	NaHCO$_3$ (pH 8)
Acid			
5-Sulfosalicyclic	Strong	0 ± 0 (2)	0 ± 0 (2)
Phenosulfonphtalein	Strong	2 ± 2 (3)	2 ± 1 (2)
5-Nitrosalicylic	2.3	52 ± 3 (2)	16 ± 2 (2)
Salicylic	3.0	61 ± 7 (4)	13 ± 1 (2)
Acetylsalicylic	3.5	35 ± 4 (3)	—
Benzoic	4.2	55 ± 3 (2)	—
Thiopental	7.6	46 ± 3 (2)	34 ± 2 (2)
p-Hydroxypropiophenone	7.8	55 ± 3 (2)	—
Barbital	7.8	4 ± 3 (4)	—
Secobarbital	7.9	30 ± 2 (2)	—
Phenol	9.9	40 ± 5 (3)	40 ± 5 (3)
Base			
Acetanilid	0.3	36 ± 3 (2)	—
Caffeine	0.8	24 ± 3 (2)	—
Antipyrine	1.4	14 ± 3 (4)	—
m-Nitroaniline	2.5	17 ± 0 (2)	—
Aniline	4.6	6 ± 4 (3)	56 ± 3 (2)
Aminopyridine	5.0	2 ± 2 (3)	—
p-Toludine	5.3	0 ± 0 (2)	47 ± 4 (2)
a-Acetylmethadol	8.3	0 ± 0 (4)	—
Quinine	8.4	0 ± 0 (2)	18 ± 2 (2)
Dextrophan, levorphanol	9.2	0 ± 2 (8)	16 ± 1 (2)
Ephedrine	9.6	3 ± 3 (2)	—
Tolazoline	10.3	7 ± 2 (4)	—
Mecamylamine	11.2	0 ± 0 (2)	—
Darstine	Cation	0 ± 0 (2)	—
Procaine amide ethobromide	Cation	0 ± 0 (2)	5 ± 1 (2)
Tetraethylammonium	Cation	0 ± 1 (2)	—

[a]The percentage absorbed in 1 hr is expressed as mean ± range (N in parentheses) (after Schanker, 1960).

The ion trapping mechanism provides a method of some forensic value for determining the presence of alkaloids (e.g., narcotics, cocaine, and amphetamines) in cases of death suspected to be due to overdosage of self-administered drugs (Table 52). Drug concentrations in gastric contents may be very high even after parenteral injection.

Absorption from the intestine has been studied by perfusing drug solutions slowly through rat intestine in situ and by varying the pH as desired. The relationships that emerge from such studies are the same as those for the stomach, the difference being that the intestinal pH is normally near neutrality.

TABLE 52   Gastric Secretion of Chemicals in the Dog[a]

	pK$_a$	Plasma protein binding (%)	Plasma concentration (total) (mg/liter)	Gastric juice concentration (mg/liter)	Gastric plasma concentration ratio	Ratio corrected for plasma binding	Theoretical ratio
Base							
Acetanilid	0.3	0	126	126	1.0	1.0	1.0
Theophyline	0.7	15	81	118	1.5	1.3	1.5
Antipyrine	1.4	0	230	938	4.1	4.2	4.2
Aniline	5.0	25	8.5	358	42		10^4
Aminopyrine	5.0	15	24	1010	42		10^4
Quinine	8.4	75	4.7	189	40		10^6
Levorphanol	9.2	50	0.2	8.3	42		10^6
Tolazoline	10.3	23	13.2	135	10		10^6
Acid							
Salicylic	3.0	75	338	0	0	0	10^{-4}
Probenecid	3.4	75	14	0	0	0	10^{-4}
Phenylbutazone	4.4	90	195	0	0	0	10^{-3}
p-Hydroxypropiophenone	7.8	75	5.5	0.62	0.11	0.5	0.6
Thiopental	7.6	75	20	2.0	0.10	0.5	0.6
Barbital	7.8	0	254	152	0.6	0.6	0.6

[a]Measurements were made 30–60 min after initiation of continuous intravenous drug infusion (from Shore et al., Tables 1 and 3).

As the pH was increased, the bases were absorbed better, the acids more poorly. Detailed studies with a great many drugs in unbuffered solutions revealed that in the normal intestine, acids with $pK_a >3.0$ and bases with $pK_a <7.8$ are very well absorbed; outside these limits the absorption of acids and bases, respectively, fell off rapidly. This behavior leads to the conclusion that the "virtual pH" in the microenvironment of the absorbing surface in the gut is about 5.3; this is somewhat more acidic than is usually considered to be the pH in the intestinal lumen.

Absorption from the buccal cavity has been shown to follow exactly the same principles as described for stomach and intestine. The pH of human and canine saliva is usually about 6. The relationship between pH, pK_a, and lipid–water partition coefficient was studied in human subjects by the following simple procedure. A known amount of a drug, usually 1 mg, in 25 ml of buffer, was placed in a subject's mouth. It was mixed by means of vigorous movements of the tongue and cheeks; care was taken not to allow any to be swallowed. After 5 min the whole volume was expectorated into a beaker, the mouth was rinsed several times with water, and the drug concentration was assayed, usually by gas–liquid chromatography. Absorption was taken to be the difference between the amount introduced and the amount remaining. These studies yielded very consistent results for a given subject on different days, with greater variability between subjects. Bases were absorbed only on the alkaline side of their pK_a, i.e., only in the nonionized form. At normal saliva pH only chlorpheniramine, the weakest base tested, was absorbed to a significant extent. In a series of n-alkyl-substituted carboxylic acids, the inverse relationship was found; all were absorbed best on the acid side of the pK_a.

The difference between the extent of availability (often designated solely as bioavailability) and the rate of availability is illustrated in Fig. 46, which depicts the concentration/time curve for a hypothetical agent formulated into three different dosage forms. Dosage forms A and B are designed so that the agent is put into the blood circulation at the same rate, but twice as fast as for dosage form C. The times at which agent concentrations reach a peak are identical for dosage forms A and B and occur earlier than the peak time for dosage form C. In general, the relative order of peak times following the administration of different dosage forms of the drug corresponds to the rates of availability of the chemical moiety from the various dosage forms. The extent of availability can be measured by using either chemical concentrations in the plasma or blood or amounts of unchanged chemical in the urine. The area under the blood concentration/time curve (area under the curve) for an agent can serve as a measure of the extent of availability. In Fig. 46, the areas under curves A and C are identical and twice as great as the area under curve B. In most cases, in which clearance is constant, the relative areas under the curves or the amount of unchanged chemical excreted in the urine will

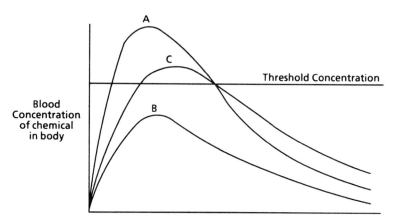

FIGURE 46   Blood concentration/time curves illustrating how changes in the rate and extent of chemical availability can influence the duration of action and the efficacy of a dose of an agent. The lines indicate the concentration (T_c) of the agent in the body. Case A is when the agent absorbed is available rapidly and completely. This product produces a prompt and prolonged response. The agent in case B is absorbed at the same rate as in case A, but is only 50% as available. There will be no response from this dose of the agent because the T_c is not reached. The agent in case C is absorbed at one-half the rate seen in cases A and B but is 100% available.

quantitatively describe the relative availability of the agent from the different dosage forms. However, even in nonlinear cases, in which clearance is dose dependent, the relative areas under the curves will yield a measurement of the rank order of availability from different dosage forms or from different routes of administration.

Because there is usually a concentration for a chemical in the blood (as shown in Fig. 46) that is necessary to elicit either a pharmacologic or toxic effect, both the rate and extent of input or availability can alter the toxicity of a compound. In the majority of cases, the duration of effects will be a function of the length of time the blood concentration curve is above the threshold concentration, and the intensity of the effect for many agents will be a function of the elevation of the blood concentration curve above the threshold concentration.

Thus, for the three different dosage forms depicted in Fig. 46 there will be significant differences in the levels of "toxicity." Dosage form B will require that twice the dose be administered to attain blood levels equivalent to those for dosage form A. Differences in the rate of availability are particularly important for agents given acutely. Dosage form A will reach the target concentration earlier than chemical from dosage form C; concentrations from A will reach a higher level and remain above the minimum effective concentration for a longer period of time. In a multiple dosing regimen, dosage forms A and C would yield the same average blood concentrations, although dosage form A will show somewhat greater maximum and lower minimum concentrations.

For most chemicals, the rate of disposition or loss from the biological system is independent of rate of input, once the agent is absorbed. Disposition is defined as what happens to the active molecule after it reaches a site in the blood circulation where concentration measurements can be made (the systemic circulations, generally). Although disposition processes may be independent of input, the inverse is not necessarily true because disposition can markedly affect the extent of availability. Agents absorbed from the stomach and the intestine must first pass through the liver before reaching the general circulation (Fig. 47). Thus, if a compound is metabolized in the liver or excreted in bile, some of the active molecule absorbed from the gastrointestinal tract will be inactivated by hepatic processes before it can reach the systemic circulation and be distributed to its sites of action. If the metabolizing or biliary excreting capacity of the liver is great, the effect on the extent of availability will be substantial. Thus, if the hepatic blood clearance for the chemical is large, relative to hepatic blood flow, the extent of availability for this chemical will be low when it is given by a route that yields first-pass metabolic effects.

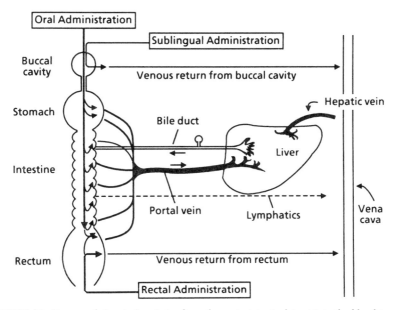

FIGURE 47 Passage of chemical moieties from the gastrointestinal tract into the bloodstream, shown in a diagrammatic fashion.

This decrease in availability is a function of the physiologic site from which absorption takes place, and no amount of dosage-form modification can improve the availability under linear conditions. Of course, toxic blood levels can be reached by this route of administration if larger doses are given.

It is important to realize that chemicals with high extraction ratios will exhibit marked intersubject variability in bioavailability because of variations in hepatic function or blood flow or both. For the chemical with an extraction ratio of 0.90 that increases to 0.95, the bioavailability of the agent will be halved, from 0.10 to 0.05. These relationships can explain the marked variability in plasma or blood drug concentrations that occurs among individual animals given similar doses of a chemical that is markedly extracted. Small variations in hepatic extraction between individual animals will result in large differences in availability and plasma drug concentrations.

The first-pass effect can be avoided, to a great extent, by use of the sublingual route and by topical preparations (e.g., nitroglycerin ointment) and can be partially avoided by using rectal suppositories. The capillaries in the lower and middle sections of the rectum drain into the interior and middle hemorrhoidal veins, which, in turn, drain into the inferior vena cava, thus bypassing the liver. However, suppositories tend to move upward in the rectum into a region where veins that lead to the liver predominate, such as the superior hemorrhoidal. In addition, there are extensive connections between the superior and middle hemorrhoidal veins, and thus probably only about 50% of a rectal dose can be assumed to bypass the liver. The lungs represent a good temporary clearing site for a number of chemicals (especially basic compounds) by partition into lipid tissues, as well as serving a filtering function for particulate matter that may be given by intravenous injection. In essence, the lung may cause first-pass loss by excretion and possible metabolism for chemicals input into the body by the nongastrointestinal routes of administration.

Biological (test subject) related factors which can influence absorption of a chemical from the gastrointestinal tract are summarized in Table 53.

The minimization of variability due to these factors rests on the selection of the appropriate animal model, by careful selection of healthy animals, and (as will be discussed later) by use of proper techniques.

There are also a number of chemical factors which may influence absorption from the GI tract. These are summarized in Table 54.

TECHNIQUES

Test materials may be administered as solutions or suspensions as long as they are homogeneous and delivery is accurate. For traditional oral administration (gavage), the solution or suspension can be administered with a suitable stom-

TABLE 53   Factors Influencing Test Subject Characteristics That Can Influence GI
Absorption

General and inherent characteristics
    General condition of the subject (e.g., starved versus well-fed or ambulatory versus supine)
    The presence of concurrent diseases (i.e., diseases may either speed or slow gastric emp-
        tying)
    Age
    Weight and degree of obesity

Physiological function
    Status of the subject's renal function
    Status of the subject's hepatic function
    Status of the subject's cardiovascular system
    Status of the subject's gastrointestinal motility and function (e.g., ability to swallow)
    pH of the gastric fluid (e.g., affected by fasting disease, food intake, or drugs)
    Gastrointestinal blood flow to the area of absorption
    Blood flow to areas of absorption for other dose forms than those absorbed through gastroin-
        testinal routes

Acquired characteristics
    Status of the subject's anatomy (e.g., previous surgery)
    Status of the subject's gastrointestinal flora
    Timing of drug administration relative to meals (i.e., the presence of food in the gastrointes-
        tinal tract)
    Body position of subject (lying on its side slows gastric emptying)
    Psychological state of subject (e.g., stress increases gastric emptying rate and depression de-
        creases rate)
    Physical exercise of subject may reduce gastric emptying rate

Physiological principles
    Food enhances gastric blood flow, which shold theoretically increase the rate of absorption.
    Food slows the rate of gastric emptying, which should theoretically slow the rate of passage
        to the intestines where the largest amounts of most agents are absorbed. This should de-
        crease the rate of absorption for most agents. Agents absorbed to a larger extent in the
        stomach will have increased time for absorption in the presence of food and should be ab-
        sorbed more completely than in fasted patients.
    Bile flow and secretion are stimulated by fats and certain other foods. Bile salts may enhance
        or delay absorption depending on whether they form insoluble complexes with drugs or
        enhance the solubility of agents.
    Changes in splanchnic blood flow as a result of food depend on direction and magnitude of
        the type of food ingested.
    The presence of active (saturable) transport mechanisms places a limit on the amount of a
        chemical that may be absorbed.

Note. The minimization of variability due to these factors rests on the selection of the appropriate
animal model, by careful selection of healthy animals, and (as will be discussed later) by use of
proper techniques.

TABLE 54   Factors Relating to Chemical Characteristics That May Influence Absorption[a]

Administration of chemical and its passage in body
    Dissolution characteristics of solid dosage forms, which depend on formulation in addition
        to the properties of the chemical itself (e.g., vehicle may decrease permeability of suspen-
        sion or capsule to water and retard dissolution and diffusion).
    Rate of dissolution in gastrointestinal fluids. Chemicals that are inadequately dissolved in
        gastric contents may be inadequately absorbed.
    Chemicals that are absorbed into food may have a delayed absorption.
    Carrier transported chemicals are more likely to be absorbed in the small intestine.
    Route of administration.
    Chemicals undergo metabolism in the gastrointestinal tract.
Physiochemical properties of chemicals
    Chemicals that chelate metal ions in food may form insoluble complexes and will not be ad-
        equately absorbed.
    pH of dosing solutions—weakly basic solutions are absorbed to a greater degree in the small
        intestine.
    Salts used.
    Hydrates or solvates.
    Crystal form of chemical (e.g., insulin).
    "Pharmaceutical" form (e.g., fluid, solid, or suspension).
    Enteric coating.
    Absorption of quatenary compounds (e.g., hexamethonium and amiloride) are decreased by
        food.
    Molecular weight of chemical (e.g., when the molecular weight of a drug is above about
        1000, absorption is markedly decreased).
    pK_a (dissociation constant).
    Lipid solubility (i.e., a hydrophobic property relating to penetration through membranes).
    Particle size of chemical in solid dosage form—smaller particle sizes will increase the rate
        and/or degree of absorption if dissolution of the chemical is the rate-limiting factor in ab-
        sorption. Chemicals that have a low dissolution rate may be made in a micronized form
        to increase their rate of dissolution.
    Particle size of the dispersed phase in an emulsion.
    Type of disintegrating agent in the formulation.
    Hardness of a solid (granule, pellet, or tablet) (i.e., related to amount of compression used
        to make tablet) or capsule if they do not disintegrate appropriately.

[a]Many of these factors are reviewed by Bates and Gibaldi (1970), and some factors could be placed
in both categories.

ach tube or feeding needle ("Popper" tube) attached to a syringe. If the dose
is too large to be administered at one time, it can be divided into equal subparts
with 2–4 hr between each administration. This subdivided dosing approach
should generally be avoided, however.

    A set of procedures which minimize technique variation and dose-to-dose
variability for rodents and other small animals follows.

Gavaging Techniques

1. Dosing should occur during the same period of the day (when possible), preferably midmorning.

2. Before beginning, the study protocol must be checked to determine the time plan and number of animals within each dose group as well as any nonroutine procedures related to dosing which may be required (e.g., urinalysis and blood sampling).

3. The animals must be weighed beforehand (if appropriate to the study design) and weights must be recorded. Doses are calculated based on body weight.

4. Doses are recorded on a form designed for the study type.

5. Sample to be gavaged should be prepared in advance and the preparation procedure documented.

GAVAGE PROCEDURE (RAT OR MOUSE)

1. Oral dosing will be done by gavage with a 3-in. stainless steel animal feeding needle attached to either a glass or disposable syringe, depending on the nature of the test suspension or solution. A different needle and syringe should be used for each dose level and material to be gavaged.

2. Choose a gavage needle of appropriate diameter as determined by the physical characteristics of the test material to be administered and the size of the animal being dosed.

3. Remove the animal from the cage by grasping it in such a manner as to immobilize the head and torso to allow insertion of the gavage needle. The method of restraint should be a recognized animal handling procedure.

4. While immobilizing the head and torso of the animal, hold the syringe barrel near its base and insert the needle into the mouth of the animal. Slide the needle along the side of the tongue until encountering resistence. Gentle pressure with the tip of the needle will facilitate passage of the needle into the esophagus. Should the needle be misdirected into the trachea, the animal may struggle and exhibit difficulty in breathing. The rings of the trachea may also be felt as the needle encounters them. Smooth passage of the needle to its full depth with the hub of the needle resting at the corner of the mouth is a good indicator of proper placement. If in doubt as to placement, remove the needle completely, allow the animal a moment to recover and reinsert the needle.

5. When the needle is all the way in, draw back slightly and slowly depress the syringe plunger, expelling the desired volume into the animal's stomach.

When administering significant volumes or viscous liquids, it is advisable to depress the plunger in stages.

6. When the complete volume has been administered slowly and gently, withdraw the needle. Observe the animal for signs of distress, respiratory difficulty, injury, or a reflux of test material through the mouth or nasal passages. If observed, these signs should be indicated on the appropriate dosing sheet and the primary investigator notified.

7. If the animal is singly caged, return it to its cage.

8. If the animal is multiple caged, place it in a separate cage until all other animals from the cage are dosed. Then return them all to their original cage.

9. Following dosing, all animals should be closely observed, paying particular attention to any signs of respiratory distress.

Test chemicals placed into any natural orifice exert local effects and, in many instances, systemic effects as well. The possibility of systemic effects occurring when local effects are of interest or of local effects occurring when systemic effects are to be evaluated should be considered.

For routes of administration in which the chemical is given orally or placed into an orifice other than the mouth, clear instructions about the correct administration of the chemical must be provided. Many cases are known of oral pediatric drops for ear infections being placed into the ear, and vice versa (ear drops being swallowed) in humans. Errors in test article administration are especially prevalent when a chemical form is being used in a nontraditional manner (e.g., suppositories that are given by the buccal route).

Many technicians may not be familiar with terms such as sublingual (under the tongue), buccal (between the cheek and gingiva), otic, and so on. A clear description of each of these nontraditional (i.e., other than gavage routes) should be discussed with technicians and instructions may also be written and given to them. Demonstrations are often useful to illustrate selected techniques of administration (e.g., to use an inhaler or nebulizer). Some chemicals must be placed by technicians into body orifices (e.g., medicated intrauterine devices such as Progestersert).

The minor routes do see some use in acute toxicity testing and at least four are briefly presented here.

THE EYE (PEROCULAR ROUTE)

The administration of drugs or accidental exposure of chemicals to the eyes is not commonly a concern in systemic toxicity. This is because the absorption of chemicals through the eyes is rarely a serious hazard due to the small surface area exposed and the efficiency of the protective mechanisms (i.e., blink reflex and tears). As long as the epithelium of the eyes remains itact, it is impermeable to many molecules but, provided that the toxicant has a suitable polar/nonpolar balance, penetration may occur (Swan and White, 1942; Kondrizer et al., 1959).

Holmstedt (1959) and Brown and Muir (1971) have reviewed perocular absorption of pesticides. Sinow and Wei (1973) have shown that the quaternary herbicide paraquat can be lethal to rabbits if applied directly to the surface of the eyes. Parathion, in particular, is exceedingly toxic when administered via the eye—a concern which must be kept in mind for the protection of pesticide applicators.

The issues pertinent to administration of materials to the eyes were addressed in the earlier chapter on ocular irritation.

RECTAL ADMINISTRATION

Because a number of therapeutic compounds are given in the form of suppositories, an indication of the toxicity after rectal administration is sometimes required. Toxicity studies and initial drug formulations of such compounds are usually performed by the oral route and the rectal formulation comes late in development and marketing. In view of the differences between laboratory animals and man in the anatomy and microflora of the colon and rectum, animal toxicity studies late in drug development are of limited value. However, in cases in which an indication of potential rectal hazard or bioavailability is required, the compound may be introduced into the rectum of the rat using an oral dosing needle to prevent tissue damage. To avoid the rapid excretion of the unabsorbed dose, anesthetized animals should be used and the dose retained with an inert plug or bung (such as a cork).

Drugs (and, therefore, test chemicals) are occasionally administered by rectum, but most are not as well absorbed here as from the upper intestine. Aminophylline, used in suppository form for the management of asthma, is one of the few drugs routinely given in this way. Inert vehicles employed for suppository preparations include cocoa butter, glycerinated vehicles, gelatin, and polyethylene glycol. Because the rectal mucosa is irritated by nonisotonic solutions, fluids administered by this route should always be isotonic with plasma (e.g., 0.9% NaCl).

VAGINAL ADMINISTRATION

Though not a common route, some materials do have routine exposure by this route (spermicides, tampons, douches, and antibiotics, for example) and, therefore, must be evaluated for irritation and toxicity by this route. The older preferred models used rabbits and monkeys (Eckstein *et al.*, 1969) but a model which uses rats has been developed (Staab *et al.*, 1987). McConnell (1973) clearly described the limitations, particularly of volume of test material involved in such tests.

NASAL ADMINISTRATION

A route which has gained increasing popularity of late for pharmaceutical administration in man is the intranasal route. The reasons for this popularity are the ease of use (and, therefore, ready patient acceptance and high compliance rate), the high degree and rate of absorption of many substances [it is reported that this is true for most substances up to 1000 mw (McMartin *et al.*, 1987)], and the avoiding of the highly acid environment in the stomach and first-pass metabolism in the liver (particularly important for some of the newer peptide moieties). The only special safety concerns are the potential for irritation of the mucous membrane and the rapid distribution of administered materials to the CNS.

A number of means may be used to administer materials nasally—nebulizers and aerosolizer pumps being the most attractive first choices. Accurate dose administration requires careful planning, evaluation of administration device, and attention to technique.

VOLUME LIMITATIONS BY ROUTE

In the strictest sense, absolute limitations on how much of a dosage form may be administered by any particular route are determined by specific aspects of the test species or dosage form. But there are some general guidelines (determined by issues of humane treatment of animals, accurate delivery of dose, and such) which can be given. These are summarized in Table 55.

The section on vehicles and formulations should, of course, be checked to see if there is any more specific guidance due to the characteristics of a particular vehicle.

SELECTION OF ROUTE

The basis for selecting routes for acute toxicity studies should be completely straightforward; the route of potential human exposure should be the route evaluated in animals, to make extrapolation of results to humans as linear as possible. Practical considerations sometimes make this impossible or unaccept-

TABLE 55   General Guidelines for Maximum Dose Volumes by Route

Route	Volume should not exceed	Notes
Oral	20 ml/kg	Fasted animals
Dermal	2 ml/kg	Limit in accuracy of dosing/available body surface
Intravenous	1 ml/kg	Over 5 min
Intramuscular	0.5 ml/kg	At one site
Perocular	0.01 ml	
Rectal	0.5 ml/kg	
Vaginal	0.2 ml in rat	
	1 ml in rabbit	
Inhalation	2 mg/liter	
Nasal	0.1 ml/nostril in monkey or dog	

ably impractical, but compromises on route should be well thought out and carefully considered. As a general rule, if the route of potential human exposure cannot be used, then a route which increases potential systemic exposure should be selected.

VEHICLES AND FORMULATION OF MATERIALS

One of the areas that is overlooked by virtually everyone in toxicology testing and research, yet is of crucial importance, is that of what vehicles are used and how one prepares test chemicals for administration to test animals (or gets them into culture media, for that matter). For a number of reasons, it is less often the case than not that a chemical of interest is administered or applied as is ("neat"). Rather, it must be put in a form that can be accurately given to animals in such a way that it will be absorbed and not be too irritating. Most laboratory toxicologists come to understand vehicles and formulation, but to the knowledge of the authors, guidance on the subject is limited to a short chapter on formulations by Fitzgerald et al. (1983).

Regulatory toxicology in the United States can be said to have arisen due to the problem of vehicles and formulation in the late 1930s, when attempts were made to formulate the new drug sulphanilamide. This drug is not very soluble in water, and a firm called Massengill in the United States produced a syrupy clear elixir formulation which was easy to take. The figures illustrate how easy it is to be misled. The drug is not very soluble in glycerol, which has an LD_{50} in mice of 31.5 g/kg, but there are other glycols which have the characteristic sweet taste and a much higher solvent capacity. Ethylene glycol has an LD_{50} of 13.7 g/kg to mice and 8.5 g/kg to rats, so it is slightly more toxic than diethylene glycol, which has an LD_{50} to rats of 20.8 g/kg, similar to that for glycerol. The drug, which is itself inherently toxic, was marketed in a 75% aqueous diethylene glycol flavored elixer. Early in 1937 came the first reports of deaths, and the situation remained obscure for about 6 months until it became clear that the toxic ingredient in the elixir was the diethylene glycol. Even as late as March 1937, Haag and Ambrose were reporting that the glycol was excreted substantially unchanged in dogs, suggesting it was likely to be safe. Within a few weeks, Holick (1937) confirmed that a low concentration of diethylene glycol in drinking water was fatal to a number of species. Hagenbusch (1937) found that necropsies on patients who had been taking 60–70 ml of the solvent per day had similar results to those seen in rats, rabbits, and dogs taking the same dose with or without the drug. This clearly implicated the solvent, although some authors considered that it was simply potentiating the toxicity of the drug. Some idea of the magnitude of this disaster may be found in the paper of Calvary and Klumpp (1939), who reviewed 105 deaths and a further 260 survivors who were affected to varying degrees, usually with progressive failure of the renal system. It is easy to be wise after the event, but the formulator fell into a classical trap, in that the difference between acute and chronic toxicity had not been adequately considered. In passing, the widespread use of ethylene glycol itself as an antifreeze has led to a number of accidental deaths which suggest that the lethal dose in man is around 1.4 ml/kg, or a volume of about 100 ml. In the Preface to the *First United States Pharmacopoeia*, published in 1820, is the statement that

> It is the object of the Pharmacopoeia to select from among substances which possess medical power, those, the utility of which is most fully established and best understood; and to form from them preparations and compositions, in which their powers may be exerted to the greatest advantage.

This suggests that the influence that formulation and preparation may have on the biological activity of a drug (and on nonpharmaceutical chemicals) has been appreciated for a considerable time.

Available and commonly used vehicles and formulating agents are reviewed, along with basic information on them, in Appendix C.

There are some basic principles to be observed in developing and preparing test material formulations. These are presented in Table 56.

Bioavailability is defined as the fraction of the dose reaching the systemic circulation as unchanged compound following administration by any route. For an agent administered orally, bioavailability may be less than unity for several reasons. The chemical may be incompletely absorbed. It may be metabolized in the gut, the gut wall, the portal blood, or the liver prior to entry into the systemic circulation (see Fig. 47). It may undergo enterohepatic cycling

TABLE 56   Desirable Characteristics of a Dosing Formulation and Its Preparation

Preparation of the formulation should not involve heating of the test material to a point anywhere near altering its chemical or physical characteristics.

If the material is a solid and is to be assessed for dermal effects, its shape and particle size should be preserved.

Multicomponent test materials (mixtures) should be formulated so that the administered form accurately represents the original mixture (i.e., components should not be selectively suspended or taken into solution).

Formulation should preserve the chemical stability and identity of the test material.

The formulation should be such as to minimize total test volumes. Use just enough solvent or vehicle.

The formulation should be as easy as possible to accurately administer.

pH of dosing formulations should be between 5 and 9, if possible.

Acids or bases should not be used to divide (for both humane reasons and to avoid pH partitioning in either that gut or the renal tubule) the test material.

If a parental route is to be employed, final solutions should be as nearly isotonic as possible.

with incomplete reabsorption following elimination into the bile. Biotransformation of some chemicals in the liver following oral administration is an important factor in the pharmacokinetic profile, as will be discussed further. Bioavailability measures following oral administration are generally given as the percentage of the dose available to the systemic circulation.

Because the components of a mixture may have very different physicochemical characteristics (solubility, vapor pressure, density, etc.) great care must be taken in preparing and administering any mixture so that what is actually tested is the mixture of interest. Examples of such procedures are making dilutions (not all components of the mixture may be equally soluble or miscible with the vehicle) and generating either vapors or respirable aerosols (not all the components may have equivalent volatility or surface tension leading to a test atmosphere that contains only a portion of the components of the mixture).

By increasing or decreasing the viscosity of a formulation, the absorption of a toxicant can be altered (Ritschel et al., 1974). Fincher (1968) has defined some of the physicochemical aspects of absorption of toxicants from particulate formulations in the gastrointestinal tract. Conversely, the use of absorbents to diminish absorption has been used as antidote therapy for some forms of intoxication. With the knowledge that rats cannot vomit, there have been serious attempts at making rodenticides safer to nontarget animals by incorporating emetics into the formulations, but this has had only a limited success. Gaines et al. (1960) used in vivo liver perfusion techniques to investigate the apparent anommaly that the carbamate Isolan was more toxic when administered to rats percutaneously than when administered orally (Gaines, 1960). It has been shown that these results, a manifestation of different formulations, have been used for the two routes of exposure and by estimating the LD_{50} values using a common solvent, n-octanol, for both routes of exposure it was found that Isolan was significantly more toxic by the oral route than by the percutaneous route, and by regression analysis it was found that at no level of lethal dose values was the reverse correct.

Although the oral route is the most convenient, there are numerous factors which make it unpredictable. Absorbtion by this route is subject to significant variation from animal to animal, and even in the individual animal at different times. Considerable effort has been spent by the pharmaceutical industry to develop drug formulations with absorption characteristics that are both more effective and more dependable. Protective enteric coatings for pharmaceuticals were introduced long ago to retard the action of gastric fluids and then disintegrate and dissolve after passage of a tablet into the human intestine. The purposes of these coatings for drugs are to protect the active ingredient which would be degraded in the stomach, to prevent nausea and vomiting caused by local gastric irritation (also a big problem in rodent studies, in which over a long period of time it frequently leads to forestomach hyperplasia), to obtain higher local concentrations of the active ingredient intended to act locally in the intestinal tract, to produce a delayed biological effect, or to deliver the active ingredient to the intestinal tract for optimal absorption there. Such coatings are generally fats, fatty acids, waxes, or other such agents, and all of these intended purposes for drug delivery can readily be made to apply for some toxicity studies. Their major drawback, however, is the marked variability in time for a substance to be passed through the stomach. In humans, this gastric emptying time can range from minutes to as long as 12 hr. One would expect the same for animals, because the limited available data suggest this is the case. Similar coating systems, including microencapsulation (see Melnick et al., 1987), are available for, and currently used in, animal toxicity studies.

The test chemical is unlikely to be absorbed or excreted unless it is first released from its formulation. It is this stage of the process which is the first and most critical step for the activity of many chemicals. If the formulation does not release the chemical, the rest of the process becomes somewhat pointless.

There have been a number of reviews of the influence that formulation may have on activity (Levi, 1963; Groves, 1966; Gibaldi, 1976; Wagner, 1971) and, in some situations, the toxicity of a chemical, especially if it is pharmacologically potent (i.e., has a steep dose–response curve), may be influenced by the manipulative process involved in getting it into the test subjects.

It might be argued that the simplest way around the formulation problem would be to administer any test chemical as a solution in water, thereby avoiding the difficulties altogether. However, because multiple, small, accurately measured doses of a chemical are required repeatedly, reproducible dilutions must be used. Also, the water itself is to be regarded as the formulation vehicle, and the test substance must be water soluble and stable in solution (many are not). If we take into account the need for accuracy, stability, and optimum performance *in vivo,* the problem can become complex.

Direct connection between observed toxicity and formulation components is not common and it is usually assumed that vehicles and other nontest chemical components are innocuous or have only transitory pharmacological effects. Historically, however, this has certainly not been the case. Even lactose may have marked toxicity in individual test animals (or humans) who may be genetically incapable of tolerating it.

The initial stage of drug release from the formulation, both in terms of the amount and the rate of release, may exercise considerable influence at the clinical response level. A close consideration of the formulation parameters of any chemical is therefore essential during the development of any new drug and, indeed, there are examples in which formulations of established drugs also appear to require additional investigation.

The effects of formulation additives on chemical bioavailability from oral solutions and suspensions have been well reviewed by Hem (1973). He pointed out how the presence of sugars in a formulation may increase the viscosity of the vehicle. However, sugar solutions alone may delay stomach-emptying time considerably when compared to solutions of the same viscosity prepared with celluloses. This may be due to an effect on osmotic pressure. Sugars of different types may also have an effect on fluid uptake by tissues, and this, in turn, correlates with the effect of sugars such as glucose and mannitol on drug transport.

Surfactants have been explored widely for their effects on drug absorption, in particular using experimental animals (Gibaldi, 1976; Gibaldi and Feldman, 1970). Surfactants act to alter dissolution rates (of lipid materials), surface areas of particles and droplets, and membrane characteristics, all of which affect absorption.

Surfactants may increase the solubility of the drug by incorporation into micelles, but the amounts of material required to increase solubility significantly are such that at least orally the laxative effects are likely to be unacceptable. The competition between the surfactant micelles and the absorption sites is also likely to reduce any useful effect and make difficult any prediction of net overall effect. However, if a surfactant has any effect at all, it is likely to be in the realm of dispersing agents which help suspensions of insoluble materials to be more readily dispersed and available for solution. Natural surfactants, in particular bile salts, may enhance absorption of poorly soluble materials.

The effective surface area of an ingested chemical is usually much smaller than the specific surface area which is an idealized *in vitro* measurement. Many drugs whose dissolution characteristics could be improved by particle size reduction are extremely hydrophobic and may resist wetting by gastro-intestinal fluids. Therefore, the gastrointestinal fluids may come into intimate contact with only a fraction of the potentially available surface area. The effective surface area of hydrophobic particles can often be increased by the addition of a surface-active agent to the formulation, which functions to reduce the contact angle between the solid and the gastrointestinal fluids. Reduction in contact angle permits more intimate contact of chemicals and fluids, thereby increasing effective surface area and dissolution rate.

Formulations for administering dermally applied toxicants present different considerations and problems. The extent and speed with which a biologically active substance penetrates the skin or other biological membranes depends on the effect which the three factors—vehicle, membrane, and chemical—exert on the diffusion process. It is now accepted that they together represent a functional unit which controls the penetration and location of the externally applied chemicals in the deeper layers of the skin or membrane layer. The importance of the vehicle for the absorption process has been neglected until recently. One of the few requirements demanded of the vehicle has been that it acts as an inert medium which incorporates the test chemical in the most homogeneous distribution possible. In addition, chemical stability and good cosmetic appearance have been desirable. Most formulations in toxicology are based on empirical experience.

The chemical incorporated in a vehicle should reach the surface of the skin at a suitable rate and concentration. If the site of action lies in the deeper layers of the epidermis or below, the substance must cross the stratum corneum, in cases in which the skin is intact. Both processes, diffusion from the dosage form and diffusion through the skin barriers, are inextricably linked. They should be considered simultaneously and can be influenced by the choice of formulation.

The thesis that all lipid-soluble compounds basically penetrate faster than water-soluble ones cannot be supported in this absolute form. A lipophilic agent can penetrate faster or slower or at the same rate as a hydrophilic agent, depending on the vehicle used.

Disregarding such chemical-specific properties as dissociation constants (in the case of ionic compounds), particle size, and polymorphism, as well as side effects of viscosity, binding to vehicle components, complex formulation, etc., the following formulation principles arise:

optimization of the concentration of chemical capable of diffusion by testing its maximum solubility;

reduction of the proportion of solvent to a degree which is adequate to
  keep the test material still in solution; and
use of vehicle components which reduce the permeability barriers.

These principles lead to the conclusion that each test substance requires
an individual formulation. Sometimes different ingredients will be required
for different concentrations in order to obtain the maximum rate of release.
No universal vehicle is available for any route, but a number of approaches
are. Any dosage preparation lab should be equipped with glassware, a stirring
hot plate, a sonicator, a good homogenizer, and a stock of the basic formulating
materials, as detailed in Appendix C.

DERMAL FORMULATIONS

Preparing formulations for application to the skin has special considerations
associated with it. For the case of human pharmaceuticals, these have even
led to a separate book (Barry, 1983).

The physical state of the skin is considerably affected by external factors
such as relative humidity, temperature, and air movement at the skin surface.
If this contact is broken, e.g., by the external application of ointments or
creams, etc., it is reasonable to assume that the skin will change in some way,
sometimes to an extent which creates new conditions of permeability for the
test material. This would be the case, for example, if the stratum corneum
becomes more hydrated or dehydrated due to the topical delivery form. Temperature might also have an effect, as is the case when any constituents of the
vehicle affect the inner structure of the skin by interaction with endogenous
skin substances. Often several of these processes occur together.

Because this is a question of interactions between the vehicle and the skin
(and the latter cannot be viewed as an inert medium), the composition of the
vehicle itself will also be altered, e.g., by incorporation of skin constituents
or through loss of volatile components.

The first contact between vehicle and skin occurs on its surface. Here the
first phase of mutual interactions undoubtedly begins with the lipid mantle
in the case of the so-called "normal" skin. If the skin has been damaged by
wounds, the surface can form a moist milieu of serous exsudate resulting in
different wetting properties. Normally it is impregnated with oily sebaceous
secretions and horny fat so that one is dealing with a hydrophobic surface
layer. Water will not spread out as a film but will form droplets, while bases
with high affinity to the skin surface constituents spread spontaneously into
a film and can wet. The degree of wetting can often be determined, in the case
of a base of a low viscosity, by measuring the angle of contact. It wets the

skin surface, is drawn by capillary action from the visible area into the large inner surface of the stratum corneum, and is transported away into the interior. It is then said that the ointment or cream penetrates well. Spreading and wetting are purely surface phenomena, not penetration in the strict sense. If the skin shows a high content of its own lipids, spreading is limited. It is also reduced if the value of the surface tension of the skin (o_s) decreases compared to the value of the interfacial ($y_{s/l}$) and the surface tension (o_l), as is the case with aqueous bases. Addition of amphiphilic compounds decreases o_l and $y_{s/l}$ and thus spreadability increases.

How much endogenous emulsifying substances of the fatty film, such as cholesterol, cholesterol esters, and fatty acid salts, can affect this spreading process is not clear. They can probably promote the emulsification of hydrophobic substances with water. Whether the sebaceous and epidermal lipids alone are sufficient to emulsify water and so form a type of emulsion film remains controversial. However, it is assumed that they, together with appropriate vehicle components, improve the spreading of the applied vehicle and that this effect can be potentiated by mechanical means such as intensive rubbing in. A good spreadability ensures that the active ingredient is distributed over a large area. High local concentrations are avoided and, at the same time, close contact is made between the chemical and the upper layers of the skin.

In grossly simplified terms, hydrogels, suspensions, and oil/water emulsions behave similarly on the skin surface to aqueous solutions. On the other hand, pastes and water/oil emulsions act like oil. The ability of an organic solvent to stick or wet depends on its specific properties, e.g., its viscosity and its surface tension.

Currently, the information concerning alterations in vehicle composition on the skin surface is sparse (Isutsumi et al., 1979). However, two possible extremes are conceivable. If the vehicle has a high vapor pressure, it often completely evaporates after a short time of application. On the other hand, the vehicle may remain on the skin surface in an almost completely unchanged composition, e.g., highly viscous vaseline or similar thick covering systems. Between these two extremes lie the remaining types of vehicle.

The first situation applies for short-chain alcohols, acetone, or ether. After their evaporation, the drug remains finely dispersed on or in the skin at 100% concentration.

If individual components evaporate, the structure of the vehicle changes and in certain circumstances, the effective drug concentration also changes. With oil/water emulsions, there is a rapid loss of water and this gives rise to the well-known cooling effect. If evaporation continues, the dispersed oil phase coalesces and forms a more or less occlusive film on the skin, together with the emulsifier and the drug. Of course, it is possible that a certain hydrophilic proportion of the drug is then present in suspended form or at least can react with charged molecules and is thus removed from the diffusion process at the start. At the same time, it is to be expected that soluble constituents of skin are incorporated so that a new system can be formed on the surface and the adjoining layers of skin. Comparable transformations probably also occur after application of water/oil (w/o) emulsions providing one realizes that the water evaporates more slowly, the cooling effect is less strong, and, due to the w/o character of the molecule, the occlusive effect can be more marked because of the affinity of the oily components for the skin.

Vaseline and similar highly viscous, lipid bases, in contrast, form from the outset a really impenetrable layer, virtually unaffected by external factors or effects emanating from the skin itself. Interactions with the skin lipids are only likely at the boundary between ointment and skin.

The evaporation of water from the skin into the atmosphere is a continual process. It can be increased or decreased by the use of suitable vehicles. The latter effect will always occur if the water vapor from the vehicle is taken away more quickly than water can diffuse from the deeper layers into the stratum corneum. This applies in principle to all hydrophilic bases, particularly for systems with an oil/water character which, after loss of most of their own water, develop a true draining effect which can lead to the drying out of the underlying tissue. How far the penetration of hydrophilic drugs can be improved with the help of oil/water systems depends on the solution properties of the rest of the components in the skin. Generally, such compounds can only seldom reach deeper layers. It is equally difficult to show an adequate release of water from hydrophilic systems to a dry skin. If any such effects do occur, they are short term, and are quickly overtaken by opposing processes. The same seems to apply to most of the traditional moisturizers such as glycerin and propylene glycol (Powers and Fox, 1957; Rieger and Deems, 1974). They can also cause a large rise in the rate of evaporation, depending on the relative humidity, and thus increase the transepidermal loss of water. It is probably not possible to prevent the drying out without preparations having some occlusive properties.

In contrast, vehicles that are immiscible with water and those with a high proportion of oils have occlusive effects. They reduce both insensible perspiration and the release of sweat. The sweat collects as droplets at the openings of the glands but does not spread as a film between hydrophobic skin surface and lipophilic base because the free surface energy of the vehicle–skin surface is smaller than that between water and skin. If a lipophilic layer of vehicle is present, this is not spontaneously replaced by the water–skin layer if sweat is secreted.

The horny layer consists of about 10% extracellular components such as lipids, proteins, and mucopolysaccharides. Around 5% of the protein and lipids form the cell wall. The majority of the remainder is present in the highly organized cell contents, predominantly as keratin fibers which are generally assigned an α-helix structure. They are embedded in a sulphur-rich amorphous matrix, enclosed by lipids which probably lie perpendicular to the protein axis. Because the stratum corneum is able to take up considerably more water than that which corresponds to its volume, it is assumed that this absorbed fluid volume is mainly located in the region of these keratin structures.

An insight into where the water molecules are absorbed can be gained from equilibrium isotherms (Ziegenmeyer, 1982), as illustrated in Fig. 48. These show a characteristic sigmoidal shape. At low relative humidity, the water is first sorbed at specific sites, probably in the region of the peptide compounds and the various polar side chains. At higher moisture content, layers of water form. By using the Zimm–Lundberg cluster theory (Zimm and Lundberg, 1956), additional information is obtained about the nature of the sorbed water.

Because of the thick intertwining of protein fibers within the cell and in the area of the cell membrane, the cell structure is rigid and remains so, but is attacked by the osmotic effect of the penetrating water. The uptake of water entails a continual shifting of the matrix, which gradually develops elastic opposing forces which increasingly resist further expansion. An equilibrium is reached if both forces balance each other out. In the case of water, it takes quite a long time until the cell is completely hydrated. This process can, however, be shortened if there are components present with a solvent effect diffusing out of the base. The duration and degree of the swelling depends on

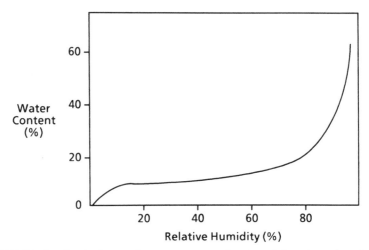

FIGURE 48 Sorption isotherms of water vapor as a function of the relative humidity and composition of constituents (%) in the stratum corneum.

the affinity of all the dissolved substances for the tissue and on the size of the maximum possible elastic reaction, which stabilize the cell structure.

INTERACTIONS BETWEEN SKIN, VEHICLE AND TEST CHEMICAL

The diffusion coefficient of the hydrated stratum corneum is larger than that of dry skin. Therefore, the rate of passage of all substances that penetrate the skin is increased. If the hydrated keratin complex is represented by a biphasic system, then it can be considered to exist as a continuous region covered with layers of water and intervening layers of lipids. Nonpolar compounds are predominantly dissolved in the nonpolar lipid matrix and diffuse through it. Polar substances, on the other hand, pass through the aqueous layers. The diffusion of water and low-molecular-weight, hydrophilic molecules through these layers of water is more difficult than a corresponding free diffusion in an aqueous solution. This could, in certain circumstances, be due to a higher degree of organization of water in the protein structures, in the sense that this water is only available as the driving force of the diffusion process to a limited degree.

The degree of hydration can be controlled by the choice of vehicle. Lipophilic paraffin bases are available, but vehicles such as water/oil emulsions are more acceptable because they are less occlusive and offer ease of formulation.

In principle, temperature can also have an effect. This may be exerted on the base if temperature-sensitive components are present, e.g., nonionic tensides. The heat derived from the room and body can be enough to change the hydrophilic–lipophilic balance and so possibly change the entire system. It has long been known that increasing temperature can considerably reduce the diffusional resistance and thereby increase the rate of penetration of substances. In practice, this effect is, however, of no importance. Of course, the skin temperature will be increased a few degrees by occlusion because of the prevention of sweating and restriction of heat radiation. However, compared to the increase in penetration achieved by the simultaneous hydration process, this effect is insignificant.

Additives aimed at accelerating penetration always attempt to enable diffusion of pharmacologically active compounds into or through the stratum corneum without damaging it and without causing undesirable systemic effects. This goal has certainly not been achieved as yet. Of course, there are numerous substances which decrease the diffusional resistance of the skin such as propylene glycol, tensides, aprotic substances such as urea, DMSO, DMF, and various other organic solvents, mostly of medium chain length. They all improve the penetration of dissolved agents, but only at the cost of the integrity of the skin structure so that the question of the degree of damage and reversibility should be raised.

If the substances have passed the stratum corneum, they also generally diffuse into the living part of the epidermis, reach the circulation, and then have systemic effects depending on the amount absorbed. These are often constituents of formulations and one generally expects them to have little direct influence on the skin penetration. However, because of their amphiphilic properties, they can form new systems with the body's constituents and even lead to a change in the physical state of water in the skin. By this means, a pathway is cleared for other hydrophilic substances into the general circulation.

Most of a permeability enhancer (such as a tenside) is bound to the stratum corneum. It is assumed that the underlying mechanism of the process involves interactions with keratin structures. Positively and negatively charged ionic groups of the proteins have been suggested as binding sites for ionic substances. Ion pairs could also form. On the other hand, hydrophobic areas are present which bind with the uncharged part of the enhancers. The total free binding energy of molecules to keratin is made up of the contributions arising from the electrostatic and nonpolar interactions. The latter increase with chain length of the molecule. This is the reason why medium-chain, predominantly anionic molecules exert stronger effects on the keratin structure than those of shorter chain length (Dominguez *et al.*, 1977).

In order to reach the interior of the tightly enmeshed keratin, the molecule must overcome the elastic energy of the polypeptide matrix. The energy necessary is proportional to the volume of the penetrating molecule. The larger the volume, the more difficult it will be for the molecule to approach the various binding sites of proteins in the interior of the keratin complex. Thus, the size of the penetrating molecule is subject to certain limits. If more molecules are present than can become bound, there is the possibility for a few of them to reach the living layers of the epidermis, as has been described for several anionic, mostly medium-chain enhancer molecules such as tensides. It remains unclear whether this is a consequence of pure saturation or if sometimes other interactions are involved, e.g., with structural lipids or hydrophilic materials from the intercellular lipids.

The extent to which the vehicle can affect the entire diffusion process can be shown by an example. In a four-component system of 40% oil, 40% water, and 20% emulsifying agent and coemulsifier, alteration of only the proportion of emulsifier and coemulsifier leads to systems of totally different colloidal–chemical structures, which can be considered as creams, gels, or microemulsions.

Dermal administration presents fewer logistic difficulties than oral administration. Liquids can be administered as supplied and powders or solids can be moistened with saline to form a thick paste or slurry or can be applied dry and moistened with saline. Solid materials (sheets or plastic, fabric, etc.) can also be administered dermally. Liquid materials or slurries are applied directly to the skin, taking care to spread the material evenly over the entire area or as much of the area as can reasonably be covered, and then covered with a strip of gauze. If a large amount of material is being administered and the abdominal skin will be exposed, it is sometimes necessary to apply material to the gauze and to the skin. Dry materials are weighed out, then placed on the gauze strip and moistened with physiological saline (generally 15 ml) so that they will adhere to the gauze. The gauze is then wrapped around the animal. This porous gauze dressing is then held in place by an additional wrapping, generally of an impervious material, to create an "occlusive" covering. This occlusion enhances penetration and prevents ingestion or evaporation of the test material.

Another recently developed approach is the use of plastic containment capsules (Modified Hill Top Chambers) for administration of well-measured doses in a moisturized microenvironment (Derelanko et al., 1987).

Finally, it should be noted that for some agents (contrary to the general rule), decreasing the concentration of chemical in a vehicle may increase its apparent intensic toxicity. This illustrates the problem associated with regulatory categorization of chemicals merely on the basis of LD_{50} values.

ORAL FORMULATIONS

The physical form of a material destined for oral administration often presents unique challenges. Liquids can be administered as supplied or diluted with an appropriate vehicle, and powders or particulates can often be dissolved or suspended in an appropriate vehicle. However, selection of an appropriate vehicle is often difficult. Water and oil (such as the vegetable oils in Appendix C) are used most commonly. Materials which are not readily soluble in either water or oil can frequently be suspended in a 1% aqueous mixture of methylcellulose. Occasionally, a more concentrated methylcellulose suspension (up to 5%) may be necessary. Materials for which appropriate solutions/suspensions cannot be prepared using one of these three vehicles often present major difficulties.

Limited solubility or suspendability of a material often dictates preparation of dilute mixtures which may require large volumes to be administered. The total volume of liquid dosing solution or suspension which can be administered to a rodent is limited by the size of its stomach. However, because rats lack a gagging reflex and have no emetic mechanism, any material administered will be retained. Guidelines for maximum amounts to be administered were given in Table 55.

Limitations on total volume, therefore, present difficulties for materials which cannot easily be dissolved or suspended. The most dilute solutions which can be administered for a limit type test (5000 mg/kg) using the maximum volume discussed previously, generally are 1% for aqueous mixtures and 50% for other vehicles.

Although vehicle control animals are not required for commonly used vehicles (water, oil, and methylcellulose), most regulations require that the biological properties of a vehicle should be known and/or that historical data be available. Unfortunately, the best solvents are generally toxic and, thus, cannot be used as vehicles. Ethanol and acetone can be tolerated in relatively high doses but produce effects which may complicate interpretation of toxicity associated with the test material alone. It is sometimes possible to dissolve a material in a small amount of one of these vehicles and then dilute the solution in water or in oil.

Gels and resins often present problems because of their viscosity at room temperature. Warming these materials in a water bath to a temperature of up to 50°C will frequently facilitate mixing and dosing. However, it is important to ascertain that no thermal degradation occurs and that actually administered formulations be at or near body temperature.

Other possibilities for insoluble materials are to mix the desired amount of material with a small amount of the animal's diet or to use capsules. The difficulty with the diet approach is the likelihood that the animal will not consume all of the treated diet or that it may selectively not consume chunks of test material. Use of the capsules, meanwhile, is labor-intensive. In rare cases, if all of these approaches fail, it may not be possible to test a material by oral administration.

If necessary, the test substance should be dissolved or suspended as a suitable vehicle, preferably in water, saline, or an aqueous suspension such as 0.5% methylcellulose in water. If a test substance cannot be dissolved or suspended in an aqueous medium to form a homogenous dosage preparation, corn oil or another solvent can be used. The animals in the vehicle control group should receive the same volume of vehicle given to animals in the highest dose group.

The test substance can be administered to animals at a constant concentration across all dose levels (i.e., varying the dose volume) or at a constant dose volume (i.e., varying the dose concentration). However, the investigator should be aware that the toxicity observed by administration in a constant concentration may be different from that observed when given in a constant dose volume. For instance, when a large volume of corn oil is given orally, gastrointestinal motility is increased, causing diarrhea and decreasing the time available for absorption of the test substance in the gastrointestinal tract. This situation is particularly true when a highly lipid-soluble chemical is tested.

If an organic solvent is used to dissolve the chemical, water should be added to reduce the dehydrating effect of the solvent within the gut lumen. The volume of water or solvent/water used to dissolve the chemical should be kept low because excess quantities may distend the stomach and cause rapid gastric emptying. In addition, large volumes of water may carry the chemical through membrane pores and increase the rate of absorption. Thus, if dose-dependent absorption is suspected, it is important that the different doses are given in the same volume of solution.

Larger volumes than those detailed earlier may be given, although nonlinear kinetics seen in such circumstances may be due to solvent-induced alteration of intestinal function. The use of water-immiscible solvents such as corn oil (which is sometimes used for gavage doses) should be avoided because it is possible that mobilization from the vehicle may be rate limiting. Magnetic stirring bars or homogenizers can be used in preparing suspensions. Sometimes a small amount of a surfactant such as Tween 80, Span 20, or Span 60 is helpful in obtaining a homogenous suspension.

A large fraction of such a material may quickly pass through the gastrointestinal tract and remain unabsorbed. Local irritation by a test substance generally decreases when the material is diluted. If the objective of the study is to establish systemic toxicity, the test substance should be administered in a constant volume to minimize gastrointestinal irritation that may, in turn, affect the absorption of the test substance. On the other hand, the test substance should be administered undiluted to assess the irritation potential of the test substance.

DOSING CALCULATIONS

One of the first things a new technician (or graduate student) must learn is how to calculate dose. Generally, administered doses in systemic toxicity studies are based on the body weight of the animal (expressed as either weight or volume—for liquids—of the test substance per kilogram of body weight of the animal), although some would maintain that surface area may be a more appropriate basis on which to gauge individual dose (as will be discussed in a later chapter). The weight (or dose) of the test substance is often expressed in mg or g of active ingredient if the test substance is not pure (that is, 100% active ingredient).

Ideally, only the 100% pure sample should be tested; however, impurity-free samples are difficult to obtain and preparation of formulations (as previously discussed) is frequently essential. The toxicity of impurities or formulation components should be examined separately if the investigator feels that they may contribute significantly to the toxicity of the test substance.

If the test substance contains only 75% active ingredient and the investigator chooses a constant dose volume of 10 ml/kg body wt across all dose levels, it will be more convenient to prepare a stock solution such that when 10 ml/kg of this stock solution is given to the animal, the dose will be the desired dose (e.g., 500 mg/kg of active ingredient). The concentration of this stock solution would be (500 mg/10 ml)/0.75 = 66.7 mg of the test substance/ml.

Aliquots of the test substance for other dose levels can then be prepared by dilution of the stock solution. For example, the solution concentration for a 250 mg/kg dose level is (200 mg/10 ml)/0.75 = 26.7 mg of the test substance/ml.

This solution can be prepared by diluting the stock solution 25 times, i.e., for each ml of the 26.7 mg/ml solution to be prepared, (26.7 mg/ml) (1 ml)/66.7 mg/ml = 0.400 ml of the stock solution should be diluted to a final volume in 1 ml with the vehicle.

The other way to express a relative dose in animals or humans is to do so in terms of body surface area. As will be discussed in the next chapter, there are many reasons for believing that the surface area approach is more accurate for relating doses between species (Schmidt-Nielson, 1984)—and especially between test animals and humans. The next chapter discusses the issue of scaling in detail and provides a table that gives a quick basis for conversion of per body weight doses to per surface area doses.

The surface area basis for dose expression and calculation is currently the accepted norm in a couple of areas—carcinogenesis and chemotherapy, for example. The reasons behind its popularity are presented and discussed in the next chapter.

COMPARISONS AND CONTRASTS OF ROUTES

Much of what needs to be said comparing the different routes used in toxicology has already been presented in this book. There are some points—and some sharp exceptions to the general rules that have already been given—that should be kept in mind for the practicing toxicologist.

The relative ranking of efficacy of routes that was presented earlier is not absolute; there can be striking exceptions. For example, though materials are usually much quicker-acting and more potent when given by the oral route than they are by the dermal, this is not always the case. In the literature, Shaffer and West (1960) reported that tetram in an aqueous solution was more toxic dermally than when given orally. LD_{50}'s reported were as follows:

	LD_{50} (mg/kg) of tetram (95% confidence limits) Oral	Percutaneous
Male	9(7–13)	2(1–3)
Female	8(6–11)	2(1–3)

In the experience of the authors, this same circumstance has come up in the past. Several materials which were relatively nontoxic orally were extremely potent by the dermal route (differences of potency of more than an order of magnitude have been seen at least twice).

A final general rule applicable to routes and vehicles should be presented here: Vehicles can mask the effects of active ingredients. Particularly for clinical signs, attention should be paid to the fact that a number of vehicles (propylene glycol, for example), as stated in Appendix C, cause transient neurobehavioral effects. These may mask similar short-lived (though not necessarily equally transient and reversible) effects of test materials.

REFERENCES

Attman, P. L., and Dittmer, D. S. (Eds.) (1971). *Respiration and Circulation*, pp. 56–59. FASEB, Bethesda, MD.

Baker, H. J., Lindsey, J. R., and Weisbroth, S. H. (1979). *The Laboratory Rat*, Vol. I, pp. 411–412. Academic Press, New York.

Barry, B. W. (1983). *Dermatological Formulations*. Dekker, New York.

Bates, T. R., and Gibaldi, M. (1970). Gastrointestinal absorption of drugs. In *Current Concepts in the Pharmaceutical Sciences: Biopharmaceutics* (J. Swarbrick, Ed.), pp. 58–99. Lea & Febiger, Philadelphia.

Blank, I. H., and Scheuplein, R. J. (1964). The epidermal barrier. In *Progress in the Biological Sciences in Relation to Dermatology* (W. Rook and I. Champion, Eds.), Vol. 2. Cambridge Univ. Press, Cambridge, UK.

Borowitz, J. L., Moore, P. F., Yim, G. K. W., and Miya, T. S. (1971). Mechanism of enhanced drug effects produced by dilution of the oral dose. *Toxicol. Appl. Pharmacol.* 19, 164–168.

Brandau, R., and Lippold, B. H. (1982). *Dermal and Transdermal Absorption*. Wissenschaftliche, Verlagsgesellschaft mbH, Stuttgart.

Bronaugh, R. L., and Maibach, H. I. (1985). *Percutaneous Absorption*. Dekker, New York.

Brown, U. K. (1980). *Acute Toxicity in Theory and Practice*. Wiley, New York.

Brown, V. K. H., and Muir, C. M. C. (1971). Some factors affecting the acute toxicity of pesticides to mammals when absorbed through skin and eyes. *Int. Pest Control* 13, 16–21.

Calvary, H. O., and Klumpp, T. G. (1939). The toxicity for human beings for diethylene glycol with sulfanilimide. *Southern Med. J.* 32, 1105.

Derelanko, M. J., Gad, S. C., Gavigan, F. A., Babich, P. C., and Rinehart, W. E. (1987). Toxicity of hydroxylamine sulfate following dermal exposure: Variability with exposure method and species. *Fundam. Appl. Toxicol.* 8, 425–431.

Dominguez, J. G., Parra, J. L., Infante, M. R., Pelejero, C. M., Balaguer, F., and Sastre, T. (1977). *J. Soc. Cosmet. Chem.* 28, 165.

Eckstein, P., Jackson, M. C. N., Millman, N., and Sobrero, A. J. (1969). Comparison of vaginal tolerance tests and spermicidal preparations in rabbits and monkeys. *J. Reprod. Fertil.* 20, 85–93.

Fincher, J. H. (1968). Particle size of drugs and its relationship to absorption and activity. *J. Pharm. Sci.* 57, 1825–1835.

Fitzgerald, J. M., Boyd, V. F., and Manus, A. G. (1983). Formulations of insoluble and immiscible test agents in liquid vehicles for toxicity testing. In *Chemistry for Toxicity Testing* (C. W. Jameson and D. B. Walters, Eds.), pp. 83–90. Butterworth, Boston.

Gad, S. C., Smith, A. C., Cramp, A. L., Gavigan, F. A., and Derelanko, M. J. (1984). Innovative designs and practices for acute systemic toxicity studies. *Drug Chem. Toxicol.* 7(5), 423–434.

Gaines, T. B. (1960). The acute toxicity of pesticides to rats. *Toxicol. Appl. Pharmacol.* 2, 88–99.

Gibaldi, M. (1976). *Biopharmaceutics in the Theory and Practice of Industrial Pharmacy* (L. Lachman, H. A. Lieberman, and J. L. Kanig, Eds.), 2nd ed. Lea & Febiger, Philadelphia.

Gibaldi, M., and Feldman, S. (1970). Mechanisms of surfactant effects on drug absorption. *J. Pharm. Sci.* 59–579.

Groves, M. (1966). The influence of formulation upon the activity of thermotherapeutic agents. *Rep. Progr. Appl. Chem.,* 51–151.

Hagenbusch, O. E. (1937). Elixir of sulfanilamide massengill. *J. Am. Med. Assos.,* 109–1531.

Hem, S. L. (1973). *Current Concepts in Pharmaceutical Sciences: Dosage Form, Design and Bioavailability* (J. Swarbrick, Ed.). Lea & Febiger, Philadelphia.

Hogben, C. A. M., Tocco, D. J., Brodie, B. B., and Schranker, L. S. (1959). On the mechanism of intestinal absorption of drugs, *J. Pharmacol. Exp. Ther.* T25;275.

Holick, H. G. O. (1937). Glycerine, ethylene glycol, prepylene glycol and diethylene glycol. *J. Am. Med. Assoc.,* 109–1517.

Holmstedt, B. (1959). Pharmacology of organophosphorus cholinesterase inhibitors. *Pharmacol. Rev.* 11, 567–688.

Houston, J. B., Upshall, D. G., and Bridges, J. W. (1974). The re-evaluation of the importance of partition coefficients in the gastrointestinal absorption of nutrients. *J. Pharmacol. Exp. Ther.* 189, 244–254.

Keberle, H. (1971). Physicochemical factors of drugs affecting absorption, distribution and excretion. *Acta Pharmacol. Toxicol.* 29(Suppl. 3), 30–47.

Kondrizer, A. A., Mayer, W. H., and Zviblis, P. (1959). Removal of sarin from skin and eyes. *Arch. Ind. Health* 20, 50–52.

Kruger, S., Greve, D. W., and Schueler, F. W. (1962). The absorption of fluid from the peritoneal cavity. *Arch. Int. Pharmacodyn.* 137, 173–178.

Levi, G. (1963). *Prescription Pharmacy* (J. B. Sprowls, Ed.), Lea & Febiger, Philadelphia.

Lien, E., Koda, R. T., and Tong, G. L. (1971). Buccal and percutaneous absorptions. *Drug Intel. Clin. Pharm.* 5, 38–41.

Lukas, G., Brindle, S. D., and Greengard, P. (1971). The route of absorption of intraperitoneally administered compounds. *J. Pharmacol. Exp. Ther.* 178, 562–566.

Marzulli, F. N. (1962). Barriers to skin penetration. *J. Invest. Dermatol.* 39, 387–393.

McConnell, R. F. (1973). Special requirements for testing spermicides. In *Meeting on Pharmaceutical Models to Assess Toxicity and Side Effects of Fertility Regulating Agents,* pp. 373–385. Geneva.

McMartin, C., Hutchinson, L. E. F., Hyde, R., and Peters, G. E. (1987). Analysis of structural requirements for the absorption of drugs and macromolecules from the nasal cavity. *J. Pharm. Sci.* 76, 535–540.

Medved, L. I., and Kundiev, Y. I. (1964). On the methods of study of penetration of chemical substances through the intact skin (Russian). *Gig. Sanit.* 29, 71–76.

Melnick, R. L., Jameson, C. W., Goehl, T. J., and Kuhn, G. O. (1987). Application of microencapsulation for toxicology studies. *Fundam. Appl. Toxicol.,* 425–431.

O'Reilly, W. J. (1972). Pharmacokinetics in drug metabolism and toxicology. *Can. J. Pharm. Sci.* **7**, 66–77.

Powers, D. H., and Fox, C. (1957). A study of the effect of cosmetic ingredients, creams and lotions on the rate of moisture loss. *Proc. Sci. Sect. Toilet Goods Skin Assoc.* **28**, 21.

Rieger, M. M., and Deems, D. E. (1974). Skin moisturizers. II. The effects of cosmetic ingredients on human stratum corneum. *J. Soc. Cosmet. Chem.* **25**, 253.

Ritschel, W. A., Siegel, E. G., and Ring, P. E. (1974). Biopharmaceutical factors influencing LD_{50}: Pt. 1 Viscosity. *Arzneim.–Forsch.* **24**, 907–910.

Schanker, L. S. (1960). On the mechanism of absorption of drugs from the gastrointestinal tract. *J. Med. Pharm. Chem.* **2**, 343–359.

Scheuplein, R. J. (1965). Mechanism of percutaneous absorption. (i) Routes of penetration and the influence of solubility. *J. Invest. Dermatol.* **45**, 334–346.

Scheuplein, R. J. (1967). Mechanism of percutaneous absorption. (ii) Transient diffusion and the relative importance of various routes of skin penetration. *J. Invest. Dermatol.* **48**, 79–88.

Schmidt-Nielsen, K. (1984). *Scaling: Why Is Animal Size so Important?* Cambridge Univ. Press, New York.

Schou, J. (1971). Subcutaneous and intramuscular injection of drugs. In *Handbook of Experimental Pharmacology* (B. B. Brodie and J. R. Gillette, Eds.), Chap. 4. Springer-Verlag, Berlin.

Schranker, L. S., Shore, P. A., Brodie, B. B., and Hogben, C. A. M. (1957). Absorption of drugs from the stomach. I. the rat. *J. Pharmacol. Exp. Ther.* **120**, 528.

Shaffer, C. B., and West, B. (1960). The acute and subacute toxicity of technical o,o-diethyl s-2-diethyl-aminoethyl phosphorothioate hydrogen oxalate (TETRAM). *Toxicol. Appl. Pharmacol.* **2**, 1–13.

Share, P. A., Brodie, B. B., and Hogben, C. A. M. (1971). The gastric secretion of drugs: A pH partition hypothesis. *J. Pharmacol. Exp. Ther.* **119**, 361.

Sinow, J., and Wei, E. (1973). Ocular toxicity of paraquat. *Bull. Environ. Contam. Toxicol.* **9**, 163–168.

Spector, W. S. (1956). *Handbook of Biological Data.* Saunders, Philadelphia.

Staab, R. J., Palmer, M. A., Auletta, C. S., Blaszcak, D. L., and McConnell, R. F. (1987). A relevant vaginal irritation/subacute toxicity model in the rabbit and ovariectomized rat. *Toxicologist* **7**, A1096.

Swan, K. C., and White, N. G. (1942). Corneal permeability; (1) Factors affecting penetration of drugs into the cornea. *Am. J. Ophthalmol.* **25**, 1043–1058.

Swenson, M. J. (Ed.) (1977). *Dukes Physiology of Domestic Animals*, p. 178. Comstock, Ithaca, NY.

Tsutsumi, H., Utsugi, T., and Hayashi, S. (1979). Study on the occlusivity of oil films. *J. Soc. Cosmet. Chem.* **30**, 345.

Wagner, J. G. (1971). *Biopharmaceutics and Relevant Pharmacokinetics.* Drug Intelligence Publications, Hamilton, IL.

Wilson, F. A., and Dietschy, J. M. (1974). The intestinal unstirred layer—Its surface area and effect on active transport kinetics. *Biochem. Biophys. Acta* **363**, 112–126.

Winne, D. (1978). Dependence of intestinal absorption *in vivo* in the unstirred layer. *Nauyn-Schmiedelberg's Arch. Pharmacol.* **304**, 175–181.

Wood, S. G., Upshall, D. G., and Bridges, J. W. (1978). The absorption of aliphatic carbamates from the rat colon. *J. Pharm. Pharmacol.* **30**, 638–641.

Ziegenmeyer, J. (1982). The influence of the vehicle on the absorption and permeation of drugs. In *Dermal and Transdermal Absorption* (R. Brandan and P. Reisen, Eds.), pp. 73–89. Wissenschaftliche Verlagsgesellschaft, Stuttgart.

Zimm, B. H., and Lundberg, J. L. (1956). Sorption of vapors by high polymers. *J. Phys. Chem.* **60**, 425.

CHAPTER 11

Considerations Specific to Animal Test Models

Just as formulations, vehicles, and routes are critical, often overlooked determinants in the design and outcome of acute toxicity studies, so too are the fundamental cornerstones for all such predictive testing, (animal models), generally overlooked. Throughout this book the authors have attempted to present some of the test-specific considerations behind selection and/or rejection of particular types of animals as models for specific tests. Indeed, we have attempted to present alternatives to animals, where currently available, and to overview in an objective manner the status of alternatives in all cases. The initial chapter of this volume presented the basic criteria by which we would present and appraise alternative models, and in the final chapter we will explore the issues limiting alternatives (and how they may be over come) in some detail.

First, however, the fundamental concepts surrounding the selection and use of animal models in acute toxicity testing must be considered. These concepts and considerations have histories which are largely unwritten and are generally (but not entirely) the same for the entire field of toxicology. But some are specific to acute toxicology as the oldest portion of the science. These concepts, and how one uses animal data to predict what might happen in humans and therefore protect them, are the subject of this chapter. To start, we must look at history in order to know something about our common models.

Animals have been used as models for centuries to predict what chemicals and environmental factors would do to humans. The earliest uses are lost in prehistory, and much of what is recorded in early history about toxicology testing indicates that humans were the test subjects. The earliest clear description of the use of animals in scientific study of the effects of environmental agents appears to be by Priestley (1772) in his study of gases. The first systematic use of animals for the screening of a wide variety of agents was published by Orfila (1814) and was described by Dubois and Geiling (1959) in their historical review. This work consisted of dosing test animals with known quantities of agents (poisons or drugs) and included the careful recording of the resulting clinical signs and gross necropsy observations. The use of animals as predictors of potential ill effects has grown since that time.

The current regulatorily required use of animal models in acute testing began by using them as a form of instrument to detect undesired contaminants. For example, canaries were used by miners to detect the presence of carbon monoxide—a case in which an animal model is more sensitive than humans (Burrell, 1912). In 1907, the Food and Drug Administration (FDA) in the United States started to protect the public by use of a voluntary testing program for new coal tar colors in foods. This was replaced by a mandatory program of testing in 1938, and such regulatorily required animal testing programs have continued to expand until recently. On what basis do the scientist and regulator then select such animal test models, and what are the characteristics of the models?

COMMON MODEL SPECIES AND THEIR CHARACTERISTICS

This section will focus on those animal species (and, indeed, strains) which are currently commonly used in predictive acute toxicology testing. It should be understood that these are animals which are commercially bred for the specific purpose of such testing, and as such are the result of extensive selective breeding programs over the past 50 years. For the two most commonly and widely used species in particular (rats and mice), these efforts have led to genetically homogeneous animals which are not found in nature.

Eight different species are currently used with any frequency in acute toxicology. These are, in approximate order of numbers of animals utilized (from most to least), the rat, mouse, rabbit, guinea pig, hamster, dog, ferret, and monkey. It should be noted that others (Schmidt-Nielsen, 1984) have reported other orders of use frequency, but the authors believe these reports to be in

TABLE 57   Equivalent Life Spans

Duration of study in days	Percentage of mean life span						
	Mouse	Hamster	Rat	Rabbit	Ferret	Dog	Monkey
15	2.7	2.8	2.1	0.75	1.0	0.4	0.27
30	5.4	5.6	4.2	1.5	2.0	0.8	0.55
60	11.0	11.2	8.3	3.0	3.8	1.5	1.1
90	16.5	16.7	12.0	4.5	5.8	2.5	1.6
180	32.9	33.3	25.0	9.0	11.5	4.9	3.3
360	65.8	66.6	49.0	18.0	23.0	9.8	6.6
720	NA	NA	99.0	36.0	46.0	20.0	13.0

Note. NA, not applicable.

error (see, for example, the 1985 and 1986 British Home Office report on animal useage, which shows the order for frequency for all animals used in research and testing to be mouse, rat, rabbit, guinea pig, hamster, dog, and monkey, with ferrets not being reported separately). The cat and frog, while common biological models, have not been used in toxicity testing for some time.

Basic physiological, reproductive, and logistical data for these eight species are presented in a comparative manner in Tables 57–62. These tables present summarized data representing much of the first line database for model selection in general studies. More detailed information about the hematology and clinical chemistry values, etc. can be found in Gad and Chengelis (1992).

There are other considerations which are more specific to particular uses in toxicology, or to personal and facility preferences or capabilities. These

TABLE 58   Physiological Data for Common Lab Animals

Species	Life span (years)	Rectal temperature (°C)	Respiration rate/min	Heart rate/min	Consumption/ 100 g BW	
					Water (ml)	Food (g)
Ferret	5–6	38–39	33–36	250	10	2–4
Guinea pig	2–5	39–40	110–160	150–160	10	8
Hamster	1–3	38–39.5	35–120	300–500	10	5–8
Monkey	15–25	38–39	40–65	150–300	7–15	20
Mouse	2–3	36.5–38	90–220	300–750	16	15
Rabbit	5–13	39–39.7	35–65	120–300	10	7
Rat	2–4	37.5–38.1	80–110	350–400	10	10
Dog	10–16	38.6	10–30	60–120	3–5	2–5

Note. Source: Collines (1979). BW, body weight.

TABLE 59   Life Spans of Common Laboratory Species and Humans

Species	Percentage of total life span			Ratio human span : animal span
	Embryonic	Gestational	Puberty	
Mouse	2.0	4.6	5.5	44
Syrian hamster	2.5	4.5	12.6	66
Rat	1.7	2.8	6.8	33
Rabbit	1.2	3.6	10.6	12
Guinea pig	1.8	4.4	4.2	17
Ferret	1.2	2.1	18.0	14.5
Dog	0.8	1.7	5.8	6.6
Monkey	0.6	3.1	20.0	4.4
Man	0.1	1.1	0.0	1.0

TABLE 60   Reproductive Data for Common Laboratory Species

Species	Puberty	Breeding age	Gestation (days)	Weaning age	Chromosome number (diploid)
Mouse	35 Days	42–56 Days	19–21	19–28 Days	40
Hamster	45–75 Days	6–8 Weeks	15–18	20–25 Days	44
Rat	37–67 Months	72–90 Days	20–22	21 Days	42
Rabbit	3–8 Months	6–9 Months	30–35	6–8 Weeks	44
Guinea pig	45–70 Days	12–14 Weeks	59–70	21–28 Days	64
Ferret	9–12 Months	1 Year	40–42	6–8 Weeks	40
Dog	6–8 Months	1 Year	52–69	42 Days	78
Monkey	3 Years	4 Years	155–170	4–6 Months	42

TABLE 61   Commonly Used Species of Primates in Toxicity Studies

Genus	Common name	Species	Place of origin
Lemur	Lemur	5–8	Madagascar
Saimiri	Squirrel monkey	2	South and Central America
Ateles	Spider monkey	12–20	South and Central America
Ceropithecus	Guenons	10–16	Africa
Macaca	Macaques	1	Southeast Asia
Pan	Chimpanzee	1	Africa

TABLE 62 Matrix of Cost and Logistical Factors in Species Selection

Species	Factor: Cost (per animal) ($)	Factor: Per diem ($)	Factor: Logistics (space/caging)	Time required to get animals	Maximum parenteral study duration[a]	Mean body weight (kg)	Test compound required (rat = 1×)[b]	Available supply of animals	Animal health concerns
Monkeys	1800	5.00	High/expensive	6 Months	Years	Cyno, 1–4; Rhesus, 8–10	Cyno, 5–20×; Rhesus, 40×	Limited	Some; Zoonoses[c]
Dogs	350	5.00	High	3 Months	Years	8–18	70×	Limited	Few
Ferrets	60	2.48	Moderate	2 Months	Month	0.5–2	5×	Limited[d]	None
Rabbits	27	1.20	Moderate	Within month	Month	1–4	5–20×	Good	Seasonal
Guinea pigs	30	1.25	Low	Within month	Month	0.2–1	1–2.5×	Good	Few
Rats	6	.50	Low	Immediate	Month	0.2–0.4	1×	Excellent	None
Hamsters	8	.60	Low	Within month	Weeks	.05–0.1	0.25×	Good	Some
Mice	1	.20	Very low	Immediate	Month	.02–.05	0.1–0.4×	Excellent	None

[a]Assuming daily dosing.
[b]For equivalent mg/kg dose.
[c]Real potential exists for transmission of disease to humans.
[d]If demand were greater, supply of ferrets would become very limited for the near term.

include handling and husbandry considerations as well as guidance on humane utilization of animals in research.

Norway Rats (*Ratus norvegicus*)

The original wild Norway rat was brown and actually originated somewhere in eastern Asia. Currently, there are four major strains commonly used in toxicology: (a) the inbred Fischer-344, originally developed for the NCI; (b) the Wistar, an albino rat originated by the Wistar Institute; (c) the Sprague–Dawley, an albino developed by the Sprague–Dawley breeding farms; and (d) the Long Evans, which is hooded with colored head and shoulders. Strains of rats and the differences between them will be covered in detail in a later section of this chapter.

The rat is considered the near-ideal species for toxicological testing and research because it grows to a weight of up to 500 g, can be easily handled, manipulated, and bled, and can be easily administered test chemicals by any of the common routes.

The male rat weighs about one and a half times as much as the female at any particular age, with specific weights varying substantially between strains. Laboratory rats are relatively docile and easy to handle, with the males being much less prone to fighting than male mice. Rats thrive well when housed singly in cages. A female with a litter will tolerate her mate but will not allow other females in the cage.

Housing

Rooms should be climate controlled to maintain mean temperatures of 22°C with variations not to exceed 3°C. Weight gain is enhanced at warmer room temperatures. Wide variations in relative humidity (40–70%) are well tolerated except by nursing females. Twelve-hour photoperiods are preferred in the rooms. Strong lights are to be avoided because the rat is nocturnal by nature.

Handling

Rats can be handled by the tail, but larger animals should be grasped near the base of the tail. An alternative procedure should be used for pregnant females. Alternative handling procedures include grasping the animal across the back with the forelimbs crossed in front of the animal's face or covering the animal with a hand towel and picking it up with only the head unwrapped.

Nutrition

Rats have long been used as models for nutrition studies for people, and a great deal of information is available on the animal's nutritional requirements. Suitable commercial diets are readily available from a number of sources. In general, laboratory diets for the rat should contain at least 15.9% protein, 3.2% fat, 0.7% phosphorus, 0.2% sodium, 0.8% calcium, 0.5% potassium, 0.3% chloride, and 5% crude fiber.

Diseases

The susceptibility of rats to mycoplasma and other pneumonias can limit their usefulness in studies of inhalation toxicology, although the improvements wrought in their husbandry and breeding have reduced the extent of this problem. The problems that arise from the use of infected animals include the obvious ones of decreased life span and resistance to stress induced by experimental manipulations, and the more subtle ones of changed susceptibility of specific organs to toxic effects, interactions of the immune system with toxins and infectious agents, and the possibility of confusing the inflammation of infection and specific tissue responses to toxicity.

MICE (*Mus musculus*)

Among all the animal species, mice are the most used in biomedical research because they are easily bred and are inexpensive. This is not the case in toxicology, however, in which the rat is somewhat more popular. As with the rat, extensive experience and commercial demand have led to the development of a large number of different strains. Some 100–200 different inbred strains are commercially available, many as models for specific disease states. The more popular strains in toxicology will be discussed later in this chapter.

The laboratory mouse is generally timid, gentle, easy to handle, somewhat photophobic, social, and more active at night than during the day. At 1 month of age, mice weigh approximately 18–22 g. Older animals can weigh as much as 50 g. Breeders will generally supply age/weight curves for their particular strains upon request. Mice do not thrive when singley caged, when they will eat and weigh less.

Mice are most commonly used in toxicology for cancer bioassays and for screening new compounds. They are particularly suitable when many animals are necessary, such as in acute systemic toxicity studies.

Mice, as we will see to be the case with almost all of the common lab animal species, do have some idiosyncrasies such as the formation of new bone within the medullary cavity and an extreme sensitivity to chloroform. It is also difficult to collect interim blood samples of sufficient size for many uses. Despite these limitations, mice still represent a comparatively good model for many uses in toxicology.

Housing

Mice, as rats, are best housed in stainless-steel cages on racks, and this is now considered the standard in toxicology. A large number of variations, such as plastic (shoebox) and disposable cages, are also available and preferable for some applications. Stock mouse cages of a $22 \times 18 \times 6$-in. size may be used to hold large numbers of animals before assignment to a study, but once allocated to a study smaller cages are usually employed to house groups of five or so animals.

Cages may have wire mesh bottoms and be suspended over a suitable medium to absorb urine and control odors. Sawdust or wood shavings may be used as bedding in solid bottom cages.

Mice should be maintained in temperature-controlled rooms within the range of $18-24°C$ and with a relative humidity in the range of $40-70\%$. Artificial lighting should be utilized to achieve a 12-hr photoperiod, and ventilation should provide from 10 to 15 air changes per hour.

Because mice are such small animals, there is a tendency to house as many as possible in as small a space as possible. This should be avoided because it contributes to the rapid development and spread of disease problems. Different strains should be kept in separate rooms.

Handling

In general, mice become more tame with handling. Technicians that are quiet and more gentle will generally be better able to handle the animals. Mice develop a tendency to bite if handled roughly and should not be provoked.

Mice can routinely be picked up by their tails, and should be held at the back of their necks between the thumb and forefinger of the researcher's left hand (if he or she is right-handed). Sufficient pressure should be used so that the animal cannot twist and bite, but not so much that the animal strangles. Intravenous injections in the mouse are best performed through the tail vein, with the animal restrained in some form of holder and the vein dilated by use of heat (such as warm water or a heat lamp).

Nutrition

Several standard diets are commercially available. Unless food consumption is being measured or test material is being delivered in the diet, pelletized food is best and should be provided in hopper-type feeders in the cage. If careful control of the quantity of food consumed is important, powdered diet in a jar-type feeder should be used. The diet should be balanced, containing 20–25% protein, 10–12% fat, 45–55% carbohydrates, 4% crude fiber, and the appropriate micronutrients (see Mitruka *et al.*, 1976). Careful attention should be addressed to the inclusion of adequate levels of minerals and vitamins.

Water and pellets should be provided *ad libitum,* but the water should not be provided in any form of open container. An automatic drip-type watering system is the method of choice, but autoclavable bottles may also be used.

Rabbits (*Oryctolagus cuniculus*)

As with rats and mice, a number of breeds of rabbits (a lagomorph, not a rodent) are available to the researcher, with the American Rabbit Breeders Association listing more than 80 varieties. However, only a few of these are commonly utilized in toxicology—most commonly the New Zealand White and the Dutch Miniature or Belted varieties.

The rabbit is a favorite model for screening chemicals for embryotoxic or developmental toxic effects, as well as almost all types of dermal testing. Unlike either the rat or the mouse, there is still no dependable supply of healthy and homogeneously responding rabbits commercially available.

Housing

In general, rabbits should be housed singly in stainless-steel cages to facilitate proper sanitation. Extreme changes of environmental conditions should be avoided. Proper artificial lighting is desirable, and windows are unnecessary. Environmental conditions in rabbit rooms should be such that temperatures are between 60 and 70°F and relative humidity is between 40 and 60%. A minimum of 10 air changes an hour are necessary, and air should not be recirculated through the room.

Cages should be mounted on movable racks to facilitate cleaning of both cages and rooms and should have wire mesh bottoms with catch pans under them. Bedding is not required, but absorbant material should be placed in the pans under the cages.

Handling

Small rabbits may be lifted and carried by grasping the fur over the back. Medium and large animals should be carried with support being provided for their body and hindlegs. Never lift a rabbit by its ears or legs.

For injection or other treatments, the animal should be restrained in a towel. During operations such as shaving, a second person should restrain the animal while the first performs the actual shaving.

Nutrition

Rabbits are herbivorous animals, and any of the traditional green foods, such as lettuce, hay, and roots, can be given. As with the other common laboratory species, high-quality diets are commercially available. Diets should contain at least 12–15% protein, 2–3.5% fat, and 20–27% crude fiber. Feed should be provided in pelletized form. Clean, fresh water should be provided *ad libitum,* preferably by an automatic system.

GUINEA PIGS (*Cavia porcellus*)

Guinea pigs have long been used as experimental animals in biomedical research because they are small, tame, and easy to control. Of the three varieties (English, Abyssinian, and Peruvian), the albino form of the short-haired English variety is the most commonly employed type in the laboratory. The Hartley strain is by far the most commonly used in toxicology.

Guinea pigs are alert, full bodied, and have smooth, shiny skin. Their coat is dense, with the hair being clean and not marked by discharge from the nose, eyes, or ears. If allowed to feed freely, guinea pigs can become quite large over time. Males will commonly reach 1 kg at 1 year and can weigh several kilos at a later age.

Guinea pigs are noteworthy because of their dietary requirement for vitamin C. As a result, diets for them are supplemented with the vitamin, and other lab animal diets cannot be substituted. The guinea pig is extremely susceptible to human tuberculosis and is an excellent model for anaphylaxis and other immunological events. In toxicology it is currently primarily used as a model for evaluating various immune-modulated events.

Housing

Guinea pigs may be housed indoors in pens on the floor, but modern practice is to cage them in small groups in drawer-type cages. These drawers have wire mesh floors and are suspended over trays containing absorbent material.

Floor pens, despite their evident disadvantages (waste of floor space, difficulty in cleaning and controlling environmental conditions, and spread of disease) are still used by some because of their simplicity and low capital cost.

Feed is generally provided as pellets and water via a drip system (either in bottles or from an automatic system). Rooms used to house guinea pigs should have temperature variations that are less than those for rodents (between 70 and 74°F is desirable) and with humidity between 40 and 60%.

Handling

Guinea pigs are very easy to handle and manipulate because of their extremely docile nature. They should be lifted by grasping the trunk gently but firmly while supporting the hindlimbs. Also, they may be immobilized simply by restraining their limbs.

Nutrition

Guinea pigs are vegetarians and thrive on a variety of diets, including many that are commercially available. Care must be taken to ensure that the selected diet provides adequate amounts of vitamins A, C, K, and E, however.

SYRIAN HAMSTER (*Mesocricetus auratus*)

The Syrian or golden hamster has several new varieties which are not gold or red at all. Typically, however, hamsters are 5 or 6 in. long and weigh from 110 to 140 g. The eyes and ears are black. Hamsters are active in the dark, irrespective of the day/night cycle. They spend a considerable amount of time grooming, and this habit should not be taken as a sign of disease.

Both the Syrian and Chinese hamster are widely used in toxicological research, though generally for different purposes. The Syrian is used in cancer bioassays as an alternative to the rat or mouse and also as a model for other toxicological testing (including acute). The Chinese is frequently used for microbiologically related tests and for genetic toxicity assays. This latter is due to their low chromosome number.

The Syrian hamster possesses a two-chamber stomach (Magalhaes, 1968), but in general its acute response to toxicants is similar to that of the rat. It has been demonstrated to be more sensitive to the toxic effects of strychnine and penicillin than either the rat or the mouse (Wills, 1968) and far less sensitive than the mouse to the acute effects of DDT (due to achieving lower brain concentrations for the same dose, which in turn is believed to be due to differences in the permiability of the blood–brain barrier). The Syrian hamster is also generally much less sensitive to the acute systemic effects of chlorinated hydrocarbon insecticides than either rats or mice (Brown, 1980).

Housing

Several types of commercial caging are available for either individual animals or for breeding and metabolic uses. Cages can be either stainless steel or autoclavable plastic (the shoebox style), with the latter being preferred. If the floors of the cage are wire mesh, the mesh size should be less than one-third of an inch (the animals are very good at escaping through small openings). Bedding, if used, should be replaced at least once a week.

Animal room temperatures should be kept at from 21 to 24°C, with a 12-hr photoperiod and relative humidity between 40 and 60%. Rooms should have at least 10 air changes per hour.

Handling

Hamsters are aggressive by nature—particularly the Syrian, which resents handling and can become difficult to handle over time. The best way to hold the hamster is by the dorsal skin behind the head with the little finger over the rear legs so that they are held between it and the thumb.

Nutrition

Any of the available commercial diets are suitable, as long as sufficient biotin, riboflavin, and fat are present (slight deficiencies in these nutrients can cause severe health problems in the hamster). Fresh water should be provided *ad libitum*.

FERRETS (*Mustela putorius furo*)

Ferrets, initially domesticated in the fourth century BC and first used in the laboratory before World War II (Pyle, 1940), are becoming an increasingly attractive species for toxicology research. As a nonrodent species which is cheaper and smaller than either the dog or the primate, they appear to offer significant advantages as a model for systemic toxicology evaluations. They have been used in such studies since the early 1960s, though primarily in developmental toxicity studies.

Ferrets reach their adult weight range at about 4 months of age, with males being about twice the size of females. Both sexes can undergo photoperiod-related fluctuations in body weight of from 30 to 40%. Subcutaneous fat increases during the fall and disappears during the spring.

Housing

Ferrets may be kept singly or in sexually distinct groups, although males can become belligerent if housed together. Cages may be constructed of heavy wire mesh, but stainless-steel cat, dog, or guinea pig cages in racks are suitable. Cages should not be solid bottomed. Bedding is not essential in cages except for bred females or when rooms are kept at lower temperatures.

Rooms should be controlled to avoid conditions of excessive heat or humidity, with sufficient air changes (10 or more) to control odors.

Nutrition

The nutritional requirements of ferrets have not been as well characterized as those of the other common laboratory species. They can be maintained using commercial dry cat food supplemented with liver or with one of the commercial chows. Ferrets will eat to the limit of their caloric needs and must, therefore, be watched carefully to make sure that they do not eat themselves into a protein deficiency. They also have little capacity to digest fiber, and food passes through the ferret in 3 or 4 hr.

It should be remembered that the ferret is a carnivore, and its diet and eating habits should be governed accordingly. Water should always be freely available to them.

Handling

Ferrets can be restrained by holding them above the shoulders, with one hand gently holding the front limbs crossed with the thumb under the animal's chin. Blood samples may be collected (with practice) by venipuncture of the caudal tail vein or by orbital bleeding.

Intramuscular injections can be given in the same manner as the dog. If the animals are handled frequently, they may be picked up with bare hands. However, such is rarely the case in acute toxicity studies and generally leather gloves should be used.

DOGS (*Canis familiaris*)

Dogs were used for physiology studies as early as the 17th century and were one of the initial test species used in formal military toxicology. They are the classical "nonrodent" species for pharmacologic and toxicologic studies. The variations on this model species have ranged across the entire span of breeds, including mongrels, but current practice in toxicology is generally that only beagles, specifically raised for research, are used. This limitation to a single breed is primarily due to the homogeneous and dependable nature of available, research-bred beagles. It is generally possible to select the age and weight of animals available from vendors within some limits.

A healthy dog is bright, attentive, and in sound bodily condition. There should be no discharge from the orifices of a healthy animal, and the skin should be free from disease with the fur shiny and well kept. Young, sexually mature animals (8–10 months of age) are to be preferred for most uses in toxicology.

Housing

This is an area where currently pending regulations make exact details as to requirements unclear, but certain general guidelines can be offered.

The dog should be provided with a clean, dry pen or cage, with the exact size being determined by the size of the animal. Stainless-steel cages in racks are preferred, but some form of exercise pen should be made available if animals are to be kept for any extended period of time.

Rooms should have good lighting and ventilation, with sufficient air changes to preclude odors from developing. Temperatures should be kept in the range of 65–72°C, and relative humidity should be maintained in the range of 20–70%.

Handling

Dogs require firm but gentle handling. A slip noose of soft rope around the neck should be utilized to lead the dog to and from its cage. Blood is traditionally collected from the cephalic or jugular vein, with iv doses being administered by the femoral artery.

Nutrition

Dogs are carnivores but can be adapted to various commercially available laboratory diets, and are traditionally maintained on such. They do take some time to adapt to a new form of food, and this should be kept in mind before or during studies.

A nutritionally adequate dry dog food should contain 22–25% protein, 3–5% fat, 16% carbohydrates, and 4–6% fiber. Wet foods should contain 13% protein, 5% fat, 16% carbohydrates, and 2–4% fiber. The actual food intake required varies considerably with animal age and size. A guide for recommended daily food intakes is as follows:

Size	Approximate weight of dog (kg)	Approximate food intake (kg)
Small	5	0.25
Medium	10	0.50
Large	18	0.90

Dogs will eat beyond their caloric needs, so feeding *ad libitum* will only lead to heavy animals. Water should always be available, and feeding should be conducted at a standard time each day, with uneaten food being removed at the end of the feeding period.

Breed

The beagle is popular for toxicity testing for a number of reasons. Their short hair and average weight of 12 kg are contributing factors. Other breeds such as spaniels have been used, but are not currently favored nor commercially available as research-bred animals.

NONHUMAN PRIMATES

Various species of nonhuman primates are frequently used in toxicologic research because of their anatomic and perceived similarities to humans. Primates are expensive, in short supply, are difficult to maintain and to use, and their use is politically sensitive. Imported animals are of uncertain quality, and their availability is decreasing. The use of these animals should be restricted to essential cases, and recent flexibility by regulatory agencies in allowing nonterminal studies and reuse of animals in scientifically justifiable cases is to be applauded.

Primates vary markedly in size, ranging from mouse lemurs weighing only a few grams to gorillas weighing up to 450 kg. Table 61 summarizes some of the more commonly used primates in toxicological testing. The most commonly used in toxicology are the cynomolgus and the rhesus.

Macaques are the most commonly used for many forms of biomedical research, partially because the similarity of their immunologic response to that of man led, early on, to their wide use in the study of human pathogens. Both the rhesus and the cynomolgus are members of this genus and are almost the only ones used for acute or short-term toxicity testing.

The male rhesus reaches puberty at 3 or 4 years, whereas the female reaches sexual maturity at 1.5–2.5 years. The adult male rhesus weighs approximately 12 kg, with the female reaching 10 kg. Cynos are smaller, being perhaps half the size of the rhesus.

Housing

Unlike the other common laboratory species, the housing of primates is complex and requires consideration of space, need for quarantine, and the intended design of experiments. Unlike all the other common lab species (with the rare exception of the hamster), primates may well carry pathogens which can be transmitted to humans (Mitruka *et al.*, 1976).

Rooms for primates should be well ventilated (with 10–15 air changes an hour) and should provide at least 1.5 m² of space for each animal weighing 3 kg or more. These rooms should have a negative air pressure relative to adjoining spaces and be maintained at a temperature of 21–24°C with a relative humidity of 50%. Rooms should always provide adequate security to prevent the escape of animals.

Cages should be stainless steel in racks, with the exact size depending on the species and age of animals caged. Cage doors should be locked such that the animals cannot open them. A 12-hr photoperiod is desirable.

Nutrition

Most primates are both physiologically and anatomically omnivorous. There are a number of commercially available laboratory diets which are to be recommended over other approaches. Fresh water should always be available to them.

Handling

There are species differences in the incidence of tuberculosis, hepatitis B virus, and other diseases/zoonoses which should be considered in animal selection and in instructions to the personnel involved in the handling of primates. Parenteral administration of test materials to primates and the collection of blood samples requires careful restraint, and the use of a device such as a primate chair is recommended in such cases. A gum elastic or other such type stomach tube is required for oral administration of test agents.

CROSS-SPECIES EXTRAPOLATION

For all the other words in this volume about the relevance of the test systems that are described, one should never forget that none of the animals we use are other than models for humans—they are not actually people. Ultimately, the continued use of animals in predictive testing must depend on how well we can use the data from these animal models to predict the outcome in people. The activity of transforming results in members of one animal species (e.g., rats) to one or more populations of another species (such as people) is called cross-species extrapolation or scaling (though, technically, scaling is actually limited to the act of making adjustments for differences in sizes or rates).

Each step in the scaling process adds an additional degree of uncertainty to the final product. Wise and prudent scientific practice calls for at least three courses of action in seeking to give the best quality (i.e., least uncertain) final product in the form of, "what does this mean to humans." These courses of action are (a) have as few steps in the prediction process as possible, (b) have as little uncertainty as possible associated with each step, and (c) understand the places and ways in which the selected model fails as a predictor. Each of these courses of action is not only an integral part of the extrapolation process but also contributes heavily to proper model (test species) selection.

Our efforts thus far have been focused primarily on step b and part of step c—performing various tests in a manner that gives us the least imprecise and most relevant data possible and understanding the associated weaknesses of the model systems we employ. As such, our efforts and resulting extrapolations to this point have generally been for the animal species in which data were being developed. Ultimately, it is necessary to predict what these data would mean in humans. With the wide range of effects we are concerned about here, what conversion factor (or factors) can we derive that would allow us to equate a dose or exposure in rats or an effect in dogs with what would be seen in humans at the same or different doses? The tools at hand for the effort consist of a collection of mathematical methods (generally based on either body weight or body surface area as a means of quantitatively bridging the gap) and a set of logical and empirical rules that have been developed over the years.

The mathematical aspects will be addressed primarily in this section, whereas the "rules" will appear in the sections that follow. Though there is some scientific basis for these mathematical conversions, it is not on a point-for-point basis and one or two orders of magnitude of uncertainty are generally involved. Such extrapolations clearly have both quantitative and qualitative aspects, and the rules seek to limit the uncertainty about the qualitative aspects. Some form of pharmacokinetic and metabolism study would seem to be the best approach to such qualitative modeling, but even these methods have both difficulties and limitations of their own (Gillette, 1979) and are expensive and generally not available for support of acute data interpretation.

The qualitative aspects of species-to-species extrapolations are best addressed by a form of classification analysis tailored to the exact problem at hand. This approach identifies the known physiological, metabolic, and other factors which may be involved in the risk-producing process in the model species (for example, the skin sensitization process in the guinea pig), establishes the similarities and differences between these factors and those in humans, and derives means to bridge the gaps between these two (or at least identifies the fact that there is no possible bridge).

Table 63 presents an overview of the classes of factors which should be considered in the initial step of a cross-species extrapolation. Examples of such actual differences which can be classified as one of these factors are almost endless.

The absorption of compound from the gastrointestinal tract and from the lungs is generally comparable among vertebrate and mammalian species. There are, however, differences between herbivorous animals and omnivorous animals due to the differences in stomach structure. The problem of distribution within the body probably relates less to species than to size and will be discussed a little later. Primarily endogenous metabolism, xenobiotic metabolism of foreign compounds, metabolic activation, or toxification/detoxification mechanisms (by whatever name) are perhaps the critical factors and these can differ widely from species to species. The increasing realization that the administered compound is not necessarily the ultimate toxicant makes the further study of these metabolic patterns critical.

In terms of excretory rates, the differences between the species are not great: Small animals tend to excrete compounds more rapidly than large animals in a rather systematic manner.

The various cellular and intracellular barriers seem to be surprisingly constant throughout the vertebrate phylum. In addition, it is becoming increasingly clear that the various receptors, such as DNA and the neurotransmitters, are comparable throughout the mammalian species.

There are life-span (or temporal) differences that are not now considered adequately in cross-species extrapolation nor have they been in the past. It takes time to develop (for example) a cellular immune response and at least some of this time may be taken up by actual cell division processes. Cell division rates appear to be significantly higher in smaller animals. Mouse and

TABLE 63 Classes of Factors to be Considered in Species-to-Species Extrapolations of Toxicity

Relative sensitivity of model (compared to humans)
  Pharmacologic
  Receptor
  Life span
  Size
  Metabolic function
  Physiological
  Anatomical
  Nutritional requirements
  Reproductive and developmental processes

rat cells turn over appreciably faster than do human cells—perhaps at twice the rate. On the other hand, the latent period for expression of many effects is also much shorter in small animals than in large ones.

Another difficulty is that the life span of man is from 4.4 to 66 times (see Table 59) that of common test species. Thus, there is generally a much longer time available for many toxicities to be expressed or developed in people than in test animals. These sorts of temporal considerations are of considerable importance, and this area of chronotoxicology has not yet really begun to be explored.

Body size, irrespective of species, seems to be important in the rate of distribution of foreign compounds throughout the body. For example, the cardiac output of the mouse is on the order of 1 ml/min, and the mouse has a blood volume of about 1 ml. The mouse is therefore turning its blood volume over every minute. In man, the cardiac output per minute is only 1/20th of the blood volume. Therefore, the mouse turns its blood over 20 times faster than man, which has clear implications for the comparative rates at which xenobiotics are systemically distributed or cleared in these two species.

Another aspect of the size difference which should be considered is that the large animal has a much greater number of susceptible cells that may interact with potential toxic agents, though there is also a proportionately increased number of "dummy" (hyporesponding) cells.

Rall (1979), Oser (1981), and Borzelleca (1984) have published articles reviewing such factors, and Calabrese (1983), and Gad and Chengelia (1992) published excellent books on the subject.

Having delineated and quantified species differences (even if only having factored in comparative body weights or relative body surface areas), one can now proceed to some form of quantitative extrapolation (or scaling).

There are currently two major approaches to scaling for use with general toxicities. These are by body weight and by body surface area (Calabrese, 1983; Schmidt-Nielsen, 1984). Both of these are single-variable or two-dimensional models and represent alternate forms of what are called allometric equations. Davidson *et al.* (1986) have presented the generalized form of such equations as

$$Y = aW^n$$

where W is body weight, n is the slope of the derived line, and a is a scaling factor. There have been proposals (Yates and Kugler, 1986) that a multidimensional model would be more accurate. Such a form of allometric equation is probably too complicated for use in acute toxicology, however, and its use would be inappropriate considering the relatively imprecise nature of the data generated.

The body weight approach is the most common general approach to scaling in toxicology—particularly in acute toxicology. There are several ways to perform a scaling operation on a body weight basis, the most often employed being to simply calculate a conversion factor (K) as

$$K = \frac{\text{Weight of human (70 kg "standard")}}{\text{Weight of average test animal}}$$

This K would be one form of scaling factor a in the general equation above. More exotic methods for doing this, such as that based on a form of linear regression, are reviewed by Calabrese (1983), who believes that the body weight method is preferable.

A difficulty with this approach is that the body weights of any population of animals or people change throughout life, and in fact even at a common age will present considerable variation. The custom, therefore, is to use an "ideal man" (70 kg for men and 50 kg for women) or "ideal" animal weight (for which there is considerably less consensus).

The alternatives are the body surface area methods, which attempt to take into account differences in metabolic rates based on the principle that these differences are in production to body surface area (because as the ratio of body surface area to body weight increases, relatively more energy is required to maintain a constant body temperature). As long ago as 1938, Benedict published a comparison of body weight versus basal metabolic rates for species from mice to elephants which showed a linear relationship between the two variables. Pinkell (1958) and Freireich et al. (1966) found a similar relationship for effective/tolerated doses for cancer chemotherapeutics. There are several methods for making such conversions, each taking the ratio of dose to the animal's body weight (in mg/kg) as a starting point, resulting in a conversion factor with mg/m^2 as the units for the product of the calculations.

The Environmental Protection Agency (EPA) version of the surface area scaling equation is generally calculated as

$$(M_{\text{human}}/M_{\text{animal}})^{1/3} = \text{surface area}$$

where M is mass in kilograms. Another form is calculated based on constants that have been developed for a multitude of species by actual surface area measurements (Spector, 1956). The resulting formula for this approach is

$$A = KW^{2/3}$$

where A is the surface area in cm^2, K is a constant specific for each species, and W is body weight in grams. A scaling factor is then simply calculated as a ratio of the surface area of man over that of the model species.

The best scaling factor is not generally agreed upon. Though the majority opinion is that surface area is preferable where a metabolic activation or deactivation is known to be both critical to the adverse effect-causing process and present in both man and the model species. These assumptions may not always be valid. Also, for the conditions under which most acute testing is performed, these facts are generally unknown. Table 64 presents a comparison of the weight and surface area extrapolation methods for the eight common laboratory animal species and humans.

Schneiderman *et al.* (1975) and Dixon (1976) have published comparisons of these methods, but Schmidt-Nielsen (1984) should be considered the primary source on scaling in interspecies comparisons.

When one is concerned about specific target organ effects, frequently the earliest indicator of such an effect is an alteration in organ weight out of proportion to what is to be expected due to changes in overall body weight (Gad *et al.*, 1984) or to changes in a standard such as brain weight. It should be pointed out that a form of scaling is involved in detecting such effects because adjustments to organ weight to account for alterations in overall body weight can take several forms. Simple ratios (Weil and Gad, 1980; Gad and Weil, 1980), analysis of covariance, or species or organ-specific allometric methods (Trieb *et al.*, 1976; Lutzen *et al.*, 1976) may be employed.

An alternative approach to achieving society's objective for the entire risk assessment process (that is, protecting the human population from unacceptable levels of involuntary risk) is the classical approach of using safety factors. This is still the methodology used in determining what acceptable risks, given the uncertainties involved, in phase I human clinical trials of a new drug, would be based on animal safety data. The presumed degree of uncertainty in these cases is instructive. In 1972, Weil summarized this approach as follows:

TABLE 64 Extrapolation of a 100 mg/kg Dose in the Mouse to Other Species

			Extrapolated dose (mg) based on		
Species	Weight (g)	Surface area[a] (cm²)	Body weight (A)	Body surface area (B)	Ratio A/B
Mouse	20	46.4	2	2.0	1.00
Rat	400	516.7	40	22.3	1.80
Hamster	50	126.5	50	5.4	1.08
Guinea pig	400	564.5	40	24.3	1.65
Ferret	500	753.9	50	32.5	1.54
Rabbit	1,500	1,272.0	150	54.8	2.74
Dog	12,000	5,766.0	1200	248.5	4.82
Monkey	4,000	2,975.0	400	128.2	3.12
Man	70,000	18,000.0	7000	775.8	9.80

[a]Surface area (except in the case of man) values calculated from the formula: surface area $(cm)^2 = K W^{2/3}$, where K is a constant for each species and W is the body weight [values of K and the surface area for man are taken from Spector (1956)].

In summary, for the evaluation of safety for man, it is necessary to: (1) design and conduct appropriate toxicological tests, (2) statistically compare the data from treated and control animals, (3) delineate the minimum effect and maximum no ill-effect levels (NIEL) for these animals, and (4) if the material is to be used, apply an appropriate safety factor, e.g., (a) 1/100 (NIEL) or 1/50 (NIEL) for some effects or (b) 1/500 (NIEL), if the effect was a significant increase in cancer in an appropriate test.

This approach has served society reasonably well over the years, once the experimental work has identified the potential hazards and quantitated the observable dose–response relationships. The safety factor approach has not generally been accepted or seriously entertained by regulatory agencies for carcinogens, mutagens, or teratogens, but is well established for other toxic effects of drugs and chemicals. It will be examined in more detail in the final chapter of this book. Until such time as the more elegant risk assessment procedures can instill greater public and scientific confidence, the use of the safety factor approach to bridge our collective uncertainty about the difference between species responses should perhaps not be abandoned so readily for other, albeit more mathematically precise and elegant, procedures.

As a final check to any multistep process of hazard assessment, the data points generated by any other studies (particularly any human exposures) of the endpoint of interest should be evaluated to determine if they fall within the range expected based on the assessment. If the available real-world data do not fit the extrapolation model at this point, then scientists have no choice but to reject such a model or assessment and start anew.

Embodied in the safety factor approach are two of the rules for cross-species extrapolation, which are actually general comparative statements of relationship between species.

In general, as animal species become larger, they also become more sensitive to short-term toxicities. This effect may be credited to a number of mechanisms (such as increases in mass of available target tissues and decreases in metabolic rate as size increases), but it is true even for nonmammalian species such as fish (Anderson and Weber, 1975) and birds (Hudson *et al.*, 1979). The rule even applies somewhat to differences in body size within the same age class of the same sex of the same species.

What this rule means is that the sensitivity of a larger species (such as a dog or man) to a short-term toxicity will be greater than that of a smaller species (such as a mouse or rat). There are, of course, exceptions and wide variations from linearity in this relationship (such as hamsters being much less sensitive to the neurotoxicity of DDT than are mice, as reported by Gingell and Wallcave in 1974). Also, those toxicities which are mediated or modulated by structurally different features [such as those toxicities associated with the skin, where general rules fall apart completely across broad ranges of structural classes (Nixon *et al.*, 1975; Campbell and Bruce, 1981)] are subject to even less certainty under this rule.

There are also those who believe that man is more sensitive than any test species, even if that species is larger than man (such as a cow or horse). Lehman (1959) published, for example, the relationships shown in Table 65.

It should be noted that much data on effects in humans are biased by man being a better (or at least more sensitive and louder) indicator of adverse effects.

As pointed out in Chapter 7, differences in sensitivity between the sexes are, in most cases, such that females are more sensitive than males. Data to support this will be reviewed later in this chapter.

Borchard *et al.* (1990) present a very broad overview of the differences in effective therapeutic doses of drug agents for a broad range of laboratory animals. The volume is also an essential resource for animal care in a vivarium.

MODEL SELECTION

Given all that has been presented on test systems, the characteristics of different species, and how one extrapolates from one species to another, the next obvious question is how are test species actually selected.

The obvious, theoretical best choice would be the species considered at risk, which would leave us with no difficulty in extrapolating from one species to another [though, as will be seen under Limitations of Models, not all members of the same species (even disregarding sex and strain differences) respond similarly]. For some applications (veterinary agents or where the concern is for the effects of potential exposures to domesticated animals or wildlife), it is possible to take this approach. But in most cases, in which the

TABLE 65   Some Relations of Drug Toxicity in Experimental Animals Compared to Man[a]

Species	Body weight	Weight ratio: animal/man	Drug dose ratio	Sensitivity: drug dose ratio/weight ratio
Man	60	1	1	1
Cow	500	8	24	Man 3× as sensitive
Horse	500	8	16	Man 2× as sensitive
Sheep	60	1	3	Man 3× as sensitive
Goat	60	1	3	Man 3× as sensitive
Swine	60	1	2	Man 2× as sensitive
Dog	10	1/6	1	Man 6× as sensitive
Cat	3	1/20	1/2	Man 10× as sensitive
Rat	0.4	1/150	1/15	Man 10× as sensitive

[a]The values in this table are averages and their validity cannot be checked against original data because Lehman (1959) only reported them as being from numerous sources.

real-life concern is potential toxicity to humans, a laboratory animal must be selected because although chemicals are still occasionally administered to people for experimental purposes, there are legal and ethical issues which make this a rare case indeed before at least some acute toxicity data have been gathered in a species other than man (NAS, 1975). Even then, initial toxicity tests carried out in man are generally at low-dose levels compared to the toxic doses predicted from animal experiments. The design of acute toxicity studies in which humans are used is commonly directed at the evaluation of alterations in blood chemistry, measurable physiological variables, and the analysis of the agent and its metabolites in the blood, urine, feces, and tissues (Nosal and Hladka, 1968; Rider *et al.*, 1969). With pesticides and a few other environmental agents, useful human acute toxicity data have been obtained by the study of accidentally exposed individuals (Brown, 1980).

What then would constitute the best choice of models? There is a set of characteristics that most would agree constitute the "ideal" animals on scientific grounds. These include (1) similarity of absorption, distribution, metabolism, and excretion in humans; (2) sensitivity of the species to the agent closely resembling that of humans; (3) evolutionary level of the animal; (4) ability of the species to express the full range of responses that humans would (such as emesis); (5) ability to make all pertinent measurements in a meaningful way; and (6) stages of the life span should correlate directly to those of humans.

However, there is also a set of desired characteristics that an ideal species should possess from a technical management point of view. These criteria are

Have a low body weight
Be easy to bleed and large enough to supply a reasonable amount of
    blood
Be easy to obtain or breed and maintain in the laboratory
Be easy to handle and to administer test agents to by the various desired
    routes
Should have a short life span
Physiology and metabolism should approximate those of humans
Should not pose a disease threat to handlers

The weight of the experimental animal is important because during the early stages of development of new commercial chemicals, only small quantities of the test material may be available.

Each of these ideal features is secondary to the desire to have a model that responds exactly as our target species. However, there is no animal species that mimics humans in all respects, so the ultimate choice depends on a balance of conflicting factors. It is all too easy to suggest that the animal of choice should fit the criteria enumerated previously, but in actuality these are empty words. Actual selections are made generally on practical and "political" grounds rather than on strict logic.

The data necessary to make decisions based on practical considerations have largely been incorporated into the tables at the beginning of this chapter. Economic considerations turn out to be among the most important. These include the cost of the animal and its upkeep, availability of test animals, housing requirements, and a host of other factors that tend to push selection toward smaller, established test animal species.

The possibilities for selection are, of course, much wider. The subkingdom of vertebrate animals alone contains a greater number of species, which can be classified into distinct categories as shown in Table 66.

Only a few of this multitude of possible species, however, have actually been employed at any time. Also, the eight species that are discussed in-depth in this chapter represent virtually all (99.9%) of the animals currently used in acute toxicology. Why is this?

How Species Are Actually Selected

There are two major sets of factors which actually drive the process of model selection in acute toxicology, with rare exceptions.

First, economic considerations, such as ease of commercial production and availability, housing, life span, etc., have, as was pointed out, favored the use of small laboratory animals. In the resulting enthusiasm for establishing rodents as satisfactory test models, toxicologists have conveniently overlooked the fact that there have been few studies correlating the toxicity of specific compounds in human and these animals species. The available information suggests a moderate to fair direct correlation (see Litchfield 1961, 1962). Difficulties in validating alternative or new test systems have tended to preclude any improvement of the model systems that are employed. There is an urgent need for a nonrodent species with a life span of up to 5 years that does not have

TABLE 66   Approximate Distribution of the Vertebrae Animal Species

Category	Number of distinct species
Fish	23,000
Amphibians	2,000
Reptiles	8,500
Mammals	4,500
All vertebrates	43,000

Note. From Rothschild (1961).

the problems inherent in the dog or primate. Ferrets, marmosets, miniature pigs, and a number of other species have been investigated during the past 15 years, but only now have people begun to use one of these (the ferret) to any extent. There is clearly an opportunity for the commercial animal breeder here, but it may be that the essential criteria are impossible to meet and the underlying societal inertia is too great. Stevenson (1979) has discussed these aspects in the wider context of general toxicology.

The second major set of factors can only be classified generally as custom or habit. What scientists and technicians have used, and what the regulators are used to interpreting data from, is generally what we tend to continue using. The resulting inertia is the greatest impediment not only to proper model selection but also to adaptation of new or improved study designs and to the development and use of in vitro models. The frequently raised issue of validation for any proposed change in what the science of toxicology does could all too often be more accurately stated as "show us that it gives us the same answers—we know how to deal with those, even if they are wrong."

To fulfill these two sets of factors, animals are actually selected for acute testing based on the following steps:

Which species will meet test design needs?

What is species availability?

How much test compound is available? If the amount is limited, the smallest (body weight) species that will meet other needs will be selected.

What species is the least expensive, both in terms of costs directly associated with the animals and indirect costs (the easier an animal is to handle, for example, the lower are the labor costs associated with the study)?

Will the species selected meet regulatory guidelines (usually easy because these either dictate a species for a particular test or simply specify rodent or nonrodent) and have regulatory "acceptance" (not so easy)?

What have we used in the past? This question usually comes first, generating a list of candidate species.

SPECIAL CASES IN SPECIES SELECTION

There are a number of routes of exposure for which a particular species is by habit (frequently based on a form of folklore) especially favored.

In inhalation, there are several special considerations of anatomy and physiology which dictate model selection. In Table 62, we presented a classification of respiratory anatomies. In addition, the following three factors should be strongly considered in species selection for inhalation studies:

Mouth (10-μ filtration) vs nose (3-μ filtration) breathers. A man versus rodent comparison, with considerable resulting differences in both particulate/droplet filtration and regional absorption.

Number of "daughter" generations of air passages. These are the number of successive times that air passages in the respiratory tree branch. There are 35 in man, but fewer than 25 in rats.

Distribution of major compartments in the respiratory tract. Humans have the following: nasopharyngeal (NP), nasal cavity and mouth; tracheobronchial (TB), larynx, trachea, and bronchials; pulmonary (P), aveolar sacs.

The rat is far and away the most common species used in inhalation, even though it is an obligatory nose breather and its respiratory morphophysiology is much different than that of humans (it has five lung lobes and a total lung surface area of 7.5 m^2—10% of that of man).

Folklore says that primates are the best inhalation model for humans. However, the closest similarity to humans in respiratory structure and function is probably found in the horse or donkey. Besides the rat, commonly used species include none of these, however. Rather, the mouse and dog are the only other commonly used species in inhalation (see Chapter 13).

Likewise, dermal studies are by custom performed on the rabbit because its dermal absorption is "greater" than that of humans, making it the most sensitive model. As discussed in Chapter 3, this in fact is not the case. Neither is it true that the dermal absorption and skin morphology of the pig most resemble humans. Rather, the answer as to which species is either most sensitive or most resembles man depends very much on the structural class of compounds in question. Recent efforts and suggestions by some that all toxicity tests be performed on a common species, such as the rat, merit wider consideration. If we as a science are not willing or able to select models on a scientific basis (what will provide us with the best prediction of what would happen in humans), then at least using a single common model, one which we understand the weaknesses of, makes greater sense.

CAUTION

Having considered the general process of model selection, one should be aware of the limitations and peculiarities of the common models and of some of the variations that occur within a species due to differences between strains of animals.

LIMITATIONS OF MODELS

Despite our best efforts, when human exposure to a chemical entity (such as a drug) occurs, the results are not always what would be expected based on animal studies. For the population as a whole, there are a number of possible explanations. Some of these are presented in Table 67.

An example of these types of problems in the extrapolation of toxicity data from one species to another can be found in published studies on fenclozic acid, which was a potential new anti-inflammatory drug (Alcock, 1971). No adverse effects were observed to occur in the mouse, rat, dog, rhesus monkey, patas monkey, rabbit, guinea pig, ferret, cat, pig, cow, or horse, but the drug caused acute cholestatic jaundice in man.

Beyond the difficulties in extrapolating from one or more test animal populations to the overall human population, there are a number of limitations to the standard model populations which are imposed by two forms of the "good scientific practice" that are employed in conducting toxicity studies. Both of these practices have as their rational the maximization of the sensitivity of the

TABLE 67   Some Reasons Why Data Obtained in Animal Studies Do Not Always Match Human Experience

---

The animal species selected differs in response from humans. The same model in a different animal species may have been more predictive.

Differences in absorption, distribution, and/or metabolism may be present.

The anatomy involved in the model may differ from that in people.

Different animal strains of the same species may generate different results.

The pathological nature of any lesions produced may differ at either macroscopic or microscopic levels that lead to different responses.

There may be critical differences between the species at subcellular, cellular, receptor, or physiological levels that lead to different responses.

Experimental conditions in the animal model may yield qualitatively different data over the course of several experiments, and it may be unclear which set is "correct."

The "dose" required to produce the observed results in animals is never achieved in humans.

The target human dose cannot be achieved in test animals.

The human population we are concerned about may differ from the population in general, and in so doing may have special characteristics which were not adequately represented in our animal model population.

---

test system, with the underlying good intention of therefore providing the greatest possible protection to people. This is not, however, always achieved.

The first of these practices is that toxicity testing has traditionally been performed at high doses. Even in acute toxicity studies which have the objective of predicting potential target organs and mechanisms of toxicity for humans at much lower doses, the study is considered suspect if all (or, for some people, any) animals survive at the highest dose level tested. This use of a maximum administerable dose and large fractions thereof is a spillover from carcinogenesis testing and times when our ability to detect effects was crude. It can frequently produce errors or difficulties in prediction of effects in people, such as those in Table 68.

The second practice is that of using test animal populations which are as homogeneous as possible. The current strategy for investigating toxicity for the most part evaluates toxicity in homogeneous populations, whether in animals or in humans, whether *in vitro* or *in vivo*. Such an approach minimizes the expression of background biological variability and therefore generates the most readily quantifiable and "sensitive" estimates of predicted toxicity in actual target populations which are more heterogeneous than the model population with respect to, among other things, susceptibility and resistance to the compound in question. The rationale may not be truly applicable to effects on humans, in which toxicity in even a relatively small susceptible population would not be acceptable. Adjustments for this wider range of susceptibility in the human population are most commonly accounted for as being part of what is involved in the use of safety factors in setting allowable limits for human exposure. This may not be either accurate or adequate.

TABLE 68 Reasons Why High-Dose Toxicity Testing Is Usually not Predictive of Human Effects

---

Solubility of the compound may be limiting.

Kinetics may be nonlinear (e.g., an enzyme may be saturated) and absorption may be decreased.

Michaelis–Menten kinetics may be applicable, and the blood levels may be greater than predicted in animals.

Metabolites formed in the animal studies may cause toxicity that would not occur with lower doses (high doses of phenacetin are one of many examples).

Detoxification mechanisms in the liver or elsewhere may be depeleted or saturated (examples are high doses of acetaminophen in the liver or of hexavalent chromium in the lungs).

Bioavailability of the dose form may be entirely different at lower doses due to local physiological effects (such as irritation) in the high-dose animal studies.

High doses in animals may overwhelm organ systems which would not be affected at lower doses, causing effects which serve to mask those seen at lower blood levels.

The underlying belief is that a potentially toxic exposure occurs with the interaction of the chemical and a model population in a particular space and time. This experimental event of exposure must be characterized by the range of "dose" type of exposure; characteristics of the exposed population (weight, sex, strain, etc.); the biologic characteristics of the effect at the molecular, cellular, tissue, organ, individual and population levels; and over a spectrum of effects from physiological through pathological and behavioral. The toxicity of the exposure must be characterized in terms of the severity of the effect, for example, clinical signs, disability, and/or death. Later, the relevance and acceptability of an observed effect to human society must be considered. As a corollary of the principles of experimental design, each variable in a protocol is rigidly fixed within a narrow range. Also, we use the "best" test population—the healthiest, most adequately fed young adult animal population possible. These laboratory animals have been carefully bred to make them as genetically defined as possible and are maintained in clean cages under narrowly controlled environmental conditions. Thus, toxicologists traditionally utilize a very robust and (at best) narrowly representative population of animals under the best of environmental conditions.

How then do we predict adverse effects for the human populations we are most concerned about, or at least allow for them in our predictions? In many cases, perhaps, one should utilize appropriate "at-risk" model populations in such tests. For example, if older individuals or those with compromised cardiovascular function are known to constitute a significant part of the potentially exposed human population, study designs should incorporate groups of animals that can serve to determine if such conditions render the animals (and therefore, potentially, people) more susceptible to toxic effects or if they change the nature of the expression of the toxic effect.

Susceptibility to an effect at any particular moment in a biological organism is determined by three sets of variables affecting the biological state of the organism at the time of exposure that are largely not apparent: genetic constitution, previous life experience, and physiological state. Genetic constitution is determined by factors of strain, species, family, congenital abnormalities, and any acquired alterations. Species factors are the result of the selection of major genetic components over the course of evolution and have already been discussed. Strain factors have largely been determined by selective breeding for concentration of genetic characteristics by the laboratory animal breeder, and considerations of strain will be presented later in this chapter.

However, there are a number of factors which are part of the other two variables (life experience and physiological state) which are not generally represented or considered in our test animal population and yet do exist in humans and do contribute to the biological outcome of a chemical exposure. These can be considered "susceptibility factors."

SUSCEPTIBILITY FACTORS

There are many factors which can alter the physiological state of an individual (or the fraction of available chemical moiety; see Table 69), and in so doing make them more (or, in some few cases, less) susceptible to the adverse effects of a chemical. These include (but are not limited to) immunological experience; psychological factors (such as stress), age, illness, conditioning factors (such as obesity and malnutrition), and sex. Immunological experience is beyond the scope of this chapter, but the others will be discussed.

SEX

Sex hormones may be the target of, or they may modify, a particular toxic response, which then may account for differential responses between the sexes to toxic materials. The current consensus is that (as was pointed out earlier) female rodents are more susceptible than males to the acute toxic effects of many chemicals, though males and females of the same strain, age, and general condition will react in a qualitatively similar manner.

As a result of reviewing the acute oral and dermal toxicities of 98 pesticides to rats, Gaines (1969) concluded that by the oral route the majority were more toxic to females than to males. He found the reverse true for only 9 of the 98 pesticides tested: aldrin, chlordane, heptachlor, abate, imidan, methyl parathion, fenchlorphos, schradan, and metepa. Pallotta et al. (1962) found the same pattern for the antibiotic acetoxycycloheximide in rats but not in dogs (where there was no sex difference).

Indeed, a review of the published literature on pesticides by Kato and Gillette (1965) found that such sex differences are common in rodents but less so in other mammals, though the information on these other species is not as definitive. Even with rodents and pesticides, however, it should be remembered that this is a general rule and not a universal truth. Steen et al.

TABLE 69 Factors Which May Increase the Fraction of Available Chemical Moiety in the Systemic Circulation

---

Renal impairment
Liver impairment
Hypoalbuminea
The presence of other moieties that displace test agent from proteins
 in circulation
Pregnancy
Immaturity of metabolism or physiologic systems

(1976) found mevinphos to be more toxic to male Mongolian gerbils than to females, while Gaines (1960) found the reverse to be the case for this compound in rats. These observations were in accord with published data on hexabarbitone sleeping times, as shown in Table 70. In general, most barbiturates cause longer sleeping times in females than in males. Likewise, as a class, organophosphates are lethal in lower doses in female rats than in males.

Shanor et al. (1961) found in humans that there is a statistically significant difference between the plasma cholinesterase levels of healthy young males and females (activity levels in females are from 64 to 74% of males), but that this difference disappeared in older people. There was no significant variation between the sexes in erythrocyte cholinesterase—a finding confirmed by Eben and Pilz (1967). Naik et al. (1970) likewise found there to be no significant difference between males and females in either total brain cholinesterase or in brain acetylcholine. These findings suggest that the distribution characteristics of toxicants working by cholinesterase inhibition mechanisms may be critical to their acute toxicity and that these distribution characteristics may be altered by the sex of the animal.

Krasovskij (1975) reviewed data on the acute toxicities of 149 chemicals and compared the results for males versus those for females. For both rats and mice, he found that the females tended to be more sensitive than the males, though not by large amounts (generally the differences were on the order of from 8 to 12%, being a little greater in rats than in mice).

Depass et al. (1984) looked at oral and dermal lethality of a number of previously studied compounds for which the results had been largely unpublished. To assess the effect of sex, they calculated the correlation coefficient (r) between the LD_{50} results for the two sexes. For 91 oral studies, r was found to be 0.93, while for 17 dermal studies with skin abrasion and 28 without, the r values were 0.73 and 0.96, respectively. The LD_{50} values between the

TABLE 70   Relative Hexobarbitone Sleeping Times for Each Sex in Two Different Rodent Species

	Mean sleeping time (min)		
Sex	Mongolian gerbil[a]	Rat[b]	Mouse[c]
Male	105 + 9.6	22 + 4	34 + 5
Female	70 + 6.9	67 + 15	31 + 5

Note. The reported sex difference did not occur in rats less than 4 weeks old.
[a]Maines and Westfall (1971).
[b]Quinn et al. (1958).
[c]Vessell (1968).

two sexes were, in other words, strongly associated. However, when the values were compared using paired t tests, there was a statistically significant trend toward higher LD_{50}'s in the males.

Similarly, Bruce (1985) reviewed studies from files on 48 chemicals and found that for only 3 of these was there evidence of lower LD_{50} values among the males than the females, and that none of these differences approached statistical significance. In 13 cases, however, the males had significantly higher LD_{50} values than the females. For these 13 studies, male LD_{50} values averaged 29% higher than those for females.

Imbalances of hormones other than those related to sexual function have also been shown to alter the susceptibility of animals to the toxic effects of chemicals. Hyperthyroidism, hyperinsulinism, adrenalectomy, and stimulation of the pituitary have all been demonstrated to be capable of modifying the effects of selected toxicants (Dauterman, 1980; Doull, 1980).

STRESS

Stress and biological rhythms (the complex interactions of physiological responses to chronologically ordered external factors) are among the least accounted for variables in acute toxicology. Though they have both been studied and identified as important determinants of sensitivity to toxicity, standard practice does not evaluate these effects or seek to consider them in predicting human effects.

Stress is a broad term for specific morphological, biochemical, physiological, and/or behavioral changes experienced by an organism in response to a stressful event or "stressor" (Vogel, 1987). Such changes can be quite drastic. Plasma levels of epinephrine in resting rats are approximately 100 pg/ml but in a stressed rat can approach 2000 pg/ml. Cessation of the stressful event usually terminates the stress response and the organism returns to its baseline homeostasis. However, if the stress response is very intense or long-lasting, a return to the original homeostasis may not occur and a new biological equilibrium may be established. The consequences of this new condition can be either beneficial (such as exercise-induced stress strengthening the heart) or detrimental (such as job-induced stress causing ulcers or hypertension) to the organism.

The typical behavioral stress responses are fear, tension, apprehension, and anxiety. Physiological stress responses can include changes in gastric secretion and motility and increases in blood pressure and heart rate. Biochemical changes are widespread during stress and include significant increases in the levels of plasma catecholamines and corticosteroids or marked changes in brain neurotransmitter concentrations. Although these are only typical response examples, most biochemical and physiological systems are probably affected during stress. Thus, potential toxicants interact with quite different physiological and/or biochemical systems during stress and the resulting outcomes of such interactions are bound to be quite different under these altered conditions.

In experimental toxicology it is customary to use nonstressed animals to evaluate the extent and modes of action of chemicals. However, animals and humans are seldom nonstressed but rather are frequently challenged by stressful events in the real world, responding to stress with some of the previously mentioned responses. Thus, agents acting at specific biochemical sites or on physiological processes will encounter different conditions during rest and stress, resulting in differences in their effects. In addition, the true action of some agents may only be revealed during stress. Thus, the variable of stress should probably be included during experimentation to better approximate (or model) various real-life situations and to predict more accurately the actions of chemicals under all types of environmental conditions.

The literature does very clearly reflect that the actions of biologically active substances can be altered during stress. Toxic effects can be increased or decreased and the results must be interpreted in this context before they can be generalized or extrapolated to the human population. Guinea pigs show an increased susceptibility to the lethal effects of ouabain during stress. Natelson *et al.* (1979) report that only 9% of nonstressed animals die, whereas 50% succumb to the same dose if the animals are stressed. Similarly, the delayed neuropathology of triorthotolyl phosphate in hens is almost tripled by stress (Ehrich and Gross, 1983), and Stockinger (1959) indicated the considerable influence that stress can have on the dose-dependent distribution of some of the elements in the body.

It has also been demonstrated that injections of adrenocorticotrophic hormone (Vaccarezza and Willson, 1964a,b) caused increases both in plasma and in cell cholinesterases in rats, but that adrenalectomy caused a progressive decline in the circulating red blood cell (RBC) cholinesterase but had no effect on plasma cholinesterase in rats. In people, injections of adrenocorticotrophic hormone also gave rise to increases in plasma and circulating cell cholinesterases (Vaccarezza and Peltz, 1960).

In reporting investigations of parathion in rats, Kling and Long (1969) demonstrated the influence that dietary stress could have on the time course of the response of cellular cholinesterase, while not altering the overall quantitative outcome. In fact, much of life (for at least the laboratory animal species) consists of a habitat that exhibits repetition of a sequence of events in an ordered manner. The effect of many biologically active agents, particularly toxicants, must interfere with these normal patterns and resulting biological cybernetics. Though Scheving *et al.* (1974) held that there was little evidence that acute toxicity displayed significant differences relative to circadian rhythms, this conclusion seems suspect. There are clear relationships between biorhythms, stress, and endocrine function.

Circadian differences in response to a range of chemicals, such as niketha-mide, ethanol, librium, methopyrapone, and ouabain, have been observed in the mouse. Halberg *et al.* (1960) demonstrated that there was a potency ratio alteration of from 3.2 to 1 for the bioassay of *Escherichia coli* endotoxin carried out at 12-hr time intervals. Also, working with rats, Lenox and Frazier (1972) demonstrated that the mortality due to methadone was influenced by a circadian cycle.

Stress due to fasting has been shown to alter the permiability of the blood–brain barrier to some chemicals (Angel, 1969). Indeed, selective starvation can also influence sensitivity—Boyd *et al.* (1970) demonstrated that feeding protein-deficient or protein-rich diets to rats could markedly alter the LD_{50} values for many pesticides.

Likewise, for some toxicants the influence of single or multiple housing can also significantly alter the results of a range of outcomes in acute toxicity tests, with marked variations in sensitivity (and even the direction of the influence) to this housing variable between different species.

AGE

Age is a factor which alters an organism's response to exposure to a test chemical. Very young or old animals may be either more or less sensitive to toxic effects than fully developed young or mature animals, and, indeed, may even have qualitatively different responses. Older rats, for example, are almost immune to the carcinogenic actions of most chemicals. Neonates are more susceptible to the actions of opiates.

Traditionally, what is used to perform tests in our studies are young adult animals. However, much of our human population is either very young or old and clearly not physiologically comparable to young adults.

Age variation may give rise to differences in susceptibility to acute intoxication by different chemicals and there is no simple rule for relating age to the sensitivity or nature of the toxic response. Goldenthal (1971) published an extensive review of the comparative acute toxicity of agents to newborn and adult animals. During the early stages of life, anatomic, physiologic, metabolic, and immunologic capabilities are not fully developed.

Substantial differences in susceptibility can sometimes even be related to small age differences. With rodents, a few months difference in age can markedly alter the response to chemicals that influence either the central nervous or immunological systems.

Biological aging is both time and species dependent (Mann, 1965). For the purposes of acute toxicology, it is generally convenient to consider the stages of biological age as being neonatal, infant, young adult, adult, and old. There is no clear dividing line between these stages in any species, though their length was loosely defined at the beginning of this chapter. Rather, development and aging are a continuum on which there is both species and individual variation. For some laboratory-bred species, however, such as the rat, there is a fairly linear relationship between the logarithm of body weight and the reciprocal of the animal's age (Gray and Addis, 1948) which can be expressed as follows:

$$\text{Log}_{10}\,[W] = \frac{-k}{d} + \log_{10} A$$

where W is weight in g, k is the slope, d is age in days, and A is the estimated asymptote or limit for W. The toxicological response to both exogenous and endogenous physiological chemicals (such as epinephrine and acetylcholine) can vary with age. Brus and Herman (1971) demonstrated that newborn mice were significantly less sensitive to epinephrine and norepinephrine than were adults, but that the reverse held true for acetylcholine. Naik et al. (1970) found that brain acetylcholine concentrations increased with body weight/age until maturity, while brain cholinesterase activity was variable at lower weights/ages and became less variable as weight/age increased. Shanor et al. (1961), using a large population sample of young adults (ages 18–35 years) and older people (ages 70–80 years), found that the plasma cholinesterase activity was approximately 24% higher in the young males than in the old males, but that no such difference existed for females or for RBC cholinesterase.

Older animals also show a large number of alterations in their response to potential toxicants when compared to young adults.

DISEASE

Disease states can modify a variety of kinetic and physiological parameters, altering the baseline homeostatic condition. Earlier, it was pointed out that a number of conditions (such as liver or renal disease) could increase the amount of available "drug" moiety in the systemic circulation. The ability to understand how pathological conditions can modify the kinetics and effects of exogenous chemicals requires an understanding of the interrelationships between these various parameters.

Stress due to infection can alter the responses of animals to biologically active chemicals. In 1972, Safarov and Aleskerov found that the dipping of sheep in an ectoparasiticide depressed antibody production and reduced the ability of the sheep to survive infections. It has been shown that some chemicals adversely affect the natural immunological defense systems, although this appears to be associated more with persistent agents retained in the organism than with those agents which are rapidly cleared. Liver (by decreasing biotransformation) and renal (by disrupting both excretory and metabolic functions) diseases associated with a preexisting condition or old age may contribute to a greater sensitivity to a toxicant. Hyperthyroid states also have been shown to increase sensitivity to the toxic effects of several classes of drugs, particularly selected psychoactive agents (Zbinden, 1963).

PHYSIOLOGICAL STATE

The influence of diet on the response of animals and humans to toxins is well established. The acute toxicity can be increased or decreased by alterations in dietary protein or the various micronutrients (an example being the decreased sensitivity of protein-deficient animals to CCl_4). Two conditions which occur in humans and are not generally recognized as diseases (obesity and subclinical malnutrition or marginal nutrition) can also alter the biological effects of chemicals and serve to increase the susceptibility of individuals to toxic actions.

Obesity may well alter the distribution and storage of a xenobiotic, especially when it is markedly lipophillic. Obesity is also generally accompanied in humans and test animals by reduced or impaired respiratory, cardiovascular, and renal function, all of which will also alter the manner and degree to which an agent may be toxic.

Subclinical malnutrition or marginal nutrition is usually at the other end of the scale from obesity, but not always or absolutely. An individual person's or animal's diet may be calorically adequate (or even oversupplied) but nutritionally marginal in terms of vitamins, proteins, minerals, and other nutrients. Any such marginal nutrient state clearly presents the possibility of an increased susceptibility to a toxic or adverse outcome of exposure to a xenobiotic, particularly if a nutritional state means limited or deficient metabolic and/or enzymatic defense mechanisms. The principal biotransformation of toxicants is performed by the microsomal mixed-function oxidase system, which is depressed by a deficiency of essential fatty acids, vitamin A, or proteins.

Boyd *et al.* (1970) and Boyd (1972) reviewed the effects of nutritional status on acute toxicity, showing alterations in the responses of rodents. Mehrle *et al.* (1973) demonstrated that the LC_{50}'s of chlordane in rainbow trout were altered by the brand of commercial diet the fish were maintained on beforehand. Furthermore, the nutritional status of animals used to prepare or provide tissues for *in vitro* studies can change the microsomal metabolism and other aspects of responsiveness of the tissue (Kato and Gillette, 1965).

Toxins also have the potential to induce nutritional deficiencies, but these are rarely of concern in acute toxicology.

Summary

If the human population we are concerned about is such that one or more of these susceptibility factors is present in a substantial portion of the members, steps should be taken to design studies so that such individuals are adequately represented by an appropriate model in the test animal population. Barring that, or in the face of having existing data on studies performed in a standard manner, consideration should be given to these factors when attempting to predict outcome of exposures in people.

SPECIES PECULIARITIES

There are a number of quirks associated with various of the common species of laboratory animals used in toxicology. Many of these are not well presented in the toxicology literature, though Oser (1981) has done his best to overview problems specific to the rat and Gralla (1986) has published a review of eight species-specific responses to toxicants (a modified form of which is presented in Table 71). Most of these peculiarities hold at least the potential to impact

TABLE 71   Species-Specific Toxic Effects

Type of toxicity	Structure	Sensitive species	Mechanism of toxicity
Ocular	Retina	Dog	Zinc chelation
Ocular	Retina	Any with pigmented retinas	Melanin binding
Stimulated basal metabolism	Thyroid	Dog	Competition for plasma binding
Porphyria	Liver	Human, rat, guinea pig, mouse, and rabbit	Estrogen-enhanced sensitivity
Tubular necrosis	Kidney	Rats (male)	Androgen-enhanced sensitivity[a]
Urolithiasia	Kidney and bladder	Rats and mice	Uricase inhibition
Teratogenesis; fetal mortality	Fetus	Rats and mice	Uricase inhibition
Cardiovascular	Heart	Rabbits	Sensitivity to microvascular constriction

[a]More sensitive than humans for many agents (such as caprolactam and halogenated solvents).

on study design and interpretation. Presented here are those that the authors believe should be considered in model selection for acute studies.

SPECIES VARIATION

Though anyone who has had to work in biological research with intact animals should be aware of the existence of wide variability between species, examples which are specific to toxicology should be pointed out along with a comparison of species sensitivities for a number of specific agents.

The rodenticide zinc phosphide is dependent on the release of phosphine by hydrochloric acid in the stomach for its activation and efficacy (Johnson and Voss, 1952). As a result, dogs and cats are considerably less sensitive than rats and rabbits because the former species secrete gastric hydrochloric acid intermittently while the latter secrete it almost continuously. That this case is not a rare one can be quickly established by examining some data sets in which we have comparative oral lethality data on several species (including humans), such as those presented in Table 72.

There are numerous additional examples of such differences in pharmacology (Tedeschi and Tedeschi, 1968).

However, just as important as these variations in general patterns or effect are the species-specific responses that are associated with the commonly employed animal models.

TABLE 72 Comparative Human Acute Lethal Doses and Animal LD_{50}'s (mg/kg via Oral Route)

Chemical	Human LD_{LO}	LD_{50} values			
		Mouse	Rat	Rabbit	Dog
Aminopyrine	220	358	685	160	150
Aniline	360	300	440		195
Amytal	43	345	560	575	
Boric acid	640	3,450	2660		
Caffeine	192	620	192	224	140
Carbofuran	11	2	5		19
Carbon tetrachloride	43	12,800	2800	6380	
Cyclohexamide		133	3		
Lindane	840		125	130	120
Fenoflurazole		1,600	283	28	50

Rat

The rat is commonly accepted as the best animal model in toxicology—the closest to our ideal (Oser, 1981). Table 73 presents a list of some of the commonly known advantages and disadvantages of the rat as a model for humans.

Calabrese (1983) has published a good comparative review of the rat as a model for man across a wide range of toxicological and biological parameters, and this should be consulted for details.

TABLE 73   Advantages and Disadvantages of the Rat as an
Experimental Model for Humans

Advantages	Disadvantages
Commonly used	Anatomic
Small size	Lack of gallbladder
Minimal housing space	Yolk sac placenta
Prolific	Multiple mammae over body surface
Short gestation	No emetic reflex
Short lactation	Fur covered
Omnivorous	Thinner stratum corneum
Dry diet acceptable	No bronchial glands
Dosing by multiple routes	Physiological
Inexpensive	Estrus and menstrual cycles
Low maintenance cost	Multiparous
Docile	Hematology
Intelligence	Obligatory nose breather
	Concentrated urine
	Limited hypersensitivity response
	Metabolic
	Purines to allantoin
	Clinical chemistry
	Enzymatic biotransformation
	High β-glucoronidase activity
	Nutritional
	Mineral requirements
	Vitamin requirements
	Ascorbic acid biosynthesis
	Histidine biosynthesis
	Behavior
	Nocturnal
	Coprophagy
	Cannibalism
	Maintenance requirements
	Temperature and humidity control
	Noise control

Mice

Mice share many advantages and disadvantages of the rats as a model for man, such as an inability to vomit (i.e., no emetic response). Additionally, their small size and high metabolic rate cause the extent of many toxic effects to be exaggerated as homeostatic mechanisms are "overshot."

Guinea Pigs

The systemic immune response in the guinea pig is exaggerated. As a result, though for many immune parameters it is the best common model for man, the animal is subject to exaggerated respiratory and cardiovascular expressions of immunologically evoked events.

Rabbits

There are no specific pathogen-free rabbits currently commercially available. Rather, the animals tend not to be as homogeneous or of as high a quality as the other common laboratory animal species. Indeed, they tend to harbor a wider range of subclinical infections which show a seasonal variation in their degree of expression (animals with a visible disease problem are more common in the spring and fall), and the stress of experimentation can cause these subclinical infections to be expressed.

Also, the alterations in dermal vascular flow which accompany the changes in phases of hair growth cause marked alterations in percutaneous absorption and in so doing may alter many dermally related responses to chemicals.

Dog

The dog is currently the first-choice, nonrodent model for toxicity studies. It is generally very cooperative. The major physiological peculiarity it has that affects toxicity testing is the ease with which it is provoked to vomit. This makes oral dosing at best impractical and at worst impossible in the case of many compounds, even if the material is encapsulated or given in diet.

CONSIDERATIONS OF STRAIN

Thus far, we have focused on the differences between the different species of common laboratory animals and on how this should influence our choice of model. But for each of the two species that are used the most in toxicology (the rat and mouse), there is the additional level of complexity caused by differences between strains.

There are three different genetic categories of strains of rodents used in toxicological research: random bred, inbred, and F-1 hybrids (or outbred). Random bred are produced in large colonies where mating occurs randomly among males and females from unrelated litters. Commercially performed random breeding should not be unplanned, but rather occur in such a manner as to minimize inbreeding. Inbred animals are the result of sister–brother or parent–offspring matings. Twenty or more generations of sister–brother and/or parent–offspring matings are necessary to establish an inbred strain. Outbred animals are the results of matings between two inbred strains and are usually more vigorous than either of the parental strains. Animals within an inbred or outbred strain are essentially identical genetically, serving to remove a significant source of biological variability.

Strains also exist in the other laboratory animal species but are generally neither as rigorously defined nor of as great a concern and have been less studied as a source of variation within toxicity studies.

That strain differences within species are a source of significant and broad differences in results has now been well established, in many cases with varying degrees of knowledge of the underlying mechanistic basis. The resistance of some strains of rabbits to atropine is believed to be due to the hydrolysis of the drug by atropinesterase, controlled by the gene A_8, belonging to the group containing the gene which governs black pigmentation. As a result, resistance to atropine and black pigmentation are often associated (Sawin and Glick, 1943). Likewise, some strains of rabbits possess a pseudococaine esterase that makes their insensitivity to this drug extreme.

There are also varieties within strains. These result from various factors which in total are labeled "genetic drift" and can lead to significant differences in response to toxicants. An example is the resistance that some wild rats have developed to the anticoagulant rodenticides (Gratz, 1973; Zimmermann and Matschiner, 1974), requiring that new forms of rodenticides be developed.

Strain variations in response to biologically active agents arise from the same general mechanistic differences as do species differences. Although these (Hilado and Furst, 1978) pharmacogenetics have been the subject of numerous reviews (Kalow, 1962, 1965; Meier, 1963a,b; Vessell, 1968; Hathway, 1970; Moore, 1972; Lang and Vessell, 1976), it is still the case that few investigators have studied the mechanisms of variation in higher animals (Becker, 1962). Also, the differences in handling characteristics have generally not appeared in the literature.

MICE

There are literally hundreds of strains of mice commercially available, and undoubtedly many of these have been used at one time or another in toxicology.

Most work, however, is performed using one of the 10 strains shown in Table 74. It should be noted that randomly bred animals are not generally used.

The differences in response to hexobarbital, discussed earlier in the between-species context, also exist between various strains of mice (though they are less marked; Jay, 1955).

Karczmar and Scudder (1967) studied the sensitivity of different strains of mice to a number of psychotropic drugs, finding qualitative and quantitative differences. Methamphetamine induced stereotypic behavior in strains in which it is normally absent, increased it markedly in strains in which it is commonly seen, and decreased it where it is normally pronounced.

Weaver and Kerley (1962) demonstrated differences in the responses of strains to d-amphetamine, whereas Brown (1961) did the same for sleeping time responses to sodium pentobarbital. Hill et al. (1975) reported that the lethal dose of chloroform was four times greater in C57BL/6 mice than in male DBA/2J strain animals, and that twice as much chloroform accumulated in the kidneys of the sensitive strain than in those of the resistant.

Miura et al. (1974) explored the acute lethality of a single batch of the pesticide BHC in five different strains of mice and discovered a wide range of sensitivities:

Strain	LD_{50} (mg/kg)
SS	411
CF1	500
AA	802
C57BL/6	1414
C3H/He	1459

Longacre et al. (1981) found significant (300%+) differences in metabolism and sensitivity to the acute toxicity of benzene between C57BL/6 and DBA/2

TABLE 74 Commonly Used Strains of Laboratory Mice (in Toxicology)

Strain	Breeding	Comments
Swiss Webster (SW)	Outbred	
CF–1	Outbred	
CD–1	Outbred	
CFW	Outbred	
nu+	Outbred	
nu/nu	Outbred	"Nude" animal
C57BL/6	Inbred	
SENCAR	Inbred	Large and aggressive
B6C3F1	Inbred	Aggressive; black[a], traditional NCI mouse
BALB/c	Inbred	

[a]Others are albino.

mice. Kawano *et al.* (1981) investigated the sensitivity of five different strains of mice to butylated hydroxytoluene and found differences of more than an order of magnitude.

Finally, Gad *et al.* (1986) evaluated 10 different strains of mice for their responsiveness to a battery of standard delayed-contact sensitivity agents and demonstrated wide variability in the responsiveness, with some strains being reproducibly either the most or least sensitive to all the agents.

RATS

Though there are not as many commercially available strains of rats as there are of mice, there are still many. Most toxicology, however, is done with one of the five strains in Table 75.

It might be assumed that any of these strains would be suitable for evaluating the acute toxicities of rodentacides, for example, but all the common laboratory rats derived from *Rattus norvegicus* respond very differently than the wild *Rattus rattus* to anticoagulant rodenticides. The response of the wild rat, on a quantitative basis, is very similar to that of man.

The effect of strain differences on the studies of the sensitivity of rats to oxygen (Robinson *et al.,* 1967), to nitrous oxide (Green, 1968), and to warfarin (Davis and Davies, 1970; Zimmermann and Matschiner, 1974) have all demonstrated significant strain differences. Similarly, differences between the effects of 3-phenylpropylaminoguanidine and phenformin on active glucose transport *in vitro* have been demonstrated not only between strains but also between rats of the same strain supplied by different breeders. As with mice, pronounced variation in the biological half-life of antipyrine was demonstrated in eight strains of rats by Quinn *et al.* (1958), with (for example) females of the M 520 strain having an average half-life of 114 min contrasted to 282 min in females of the Buffalo rat strain.

Powers *et al.* (1984) demonstrated significant differences in the renal responses of three strains of rats (Wistar, Sprague–Dawley, and Fischer-344) to

TABLE 75   Commonly Used Strains of Laboratory Rats

Strain	Breeding	Notes
Sprague–Dawley (SD)	Outbred	Larger
Wistar (WI)	Outbred	
Long–Evans (LE)	Outbred	Hooded; more difficult to handle
Holtzman (CDH[SD])	Outbred	
Fischer 344 CDF (F—344)	Inbred	NCI animal of choice; smaller

caprolactam, showing the latter two to be more sensitive. Likewise, Derelanko (1987) published a report of measurable differences in the life span of erythrocytes of three of the most common strains of laboratory rats.

SUMMARY

Strains of rodents are usually selected on the basis of local custom—what has been used in the past will be used again. Clearly, this should not be the case if comparability of data between different laboratories is a major concern. The powerful argument can be made, however, that experience in handling and observing a particular strain of animal significantly increases the ability of researchers to detect abnormal activities or clinical signs.

BIOLOGICAL VARIATION

There are also individual animal-to-animal variations in temperature, health, and sensitivity to toxicities which are recognized and expected by experienced animal researchers but are only broadly understood. The resulting differences in response are generally accredited to "individual biological variation." This same phenomenon has been widely studied and observed among humans and is expected by any experienced clinician. Examples of such individual variations in humans include isoniazid, succinylcholoine, and glucose-6-phosphate levels and/or activities. In the first of these, "slow inactivators" who are deficient in acetyltransferase, and therefore acetylate agents such as isoniazid, only slowly and are thus more liable to suffer from the peripheral neuropathy caused by an accumulation of isoniazid. At the same time, people with more effective acetyltransferase require larger doses of isoniazid to benefit from its therapeutic effects, but in so doing are more likely to suffer liver damage.

Likewise, individuals with low levels of serum cholinesterase may exhibit prolonged muscle relaxation and apnea following an injection of a standard dose of the muscle relaxant succinylcholoine, and glucose-6-phosphate dehydrogenase deficiency is responsible for the increased probability of some individuals given primaquine or antipyrine to suffer from a hemolytic anemia.

ANIMAL CARE, HUSBANDRY, AND WELFARE

It should go without saying that the quality and integrity of any toxicity study requires that healthy animals of a defined nature and background be used for such studies, and that the animals be maintained in a controlled environment which excludes environmental variables which would influence the biological processes of interest.

It serves no purpose either to purchase a low-quality, microbially undefined animal for use in a barrier-type facility or to place the best available germ-free animals in poorly maintained conventional facilities. The nature and risks of the planned experiment dictate the absolute minimum acceptable quality for both animal and facility.

Also, the economics of modern research are such that animals are a minimal part of the cost of doing toxicologic research—the cost of the skilled labor and capital equipment involved is much greater.

Operational and extraneous factors can have a dramatic influence on the outcome of even an acute test as well as on the interpretation and usefulness of the results. Contaminants in the water, diet, bedding, or air can introduce undesired (and frequently undetected) variables or modifiers to the toxicity of chemicals under test. Other factors, such as subclinical infections, can reduce the effective number of animals in a study.

FACILITIES

Good physical design and maintenance of the vivarium are required to provide for the desired high standards of animal care, for a safe working environment, and for an efficient research organization. The animal facilities should be separated from the rest of the laboratories and offices, with access restricted to essential personnel only. A separate quarantine area should be available to hold newly arrived animals for observation until their health can be assured.

Small rooms are recommended for acute toxicity studies, allowing for separate rooms for different species (while still making it possible to economically use different species as "best model" considerations require) and flexibility in managing work flow can be maintained. This also allows for better prevention and easier containment of any disease outbreaks and reduces the possibility of errors due to many studies going on in a single room. The increased fixed costs incurred by using separate rooms are thus considered warranted.

All air entering and leaving the animal facility should be adequately filtered and otherwise preconditioned, with rooms receiving 10–15 air changes an hour. Automatic monitoring, control, and recording of temperature and humidity in individual rooms is desirable.

OPERATIONS

The essential feature to any successful animal care operation is a well-trained and motivated staff interested and concerned with both the health of individual animals and their contribution to the overall research effort. Work practices are very commonly overlooked as a source of variability and low productivity in toxicological research and yet are one of the major components under the daily control of management.

Lack of, or improper quarantine can inadvertently introduce disease into a facility and endanger studies in progress and even those yet to come. Animals should be taken directly to the quarantine area upon arrival and before their shipping containers are opened. If an epizootic disease is discovered in any animals of a shipment during quarantine, all should be returned or disposed of.

Both professional and technical staff involved directly in handling animals and in using them in research should receive training in proper techniques of humane animal usage and in personal hygiene. Training should also cover means of alleviating and/or avoiding pain in animals. Those individuals with disease conditions that could affect the animals' health should not be permitted in the vivarium.

EQUIPMENT AND SUPPLIES

To complement a well-designed and constructed facility, equipment and supplies should be of appropriate construction and nature to facilitate efficient maintenance, sanitation, and use. If at all possible, key equipment such as heaters and air conditioners should have both a primary and a backup unit.

Most current commercially available caging and rack systems are designed for easy and proper sanitation. Plastic or stainless-steel cages are now the norm, and they provide for effective chemical and disease control and containment.

Care should be taken in selecting feeders, with consideration of intended feed type (pellet, block, or powder), ease of filling and cleaning, and animal eating and living habits in mind. An automatic watering system which provides a continuous supply of fresh, contaminant (both chemical and biological)-free water to each cage on a dependable basis is now the standard. If a plastic shoebox-style cage is to be used, however, consideration should be given to using either a cage with a mesh bottom or a water bottle arrangement, to avoid the possibility of flooding and drowning animals. Each water outlet should be checked at least twice a day to ensure proper operation.

ENVIRONMENTAL FACTORS

Temperature

Changes in temperature may alter the toxicity of a compound. For example, at ambient temperatures colchicine and digitalis are more lethal to the rat than to the frog. But the sensitivity of the frog can be increased by raising the environmental temperature of the two species. The duration of response also decreases as the temperature is raised, suggesting that a temperature-dependent biotransformation of these compounds is involved.

Temperature may include both the background environmental temperature and the internal, physiologically regulated temperature of the animal itself. Many chemicals can profoundly alter body temperature (Cremer and Bligh, 1969). Environmental temperature and humidity are generally closely related and as such have frequently been considered together (Lang and Vessel, 1976). Understanding the basis for the temperature dependence of many of the actions of biologically active compounds has been an area of significant progress over the past 20 years. Belehradek (1957) successfully combined his own and other investigators research to produce a unified theory of cellular rate processes based on an analysis of the actions of temperature. He concluded that the rate of biological processes is primarily dependent on the resistance of cellular matter to the free movement of molecules within the cells rather than the rate of actual chemical reactions themselves. He was enthusiastic about the relationship between the rate responses of cellular systems and Slotte's temperature–viscosity relationship formula. Brody (1964) has, however, reviewed the applicability of this last theory to vertebrate animals and pointed out its shortcomings.

The relationship between responses to toxicants and ambient temperature in animals is sometimes paradoxical. Usinger (1957) investigated this in mice and found a series of biphasic relationships with "optimal" or peak ranges. Mean oxygen consumption per unit body weight diminishes as temperature increases from 25 to 30°C, then rises again as ambient temperature is increased further. Likewise, he measured the rectal temperature when the ambient temperature was 25°C, which increased on either side of this temperature.

Ahdaya et al. (1976) investigated thermoregulation in mice exposed to parathion, carbaryl, and DDT at temperatures of 1, 27, and 38°C. All three of the pesticides were found to be least toxic at 27°C. Doull (1972) has reviewed these temperature-dependent responses for many chemicals and presented the hypothesis that temperature is directly correlated with the magnitude and inversely correlated with the duration of the biological response to biologically active xenobiotics in many organisms. Though this temperature dependence stands as a general rule, there are a number of special-case exceptions. Also, it is clear that the effect of temperature on one response variable may not necessarily be predictive of effects on other biological response variables.

Baetjer and Smith (1956) found that the onset of death, rate of dying, and rate of recovery due to parathion in mice were more rapid, while the mortality was higher, at 35.6°C than at 22.8°C. At 15.5°C, the onset of death was delayed and the total mortality was greater than that at 22.8°C. They also investigated the influence of both pre- and postexposure temperatures on the response of the mice and determined that mortality varied directly with the preexposure and inversely with the postexposure ambient temperatures. Their conclusion was that the results could not be attributed to the acceleration of reaction rates but rather were due to alterations in the rates of physical factors, such as the absorption rate.

Keplinger and Deichmann (1967) investigated the toxicity of 58 chemicals under different ambient conditions, including temperature. They found that many of the patterns of acute toxicity response were biphasic relative to ambient temperature, with some temperature in the ambient range being associated with a peak sensitivity in many cases.

Humidity

Selisko *et al.* (1963) investigated the effects of a number of environmental factors on the acute ip toxicity of nicotine to mice and found only humidity to have a significant influence. Humidity does not have a marked influence on absorption through the skin except at the extreme limits of its range (Neely *et al.*, 1967), and the relationship between humidity and transdermal water loss in sweating animal species is not linear (Grice *et al.*, 1972). The relationship in nonsweating species (which include all of our common laboratory species) is even more complex (Neely *et al.*, 1967).

The physiological status of the test animal in terms of hydration can markedly influence its response to toxicants. Muller and Vernikos-Danelis (1968) showed that the LD_{50}'s of caffeine and dextroamphetamine in mice were markedly affected by both ambient temperature and the animals' hydration, with caffeine showing a large potentiation of toxicity at 30°C while dextroamphetamine showed much less change. At lower temperatures (22 and 15°C) the acute toxicity of both compounds was much less influenced by hydration.

Barometric Pressure

Interest in the effect of atmospheric pressure on the toxicity of chemicals is fairly recent, arising from human activities in space and deep sea diving vessels. At high altitudes, the toxicities of digitalis and strychnine are decreased while that of amphetamine is increased. The influence of atmospheric pressure seems to be mainly (but not entirely) attributable to altered physiological oxygen tension rather than a direct pressure effect (Brown, 1980). Recently this interest has taken a new turn as concern as to the possible hazard of fires and atmospheric contaminants on submarines has surfaced.

Light

Whole body irradiation with electromagnetic radiation, including light, increases the toxicity of CNS stimulants and decreases that of CNS depressants. The toxicity of analgesics such as morphine does not seem to be altered. Many toxicants do exhibit a diurnal pattern of response in animals that is generally related to the light pattern. In rats and mice, P450 enzyme activity is at its greatest at the beginning of the dark phase of the cycle.

Social Factors

A variety of social factors (interactions between individual animals and between animals and research workers) can modify the toxicities of chemicals in animals and undoubtedly also in humans. Animal handling, housing (singly or in groups), types of cages, and laboratory routine are all important components of such considerations.

Edwards (1982) should be consulted for a good overview of the factors to be considered in the design and operation of a laboratory, in terms of both good science and economic and regulatory considerations.

REGULATIONS

The basic role of animals in biomedical research, and even more so of their use in toxicity testing, has in recent years been called into question. This wide discussion and debate is beyond the scope of this book, and the reader is referred to the volumes by Sperlinger (1981), Sechzer (1983), and Fox (1986) regarding relevance in that area. The reasons for the debate, however, include both questions as to the relevance of findings in our current models (or, indeed, in any animal models; see Garattini, 1985) and well-founded concern arising from abuses (both real and perceived) of research animals.

The use of animals in research is becoming an increasingly regulated undertaking. The two most important of such regulations in the United States are the 1987 Animal Welfare Act and the NIU "guide," which, due to the manner of its use by many organizations, is, in effect, a regulation. It is beyond the scope of this volume to attempt to summarize these regulations, and the original documents should be consulted.

A great deal of information and guidance can also be found in the AALAS *Manual for Laboratory Animal Technicians* (Collins, 1979).

HUMANE CARE AND USE

Of greatest importance to the practicing toxicologist should be that all animal research be carried out in as humane a manner as possible, using as few animals as necessary to satisfactorily perform the job at hand. Toward helping its members pursue this goal, in 1986 the Society of Toxicology adopted a position statement regarding the use of animals in toxicology:

> The Society of Toxicology is dedicated to acquiring knowledge for the improvement of the health and safety of humans and other animals and the protection of their environment.
>
> To fulfill this objective, the Society is committed to the design and conduct of the best possible scientific research. To ensure this, the Society views as necessary the use of laboratory animals in toxicological research and testing except in those procedures where valid, scientific alternative techniques are available. The code of ethics of the Society of Toxicology states that each member shall "observe the spirit as well as the letter of the laws, regulations, and ethical standards with regard to the welfare of humans and animals involved in any experimental procedures." The Society supports careful consideration of the number of animals used and encourages reduction where scientifically feasible. The Society strongly encourages and supports the development of valid scientific alternatives to current animal research testing procedures.

The society is also working on a set of guiding principles for animal usage, but these will take some time to finish and adopt. The set prepared and proposed by the New York Academy of Science is good, and should be consulted not only for guidance but also for the great deal of information that it provides.

REFERENCES

Ahdaya, S. M., Shah, P. V., and Guthrie, F. E. (1976). Thermoregulation in mice treated with parathion, carbaryl or DDT. *Toxicol. Pharmacol.* **35**, 575–580.

Alcock, S. J. (1971). An anti-inflammatory compound: Non-toxic to animals, but with an adverse action in man. *Proc. Eur. Soc. Stud. Drug. Toxicol.* **12**, 184–190.

Anderson, P. D., and Weber, L. J. (1975). Toxic response as a quantitative function of body size. *Toxicol. Appl. Pharmacol.* **33**, 471–481.

Angel, G. (1969). Starvation, stress and the blood brain barrier. *Dis. Nerv. Syst.* **30**, 94–97.

Animal Welfare Act of 1987, PL 99–198, CFR 9 (Vol 52, No. 61, 10292–10322).

Baetjer, A. M., and Smith, R. (1956). Effect of environmental temperature on reaction of mice to parathion, an anticholinesterase agent. *Am. J. Physiol.* **186**, 39–46.

Baker, H. J., Lindsey, J. R., and Weisbroth, S. H. (1979). *The Laboratory Rat,* Vol. I, pp. 411–412. Academic Press, New York.

Becker, W. A. (1962). Choice of animals and sensitivity of experiments. *Nature* **193**, 1264–1266.

Belehradek, J. (1957). A unified theory of cellular rate processes based upon an analysis of temperature action. *Protoplasma* **48**, 53–71.

Benedict, F. C. (1938). *Vita Energetics: A Study in Comparative Basal Metabolism,* Vol. 503, pp. 1–215. Carnegie Press, Madison, NJ.

Borchard, R. E., Barnes, C. D., and Eltherington, L. G. (1990). *Drug Dosage in Laboratory Animals: A Handbook,* 3rd ed. Telford Press, Caldwell, NJ.

Borzelleca, J. F. (1984). Extrapolation of animal data to man. In *Concepts in Toxicology* (A. S. Tegeris, Ed.), Vol. I, pp. 294–304. Krager, New York.

Boyd, E. M., Dodos, I., and Krijnen, C. J. (1970). Endosulfan toxicity and dietary protein. *Arch. Environ. Health* **21**, 15–19.

Brody, S. (1964). *Bioenergetics and Growth.* Hafner, New York.

Brown, A. M. (1961). Sleeping time response of time-random bred, inbred and F1-hybrids to pentobarbitone sodium. *J. Pharm. Pharmacol.* **13**, 679–687.

Brown, V. K. (1980). *Acute Toxicity in Theory and Practice.* Wiley, New York.

Bruce, R. D. (1985). An up-and-down procedure for acute toxicity testing. *Fundam. Appl. Toxicol.* **5**, 151–157.

Brus, R., and Herman, Z. S. (1971). Acute toxicities of adrenaline, noradrenaline and acetylcholine in adult and neo-natal mice. *Diss. Pharm. Pharmacol.* **23**, 435–437.

Burrell, G. A. (1912). The use of mice and birds for detecting carbon monoxide after mine fire and explosions. *Technical Paper 11,* pp. 3–16. Department of Interior, Bureau of Mines Washington, D.C.

Calabrese, E. J. (1983). *Principles of Animal Extrapolation.* Wiley, New York.

Campbell, R. L., and Bruce, R. D. (1981). Comparative dermatotoxicology. *Toxicol. Appl. Pharmacol.* **59**, 555–563.

Collins, G. R. (1979). *Manual for Laboratory Animal Technicians,* Publ. 67–3. American Association for Laboratory Animal Science, Joliet, IL.

Cremer, J. E., and Bligh, J. (1969). Body temperature and responses to drugs. *Br. Med. Bull.* **23**, 299–306.

Dauterman, W. C. (1980). Physiological factors affecting metabolism of xenobiotics. In *Introduction to Biochemical Toxicology* (E. Hodgson and F. E. Guthrie, Eds.). Elsevier, New York.

Davidson, I. W. F., Parker, J. C., and Beliles, R. P. (1986). Biological basis for extrapolation across animal species. *Regul. Toxicol. Pharmacol.* **6**, 211–237.

Davis, R. J., and Davies, B. H. (1970). The biochemistry of warfarin resistance in the rat. *Biochem. J.* **118**, 44P–45P.

Depass, L. R., Myers, R. C., Weaver, E. V., and Weil, C. S. (1984). *Alternative Methods in Toxicology, Vol. 2. Acute Toxicity Testing,* pp. 141–153. Liebert, New York.

Derelanko, M. J. (1987). Determination of erythrocyte life span in F-344, Wistar, and Sprague–Dawley rats using a modification of the [³H]diisopropylfluorophosphate ([³]DFP) method. *Fundam. Appl. Toxicol.* **9**, 271–276.

Dixon, R. L. (1976). Problems in extrapolating toxicity data from laboratory animals to man. *Environ. Health Perspect.* **13**, 43–50.

Doull, J. (1972). The effect of physical environmental factors on drug response. In *Essays in Toxicology* (W. J. Hayes, Ed.), Vol. 3. Academic Press, New York.

Doull, J. (1980). Factors influencing toxicology. In *Casarett and Doull's Toxicology* (J. Doull, C. D. Klaassen, and M. O. Amdur, Eds.). Macmillan, New York.

Dubois, K. P., and Geiling, E. M. K. (1959). *Textbook Toxicology,* pp. 11–12. Oxford Univ. Press, New York.

Eben, A., and Pilz, W. (1967). Abhangigbeit der Acetylcholinesterase-acktivatat in Plasma and Erythrocyten von der alter und geschlecht der Ratte. *Arch. Toxicol.* **23**, 27–34.

Edwards, A. G. (1982). Animal care and maintenance. In *Principles and Methods of Toxicology* (A. W. Hayes, Ed.), pp. 321–345. Raven Press, New York.

Ehrich, M., and Gross, W. B. (1983). Modification of triorthotolyl phosphate toxicity in chickens by stress. *Toxicol. Appl. Pharmacol.* **70**, 249–254.

Ensminger, M. E., and Olentine, C. J. (1978). Mink nutrition. In *Feeds and Nutrition-Complete,* pp. 997–1017. Ensminger, Clovis, CA.

Evans, R. H. (1982). Ralston Purina Co., St. Louis, MO.

Freireich, E. J., Gehan, E. A., Rall, D. P., Schmidt, L. H., and Skipper, H. E. (1966). Quantitative comparison of toxicity of anticancer agents in mouse, rat, hamster, dog, monkey and man. *Cancer Chemother. Rep.* 50, 219–244.

Fox, M. A. (1986). *The Case for Animal Experimentation.* Univ. of California Press, Berkeley.

Gad, S. C., and Chengelis, C. P. (1992). *Animal Models in Toxicology.* Dekker, New York.

Gad, S. C., and Weil, C. S. (1980). Statistical analysis of body weight—A reply. *Toxicol. Appl. Pharmacol.* 57, 335–337.

Gad, S. C., Smith, A. C., Cramp, A. L., Gavigan, F. A., and Derelanko, M. J. (1984). Innovative designs and practices for acute systemic toxicity studies. *Drug Chem. Toxicol.* 7, 423–434.

Gad, S. C., Dunn, B. J., Dobbs, D. W., and Walsh, R. D. (1986). Development and validation of an alternative dermal sensitization test: The mouse ear swelling test (MEST). *Toxicol. Appl. Pharmacol.* 84, 93–114.

Gaines, T. B. (1960). The acute toxicity of pesticides to rats. *Toxicol. Appl. Pharmacol.* 2, 88–99.

Gaines, T. B. (1969). Acute toxicology of pesticides. *Toxicol. Appl. Pharmacol.* 14, 515–534.

Garattini, S. (1985). Toxic effects of chemicals: Difficulties in extrapolating data from animals to man. *Crit. Rev. Toxicol.* 16, 1–29.

Gillette, J. R. (1979). Extrapolating from microsomes to mice to men. *Drug Metab. Dispos.* 7, 121–123.

Gingell, R., and Wallcave, L. (1974). Species differences in the acute toxicity and tissue distribution of DDT in mice and hamsters. *Toxicol. Appl. Pharmacol.* 28, 385–394.

Goldenthal, E. I. (1971). A compilation of LD_{50} values in newborn and adult animals. *Toxicol. Appl. Pharmacol.* 18, 185–207.

Gralla, E. J. (1986). Species specific toxicoses with some underlying mechanisms. In *Safety Evaluation of Drugs and Chemicals* (W. E. Lloyd, Ed.), pp. 55–81. Hemisphere, New York.

Gratz, N. G. (1973). A critical review of currently used single dose rodenticides. *Bull. World Health Org.* 48, 469–477.

Gray, H., and Addis, T. (1948). Rat colony testing by Zucker's weight-age relation. *Am. J. Physiol.* 153, 35–40.

Green, C. D. (1968). Strain sensitivity of rats to nitrous oxide. *Anes. Analg.* 47, 509–514.

Grice, K., Sattar, H., and Baker, H. (1972). The effect of ambient humidity on transepidermal water loss. *J. Invest. Dermatol.* 58, 343–346.

Halberg, F., Johnson, E. A., Brown, B. W., and Bittner, J. J. (1960). Susceptibility rhythm to *E. coli* endotoxin and bioassay. *Proc. Soc. Exp. Biol. Med.* 103, 142–144.

Haley, T. J., Dooley, K. L., and Harmon, J. R. (1973). Acute oral toxicity of N-2-fluorenlyacetamide (2FAA) in several strains of mice. *Proc. Soc. Exp. Biol. Med.* 143, 1117–1119.

Hathway, D. E. (1970). Species, strain and sex differences in metabolism. In *Foreign Compound Metabolism in Mammals* (D. E. Hathway, Ed.). The Chemical Society, London.

Hilado, C. J., and Furst, A. (1978). Reproducibility of toxicity data as a function of mouse strain, animal lot and operator. *J. Combust. Toxicol.* 5, 75–80.

Hill, R. N., Clemens, T. L., Liv, D. K., Vesell, E. S., and Johnson, W. D. (1975). Genetic control of chloroform toxicity in mice. *Science* 190, 159–161.

Hudson, R. H., Haegele, M. A., and Tucker, R. K. (1979). Acute oral and percutaneous toxicity of pesticides to mallards: Correlations with mammalian toxicity data. *Toxicol. Appl. Pharmacol.* 47, 451–460.

Jay, G. E., Jr. (1955). Variation in response of various mouse strains to hexobarbital (Evipal). *Proc. Soc. Exp. Biol. Med.* 90, 378–380.

Johnson, H. D., and Voss, E. (1952). Toxicological studies of zinc phosphide. *J. Am. Pharm. Assoc.* 41, 468–472.

Kalow, W. (1962). *Pharmacogenetics—Heredity and the Response to Drugs.* Saunders, Philadelphia.

Kalow, W. (1965). Dose–response relationship and genetic variation. *Ann. N.Y. Acad. Sci.* 123, 212–218.

Karczmar, A. G., and Scudder, C. L. (1967). Behavioral responses to drugs and catecholamine levels in mice of different strains and genera. *Fed. Proc.* **26**, 1189–1191.

Kato, R., and Gillette, J. R. (1965). Sex difference in the effects of abnormal physiological states on the metabolism of drugs by rat liver microsomes. *J. Pharmacol. Exp. Ther.* **150**, 2285–2291.

Kawano, S., Nakao, T., and Hirage, K. (1981). Strain differences in butylated hydroxytoluene—induced deaths in male mice. *Toxicol. Appl. Pharmacol.* **61**, 475–479.

Keplinger, M. L., and Deichmann, W. B. (1967). Acute toxicity of combinations of pesticides. *Toxicol. Appl. Pharmacol.* **10**, 586–595.

Krasovskij, G. N. (1975). Species and sex differences in sensitivity to toxic substances. In *Methods Used in the USSR for Establishing Biologically Safe Levels of Toxic Substances*. WHO, Geneva.

Lang, C. M., and Vessell, E. S. (1976). Environmental and genetic factors affecting laboratory animals: Impact on biomedical research. *Fed. Proc.* **35**, 1123–1124.

Lehman, A. J. (1959). Some relations of drug toxicities in experimental animals compared to man. In *Appraisal of Safety of Chemicals in Foods, Drugs and Cosmetics*. Association of Food and Drug Officials of the United States, Washington, D.C.

Lenox, R. H., and Frazier, T. W. (1972). Methadone induced mortality as a function of the cirdadian cycle. *Nature* **239**, 397–398.

Litchfield, J. T. (1961). Forecasting drug effects in man from studies in laboratory animals. *J. Am. Med. Soc.* **177**, 34.

Litchfield, J. T. (1962). Symposium on clinical drug evaluation and human pharmacology. *Clin. Pharmacol. Ther.* **3**, 665.

Longacre, S. L., Kocsis, J. J., and Snyder, R. (1981). Influence of strain differences in mice on the metabolism and toxicity of benzene. *Toxicol. Appl. Pharmacol.* **60**, 398–409.

Lutzen, L., Trieb, G., and Pappritz, G. (1976). Allometric analysis of organ weights: II. Beagle dogs. *Toxicol. Appl. Pharmacol.* **35**, 543–551.

Maines, M. D., and Westfall, B. A. (1971). Sex difference in the metabolism of hexabarbitone in the Mongolian gerbil. *Proc. Soc. Exp. Biol. Med.* **138**, 820–822.

Meier, H. (1963a). Potentialities for and present status of pharmacological research in genetically controlled mice. In *Advances in Pharmacology* (S. Garattini and P. A. Shore, Eds.), Vol. 2. Academic Press, New York.

Meier, H. (1963b). *Experimental Pharmacogenetics: Physiopathology of Heredity and Pharmacologic Responses*. Academic Press, New York.

Mitruka, B. M., Rawnsley, H. M., and Dharam, V. V. (1976). *Animals for Medical Research*. Wiley, New York.

Miura, K., Ino, T., and Izuka, S. (1974). Comparison of susceptibilities to the acute toxicity of BHC in strains of experimental mice. *Jikken Dodutsu* **2**, 198.

Moore, D. H. (1972). Species, sex and strain differences in metabolism. In *Foreign Compound Metabolism in Mammals* (D. E. Hathway, Ed.). The Chemical Society, London.

Muller, P. J., and Vernikos-Danellis, J. (1968). Alteration in drug toxicity by environmental variables. *Proc. Western Pharmacol. Soc.* **11**, 52–53.

Naik, S. R., Anjaria, R. J., and Sheth, U. K. (1970). Studies on rat brain acetylcholine and cholinesterase, Pt 1. Effect of body weight, sex, stress and CNS depressant drugs. *Indian J. Med. Res.* **58**, 473–479.

Natelson, B. H., Hoffman, S. L., and Cagin, N. A. (1979). A role for environmental factors in the production of digitalis toxicity. *Pharmacol. Biochem. Behav.* **12**, 235–237.

National Academy of Sciences (NAS) (1975). *Experiments and Research with Humans: Values in Conflict*, Academy Forum, 3rd in series. NAS, Washington, DC.

National Institutes of Health (NIH) (1985). *Guide for the Care and Use of Laboratory Animals*, HHS, NIH Publ. No. 85–23. NIH, Washington, DC.

Neely, W. A., Turner, M. D., and Taylor, A. E. (1967). Bidirectional movement of water through the skin of a non-sweating animal. *J. Surgical Res.* 7, 323–328.

Nixon, G. A., Tyson, C. A., and Wertz, W. C. (1975). Interspecies comparisons of skin irritancy. *Toxicol. Appl. Pharmacol.* 31, 481–490.

Nosal, M., and Hladka, A. (1968). Determination of the exposure to fenitrothion on the basis of the excretion of p-nitro-m-cresol by the urine of persons tested. *Arch. Gewerbepath. Gewerbehyg.* 25, 28–38.

Orfila, M. J. B. (1814). *Traite de toxicologie.*

Oser, B. L. (1981). The rat as a model for human toxicology evaluation. *J. Toxicol. Environ. Health* 8, 521–542.

Pallotta, A. J., Kelly, M. J., Rall, D. P., and Ward, J. W. (1962). Toxicology of acetoxycycloheximide as a function of sex and body weight. *J. Pharmacol.* 136, 400–405.

Pinkel, D. (1958). The use of body surface area as a criterion of drug dosage in cancer chemotherapy. *Cancer Res.* 18, 853–856.

Powers, W. J., Peckham, J. C., Siino, K. M., and Gad, S. C. (1984). Effects of subchronic dietary caprolactam on renal function. In *An Industry Approach to Chemical Risk Assessment*, pp. 77–96. Industrial Health Foundation, Pittsburgh.

Priestley, J. (1772). On different kinds of air. *Philos. Trans.*

Pyle, N. J. (1940). Use of ferrets in laboratory work and research investigations. *Am. J. Public Health* 30, 787–796.

Quinn, G. P., Axelrod, J., and Brodie, B. B. (1958). Species, strain and sex differences in metabolism of hexabarbitone, amidopyrine, antipyrine and aniline. *Biochem. Pharmacol.* 1, 152–159.

Rall, D. P. (1979). Relevance of animal experiments to humans. *Environ. Health Perspect.* 32, 297–300.

Rider, J. A., Moeller, H. C., Puletti, E. J., and Swader, J. I. (1969). Toxicity of parathion, systox, octamethyl pyrophosphoramide and methyl parathion in man. *Toxicol. Appl. Pharmacol.* 14, 603–611.

Robinson, F. R., Harper, D. T., and Kaplan, H. P. (1967). Comparison of strains of rats exposed to oxygen at various pressures. *Lab. Anim. Care* 17, 433–441.

Rothschild, Lord (1961). *A Classification of Living Animals.* Longmans, London.

Sawin, P. B., and Glick, D. (1943). Atropinesterase, a genetically determined enzyme in the rabbit. *Proc. Natl. Acad. Sci.* 29, 55–59.

Scheving, L. E., Mayerbach, H. V., and Pauly, J. E. (1974). An overview of chronopharmacology. *J. Eur. Toxicol.* 7, 203–227.

Schmidt-Nielsen, K. (1984). *Scaling: Why Is Animal Size so Important?* Cambridge Univ. Press, New York.

Schneiderman, M. A., Mantel, N., and Brown, C. C. (1975). *Ann. N.Y. Acad. Sci.* 246, 237–248.

Sechzer, J. A. (1983). The role of animals in biomedical research. *Ann. N.Y. Acad. Sci.* 406.

Selisko, O., Hentschel, G., and Ackermann, H. (1963). Uber die abhangigkeit der mittleren Todlichen Dosis (LD$_{50}$) von exogenen Faktoren. *Arch. Int. Pharmacodyn. Ther.* 45, 51–69.

Shanor, S. P., van Hees, G. R. Baart, N., Erdos, E. G., and Foldes, E. F. (1961). The influence of age and sex on human plasma and red cell cholinesterase. *Am. J. Med. Sci.* 242, 357–361.

Smith, R. L. (1974). The problem of species variations. *Ann. Nutr. Alim.* 28, 335.

Spector, W. S. (1956). *Handbook of Biological Data.* Saunders, Philadelphia.

Sperlinger, D. (1981). *Animals in Research: New Perspectives in Animal Experimentation.* Wiley, New York.

Steen, J. A., Hanneman, G. D., Nelson, P. L., and Folk, E. D. (1976). Acute toxicity of mevinophos to gerbils. *Toxicol. Appl. Pharmacol.* 35, 195–198.

Stevenson, D. E. (1979). Current problems in the choice of animals for toxicity studies. *J. Toxicol. Environ. Health* 5, 9–15.

Stockinger, H. E. (1953). Size of dose; its effect on distribution in the body. *Nucleonics* **11**, 24–27.

Tedeschi, D. H., and Tedeschi, R. E. (1968). *Importance of Fundamental Principles in Drug Evaluation.* Raven Press, New York.

Trieb, G., Pappritz, G., and Lutzen, L. (1976). Allometric analysis of organ weights. I. Rats. *Toxicol. Appl. Pharmacol.* **35**, 531–542.

Usinger, W. (1957). Respiratorischer Stoffweschel und Korpertemperatur der weissen Mans in thermoindifferenter Umgebung. *Pflugers Archiv.* **264**, 520–535.

Vaccarezza, J. R., and Peltz, L. (1960). Effect of ACTH on blood cholinesterase activity in normal subjects and respiratory–allergy patients. *Presse. Med.* **68**, 723–724.

Vaccarezza, J. R., and Willson, J. A. (1964a). The effect of ACTH on cholinesterase activity in plasma, whole blood and blood cells of rats. *Experientia* **20**, 23.

Vaccarezza, J. R., and Willson, J. A. (1964b). The relationship between corticosterone administration and cholinesterase activity in rats. *Experientia* **21**, 205.

Vessell, E. S. (1968). Genetic and environmental factors affecting hexobarbital metabolism in mice. *Ann. N.Y. Acad. Sci.* **151**, 900–912.

Vessell, E. S. (1969). Recent progress in pharmacogenetics. In *Advances in Pharmacology and Chemotherapy, Vol. 7* (S. Garattini, A. Goldin, F. Hawking, and I. J. Koplin, Eds.), Academic Press, New York.

Vogel, W. H. (1987). Stress—The neglected variable in experimental pharmacology and toxicology. *Trends Pharmacol. Sci.* **7**, 35–37.

Weaver, L. S., and Kerley, T. L. (1962). Strain differences in response of mice to d-amphetamine. *J. Pharm. Exp. Ther.* **135**, 240–245.

Weil, C. S., and Gad, S. C. (1980). Applications of methods of statistical analysis to efficient repeated dose toxicology tests 2. Powerful methods for analysis of body liver and kidney weight data. *Toxicol. Appl. Pharmacol.* **52**, 214–226.

Wills, J. H. (1968). Pharmacology. In *The Golden Hamster—Its Biology and Use in Medical Research* (R. A. Hoffman, P. F. Robinson, and H. Magalhaes, Eds.). Iowa State Univ. Press, Ames.

Yates, F. E., and Kugler, P. N. (1986). Similarity principles and intrinsic geometries: Contrasting approaches to interspecies scaling. *J. Pharm. Sci.* **75**, 1019–1027.

Zbinden, G. (1963). Experimental and clinical aspects of drug toxicity. In *Advances in Pharmacology* (S. Garratini and P. A. Shore, Eds.), pp. 1–112. Academic Press, New York.

Zimmermann, A., and Matschiner, J. T. (1974). Biochemical basis of hereditary resistance to warfarin in the rat. *Biochem. Pharmacol.* **23**, 1033–1040.

CHAPTER 12

Statistical Analysis of Acute Toxicology and Safety Studies

Recognition of the importance of acute tests in the overall scheme of things has recently caused more attention to be paid to their performance and results, leading to both better day-to-day performance of the tests and closer scrutiny of their designs. At the same time, increased concern as to both reducing the numbers of animals used in research and testing and ensuring the use of humane methods in such testing has created additional reasons for critical review of study design and conduct.

The first (and most important) step in designing any toxicity study is developing a clear statement of the objective for the study; that is, what question is to be answered. In acute studies, this is more complex because there are generally three distinct levels or types of answers sought and therefore of degree of effort merited in performing a study. The simplest level is the screen, which is designed purely to identify compounds which give such extreme results (such as lethality at very low dosage levels) that no data are desired on other aspects of toxicity. The intermediate category is the probe, which is intended to give enough information to either perform a more definitive study or to be able to compare and rank order a set of compounds (prioritizing them for further study). The most complicated acute study is intended to provide as much information as possible and is frequently used when it is intended to be the "definitive" toxicology study for the foreseeable future.

Each of these three levels may apply to each of the two major categories of acute studies (in terms of the scope of question asked). These are single-endpoint studies (which assess dermal and ocular irritation and corrosion, sensitization, photosensitization, and lethality) and shotgun studies (which assess or identify systemic effects such as target organs and no-observable-effect levels). In this volume we have presented each of the common designs for these tests, their objectives, the types of data they generate, and some current alternative test designs and models. Here we present some of the problems associated with test design and analysis and suggest some solutions.

BASICS

Each measurement we make—each individual piece of experimental information we gather—is called a datum. It is extremely unusual, however, to either obtain or attempt to analyze a datum. Rather, we generally gather and analyze multiple pieces at one time, the resulting collection being called data.

Data are collected on the basis of their association with a treatment (intended or otherwise) as an effect (a property) that is measured in the experimental subjects of a study, such as body weights. These identifiers (that is, treatment and effect) are termed variables. Our treatment variables (those that the researcher or nature control and which can be directly controlled) are termed independent, while our effect variables (such as weight, life span, and number of neoplasms) are termed dependent variables—their outcome is believed to depend on the "treatment" being studied.

All the possible measures of a given set of variables in all the possible subjects that exist is termed the population for those variables. Such a population of variables cannot be truly measured. For example, one would have to obtain, treat, and measure the weights of all the Fischer-344 rats that were, are, or ever will be. Instead, we deal with a representative group—a sample. If our sample of data is appropriately collected and of sufficient size, it serves to provide good estimates of the characteristics of the parent population from which it was drawn.

Two terms refer to the quality and reproducibility of measurements of variables. The first, accuracy, is an expression of the closeness of a measured or computed value to its actual or "true" value in nature. The second, precision, reflects the closeness or reproducibility of a series of repeated measurements of the same quantity.

If we arrange all of our measurements of a particular variable in order as a point on an axis marked as to the values of that variable, and if our sample were large enough, the pattern of distribution of the data in the sample would begin to become apparent. This pattern is a representation of the frequency distribution of a given population of data—that is, of the incidence of different measurements, their central tendency, and dispersion.

The most common frequency distribution in nature is the normal (or Gaussian) distribution. This distribution is such that two-thirds of all values are within one standard deviation (to be defined below) of the mean (or average value for the entire population) and 95% are within 1.96 standard deviations of the mean. The mathematical equation for the normal curve is

$$y = \frac{1}{\sigma\sqrt{2\pi}} e^{-\frac{(x-\mu)^2}{2\sigma^2}}$$

where μ is the mean and σ is the standard deviation.

There are other frequency distributions, such as the binomial, Poisson, and chi-square.

In all areas of biological research, optimal design and appropriate interpretation of experiments require that the researcher understand both the biological and technological underpinnings of the system being studied and of the data being generated. From the point of view of the statistician, it is vitally important that the experimenter both know and be able to communicate the nature of the data and understand its limitations. One classification of data type is presented in Table 76.

The nature of the data collected is determined by three considerations. These are the biological source of the data (the system being studied), the instrumentation and techniques being used to make measurements, and the design of the experiment. The researcher has some degree of control over each

TABLE 76 Types of Variables (DATA) and Examples of Each Type

Classified by	Type	Example
Scale		
Continuous	Scalar	Body weight
	Ranked	Severity of irritation
Discontinuous	Scalar	Days until the first observation of recovery from skin lesion
	Ranked	Clinical observations in animals
	Attribute	Eye colors in fruit flies
	Quantal	Dead/alive or present/absent
Frequency distribution	Normal	Body weights
	Bimodal	Some clinical chemistry

of these—with the least over the biological system (he/she normally has a choice of only one of several models to study) and most over the design of the experiment or study. Such choices, in fact, dictate the type of data generated by a study.

Statistical methods are based on specific assumptions. Parametric statistics—those that are most familiar to the majority of scientists—have more stringent underlying assumptions than do nonparametric statistics. Among the underlying assumptions for many parametric statistical methods (such as the analysis of variance) is that the data are continuous. The nature of data associated with a variable (as described previously) imparts a "value" to that data, the value being the power of the statistical tests which can be employed.

Continuous variables are those which can, at least theoretically, assume any of an infinite number of values between any two fixed points (such as measurements of body weight between 2.0 and 3.0 kg). Discontinuous variables, meanwhile, are those which can have only certain fixed values, with no possible intermediate values (such as counts of five and six dead animals, respectively).

Limitations on our ability to measure constrain the extent to which the real-world situation approaches the theoretical, but many of the variables studied in toxicology are in fact continuous. Examples of these are lengths, weights, concentrations, temperatures, periods of time, and percentages. For these continuous variables, we may describe the character of a sample with measures of central tendency and dispersion that we are most familiar with— the mean, denoted by the symbol $\overline{X}$ and also called the arithmetic average, and the standard deviation (SD), which is denoted by the symbol σ and is calculated as being equal to

$$\sqrt{\frac{\Sigma X^2 - \frac{(X)^2}{N}}{N-1}}$$

where X is the individual datum and N is the total number of data in the group.

Contrasted with these continuous data, however, we have discontinuous (or discrete) data, which can only assume certain fixed numerical values. In these cases our choice of statistical tools or tests is, as we will find, more limited.

PROBABILITY

Probability is simply the likelihood that in a sufficiently large sample a particular event will occur or a particular value will be found. Hypothesis testing, for example, is generally structured so that the likelihood of a treatment group being the same as a control group (the so-called "null hypothesis") can be assessed as being less than a selected low level (very frequently 5%), which implies that we are 1.0 (that is, 1.0–0.05 or 95% sure) that the groups are not equivalent.

SIGNIFICANCE AND ERROR IN BIOMEDICAL SCIENCES

Statistics are used in the biomedical sciences as a tool to try to understand data and nature. The most common use of this tool is to ask the question—does this really mean something? The question of significance is the objective of the function of statistics called hypothesis testing.

Statistical significance is expressed in terms of probability (or level of confidence in a result) and has associated with it two kinds of possible outcomes. One evaluates the probability of the two possibilities assuming a determination of statistical significance and the types of error associated with these possibilities. In one of these (the "false positive"), we have a circumstance in which there is a statistical significance in the measured difference between treated and control groups, but there is no true biological significance to the finding. This is not an uncommon happening, for example, in the case of clinical chemistry parameters. This is called type I error by statisticians, and the probability of this happening is called the α level. In the other possibility (the "false negative"), we have no statistical significance, but the differences between groups are biologically/toxicologically significant. This is called type II error by statisticians, and the probability of such an error happening by random chance is called the β level.

Thus, a type I error is committed when our statistical tests tell us we have a significant result when, in fact, we do not. In statistical terminology, this is stated as "when a true null hypothesis is rejected incorrectly." If a single hypothesis is being statistically evaluated, then the investigator simply assumes that the probability of making a type I error is some predetermined level of confidence, traditionally 0.05. The per comparison error for this one contrast is fixed at, for example, 0.05, and the researcher is thus assured that the probability of a finding occurring by chance is less than 5%. With multiple hypotheses, however, other types of error rates should be considered—specifically, the experiment-wise error rate (EW) and the per-comparison error rate (EP).

The overall error rate is the probability of making at least one type I error while collecting data in an experiment. This EW can never be smaller than the error rate per comparison and often is much larger. The relation of per-comparison and EW error rates depends on the degree of statistical dependence of the tests. For totally independent tests, the EW can be expressed in the following equation:

$$EW = 1 - (1 - \alpha)^c$$

where c is the number of independent tests and α is the error rate per test. This equation shows that the EW increases rapidly with the number of hypotheses statistically evaluated.

The relationship between per-comparison and experiment-wise error rates is complex when dependent tests are conducted, a condition that one may say always exists to some degree when more than one dependent variable is statistically evaluated in one study. The more nearly independent the tests, the closer the EW approaches the previous equation. The more highly related the tests, the closer the EW is to the error rate specified for an individual comparison. When completely dependent tests are conducted in which the variables considered are perfectly correlated, the per-comparison and experiment-wise error rates are identical.

The per-experiment error rate is the expected number of type I errors for a particular group of significance tests, and it can be computed using the following equation:

$$EP = c_\alpha$$

where α is the significance level—which remains constant for all tests—and c is the number of comparisons. In the case of 20 comparisons at the 0.05 confidence level, EP = 20 (0.05). This means that for the 0.05 level one would expect exactly one type I error to occur in the long run for any 20 tests of significance. One should note that the EP is an expected value, whereas the EW is the probability of at least one type I error occurring with a set of comparisons. The EW for 20 comparisons at the 0.05 significance level is $1 - (1 - 0.05)^{20}$, or 0.64, indicating that the probability of at least one type I error occurring among those tests reported as significant at the 0.05 level is 0.64. These calculations assume that the tests are independent of one another. For nonorthogonal comparisons in which some degree of correlations exists between the data sets on successive tests, the formulas provided previously overestimate the error rates.

A variation of the EW and EP, referred to as the percentage error rate (PE), may provide even more useful information than the traditional EW and EP. The computation of the PE includes both the number of tests expected to be significant and the number that actually turn out to be statistically significant at a given α level. The following formula computes the percentage error rate:

$$PE = 100c\alpha/M$$

where α is the α level for a set of comparisons, c is the total number of comparisons, and M is the number of tests found to be significant at or beyond the specified significance level.

The PE indicates the proportion of results labeled statistically significant that are likely to occur by chance. As the ratio approaches 1.00 (100%), this indicates that the number of tests found to be significant is approximately equal to the number of tests one would expect to find significant purely by chance. As the ratio decreases and approaches the individual α level for a set of comparisons, it indicates the particular percentage of the results likely to occur by chance, whereas 100—PE indicates the percentage of the results likely to occur because of "nonchance" effects. For example, if 1 of 20 comparisons evaluated at the 0.05 level is statistically significant, the PE = 100 (20) (0.05)/ 1 = 100%, suggesting that the number of tests found to be significant—1—is the number expected to be significant by chance. If, however, 4 of 20 comparisons conducted at the 0.05 confidence level are found to be statistically significant, the PE = 100 (20) (0.05)/4 = 25%, indicating that approximately 25% of the results—1 of 4—occurred by chance, whereas the remaining 75%—3 of 4—likely did not.

The PE may be applied to all tests of significance, including both parametric and nonparametric procedures. One may apply it to all the tests in a given research project or to families of tests within a study. The PE is a broad general notion, whereas such α protections as those of Tukey, Duncan, Scheffe, and the like are limited in their applications to certain parametric techniques. The PE standardizes procedures and clearly defines the meaning of a statistically significant difference across studies and situations calling for diverse statistical approaches.

In a toxicology study, however, it is arguable that the major interest lies in the false negative error rate (that is, in type II error). If a treatment has an effect of a given magnitude, what is the chance of an experiment failing to detect this effect as statistically significant? Unlike the false positive error rate, this chance does not remain fixed and it depends on a number of factors, the most important of which are

number of animals/treatment group;
the magnitude of the toxic effect;
the variability of the experimental material;
the false positive error rate selected.

The problems of false positive results in toxicology, and to a lesser extent of false negative results, have been widely discussed in the context of carcinogenicity studies. However, for shorter-term toxicity experiments, little attention appears to have been paid to the problem of false negative results. This correspondence stops short of indicating what the false negative error rates are likely to be in practice.

The situation in toxicology has some similarities with that in clinical trials, where the failure to detect an adverse drug reaction would have potentially important consequences. In clinical trials, however, it is common practice to choose the study size to achieve a particular false negative error rate, whereas in toxicology the size of the study is usually fixed according to regulatory guidelines and logistical considerations.

It should be noted that the methods described here are better suited to analyzing data when the interest is truly in detecting the absence of an effect with little chance of false negatives. Anderson and Hauck (1983) should be consulted for a more thorough discussion of considerations involved in cases in which the desire is to have few false positives (that is, when the direction of the hypothesis test has been reversed). There are also many forms of graphical analysis methods available (see Chambers *et al.*, 1983, for example), including some newer forms which are particularly well suited to multivariate data (the type that is common in more complicated screening test designs).

To further complicate the situation, in biomedical research in general (and toxicology in particular), we are concerned about two forms of significance—statistical, which we have just discussed, and biological, which is more of a question of relevance. These two forms are not identical nor equivalent. It is quite possible for something to be statistically significant but not biologically significant.

The reasons that biological and statistical significance are not identical are multiple, but a central one is certainly causality. Through our consideration of statistics, we should keep in mind that just because a treatment and a change in an observed organism are seemingly or actually associated with each other does not "prove" that the former caused the latter. Though this fact is now widely appreciated for correlation (for example, that fact that the number of storks' nests found each year in England is correlated with the number of human births that year does not mean that storks bring babies), it is just as true in the general case of significance. Timely establishment and proof that treatment causes an effect requires an understanding of the underlying mechanism and proof of its validity. At the same time, it is important to realize that not finding a good correlation or suitable significance associated with a treatment and an effect likewise does not prove that the two are not associated—that a treatment does not cause an effect. At best, it gives us a certain level of confidence that under the conditions of the current test, these items are not associated. This is complicated further in toxicology by the phenomenon of variance inflation (illustrated in Fig. 49), which serves to further reduce the sensitivity of tests (Gad and Weil, 1988).

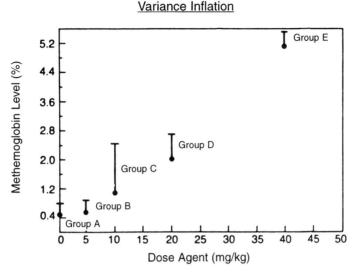

FIGURE 49   A graph illustrating the concept of variance inflation in toxicology. As an effect is approached in the dose–response curve, the more sensitive individuals respond before the bulk of the population, increasing the variance (dispersion) of group parameters and therefore decreasing the sensitivity of traditional tests for significance. Points are means; error basis are +1 SD.

FUNCTIONS OF STATISTICS

Statistical methods may serve to do any combination of three possible tasks. The one we are most familiar with is hypothesis testing—that is, determining if two (or more) groups of data differ from each other at a predetermined level of confidence. A second function is the construction and use of models which may be used to predict future outcomes of chemical—biological interactions. This is most commonly seen in linear regression or in the derivation of some form of correlation coefficient. Model fitting allows us to relate one variable (typically a treatment or "independent" variable) to another. The third function, reduction of dimensionality, continues to be less commonly utilized than the first two (particularly in acute toxicology). This final category includes methods for reducing the amount of information, therefore making a problem easier to visualize and to understand. A subset of this last function, discussed under Descriptive Statistics, is the reduction of raw data to single expressions of central tendency and variability (such as the mean and standard deviation).

There is also a special subset of statistical techniques which is part of both the second and the third functions of statistics. This is data transformation, which includes such things as the conversion of numbers to log or probit values.

As a matter of practicality, this chapter is primarily designed to address the first of the three functions of statistical methods that we presented (hypothesis testing). The second function, modeling—especially in the form of dose response—is becoming increasingly important as the science continues to evolve from the descriptive phase to a mechanistic phase (i.e., the elucidation of mechanisms of action) and as we try to develop alternative methods.

DESCRIPTIVE STATISTICS

Descriptive statistics are used to convey, in summary, the general nature of the data. As such, the parameters describing any single group of data have two components. One of these describes the location of the data, while the other gives a measure of the dispersion of the data in and about this location. Often overlooked is the fact that the choice of which parameters are used to give these pieces of information implies a particular type of distribution for the data.

Most commonly, location is described by giving the (arithmetic) mean and dispersion by giving the SD or the standard error of the mean (SEM). The calculation of the first two has already been described. If we again denote the total number of data in a group as N, then the SEM would be calculated as

$$\text{SEM} = \frac{\text{SD}}{\sqrt{N}}$$

The use of the mean with either the SD or SEM implies, however, that one has reason to believe that the data being summarized are from a population which is at least approximately normally distributed. If this is not the case, then we should use a set of statistical descriptors which do not require a normal distribution. These are the median (for location) and the semiquartile distance (for a measure of dispersion). These somewhat less familiar parameters are characterized as follows.

Median

When all the numbers in a group are arranged in a ranked order (that is, from smallest to largest), the median is the middle value. If there is an odd number of values in a group then the middle value is obvious (in the case of 13 values, for example, the seventh largest is the median). When the number of values in the sample is even, the median is calculated as the midpoint between the $(N/2)$th and the $([N/2] + 1)$th number. For example, in the series of numbers 7, 12, 13, and 19, the median value would be the midpoint between 12 and 13, which is 12.5.

Semiquartile Distance

When all the data in a group are ranked, the space between any two quartiles of the data contains one ordered quarter of the values. Typically, we are most interested in the borders of the middle two quarters of the data defined by the quartiles Q_1 and Q_3, which together represent the semiquartile distance and which contain the median as their center. Given that there are N values in an ordered group of data, the upper limit of the jth quartile (Q_j) may be computed as being equal to the $[j(N + 1)/4th]$ value. Once we have used this formula to calculate the upper limits of Q_1 and Q_3, we can then compute the semiquartile distance [which is also called the quartile deviation (QD)] with the formula $QD = (Q_3 - Q_1)/2$.

For example, for the 15-value data set 1, 2, 3, 4, 4, 5, 5, 5, 6, 6, 6, 7, 7, 8, 9, we can calculate the upper limits of Q_1 and Q_3 as

$$Q_1 = \frac{1(15 + 1)}{4} = \frac{16}{4} = 4$$

$$Q_3 = \frac{3(15 + 1)}{4} = \frac{48}{4} = 12$$

The 4th and 12th values in this data set are 4 and 7, respectively. The semiquartile distance can then be calculated as

$$QD = \frac{7 - 4}{2} = 1.5$$

One final sample parameter which sees some use in toxicology (primarily in inhalation studies) is the geometric mean, denoted by the term $\overline{X}_g$. This is calculated as

$$\overline{x}_g = (x_1 \cdot x_2 \cdots x_N)^{1/N}$$

and has the attractive feature that it does not give excessive weight to extreme values (or "outliers"), such as the mass of a single very large particle in a dust sample. In effect, it "folds" extreme values in toward the center of the distribution, decreasing the sensitivity of the parameter to the undue influence of the outlier. This is particularly important, for example, in the case of aerosol samples in which a few very large particles would cause the arithmetic mean of particle diameters to present a misleading picture of the nature of the "average" particle.

There are times when it is desired to describe the relative variability of one or more sets of data. The most common way of doing this is to compute the coefficient of variation (CV), which is calculated simply as the ratio of the standard deviation to the mean:

$$CV = \frac{SD}{\overline{X}}$$

A CV of 0.2 (or 20%) thus means that the standard deviation is 20% of the mean. In toxicology the CV is frequently between 20 and 50% and may at times exceed 100%. Note that if it is desired to express the CV as a percentage, the results of the previous equation should be multiplied by 100.

EXPERIMENTAL DESIGN

Toxicological experiments generally have a twofold purpose. The first question is whether or not an agent results in an effect on a biological system. The second question is how much of an effect is present. Both the cost to perform research to answer such questions and the value that society places on the results of such efforts have continued to increase rapidly. Additionally, it has become increasingly desirable that the results and conclusions of studies aimed at assessing the effects of environmental agents be as clear and unequivocal as possible. It is essential that every experiment and study yield as much information as possible in terms of the question being asked, and that (more specifically) the results of each study have the greatest possible chance of answering the questions it was conducted to address. The statistical aspects of such efforts, as far as they are aimed at structuring experiments to maximize the possibilities of success, are called experimental design.

The concept of censoring and its understanding are essential to the design of acute toxicity studies. Censoring is the exclusion of measurements from certain experimental units, or indeed of the experimental units themselves, from consideration in data analysis or inclusion in the experiment at all. Censoring may occur prior to initiation of an experiment (where, in modern toxicology, this is almost always a planned procedure), during the course of an experiment (when they are almost universally unplanned, resulting from such problems as the death of animals on test), or after the conclusion of an experiment (when usually data are excluded because of being identified as some form of outlier).

In practice, a priori censoring in toxicology studies occurs in the assignment of experimental units (such as animals) to test groups. The most familiar example is in the common practice of assignment of test animals to acute, subacute, subchronic, and chronic studies, in which the results of otherwise random assignments are evaluated for body weights of the assigned members. If the mean weights are not found to be comparable by some preestablished criterion (such as a 90% probability of difference by analysis of variance), then members are reassigned (censored) to achieve comparability in terms of starting body weights. Such a procedure of animal assignment to groups is known as a censored randomization.

There are number of aspects of experimental design which are specific to the practice of toxicology. Before we look at a suggestion for step-by-step development of experimental designs, these aspects should be considered as follows.

1. Frequently, the data gathered from specific measurements of animal characteristics are such that there is wide variability in the data. Often, such wide variability is not present in a control or low-dose group, but in an intermediate dosage group variance inflation may occur. That is, there may be a large standard deviation associated with the measurements from this intermediate group. In the face of such a set of data, the conclusion that there is no biological effect based on a finding of no statistically significant effect might well be erroneous.

2. In designing experiments, a toxicologist should keep in mind the potential effect of involuntary censoring on sample size. In other words, though a study might start with five dogs per group, this provides no margin should any die before the study is ended and blood samples are collected and analyzed. Just enough experimental units per group frequently leaves too few at the end to allow meaningful statistical analysis, and allowances should be made accordingly in establishing group sizes.

3. It is certainly possible to pool the data from several identical toxicological studies. For example, after first having performed an acute inhalation study in which only three treatment group animals survived to the point at which a critical measure (such as analysis of blood samples) was performed, we would not have enough data to perform a meaningful statistical analysis. We would then repeat the protocol with new control and treatment group animals from the same source. At the end, after assuring ourselves that the two sets of data are comparable, we could combine (or pool) the data from survivors of the second study with those from the first. The costs of this approach, however, would then be both a greater degree of effort expended (than if we had performed a single study with larger groups) and increased variability in the pooled samples (decreasing the power of our statistical methods).

4. Another frequently overlooked design option in toxicology is the use of an unbalanced design—that is, of different group sizes for different levels of treatment. There is no requirement that each group in a study (control, low dose, intermediate dose, and high dose) have an equal number of experimental units assigned to it. Indeed, there are frequently good reasons to assign more experimental units to one group than to others, and all the major statistical methodologies have provisions to adjust for such inequalities, within certain limits. The two most common uses of the unbalanced design have larger groups

designed to either the highest dose, to compensate for losses due to possible deaths during the study, or to the lowest dose, to give more sensitivity in detecting effects at levels close to an effect threshold—or more confidence to the assertion that no effect exists.

5. We are frequently confronted with the situation in which an undesired variable is influencing our experimental results in a nonrandom fashion. Such a variable is called a confounding variable—its presence, as discussed earlier, makes the clear attribution and analysis of effects at best difficult and at worst impossible. Sometimes such confounding variables are the result of conscious design or management decisions, such as the use of different instruments, personnel, facilities, or procedures for different test groups within the same study. Occasionally, however, such confounding variables are the result of unintentional factors or actions, in which case it is called a lurking variable. Examples of such variables are almost always the result of standard operating procedures being violated—water not being connected to a rack of animals over a weekend, a set of racks not being cleaned as frequently as others, or a contaminated batch of feed being used.

6. Finally, some thought must be given to the clear definition of what is meant by experimental unit and concurrent control. The experimental unit in toxicology encompasses a wide variety of possibilities. It may be cells, plates of microorganisms, individual animals, litters of animals, etc. The importance of clearly defining the experimental unit is that the number of such units per group is the "N" which is used in statistical calculations or analyses, and critically affects such calculations. A true concurrent control is one that is identical in every manner with the treatment groups except for the treatment being evaluated. This means that all manipulations, including gavaging with equivalent volumes of vehicles or exposing to equivalent rates of air exchanges in an inhalation chamber, should be duplicated in control groups just as they occur in treatment groups.

The goal of the six principles of experimental design is statistical efficiency and the economizing of resources. It is possible to think of design as a logic flow analysis. Such an analysis is conducted in three steps and should be performed every time any major study or project is initiated or, indeed, at regular periods during the course of conduct of a series of "standard" smaller studies. These steps are detailed below.

1. Define the objective of the study—get a clear statement of what questions are being asked.

> Can the question, in fact, be broken down into a set of subquestions?
> Are we asking one or more of these questions repeatedly? For example, does "X" (an event or effect) develop at 1, 7, or 14 days past treatment, and/or does it progress/regress or recover?

What is our model to be in answering this/these questions? Is it appropriate and acceptably sensitive?

2. For each subquestion (i.e., separate major variable to be studied):

How is the variable of interest to be measured?

What is the nature of the data generated by the measure? Are we getting an efficient set of data? Are we buying too little information (would another technique improve the quality of the information generated to the point that it becomes a higher "class" of data?) or too much information—i.e., does some underlying aspect of the measure limit the class of data obtainable within the bounds of feasibility of effort?

Are there possible interactions between measurements? Can they be separated/identified?

Is our N (sample size) both sufficient and efficient?

What is the control—formal or informal? Is it appropriate?

Are we needlessly adding confounding variables (asking inadvertent or unwanted questions)?

Are there "lurking variables" present? These are undesired and not readily recognized differences which can affect results, such as different technicians observing different groups of animals.

How large an effect will be considered biologically significant? This is a question which can only be resolved by reference to experience or historical control data.

3. What are the possible outcomes of the study—i.e., what answers are possible to both our subquestions and our major question?

How do we use these answers?

Do the possible answers offer a reasonable expectation of achieving the objectives that caused us to initiate the study?

What new questions may these answers cause us to ask? Can the study be redesigned, before it is actually started, so that these "revealed" questions may be answered in the original study?

When considering the last portion of our logic analysis, however, we must start by considering each of the things which may go wrong during the study. These include the occurrence of an infectious disease, the finding that an incorrect vehicle or concentration of test material had been used, or the uncovering of a hidden variable. Do we continue or stop the study? How will we now separate those portions of observed effects which are due to the chemical under study and those portions which are due to the disease process? Can we preclude (or minimize) the posibility of a disease outbreak by doing a more extensive health surveillance and quarantine on our test animals prior to the start of the study? Could we select a better test model—one that is not as sensitive to upper respiratory or nasal irritation?

For the reader who would like to further explore experimental design, there are a number of more detailed texts available which include more extensive treatments of the statistical aspects of experimental design. Among those recommended are Cochran and Cox (1975), Diamond (1981), Federer (1955), Hicks (1982), and Myers (1972). Gad and Weil (1988) focus on experimental design in toxicology.

METHODS

One approach for the selection of appropriate statistical techniques to employ in a particular situation is by the use of a decision tree methodology. The methods presented here were selected with one such decision tree (Gad & Weil, 1988) in mind.

BARTLETT'S TEST FOR HOMOGENEITY OF VARIANCE

Bartlett's test (see Sokal and Rohlf, 1981, pp. 403–407) is used to compare the variances (values reflecting the degree of variability in data sets) among three or more groups of data, where the data in the groups are continuous sets (such as body weights, organ weights, red blood cell counts, or diet consumption measurements). It is expected that such data will be suitable for parametric methods, and Bartlett's is frequently used as a test for the assumption of equivalent variances.

Bartlett's is based on the calculation of the corrected χ^2 value by the formula:

$$\chi^2_{corr} = 2.3026 \frac{\Sigma df \left(\log_{10} \left[\frac{\Sigma[df(S^2)]}{\Sigma df} \right] \right) - \Sigma[df(\log_{10}S^2)]}{1 + \frac{1}{3(K-1)} \left[\Sigma \frac{1}{df} - \frac{1}{\Sigma df} \right]}$$

where S^2 is the variance $= [N(\Sigma X)^2 - (\Sigma X)^2/N]/N - 1$, X is the individual datum within each group, N is the number of data within each group, K is the number of groups being compared and df is the degrees of freedom for each group $= (N - 1)$.

The corrected χ^2 value yielded by the above calculations is compared to the values listed in the χ^2 table according to the numbers of degrees of freedom (such as found in Snedecor and Cochran, 1980, pp. 470–471).

If the calculated value is smaller than the table value at the selected p level (traditionally 0.05), the groups are accepted to be homogeneous and the use of analysis of variance (ANOVA) is assumed proper. If the calculated χ^2 is greater than the table value, the groups are heterogeneous and other tests are necessary.

RANDOMIZATION

Randomization is the act of assigning a number of items (plates of bacteria or test animals, for example) to groups in such a manner that there is an equal chance for any item to end up in any one group. This is a control against any possible bias in assignment of subjects to test groups. A variation on this is censored randomization, which ensures that the groups are equivalent in some aspect after the assignment process is complete. The most common example of a censored randomization is one in which it is ensured that the body weights of test animals in each group are not significantly different from those in the other groups. This is done by analyzing group weights for homogeneity of variance and by analysis of variance after animal assignment, then rerandomizing if there is a significant difference at some nominal level, such as $p \leq 0.10$. The process is repeated until there is no difference.

There are several methods for actually performing the randomization process. The three most commonly used are card assignment, use of a random number table, and use of a computerized algorithm.

For the card-based method, individual identification numbers for items (plates or animals, for example) are placed on separate index cards. These cards are then shuffled and placed one at a time in succession into piles corresponding to the required test groups. The results are a random group assignment.

The random number table method requires only that one have unique numbers assigned to test subjects and access to a random number table. One simply sets up a table with a column for each group to which subjects are to be assigned. We start from the head of any one column of numbers in the random table (each time the table is used, a new starting point should be utilized). If our test subjects number less than 100, we utilize only the last two digits in each random number in the table. If they number more than 99 but less than 1000, we use only the last three digits. To generate group assignments, we read down a column, one number at a time. As we come across digits which correspond to a subject number, we assign that subject to a group (enter its identifying number in a column), proceeding to assign subjects to groups from left to right filling one row at a time. After a number is assigned to an animal, any duplication of its unique number is ignored. We use as many successive columns of random numbers as we may need to complete the process.

The third (and now most common) method is to use a random number generator that is built into a calculator or computer program. Procedures for generating these are generally documented in user manuals.

TRANSFORMATIONS

If our initial inspection of a data set reveals it to have an unusual or undesired set of characteristics (or to lack a desired set of characteristics), we have a choice of three courses of action. We may proceed to select a method or test appropriate to this new set of conditions, abandon the entire exercise, or transform the variable(s) under consideration in such a manner that the resulting transformed variates (X' and Y', for example, as opposed to the original variates X and Y) meet the assumptions or have the characteristics that are desired.

The key to all this is that the scale of measurement of most (if not all) variables is arbitrary. That is, although we are most familiar with a linear scale of measurement, there is nothing which makes this the "correct" scale on its own, as opposed to a logarithmic scale [familiar logarithmic measurements are that of pH values or earthquake intensity (Richter scale)]. Transforming a set of data (converting X to X') is really as simple as changing the scale of measurement.

There are at least four good reasons to transform data:

1. To normalize the data, making them suitable for analysis by our most common parametric techniques such as ANOVA. A simple test of whether a selected transformation will yield a distribution of data which satisfies the underlying assumptions for ANOVA is to plot the cumulative distribution of samples on probability paper (that is, a commercially available paper which has the probability function scale as one axis). One can then alter the scale of the second axis (that is, the axis other than the one which is on a probability scale) from linear to any other (logarithmic, reciprocal, square root, etc.) and see if a previously curved line indicating a skewed distribution becomes linear to indicate normality. The slope of the transformed line gives us an estimate of the standard deviation. Also, if the slopes of the lines of several samples or groups of data are similar, we accordingly know that the variances of the different groups are homogeneous.

2. To linearize the relationship between a paired set of data, such as dose and response. This is the most common use in toxicology for transformations and is demonstrated under Probit/Log Transforms and Regression.

3. To adjust data for the influence of another variable. This is an alternative in some situations to the more complicated process of analysis of covariance. A ready example of this usage is the calculation of organ weight to body weight

ratios in *in vivo* toxicity studies, with the resulting ratios serving as the raw data for an analysis of variance performed to identify possible target organs. This use is discussed in detail later in this chapter.

4. To make the relationships between variables clearer by removing or adjusting for interactions with third, fourth, etc. uncontrolled variables which influence the pair of variables of interest.

Common transformations are presented in Table 77.

FISHER'S EXACT TEST

Fisher's exact test should be used to compare two sets of discontinuous, quantal (all or none) data. Small sets of such data can be checked by contingency data tables, such as those of Finney *et al.* (1963). Larger sets, however, require computation. These include frequency data such as incidences of mortality or certain histopathological findings, etc. Thus, the data can be expressed as ratios. These data do not fit on a continuous scale of measurement but usually involve numbers of responses classified as either negative or positive—that is, a contingency table situation (Sokal and Rohlf, 1981, pp. 738–743).

The analysis is started by setting up a 2 × 2 contingency table to summarize

TABLE 77 Common Data Transformations

Transformation	Calculated[a]	Example of use
Arithmetic	$x' = \dfrac{x}{y}$ or $x' = x + c$	Organ weight/body weight
Reciprocals	$x' = \dfrac{1}{x}$	Linearizing data, particularly rate phenomena
Arcsine (also called angular)	$x' = $ arcsine	Normalizing dominant lethal and mutation rate data
Logarithmic	$x' = \log x$	pH values
Probability (probit)	$x' = $ probability X	Percentage responding
Square roots	$x' = \sqrt{x}$	Surface area of animal from body weight
Box cox	$x' = (x^v - 1)$; for $v \neq 0$ $x' = 1nx^v$; for $v = 0$	A family of transforms for use when one has no prior knowledge of the appropriate transformation to use

[a]x and y are original variables, x' and y' are transformed values. c, a constant.

[b]Plotting a double reciprocal (that is, $\dfrac{1}{x}$ vs $\dfrac{1}{y}$ will linearize almost any data set; so will plotting the log transforms of a set of variables.

the numbers of "positive" and "negative" responses as well as the totals of these as follows:

	Positive	Negative	Total
Group I	A	B	A + B
Group II	C	D	C + B
Total	A + C	B + D	A + B + C + D = N total

Using the above set of symbols, the formula for probability (p) appears as follows:

$$P = \frac{(A + B)!(C + D)!(A + C)!(B + D)!}{N!A!C!D!}$$

The exact test produces a p which is the sum of the above calculation repeated for each possible arrangement of the numbers in the above cells (that is, A, B, C, and D) showing an association equal to or stronger than that between the two variables.

The p resulting from these computations will be the exact one- or two-tailed probability depending on which of these two approaches is being employed. This value tells us if the groups differ significantly (e.g., with a probability less than 0.05) and the degree of significance of any such differences.

2 × 2 CHI-SQUARE

Though Fisher's exact test is preferable for analysis of most 2 × 2 contingency tables in toxicology, the chi-square test is still widely used and is preferable in a few unusual situations (particularly if cell sizes are large but only limited computational support is available).

The formula is simply:

$$\chi^2 = \frac{(0_1 - E_1)^2}{E_1} + \frac{(0_2 - E_2)^2}{E_2} = \Sigma \frac{(0_i - E_i)^2}{E_i}$$

where 0 are observed numbers (or counts) and E are expected numbers. The common practice in toxicology is for the observed figures to be test or treatment group counts. The expected figure for each box or cell in a contingency table is calculated as follows:

$$E = \frac{(\text{Column total})(\text{Row total})}{\text{Grand total}}$$

R × C CHI-SQUARE

The R×C chi-square test can be used to analyze discontinuous (frequency) data as in the Fisher's exact 2×2 chi-square tests. However, in the R×C test (R, row; C, column) we wish to compare three or more sets of data. An example would be comparison of the incidence of seizures among mice on three or more oral dosage levels. We can consider the data as positive (seizures) or negative (no seizures). The expected frequency for any box is equal to (row total) (column total)/(N_{total}).

As in the Fisher's exact test, the initial step is setting up a table (a R×C contingency table). This table would appear as follows:

	Positive	Negative	Total
Group	A_1	B_1	$A_1 + B_1 = N_1$
Group II	A_2	B_2	$A_2 + B_2 = N_2$
	↓	↓	↓
Group R	A_R	B_R	$A_R + B_R = N_R$
Total	N_A	N_B	N_{total}

Using these symbols, the formula for χ^2 is

$$\chi^2 = \frac{N_{tot}^2}{N_A N_B N_K}\left(\frac{A_1^2}{N_1} + \frac{A_2^2}{N_2} + \frac{A_K^2}{N_K} - \frac{N_A^2}{N_{tot}}\right)$$

This resulting χ^2 value is compared to table values (as in Snedecor and Cochran, 1980, pp. 470–471) according to the number of degrees of freedom, which is equal to $(R - 1)(C - 1)$. If χ^2 is smaller than the table value at the 0.05 probability level, the groups are not significantly different. If the calculated χ^2 is larger, there is some difference among the groups and 2 × 2 chi-square or Fisher's exact tests will have to be computed to determine which group(s) differs from which other group(s).

WILCOXON'S RANK-SUM TEST

The Wilcoxon rank-sum test is commonly used for the comparison of two groups of nonparametric (interval or not normally distributed) data, such as those which are not measured exactly but rather as falling within certain limits (for example, how many animals died during each hour of an acute study). The test is also used when there is no variability (variance = 0) within one or more of the groups we wish to compare (Sokal and Rohlf, 1981, pp. 432–437).

The data in both groups being compared are initially arranged and listed in order of increasing value. Then each number in the two groups must receive a rank value. Beginning with the smallest number in either group (which is given a rank of 1.0), each number is assigned a rank. If there are duplicate numbers (called "ties"), then each value of equal size will receive the median rank for the entire identically sized group. Thus, if the lowest number appears twice, both figures receive the rank of 1.5. This, in turn, means that the ranks of 1.0 and 2.0 have been used and that the next highest number has a rank of 3.0. If the lowest number appears three times, then each is ranked as 2.0 and the next number has a rank of 4.0. Thus, each tied number gets a "median" rank. This process continues until all the numbers are ranked. Each of the two columns of ranks (one for each group) is totalled giving the "sum of ranks" for each group being compared. As a check, we can calculate the value:

$$\frac{(N)(N + 1)}{2}$$

where N is the total number of data in both group. The result should be equal to the sum of the sum of ranks for both groups.

The sum of rank values are compared to table values (such as Beyer, 1976, pp. 409–413) to determine the degree of significant differences, if any. These tables include two limits (an upper and a lower) that are dependent on the probability level. If the number of data are the same in both groups ($N_1 = N_2$), both of the calculated sums of ranks must fall within the two limit values. If this is the case, the two groups are not statistically different. If one or both of the sums of ranks is equal to or falls outside the table limits, the groups are different at that probability level. If the numbers of data in the two groups are not equal ($N_1 \neq N_2$), then the lesser sum of ranks (smaller N) is compared to the table limits to find the degree of significance. Normally the comparison of the two groups ends here and to the degree of significant difference can be reported.

KRUSKAL–WALLIS NONPARAMETRIC ANOVA

The Kruskal–Wallis nonparametric one-way analysis of variance should be the initial analysis performed when we have three or more groups of data which are by nature nonparametric (not a normally distributed population, of a discontinuous nature, or all the groups being analyzed are not from the same population) but not of a categorical (or quantal) nature. Commonly these will be either rank-type evaluation data (such as behavioral toxicity observation scores) or reproduction study data. The analysis is initiated (Pollard, 1977, pp. 170–173) by ranking all the observations from the combined groups to be analyzed. Ties are given the average rank of the tied values (that is, if two values which would tie for 12th rank—and therefore would be ranked 12th and 13th—both would be assigned the average rank of 12.5).

The sum of ranks of each group (r_1, r_2, $\cdots$ r_k) is computed by adding all the rank values for each group. The test value H is then computed as

$$H = \frac{12}{n(n + 1)} \Sigma(r_1^2/n_1 + r_2^2/n_2 + \cdots + r_k^2/n_k) - 3(n + 1)$$

where n_1, n_2, $\cdots$ n_k are the number of observations in each group. The test statistic is then compared with a table of H values (such as in Gad and Weil, 1986). If the calculated value of H is greater than the table value for the appropriate number of observations in each group, there is a significant difference between the groups, but further testing (using the distribution-free multiple comparisons method) is necessary to determine where the difference lies.

STUDENT'S t TEST (UNPAIRED t TEST)

Pairs of groups of continuous, randomly distributed data are compared via this test. We can use this test to compare three or more groups of data, but they must be intercompared by examination of two groups taken at a time and are preferentially compared by ANOVA. Usually this means comparison of a test group versus a control group, although two test groups may be compared as well. To determine which of the three types of t tests described in this chapter should be employed, the Bartlett's and F test are usually performed first. These will tell us if the variances of the data are approximately equal, which is a requirement for the use of a parametric method. If the F test indicates homogeneous variances and the numbers of data within the groups (N) are equal, then the Student's t test is the appropriate procedure (Sokal and Rohlf, 1981, pp. 226–231). If the F is significant (the data are heterogeneous) and the two groups have equal numbers of data, the modified Student's t test is applicable (Diem and Lentner, 1975).

The value of t for Student's t test is calculated using the formula:

$$t = \frac{\overline{X}_1 - \overline{X}_2}{\sqrt{\Sigma D_1^2 + \Sigma D_2^2}} \sqrt{\frac{N_1 N_2}{N_1 + N_2}} (N_1 + N_2 - 2)$$

where the value of $\Sigma D^2 = [N\Sigma X^2 - (\Sigma X)^2]/N$.

The value of t obtained from the calculations is compared to the values in a t distribution table according to the appropriate number of degrees of freedom (df). If the F value is not significant (i.e., variances are homogeneous), the $df = N_1 + N_2 - 2$. If the F was significant and $N_1 = N_2$, then the $df = N - 1$. Although this case indicates a nonrandom distribution, the modified t test is still valid. If the calculated value is larger than the table value at $p = 0.05$, it may then be compared to the appropriate other table values in order of decreasing probability to determine the degree of significance between the two groups.

Cochran's t Test

The Cochran test should be used to compare two groups of continuous data when the variances (as indicated by the F test) are heterogenous and the numbers of data within the groups are not equal ($N_1 \neq N_2$). This is the situation, for example, when the data, though expected to be randomly distributed, were found not to be (Cochran and Cox, 1975, pp. 100–102).

Two t values are calculated for this test, the "observed" t (t_{obs}) and the "expected" t (t'). The observed t is obtained by

$$t_{obs} = \frac{\overline{X}_1 - \overline{X}_2}{W_1 + W_2}$$

where $W = SEM^2 = S^2/N$, where S (variance) can be calculated from

$$S = \frac{\dfrac{N\Sigma X^2 - (\Sigma X)^2}{N}}{N - 1}$$

The value for t' is obtained from

$$t' = \frac{t_1' W_1 + t_2' W_2}{W_1 + W_2}$$

where t_1' and t_2' are values for the two groups taken from the t distribution table corresponding to $N - 1$ degrees of freedom (for each group) at the 0.05 probability level (or such level as one may select).

The calculated t_{obs} is compared to the calculated t' value (or values, if t' values were prepared for more than one probability level). If t_{obs} is smaller than a t', the groups are not considered to be significantly different at that probability level.

Analysis of Variance

ANOVA is used for the comparison of three or more groups of continuous data when the variances are homogeneous and the data are independent and normally distributed.

A series of calculations are required for ANOVA, starting with the values within each group being added (ΣX) and then these sums being added ($\Sigma\Sigma X$).

Each figure within the groups is squared, and these squares are then summed (ΣX^2) and these sums are totalled ($\Sigma\Sigma X^2$).

Next the correction factor (CF) can be calculated from the following formula:

$$CF = \frac{\left(\displaystyle\sum_1^K \sum_1^N X\right)^2}{N_1 + N_2 + \cdots N_k}$$

where N is the number of values in each group and K is the number of groups. The total sum of squares (SS) is then determined as follows:

$$SS_{total} = \sum_1^K \sum_1^N X^2 - CF$$

In turn the sum of squares between groups (bg) is found from

$$SS_{bg} = \frac{(\Sigma X_1)^2}{N_1} + \frac{(\Sigma X_2)^2}{N_2} + \cdots \frac{(\Sigma X_k)^2}{N_k} - CF$$

The sum of squares within group (wg) is then the difference between the last two figures, or:

$$SS_{wg} = SS_{total} - SS_{bg}$$

Now, there are three types of degrees of freedom to determine. The first, total df, is the total number of data within all groups under analysis minus one ($N_1 + N_2 + \cdots N_k - 1$). The second figure (the df between groups) is the number of groups minus one ($K - 1$). The last figure (the df within groups or "error df") is the difference between the first two figures ($df_{total} - df_{bg}$).

The next set of calculations requires determination of the two mean squares (MS_{bg} and MS_{wg}). These are the respective sum of square values divided by the corresponding df figures ($MS = SS/df$). The final calculation is that of the F ratio. For this, the MS between groups is divided by the MS within groups ($F = MS_{bg}/MS_{wg}$).

A table of the results of these calculations from Example 15 in Gad and Weil (1986) would appear as follows:

	df	SS	MS	F
Bg	3	0.04075	0.01358	4.94
Wg	12	0.03305	0.00275	
Total	15	0.07380		

For interpretation, the F ratio value obtained in the ANOVA is compared to a table of F values. If $F \leq 1.0$, the results are not significant and comparison with the table values is not necessary. The dfs for the greater mean square

(MS_{bg}) are indicated along the top of the table. Read down the side of the table to the line corresponding to the *df* for the lesser mean square (MS_{wg}). The figure shown at the desired significance level (traditionally 0.05) is compared to the calculated *F* value. If the calculated number is smaller, there are no significant differences among the groups being compared. If the calculated value is larger, there is some difference but further (post hoc) testing will be required before we know which groups differ significantly.

LINEAR REGRESSION

Foremost among the methods for interpolating within a known data relationship is regression—the fitting of a line or curve to a set of known data points on a graph, and the interpolation ("estimation") of this line or curve in areas where we have no data points. The simplest of these regression models is that of linear regression (valid when increasing the value of one variable changes the value of the related variable in a linear fashion, either positively or negatively). This is the case we will explore here, using the method of least squares.

Given that we have two sets of variables, *x* (e.g., mg/kg of test material administered) and *y* (e.g., percentage of animals so dosed that die), what is required is solving for *a* and *b* in the equation $Y_i = a + bx_i$, where Y_i is the fitted value of Y_i at x_i, and we wish to minimize $(Y_i - Y_i)^2$. We solve the equations

$$b = \frac{\Sigma x_1 y_1 - nx\bar{y}}{\Sigma x_1^2 - n\bar{x}^2}$$

$$a = \bar{y} - b\bar{x}$$

where *a* is the *y* intercept, *b* is the slope of the time, and *n* is the number of data points.

Note that in actuality, dose–response relationships are often not linear and instead we must use either a transform (to linearize the data) or a nonlinear regression method (a good discussion of which may be found in Gallant, 1975).

Note also that one can use the correlation test statistic to determine if the regression is significant (and, therefore, valid) at a defined level of certainty. A more specific test for significance would be the linear regression analysis of variance (Pollard, 1977).

PROBIT/LOG TRANSFORMS AND REGRESSION

As we noted in the preceding section, dose–response problems (among the most common interpolation problems encountered in toxicology) rarely are straightforward enough to make a valid linear regression directly from the raw data. The most common valid interpolation methods are based on probability ("probit") and logarithmic ("log") value scales, with percentage responses (death, tumor incidence, etc.) being expressed on the probit scale while doses (Y_i) are expressed on the log scale. There are two strategies for such an approach. The first is based on transforming the data to these scales, then doing a weighted linear regression on the transformed data (if one does not have access to a computer or a high-powered programmable calculator, the only practical strategy is not to assign weights). The second requires the use of algorithms (approximate calculation techniques) for the probit value and regression process and is extremely burdensome to perform manually.

One approach to the first strategy requires that a table be constructed with pairs of values of x_i and Y_i listed in order of increasing values of Y_i (percentage response). Beside each of these columns a set of blank columns should be left so that the transformed values may be listed. We then simply add the columns described in the linear regression procedure. Log and probit values may be taken from any of a number of sets of tables and the rest of the table is then developed from these transformed x_i' and y_i' values (denoted as x_i' and y_i''). A standard linear regression is then performed.

The second strategy we discussed has been broached by a number of authors (Bliss, 1935; Finney, 1977; Litchfield and Wilcoxon, 1949; Prentice, 1976). All these methods, however, are computationally cumbersome. It is possible to approximate the necessary iterative process using the algorithms developed by Abramowitz and Stegun (1964), but even this merely reduces the complexity to a point where the procedure may be readily programmed on a small computer or programmable calculator.

MOVING AVERAGES

An obvious drawback to the interpolation procedures we have examined to date is that they do take a significant amount of time (though they are simple enough to be done manually, especially if the only result we desire is an LD_{50}, LC_{50}, or LT_{50}.

The method of moving averages (Thompson and Weil, 1952; Weil, 1962) gives a rapid and reasonably accurate estimate of this "median-effective dose" (m) and the estimated standard deviation of its logarithm.

Such methodology requires that the same number of animals be used per dosage level and that the spacing between successive dosage exposure levels be geometrically constant (i.e., levels of 1, 2, 4, and 8 mg/kg or 1, 3, 9, and 27 ppm). Given this and access to a table for the computation of moving averages (such as found in Appendix B), one can readily calculate the median effective dose with the formula (illustrated for dose):

$$\log m = \log D + d\ (K - 1)/2 + df$$

where m is the median effective dose or exposure, D is the lowest dose tested, d is the log of the ratio of successive doses/exposures, and f is a table value taken from Gad and Weil (1988) for the proper K (the total number of levels minus 1).

APPLICATIONS

MEDIAN LETHAL AND EFFECTIVE DOSES

For many years, the starting point for evaluating the toxicity of an agent was to determine its LD_{50} or LC_{50}, which are the dose or concentration of a material at which half of population of animals would be expected to die. These figures are analogous to the ED_{50} (effective dose for half a population) used in pharmacologic activities and are derived by the same means.

To calculate either of these figures we need, at each of several dosage (or exposure) levels, the number of animals dosed and the number that died. If we seek only to establish the median effective dose in a range-finding test, then 4 or 5 animals per dose level, using Thompson's method of moving averages, is the most efficient methodology and will give a sufficiently accurate solution. With two dose levels, if the ratio between the high and low dose is two or less, even total or no mortality at these two dose levels will yield an acceptably accurate median lethal dose, although a partial mortality is desirable. If, however, we wish to estimate a number of toxicity levels (LD_{10} and LD_{90}) and are interested in more precisely establishing the slope of the dose/lethality curve, the use of at least 10 animals per dosage level with the previously described log/probit regression technique would be the most common approach (though one that will hopefully be discontinued). Note that in the equation $Y_i = a + bx_i$, b is the slope of the regression line and our method already allows us to calculate 95% confidence intervals about any point on this line. Note also that the confidence interval at any one point will be different from the interval at other points and must be calculated separately. Additionally, the nature of the probit transform is such that toward the extremes—LD_{10} and LD_{90}, for example—the confidence intervals will "balloon." That is, they become very wide. Because the slope of the fitted line in these assays has a very large uncertainty, in relation to the uncertainty of the LD_{50} itself (the midpoint of the distribution), much caution must be used with calculated LD_x's other than LD_{50}'s. The imprecision of the LD_{35}, a value close to the LD_{50}, is discussed by Weil (1972), as is that of the slope of the log dose–probit line (Weil, 1975). Debanne and Haller (1983) reviewed the statistical aspects of different methodologies for estimating a median effective dose.

BODY AND ORGAN WEIGHTS

Among the sets of data commonly collected in studies in which animals are dosed with (or exposed to) a chemical are body weight and the weights of selected organs. In fact, body weight (or the rate of gain of body weight) is frequently the most sensitive indication of an adverse effect. How to best analyze this and in what form to analyze the organ weight data (as absolute weights, weight changes, or percentages of body weight) have been the subject of a number of articles (Jackson, 1962; Weil, 1962, 1970; Weil and Gad, 1980).

Both absolute body weights and rates of body weight change (calculated as changes from a baseline measurement value which is traditionally the animal's weight immediately prior to the first dosing with or exposure to test material) are almost universally best analyzed by ANOVA followed, if called for, by a post hoc test. Even if the groups were randomized properly at the beginning of a study (no group being significantly different in mean body weight from any other group, and all animals in all groups within two standard deviations of the overall mean body weight), there is an advantage to performing the computationally slightly more cumbersome (compared to absolute body weights) analysis of changes in body weight. The advantage is an increase in sensitivity because the adjustment of starting points (the setting of initial weights as a "zero" value) acts to reduce the amount of initial variability. In this case, Bartlett's test is performed first to ensure homogeneity of variance and the appropriate sequence of analysis follows.

With smaller sample sizes, the normality of the data becomes increasingly uncertain, and nonparametric methods such as Kruskal–Wallis may be more appropriate (see Zar, 1974).

The analysis of relative (to body weight) organ weights is a valuable tool for identifying possible target organs (Gad et al., 1984). How to perform this analysis is still a matter of some disagreement, however.

Weil (1962) presented evidence that organ weight data expressed as percentages of body weight should be analyzed separately for each sex. Furthermore, because the conclusions from organ weight data of males differ often from those of females, data from animals of each sex should be used in this measurement. Also, Weil (1970, 1973), Boyd and Knight (1963), and Boyd (1972) have discussed in detail other factors which influence organ weights and must be taken into account.

The two competing approaches to analyzing relative organ weights call for either (1) calculating organ weights as a percentage of total body weight (at the time of necropsy) and analyzing the results by ANOVA, or (2) analyzing results by ANCOVA, with body weights as the covariates as discussed by Weil and Gad (1980).

A number of considerations should be kept in mind when these questions are addressed. First, one must keep a firm grasp on the difference between biological significance and statistical significance. In this particular case, we are especially interested in examining organ weights when an organ weight change is not proportional to changes in whole body weights. Second, we are now required to detect smaller and smaller changes while still retaining a similar sensitivity (i.e., the $p < 0.05$ level).

There are several devices to attain the desired increase in power. One is to use larger sample sizes (number of animals) and the other is to utilize the most powerful test we can. However, the use of even currently employed numbers of animals is being vigorously questioned and the power of statistical tests must, therefore, now assume an increased importance in our considerations.

The biological rationale behind analyzing both absolute organ weight and the organ weight to body weight ratio (this latter as opposed to a covariance analysis of organ weights) is that in the majority of cases, except for the brain, organs change weight (except in extreme cases of obesity or starvation) in proportion to total body weight. We are particularly interested in detecting cases in which this is not so. Analysis of actual data from several hundred studies (unpublished data) has shown no significant difference in rates of weight change of target organs (other than the brain) compared to total body weight for healthy animals in those species commonly used for acute and repeated dose studies (rats, mice, rabbits, and dogs). Furthermore, it should be noted that analysis of covariance is of questionable validity in analyzing body weight and related organ weight changes because a primary assumption is the independence of treatment—that the relationship of the two variables is the same for all treatments (Ridgeman, 1975). Plainly, in toxicology this is not true.

In cases in which the differences between the error mean squares are much greater, the F ratios will diverge in precision from the result of the efficiency of covariance adjustment. In these cases, either sample sizes are much larger or the differences between means themselves are much larger. This latter case is one which does not occur in the designs under discussion in any manner that would leave analysis of covariance as a valid approach because group means start out being very similar and cannot diverge markedly unless there is a treatment effect. As we have discussed earlier, a treatment effect invalidates a prime underpinning assumption of analysis of covariance.

BEHAVIORAL TOXICOLOGY

A brief review of the types of studies/experiments conducted in the area of behavioral toxicology, and a classification of these into groups, is in order. Although there are a small number of studies which do not fit into the following classification, the great majority may be fitted into one of the following four groups. Many of these points were first covered by one of the authors in an earlier article (Gad, 1982a).

Observational score-type studies are based on observing and grading the response of an animal to its normal environment or to a stimulus which is imprecisely controlled. This type of result is generated by one of two major types of studies. Open-field studies involve placing an animal in the center of a flat, open area and counting each occurrence of several types of activities (grooming, moving outside a designated central area, rearing, etc.) or timing until the first occurrence of each type of activity. The data generated are scalar of either a continuous or discontinuous nature but frequently are not of a normal distribution. Tilson *et al.* (1980) presented some examples of this type.

Observational screen (or "functional observational battery") studies involve a combination of observing behavior and evoking a response to a simple stimulus, the resulting observation being graded as normal or as deviating from normal on a graded scale. Most of the data so generated are rank in nature, with some portions being quantal or interval. Irwin (1968) and Gad (1982b) have presented schemes for the conduct of such studies. Table 78 gives an example of the nature (and of one form of statistical analysis) of such data generated after exposure to one material.

The second type of study is one which generates rates of response as data. The studies are based on the number of responses to a discrete controlled stimulus or are free of direct connection to a stimulus. The three most frequently measured parameters are licking of a liquid (milk, sugar water, ethanol, or a psychoactive agent in water), gross locomotor activity (measured by a photocell or electromagnetic device), or lever pulling. Work presenting examples of such studies has been published by Annau (1972) and Norton (1973). The data generated are most often of a discontinuous or continuous scalar nature and are often complicated by underlying patterns of biological rhythm.

The third type of study generates a variety of data which are classified as error rate. These are studies based on animals learning a response to a stimulus or memorizing a simple task (such as running or swimming a maze or a Skinner box-type shock avoidance system). These tests or trials are structured so that animals can pass or fail on each of a number of successive trials. The resulting data are quantal, though frequently expressed as a percentage.

The final major type of study is that which results in data which are measures of the time to an endpoint. They are based on animals being exposed to or

TABLE 78   Irwin Screen Parameters Showing Significant Differences between Treated and Control Groups

| | Rats (18-crown-6 animals given 5.0 mg/kg ip) | | | |
Parameter	Control sum of ranks	N_c	18-crown-6 treated sum of ranks	N_t	Observed difference in treated animals (compared to controls)
Twitches	55.0	10	270.0	15	Involuntary muscle twitches
Visual placing	55.0	10	270.0	15	Less aware of visual stimuli
Grip strength	120.0	10	205.0	15	Considerable loss of strength, especially in hindlimbs
Respiration	55.0	10	270.0	15	Increased rate of respiration
Tremors	55.0	10	270.0	15	Marked tremors

Note. All parameters are significant at $p < 0.05$ (Gad et al., 1978).

dosed with a toxicant and the time taken for an effect to be observed is measured. The endpoint is usually failure to continue to be able to perform a task and can, therefore, be death, incapacitation, or the learning of a response to a discrete stimulus. Burt (1972) and Johnson et al. (1972) have presented data of this form. The data are always of a censored nature—that is, the period of observation is always artificially limited as in measuring time to incapacitation in combustion toxicology data, where animals are exposed to the thermal decomposition gases of test materials for a period of 30 min. If incapacitation is not observed during these 30 min, it is judged not to occur. The data generated by these studies are continuous, discontinuous, or rank in nature. They are discontinuous because the researcher may check or may be restricted to checking for the occurrence of the endpoint only at certain discrete points in time. On the other hand, they are rank if the periods to check for occurrence of the endpoint are far enough apart, in which case one may actually know only that the endpoint occurred during a broad period of time—but not at what point in that period.

Most, if not all, behavioral toxicology studies depend on at least some instrumentation. Very frequently overlooked here (and, indeed, in most research) is that instrumentation, by its operating characteristics and limitation, goes a long way toward determining the nature of the data generated by it. An activity monitor measures motor activity in discrete segments. If it is a "jiggle cage"-type monitor, these segments are restricted so that only a distinctly limited number of counts can be achieved in a given period of time and then only if they are of the appropriate magnitude. Likewise, technique can also readily determine the nature of data. In measuring response to pain, for example, one could record it as a quantal measure (present or absent), a rank score (on a scale of 1–5 for decreased to increased responsiveness, with 3 being "normal"), or as scalar data (by using an analgesia meter which determines how much pressure or heat is required to evoke a response).

Study design factors are probably the most widely recognized of the factors which influence the type of data resulting from a study. Number of animals used, frequency of measures, and length of period of observation are three obvious design factors which are readily under the control of the researcher and which directly help to determine the nature of the data.

SCREENING

One major set of activities in toxicology and pharmacology is the screening for the presence or absence of an effect. Such screens are almost always focused on detecting a single endpoint of effect (such as mutagenicity, lethality, neuro or developmental toxicity, etc.) and have a particular set of operating characteristics in common.

1. A large number of compounds are to be evaluated so that ease and speed of performance (which may also be considered efficiency) is a major desirable characteristic.

2. The screen must be very sensitive in its detection of potential effective agents. An absolute minimum of effective agents should escape detection—that is, there should be very few false negatives (in other words, the type II error rate or β-level should be low). Stated another way, the signal "gain" should be way up.

3. It is desirable that the number of false positives be small (that is, that there be a low type I error rate or α level).

4. Items 1–3 are all to some degree contradictory, requiring the involved researchers to agree on a set of compromises. These typically start with acceptance of a relatively high α level (0.10 or more)—a higher "noise" level.

5. In an effort to better serve Item 1, such screens are frequently performed in batteries such that multiple endpoints are measured in the same operation. Additionally, such measurements may be repeated over a period of time in each model as a means of supporting Item 2.

6. The screen should use small amounts of compound to enable Item 1 and allow evaluation of materials which have limited availability (such as novel compounds early on in development).

In an early screen, a relatively large number of compounds will be tested. It is unlikely that one will stand out so much as to be statistically significantly more important than all the other compounds. A more or less continuous range of activities will be found. Compounds showing the highest activity will proceed to the next assay or tier in the series and may be used as lead compounds in a new cycle of testing and evaluation.

Each assay can have an associated activity criterion (see Chapter 9). If the result for a particular test compound meets this criterion, the compound may pass to the next stage. This criterion could be based on statistical significance (i.e., all compounds with observed activities significantly greater than the control at the 5% level could be tagged). However, for early screens such a criterion may be too strict and few compounds may go through to further testing.

A useful indicator of the efficiency of an assay series is the frequency of discovery of truly active compounds. This is related to the probability of discovery and to the degree of risk associated with a compound. These two factors in turn depend on the distribution of activities in the test series and the changes at each stage of rejecting and accepting compounds with given activities.

Statistical modeling of the assay system may lead to the improvement of the design of the system to reduce the interval between discoveries. The objectives behind a screen and considerations of (1) costs for producing compounds and testing and of (2) the degree of uncertainty about test performance will determine desired performance characteristics of specific cases. Preliminary results suggest that in the most common case of early toxicity screens performed to remove possible problem compounds, it may be beneficial to increase the number of compounds tested, decrease the numbers of animals per group, and increase the range and number of doses. The result will be less information on more structures but an overall increase in the frequency of discovery (assuming that truly active compounds are entering the system at a steady rate).

It should be noted that the methodologies are better suited to analyzing screening data when the interest is truly in detecting the absence of an effect with little chance of a type II error (i.e., a low rate of false negatives). Anderson and Hauck (1983) should be consulted for a more thorough discussion of considerations involved in cases in which type I error is to be minimized (that is, where the desire is to have few false positives).

The design of each assay and the choice of the activity criterion should therefore be adjusted bearing in mind the relative costs of retaining false positives and rejecting false negatives. Decreasing the group sizes in the early assays reduces the chance of obtaining significance at any particular level (such as 5%) so that the activity criterion must be relaxed, in a statistical sense, to allow more compounds through. At some stage, however, it becomes too expensive to continue screening many false positives and the criteria must be tightened accordingly.

Screening systems may be approached by one of at least three different formats. These are single stage, sequential, and tier. For purposes of this presentation, we will consider only the single-stage case.

An excellent introduction to this subject is Redman's (1981) interesting approach which identifies four characteristics of an assay. It is assumed that a compound is either active or inactive, and that the proportion of actives can be estimated from past experience. After testing, a compound will be classified as positive or negative. It is then possible to design the assay so as to optimize the following characteristics:

"Sensitivity"—the ratio of true positives to total actives
"Specificity"—the ratio of true negatives to total inactives
"Positive accuracy"—the ratio of true to observed positives
"Negative accuracy"—the ratio of true to observed negatives
Capacity
Reproducibility

An advantage of testing more compounds is that it gives the opportunity to average activity evidence over structural classes or to study quantitative structure–activity relationships (QSARs). QSARs can be used to predict the activity of new compounds and thus reduce the chance of *in vivo* testing on negative compounds. They can increase the proportion of truly active compounds passing through the system.

It should be remembered that maximization of the performance of a series of screening assays requires close collaboration between the biologist, chemist, and statistician. It should be noted, however, that screening forms only part of a much larger research and development context.

Screens may thus truly be considered the biological equivalent of exploratory data analysis (EDA). EDA methods, if fact, provide a number of useful possibilities for less rigid and yet quite utilitarian approaches to the statistical analysis of the data from screens and are one of the alternative approaches presented and evaluated in this presentation.

Over the years the author has conducted, presented, published (Gad *et al.*, 1978, 1979, 1985, 1987; Gad, 1982,ab) or consulted on a large number of screening studies. These have usually been directed at detecting or identifying potential behavioral or neurotoxicants, but they have also been directed at pharmacologic, immunotoxic, and genotoxic agents. Two alternative approaches to analysis of the data resulting from screens have been proposed (Gad, 1988).

These were a control chart approach and a semigraphical exploratory data analysis method. These are summarized below.

CONTROL CHARTS

The control chart approach, commonly used in manufacturing quality control for another form of screening (Redman, 1981), offers some desirable characteristics.

During the development of screen methodology, for example, by keeping records of cumulative results, an initial estimate of the variability (such as standard deviation) of each assay is available when full-scale use of the screen starts. The initial estimates can then be revised as more data is generated (i.e., as we become more familiar with the screen).

The following example shows the usefulness of control charts for control measurements in a screening procedure. Our example test for screening potential muscle strength suppressive agents measures reduction of grip strength by test compounds compared to a control treatment. A control chart was established to monitor the performance of the control agent (a) to establish that the mean and variability of control for a given experiment are within reasonable limits (a validation of the assay procedure). The average grip strengths and the average range for a series of experiments are shown below along with a control chart.

As in control charts for quality control, the mean and average range of the assay were determined from previous experiments. In this example, the screen had been run 20 times previous to the data shown. These initial data showed a mean grip strength of 400 g and a mean range (R) of 90. These values were used for the control chart, with the starting data shown in Table 79. The subgroups are of size 5. The action limits for the $\overline{X}$ and range charts were calculated as follows: $\overline{X} \pm 0.58 R = 400 \pm 0.58(90) = 348$ to 452 ($\overline{X}$ chart) $R(2.11) = 90(2.11) = 190$, the upper limit for the range.

Note that the range limit actually establishes a limit for the variability of our data—that it is, in fact, a "detector" for the presence of outliers (extreme values). This data set in a control chart format is shown in Fig. 50.

Such charts may also be constructed and used for proportion- or count-type data. By constructing such charts for the range of control data, we may then use them as rapid and efficient tools for detecting effects in groups being assessed for that same screen endpoint.

CENTRAL TENDENCY PLOTS

The objective behind our analysis of neurobehavioral screen data is to have a means of efficiently, rapidly, and objectively identifying those agents which

TABLE 79   Average Grip Strengths (in g) and Ranges for Screening Procedures

Test number	Mean	Range	Test number	Mean	Range
1	380	40	11	280	120
2	430	30	12	410	100
3	340	30	13	400	220
4	480	60	14	340	50
5	380	240	15	370	40
6	450	40	16	430	140
7	490	50	17	370	60
8	320	90	18	450	80
9	480	50	19	320	70
10	340	80	20	420	130

Values for determining upper and lower limits for mean ($\bar{X}$) and range charts

Sample size of subgroup (N)	A: Factor for X chart	Range chart factors	
		Lower limit (D_L)	Upper limit (D_u)
2	1.88	0	3.27
3	1.02	0	2.57
4	0.73	0	2.28
5	0.58	0	2.11
6	0.48	0	2.00
7	0.42	0.08	1.92
8	0.37	0.14	1.86
9	0.34	0.18	1.82
10	0.31	0.22	1.78
20	0.18	0.41	1.59

have a reasonable probability of being neurotoxicants. Any materials that we so identify will be further data that can be analyzed by traditional means. In other words, we want a method which makes results that are out of the ordinary stand out. To do this we must first set the limits on "ordinary" and then overlay a scheme which causes those things which are not ordinary to become readily detected.

If we proceed to collect a set of control data on a variable (e.g., our observation of righting reflex scores) from some number of ordinary animals, and then plot it as a set of two histograms (one for individual animals and the second for the highest score in each randomly assigned group of 5 animals), we would have two histograms as shown in Fig. 51 (data derived from 200 control animals).

Such a plot then acts to identify the nature of our data, visually classifying it into those that will not influence our analysis (in the set shown, clearly

CONTROL CHART FOR MEANS AND RANGE FOR CONTROL GROUP IN SCREENING PROCEDURE FOR AGENTS AFFECTING RAT GRIP STRENGTH.

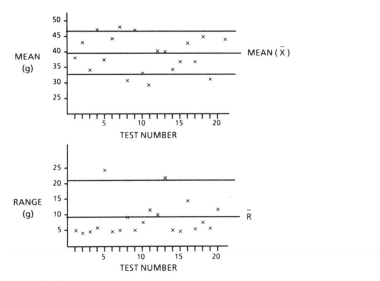

FIGURE 50   Example of control chart used to "prescreen" (actually, explore and identifying influential) data from a portion of a functional observational battery. The control chart is for means and range for control group in screening procedure for agents affecting rat grip strength. Possible individual scores range from 0 to 8. Group total scores would thus range from 0 to 40 (shown are the number of groups which contain individual scores in the indicated categories).

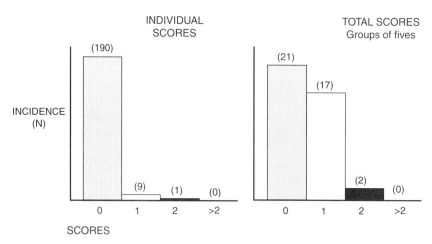

FIGURE 51   Example of a "central tendency" plot. Possible individual scores range from 0 to 8. Group total scores would thus range from 0 to 40 (shown are the number of groups which contain individual scores in the indicated categories).

TABLE 80   Identification Performance of Statistical Approaches

Data set	ANOVA	Contingency table	Rank sum	Control chart	Central tendency
		Results of analysis by method			
		Positives (truly neurologically active materials)			
1	−	−	−	+	+
2	−	−	−	+	+
3	−	−	−	+	+
4	−	−	−	+	+
5	−	−	−	+	+
6	−	−	−	+	+
7	−	−	−	+	+
8	+	−	+	+	+
9	−	−	−	+	+
10	−	−	−	+	+
11	−	+	+	+	+
12	−	−	−	+	+
13	−	+	+	+	+
14	+	+	+	+	+
15	−	+	+	+	+
16	−	+	+	+	+
17	−	−	−	+	+
18	−	−	−	+	+
19	−	−	−	+	+
20	−	−	−	+	+
21	−	−	−	+	+
		Negatives (materials for which no evidence of neurotoxicity was found)			
22	−	−	−	+	−
23	−	−	−	−	−
24	−	−	−	−	−
25	−	−	−	−	−
26	−	−	−	−	+

Note. +, Test detected effect; −, test did not detect effect.

scores of "0" fit into this category) and those that do critically influence the outcome of an analysis.

We can (and should) develop such plots for each of our variables. Simple inspection makes clear that "no effect" answers (0 values in the example central tendency plot) do not interest us or influence our identifying of an outlier in a group and should simply be set aside before continuing with analysis.

One can then focus on the rest of the data. In the 26 data set studied (Gad, 1988), a little over 50%, the number of data points was reduced from 174,750 to 10,403 (a reduction of ~94%). The summary results are shown in Table 80.

Focusing our efforts on the remainder, it becomes clear that though the incidence of a single nonzero observation in a group means nothing (that is, it occurs 40% of the time by chance), group scores of two or more occurred only 5% of the time by chance.

The approach of this method is then to develop a histogram for each ranked or quantal variable, both by individual and group. "Useless" data (that which will not influence the outcome of the analysis) is then identified and dropped from analysis. Group scores may then be simply evaluated against the baseline histograms to identify those groups with scores divergent enough from control to either be true positives or an acceptably low-incidence false positive. Additional control data can continue to be incorporated in such a system over time, both increasing the power of the analysis and providing a check on screen performance.

REFERENCES

Abramowitz, M., and Stegun, I. A. (1964). *Handbook of Mathematical Functions,* pp. 925–964. National Bureau of Standards, Washington, DC.

Anderson, S., and Hauck, W. W. (1983). A new procedure for testing equivalence in comparative bioavailability and other clinical trials. *Commun. Stat. Theor. Methods* 12, 2663–2692.

Annau, Z. (1972). The comparative effects of hypoxia and carbon monoxide hypoxia on behavior. In *Behavioral Toxicology,* (B. Weiss and V. G. Laties, Eds.), pp. 105–127. Plenum, New York.

Beyer, W. H. (1976). *Handbook of Tables for Probability and Statistics.* Chemical Rubber Co., Boca Raton, FL.

Bliss, C. I. (1935). The calculation of the dosage–mortality curve. *Ann. Appl. Biol.* 22, 134–167.

Boyd, E. M. (1972). *Predictive Toxicometrics.* Williams & Wilkins, Baltimore.

Boyd, E. M., and Knight, L. M. (1963). Postmortem shifts in the weight and water levels of body organs. *Toxicol. Appl. Pharmacol.* 5, 119–128.

Bruce, R. D. (1985). An up-and-down procedure for acute toxicity testing. *Fundam. Appl. Toxicol.* 5, 151–157.

Burt, G. S. (1972). Use of behavioral techniques in the assessment of environmental contaminants. In *Behavioral Toxicology* (B. Weiss and V. G. Laties, Eds.), pp. 241–263. Plenum, New York.

Chambers, J. M., Cleveland, W. S., Kliner, B., and Tukey, P. A. (1983). *Graphical Methods for Data Analysis.* Duxbury Press, Boston.

Debanne, S. M., and Haller, H. S. (1983). Evaluation of statistical methodologies for estimation of median effective dose. *Toxicol. Appl. Pharmacol.* 79, 274–282.

DePass, L. R., Myers, R. C., Weaver, E. V., and Weil, C. S. (1984). An assessment of the importance of number of dosage levels, number of animals per dosage level, sex and method of LD_{50} and slope calculations in acute toxicity studies. *Alternate Methods in Toxicology, Vol. 2: Acute Toxicity Testing: Alternate Approaches* (A. M. Goldberg, Ed.), pp. 139–154. Liebert, New York.

Diem, K., and Lentner, C. (1975). *Documenta Geigy Scientific Tables,* pp. 158–159. Geigy, New York.

Finney, D. K. (1977). *Probit Analysis,* 3rd ed. Cambridge Univ. Press, Cambridge, UK.

Gad, S. C. (1982a). Statistical analysis of behavioral toxicology data and studies. *Arch. Toxicol. Suppl.* 5, 256–266.

Gad, S. C. (1982b). A neuromuscular screen for use in industrial toxicology. *J. Toxicol. Environ. Health* 9, 691–704.

Gad, S. C. (1988). An approach to the design and analysis of screening studies in toxicology. *J. Am. Coll. Toxicol.* **8**, 127–138.

Gad, S. C., and Weil, C. S. (1988). *Statistics and Experimental Design for Toxicologists,* 2nd ed. CRC Press, Boca Raton, FL.

Gad, S. C., Conroy, W. J., McKelvey, J. A., and Turney, R. A. (1978). Behavioral and neuropharmacological toxicology of the macrocyclic ether 18-crown 6. *Drug Chem. Toxicol.* **1**, 339–354.

Gad, S. C., Smith, A. C., Cramp, A. L., Gavigan, F. A., and Derelanko, M. J. (1984). Innovative designs and practices for acute systemic toxicity studies. *Drug Chem. Toxicol.* **7**, 423–434.

Gad, S. C., Reilly, C., Siino, K. M., and Gavigan, F. A. (1985). Thirteen cationic ionophores: Their acute toxicity neurobehavioral and membrane effects. *Drug Chem. Toxicol.* **8**(6), 451–468.

Gad, S. C., Dunn, B. J., Gavigan, F. A., Reilly, C., and Peckham, J. C. (1997). Acute and neurotoxicity of 5,7,11-dodecariyn-1-ol and 5,7,11,13-octadecatetrayne-1, 18-diol. *J. Appl. Toxicol.* in press.

Gallant, A. R. (1975). Nonlinear regression. *Am. Stat.* **29**, 73–81.

Irwin, S. (1968). Comprehensive observational assessment. *Psychopharmacologia* **13**, 222–257.

Jackson, B. (1962). Statistical analysis of body weight data. *Toxicol. Appl. Pharmacol.* **4**, 432–443.

Johnson, B. L., Anger, W. K., Setzer, J. V., and Xinytaras, C. (1972). The application of a computer controlled time discrimination performance to problems. In *Behavioral Toxicology* (B. Weiss and V. G. Laties, Eds.), pp. 129–153. Plenum, New York.

Litchfield, J. T., and Wilcoxon, F. (1949). A simplified method of evaluating dose effect experimenta. *J. Pharmacol. Exp. Ther.* **96**, 99–113.

Norton, S. (1973). Amphetamine as a model for hyperactivity in the rat. *Physiol. Behav.* **11**, 181–186.

Pollard, J. H. (1977). *Numerical and Statistical Techniques.* Cambridge Univ. Press, New York.

Prentice, R. L. (1976). A generalization of the probit and logit methods for dose response curves. *Biometrics* **32**, 761–768.

Redman, C. (1981). Screening compounds for clinically active drugs. In *Statistics in the Pharmaceutical Industry* (C. R. Buncher and J. Tsay, Eds.), pp. 19–42. Dekker, New York.

Snedecor, G. W., and Cochran, W. G. (1980). *Statistical Methods,* 7th ed. Iowa State Univ. Press, Ames.

Sokal, R. R., and Rohlf, E. J. (1981). *Biometry.* Freeman, San Francisco.

Thompson, W. R., and Weil, C. S. (1952). On the construction of tables for moving average interpolation. *Biometrics* **8**, 51–54.

Tilson, H. A., Cabe, P. A., and Burne, T. A. (1980). Behavioral procedures for the assessment of neurotoxicity. In *Experimental and Clinical Neurotoxicology* (P. S. Spencer and N. H. Schaumburg, Eds.), pp. 758–766. Williams & Wilkins, Baltimore.

Weil, C. S. (1962). Applications of methods of statistical analysis to efficient repeated-dose toxicological tests. I. General considerations and problems involved. Sex differences in rat liver and kidney weights. *Toxicol. Appl. Pharmacol.* **4**, 561–571.

Weil, C. S. (1970). Selection of the valid number of sampling unit and a consideration of their combination in toxicological studies involving reproduction, teratognesis or carcinogenesis. *Fd. Cosmet. Toxicol.* **8**, 177–182.

Weil, C. S. (1972). Statistics vs. safety factors and scientific judgement in the evaluation of safety for man. *Toxicol. Appl. Pharmacol.* **21**, 459–472.

Weil, C. S. (1973). Experimental design and interpretation of data from prolonged toxicity studies. In *Proc. 5th Int. Congr. Pharmacol.,* Vol. 2, pp. 4–12. Beacon Press, San Francisco.

Weil, C. S. (1975). Toxicology experimental design and conduct as measured by interlaboratory collaboration studies. *J. Assoc. Off. Anal. Chem.* **58**, 687–688.

Weil, C. S., and Gad, S. C. (1980). Applications of methods of statistical analysis to efficient repeated-dose toxicologic tests. 2. Methods for analysis of body, liver and kidney weight data. *Toxicol. Appl. Pharmacol.* **52**, 214–226.

Weil, C. S., Carpenter, C. P., and Smyth, H. J. (1953). Specifications for calculating the median effective dose. *Am. Ind. Hyg. Assoc. Q.* **14**, 200–206.

Zar, J. H. (1974). *Biostatistical Analysis*, p. 50. Prentice-Hall, Englewood Cliffs, NJ.

Zbinden, G., and Flury-Roversi, M. (1981). Significance of the LD_{50} test for the toxicological evaluation of chemical substances. *Arch. Toxicol.* **47**, 77–99.

CHAPTER 13

Acute Inhalation

Inhalation is, in many senses, a special-case route of administration for toxicology as a whole and for acute toxicology in particular. As will be reviewed here, animal inhalation studies are difficult and complex to perform correctly. Generally, only two broad types of acute studies are performed using this route (the acute systemic exposure and the pulmonary sensitization/irritation study), and, typically, such acute toxicology studies are not performed well. The complexity and cost of such studies firmly dictates that they be performed only when there are substantial opportunities for human inhalation exposure. Such opportunities occur under three broad categories. In order of decreasing occurrence or importance, these are occupational (from the workplace, either in the normal course of operations or during maintenance or accident situations), environmental (a spectacular example being Bhophal), or when the material is to be used as a therapeutic by this route.

GENERAL PRINCIPLES

Types of Exposure

All inhalation studies, including acute ones, can be classified in two ways—either by the pattern of exposure or by the physical nature of the test atmosphere. Both of these classifications are important because they dictate equipment, animal selection, and details of study design.

Pattern refers to how (or how much of) a test animal is exposed to the atmosphere of interest. In practice, there are only very limited situations in which exposure to a toxicant is purely by inhalation (these cases are with therapeutics when an individual has a material administered directly into the nasal or oral cavity and with an inhalation test system, where only nose exposure is truly achieved). Rather, both in the real world and in the laboratory, inhalation exposure is accompanied by certain degrees of dermal and oral exposure. How concerned one is with the possible confounding effects of such other route exposures on the evaluation of biological outcome dictates selection of pattern of exposure.

The three major categories of exposure patterns used for acute studies are nose only, head only, and whole body. There are also minor routes (intratracheal or lung only and partial lung) which will not be discussed here because they are not routinely used in acute toxicity studies. They see use only in special research settings, allowing precise delivery of doses of test material directly to the lungs.

In "nose only," the test animal is situated so that only its nasal region (or, for dogs and primates, where a mask is used to administer test compound, only the mouth and nasal region) is exposed to a test atmosphere. This can be achieved by having the animal restrained with only its nose poking into a small stream of test atmosphere such as the rat shown in Fig. 52 or with a breathing mask fitted over the nose and mouth region. There is still some small amount of oral exposure in such a system because animals will swallow any material deposited on the surface of their mouths or "cleared" from the nasal region or lungs back into the trachea.

Head-only exposure, which is somewhat more common, allows a bit more potential for oral and dermal exposure. In such a system, the animal's entire head, "airlocked" off from the rest of its body by some form of elastic barrier or collar, is in a chamber into which a test atmosphere is introduced (as illustrated by the rat in Fig. 52). Dogs and monkeys can be trained to accept exposure via a face mask, but these species are rarely used for acute toxicology studies.

Whole body exposure, in which the entire animal is in a chamber into which a test atmosphere is introduced, is the least complicated pattern of

HEAD AND NOSE ONLY INHALATION CHAMBER DESIGNS

Bell Jar:

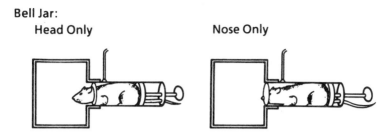

Head Only   **Nose Only**

Pulmonary Irritation/Sensitization "tube":

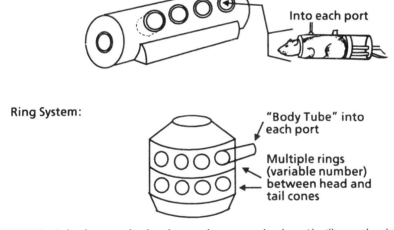

Into each port

Ring System:

"Body Tube" into each port

Multiple rings (variable number) between head and tail cones

FIGURE 52 Stylized common head- and nose-only exposure chambers. Also illustrated are head- and nose-only exposure in the rat.

exposure. As will be seen later, there are a wide variety of chamber designs available such that all common laboratory species can be exposed using this methodology. There will be extensive dermal and oral administration in animals exposed whole body (particularly oral in rodents and rabbits which carefully "preen" themselves after an exposure). For gases and vapors, of course, such considerations have minimal impact.

The advantages and disadvantages associated with each of these exposure patterns are summarized in Table 81.

The other manner of classifying inhalation studies is in terms of the exposure

TABLE 81   Advantages, Disadvantages, and Considerations Associated with Patterns of Inhalation Exposure

Mode of exposure	Advantages	Disadvantages	Design considerations
Whole body	Variety and number of animals Chronic studies possible Minimum restraint Large historical database Controllable environment Minimum stress Minimum labor	Messy Multiple routes of exposure: skin, eyes, oral Variability of "dose" Cannot pulse exposure easily Poor contact between animals and investigators Capital intensive Inefficient compound usage Difficult to monitor animals during exposure	Cleaning effluent air Inert materials Losses of test material Even distribution in space Sampling Animal care Observation Noise, vibration, humidity Air temperature Safe exhaust Loading Reliability
Head only	Good for repeated exposure Limited routes of entry into animal More efficient dose delivery	Stress to animal Losses can be large Seal around neck Labor in loading/unloading	Even distribution Pressure fluctuations Sampling and losses Air temperature, humidity Animal comfort Animal restraint
Nose/mouth only	Exposure limited to mouth and respiratory tract Uses less material (efficient) Containment of material Can pulse the exposure	Stress to animal Seal about face Effort to expose large number of animals	Pressure fluctuations Body temperature Sampling Airlocking Animals comfort Losses in plumbing/masks
Lung only (Tracheal administration)	Precision of dose One route of exposure Uses less material (efficient) Can pulse the exposure	Technically difficult Anesthesia or tracheostomy Limited to small numbers Bypasses nose Artifacts in deposition and response Technically more difficult	Air humidity/temperature Stress to the animal Physiologic support
Partial lung	Precision of total dose Localization of dose Can achieve very high local doses Unexposed control tissue from same animal	Anesthesia Placement of dose Difficulty in interpretation of results Technically difficult Possible redistribution of material within lung	Stress to animal Physiologic support

Note. Modified after Phalen (1976).

"media"—that is, the physical nature of the contaminant atmosphere that is being evaluated. Though several of these categories can be subdivided or defined somewhat differently, for our purposes in this chapter the types of possible test atmosphere are gases, aerosols, and dusts (with the special case of smokes being presented separately as part of the last chapter in this book).

Gases are generally the easiest type of exposures to perform because the contaminants in the test atmosphere are in the gaseous phase. This makes handling and manipulating the atmosphere relatively easy. There are two subcategories, however (based on the predominant physical state of test material under "ambient" conditions). These are "true" gases (which can be metered from tanks or generated simply from a highly volatile liquid) and vapors (where the test material is a liquid of low volability). Generating vapors can be a very difficult problem.

Technically, aerosols include any liquid or solid-phase material which forms a stable suspension in air. Using this definition, and depending on the size of the particles or droplets involved, there is a wide range of subcategories and materials that can be of concern (as illustrated in Figure 53). For our purposes here, however, aerosols mean only liquid-phase materials. These are generally more difficult to properly conduct an exposure of but not as difficult as the final category.

Dusts are solid-phase (contaminant) particles suspended into a gaseous

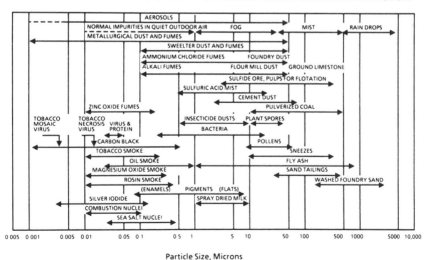

AERODYNAMIC PARAMTERS OF COMMON ENVIRONMENTAL AIRBORNE AEROSOLS

Particle Size, Microns

FIGURE 53 Classes of particles and liquid aerosols with potential for inhalation, displayed in order of relative sizes.

(atmosphere) phase. They are generally the most difficult to conduct a proper study with for reasons which will become obvious. Fibers represent a subcategory of dusts which represent an even more difficult special case.

BASIC STEPS

A technically good inhalation exposure can be broken into four major basic steps. One can consider these four problems which must be solved before an actual study is undertaken. In fact, it is this aspect of inhalation which makes the proper conduct of such studies difficult and expensive. The steps are

Generation of a test atmosphere
Containment, mixing, and movement of test atmosphere and animals (both before and after exposure)
Measurement and characterization of what animals have been exposed to (dosimetry)
Cleanup and disposal of resulting "wastes" (gaseous, solid, and liquid)

Each of the first three of these steps will be discussed in further detail in this chapter, while the fourth is beyond the scope of the objectives of this book (the reader is referred to Leong, 1981, and Nelson, 1971, for the subject of cleanup and disposal).

First, however, some basic information on the behavior of gases (and of other phases suspended in gases) and of respiratory physiology should be reviewed.

GAS LAWS

Gases are generally the easiest materials to handle. Supplied as either tanks of pressurized gas or as a readily volatilized liquid, it is easy to achieve the desirable characteristics of a generation system (discussed later) usually by simply metering the gas into an airstream, ensuring mixing, and feeding the result into an inhalation chamber.

The behavior of gases is generally characterized by the gas laws, which assume the gas acts as an ideal gas. Under laboratory conditions, such predictions are usually so close to the actual behavior of gases that any variation is minor.

Pressure, Temperature, and Volume

The relationship between the pressure and volume of a gas at a constant temperature is described by Boyle's law, which states that the volume, V, is inversely proportional to the pressure, P:

$$V = K(1/P) \tag{A}$$

where K is a proportionality constant, or

$$P_1V_1 = P_2V_2 \tag{B}$$

The relationship between the temperature and volume of a gas at a constant pressure is described by Charles' law, which states that the volume is directly proportional to the absolute temperature, T:

$$V = KT \tag{C}$$

A more general equation involving all three variables can be obtained by combining Eqs. (A) and (C):

$$PV = KT \tag{D}$$

or

$$\frac{P_1V_1}{T_1} = \frac{P_2V_2}{T_2} \tag{E}$$

if K is proportional to the number of moles of gas, n, then

$$PV = nRT \tag{F}$$

which is the well-known ideal gas law. The most commonly used values of the molar gas constant, R, can be found in handbooks or in Nelson (1971).

Density

The calculation of gas density is important both for correcting flow rates and for determining how well gases conform to the ideal gas law. If W is the weight and M is the molecular weight, then

$$n = W/M \tag{G}$$

Equation F then becomes

$$PV = WRT/M \tag{H}$$

or

$$W/V = PM/RT \tag{I}$$

where W/V is the ideal gas density. The calculated densities of some of the more common gases can be found in handbooks or in Nelson (1971).

Concentration

The concentrations of gas and vapor mixtures are almost always expressed in units of percentage or parts per million of volume, although in some air pollution, industrial hygiene, and animal toxicology work the most convenient unit may be weight per unit volume. For concentrations above 0.1%, the concentration, C, is usually expressed in percentage. This can be calculated for ideal gases by

$$C\% = \frac{10^2\, v_a}{v_a + v_b + \cdots = v_n} = \frac{10^2\, p_a}{p_a + p_b + \cdots p_n} \qquad (J)$$

where $v_{a,b}\cdots_n$ and $p_{a,b}\cdots_n$ are the volumes and partial pressures of components, a, b, $\cdots$, n at a constant temperature. For concentrations below 0.1%, the concentration is usually expressed in parts per million by volume (i.e., the number of parts by volume of trace gas in a million parts of gas mixture). This can be calculated for ideal gases by

$$C_{ppm} = \frac{10^6\, v_a}{v_D + v_a} = \frac{10^6\, p_a}{p_D + p_a} \qquad (K)$$

where v_D and p_D are the volume and pressure of the diluent gas. The v_a and the p_a terms are usually neglected when dealing with concentrations below 5000 parts per million because their contribution to the total volume is usually insignificant. However, above 5000 parts per million, the contaminant gas becomes more dominant and its volume must be included in the total gas volume. Table 82 illustrates how the numerical value of the concentration is

TABLE 82   Concentration by Volume of Gas A in a Mixture of Gases A and B

Based on total volume of gases A and B $(v_D + v_a)$		Based on volume of gas B (v_D) only	
%	ppm	%	ppm
0.0001	1	0.0001000001	1.000001
0.001	10	0.00100001	10.0001
0.01	100	0.010001	100.01
0.1	1,000	0.1001	1,001
0.5	5,000	0.5025	5,025
1	10,000	1.010	10,100
10	100,000	11.11	111,100
20	200,000	25	250,000
50	500,000	100	1,000,000
100	1,000,000	—	—

altered depending on whether or not the trace-gas volume is included in the denominator of Eq. (K).

Concentration can also be calculated when a known weight or volume of a liquid is vaporized in a known volume of a diluent gas. If the liquid has a weight, W, and a molecular weight, M, and if it is evaporated at a pressure, P, and a temperature, T, then the volume of vapor produced is given by

$$v_a = \frac{WRT}{MP} \tag{L}$$

If v_a is diluted with v_p, then the resulting concentration on a volume percentage basis is determined by the equation

$$C\% = \frac{10^2 v_a}{v_a + v_d} = \frac{10^2 \dfrac{WRT}{MP}}{WRT + v_d/MP} = \frac{10^2}{v_d{}^m/1 + WRT} \tag{M}$$

Similarly, the concentration in parts per million by volume is determined as

$$C_{ppm} = \frac{10^6 v_a}{v_D} = \frac{10^6 \dfrac{WRT}{MP}}{v_D} \tag{N}$$

Usually, W is expressed in terms of the volume of liquid, v_L, and density, D_L. Equation (N) then becomes

$$C_{ppm} = \frac{10^6 v_L D_L RT}{v_D MP} \tag{O}$$

At room temperature (25°C) and pressure (760 mm Hg), this reduces to

$$C_{ppm} = \frac{24.5 \times 10^6 v_L D_L}{v_D M} \tag{P}$$

Concentration is sometimes expressed in units of weight per unit volume (weight per unit volume is usually given in units of milligrams per cubic meter) when the concentration of aerosols such as metal fumes, mists, or dusts in air or some other supporting gas is being measured. Copper, lead, and iron fumes are prime examples. Such concentration is calculated by

$$C_{w/v} = \frac{W}{v_D} \tag{Q}$$

which is related to concentration in parts per million by

$$C_{w/w} = \frac{10^{-6}C_{ppm}MP}{RT} \tag{R}$$

and to vapor pressure by

$$C_{w/v} = \frac{p_a MP}{p_D RT} \tag{S}$$

Usually, however, P_D closely approximates P. Equation S, therefore, simplifies to

$$C_{w/v} = \frac{P_a M}{PT} \tag{T}$$

Nonideal Pressure

Most gases adhere closely to the ideal gas law at room temperature and atmospheric pressure. However, for the best accuracy with mixed gases, deviations from ideality must be taken into account, especially at high pressures. This is accomplished by comparing the actual gas density, D_A, with the ideal density, D_i, and the actual gas volume, v_A, with the ideal density, D_p, under the same conditions. The actual gas volume, v_A, can then be corrected to the ideal volume, v_i, and can be used to make precise gas mixtures using the equation

$$v_i = Kv_A = \frac{D_A}{D_i} v_A \tag{U}$$

At 0°C and 760 mm Hg, D_i can be found from

$$D_i = \frac{M}{22.414} \tag{V}$$

Tables of values for D_A, D_i, and D_A/D_i under standard conditions can be found in Nelson (1971).

Behavior of the Secondary Phase in a Gas

Aerosol and dust behavior can be described similarly for our purposes here. The two most important characteristics of an aerosol or dust are aerodynamic size (Stoke's diameter) and density. Particle shape, in the special case of fibers (a fiber being defined as a particle with a length greater than three times its width), is also important, as is hydroscopic behavior when it is extreme.

The importance of these characteristics arises from the fact that deep lung penetration is generally important to ensure maximum biological effect, and these characteristics help determine how deep penetration will be. The respira-

COMPARTMENTAL MODEL OF THE RESPIRATORY TRACT
(HUMAN)

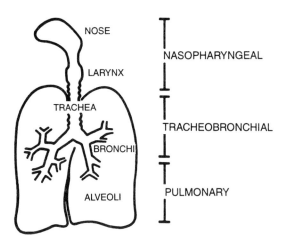

FIGURE 54   Comparative model of human respiratory tract, showing the three major divisions and their structural components.

tory tract is generally broken down into three regions—the nasopharynx (NP), tracheobronchial region (TB), and pulmonary region (or deep lung). There are five general mechanisms for the deposition of particles in the respiratory tract; three of these are illustrated schematically in Fig. 54.

The five mechanisms of particle deposition in the respiratory tract are presented in Table 83.

Some important interrelationships between these mechanisms and secondary considerations are presented in Table 84 (after Morrow, 1960).

When a particle comes in contact with the surface of the respiratory tract,

TABLE 83   Mechanism of Respiratory Deposition of Particles

Direct interception	When a particle physically cannot transit a portion of the respiratory tract
	Important only for fibers as they pass from one tube to another
Inertial impaction	Particularly important for dense particle
	Usually occurs near tube bifurcations (i.e., where passages divide)
Sedimentation	Primarily a gravity effect
Diffusion	Particles less than 0.5 μ in diameter and of medium to low density
	Primarily deep pulmonary
Electrostatic	Special case for unusual particles that accumulate charges

TABLE 84 Primary Factors Involved in the Respiratory Toxicology of Particulate Matter

Factor	Particles involved (in humans)	Related factors	Deposition factors	Special considerations
Sedimentation	>0.1 to <50 μm	Particle shape and density, particulate concentration (aggregation), "slip," hygroscopicity	To cause dust deposition in nasal pharynx and tracheal–bronchial tree	Highly significant in toxicological studies, probably the most important deposition factor
Inertia	<50 μm	Same as above plus relative velocities of particle and air	Same as above with tendency to promote earlier deposition	Especially significant with soluble or absorbable dusts
Diffusion	>0.002 to <0.5 μm	Electric charge, hygroscopicity, particle concentration (aggregation), thermal gradients	Dust deposition where large and intimate surfaces involved, viz. lung bronchioles and parenchyma	Most important when dust is insoluble and submicron in size. Also significant when these dusts serve as "carriers"
Respiratory frequency	All sizes	Air velocities, residence times, turbulence, dead space ventilation	Increasing tends to decrease deposition (possible very high rates, e.g., >20 may increase deposition)	Exercise, physical labor, and heated environs will have variable effects on subjects but, in general, will tend to increase both these factors together
Tidal volume	All sizes	Number of particles, alveolar ventilation, residence time	Increasing tends to increase deposition (even at constant minute volume)	

TABLE 85 Relative Importance of Mechanisms

Region	Process			
	Interception	Impaction[a]	Sedimentation	Diffusion
NP	+++		+	
TB	++	+	++	++
Pulmonary		++	++	+++

[a]Primarily for fibers.

the moist surface (and surface tension associated with that surface) prevents the particle (or droplet) from rejoining the airstream and, therefore, makes contact synonomous with deposition. The importance of the four major factors in deposition of particles in the different regions of the respiratory tract is presented in Table 85.

The three major regions of the respiratory tract referred to in Table 85 are illustrated (as they occur in humans) in Fig. 54. Figure 55 gives a graphic display of the distribution of deposition of particles/droplets of a range of sizes in each of the three regions.

BASICS OF RESPIRATORY PHYSIOLOGY

It is the need for oxygen in the final steps of cellular oxidation–reductions of the cytochrome system that makes it such an essential material for all animals.

PARTICLE SIZE DEPOSITION PROBABILITIES FOR PARTICLES OF VARYING SIZES

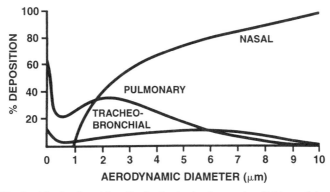

FIGURE 55 Particle size deposition distribution in the three major divisions of the respiratory tract of humans.

Carbon dioxide is a gaseous by-product of the oxidation of protein, carbohydrate, and lipids. Oxygen consumption and carbon dioxide production are nearly inseparable activities, and together they constitute animal respiration.

Animal respiration is divided into three phases: (1) external respiration—the mechanisms by which an animal obtains oxygen from the external environment and the mechanisms by which carbon dioxide is eliminated to the external environment; (2) gas transport—the mechanisms used to distribute oxygen to all of the body cells of an animal after it has been extracted from the external environment by the respiratory organs and also the mechanisms by which carbon dioxide is transported from body cells to sites of elimination; and (3) internal respiration—the metabolic reactions of oxidation–reduction in which oxygen is consumed and carbon dioxide (and energy) is produced. For our purposes, we are concerned only with the first two of these phases.

To understand animal respiration, we must consider not only the nature of the respiratory organs but also the mechanisms used to control respiration and the nature of respiratory system adaptations to different environments. As with other homeostatic functions, respiration in the animal must be integrated with and coordinated to all of other regulatory activities. Gas transport mechanisms, in addition to providing a route by which oxygen and carbon dioxide may be transported, also in many animals serve as part of the pH regulating mechanism.

As is true of other homeostatic systems, the respiratory organs and their controls have received the most attention in the vertebrates and especially in mammals. Thus, much of the detail of this discussion will be based on respiration in these groups.

OXYGEN DIFFUSION AND SOLUBILITY

Oxygen diffuses only very slowly through aqueous media, and diffusion alone is an unsatisfactory mechanism for removing oxygen from the external environment and supplying it to all body cells. Only if the organism is smaller than about 1 mm in diameter is diffusion adequate to supply its oxygen requirements. This does not mean that diffusion of respiratory gases is not an important part of respiratory activity. Diffusion is the basic mechanism by which oxygen or carbon dioxide cross respiratory membranes or move from body fluids into cells; however, diffusion must be aided by other mechanisms that ensure a constant supply of oxygen for the animal and removal of carbon dioxide. In all larger organisms there is a need for specialized vascular surfaces for extracting oxygen from the environment and mechanisms for moving the medium so that the greatest possible oxygen supply is available.

The amount of oxygen required by an animal depends on its size—smaller animals have a higher metabolic rate per unit of body weight and therefore usually require more oxygen on a unit weight basis than do larger animals). However, the activity of an animal also determines its oxygen needs. Table 86 illustrates this point.

Oxygen diffusion is relatively slow in water compared with its diffusion in air. The diffusion coefficient at 20°C for oxygen in air is about 11; in water the diffusion coefficient is about 0.00003; in a tissue such as muscle the diffusion coefficient is about 0.00001.

The solubility of oxygen in water is much less than its concentration in the atmosphere. The atmosphere contains about 20 times as much oxygen as can be dissolved in a similar volume of water. This means that, compared with an air-breather, an aquatic animal must pass a much greater volume of the medium over its respiratory surfaces in order to obtain a given volume of oxygen. In addition, the density and viscosity of aqueous media are greater than those of air, and thus more work must be done to move the aqueous medium in order to obtain oxygen.

The carbon dioxide content of natural water is very low, often zero; and because carbon dioxide is very soluble in water and has a much higher rate of diffusion than oxygen, the concentration gradient of carbon dioxide between the animal and its environment is favorable for the diffusion of carbon dioxide from the animal. Because the terrestrial atmosphere also contains only a very low carbon dioxide concentration, about 0.04%, the elimination of carbon dioxide from an animal is generally not as much of a problem as the obtaining of oxygen. Carbon dioxide in water is converted to carbonic acid via the enzyme carbonic anhydrase, then almost immediately breaks down to bicarbonate and hydrogen ion, and this buffering action serves to maintain a higher pH of aqueous media compared with the pH that would result from the presence of the acidic carbon dioxide itself. The conversion of carbon dioxide to bicarbonate also serves to lower the carbon dioxide concentration of aqueous environments, thus maintaining a favorable concentration gradient for diffusion from the animal.

TABLE 86 Oxygen Consumption of Some Animals

Organism	Weight	Temperature (°C)	Oxygen consumption (ml/g wet weight/hour)
Vertebrates (homeothermic)			
Mouse	20 g	37	2.5 (rest)
			20 (running)
Man	70 kg	37	0.2 (rest)
			4.0 (max. work)

The oxygen content of water varies according to both temperature and salt concentration. A 2.9% NaCl solution can contain, maximally, 40 ml O_2 per liter when equilibrated with oxygen at 0°C and at 1 atm; pure water under these same conditions can hold 50 ml O_2 per liter.

The higher the temperature, the less the amount of oxygen (or other gas) a given volume of water can contain. This means that at higher temperatures, the amount of oxygen available to aquatic animals decreases. Tables 87 and 88 illustrate the relations between gas concentrations, temperature, and salinity. Concentrations are expressed in terms of the absorption coefficient—that is, the amount of gas which could dissolve in a given volume of water when the pressure of the gas is 1 atm. The volumes are given in terms of normal temperature (0°C) and pressure (1 atm = 760 mm Hg). The volume of gas that can dissolve decreases in proportion to decreases in its pressure. This is true regardless of the presence of other gases (see Table 87).

GAS VOLUMES AND PRESSURES

Normal atmospheric pressure at sea level can support a column of mercury 760 mm in height (760 mm Hg pressure = 1 atm). The atmosphere is composed of 78.09% nitrogen, 20.95% oxygen, 0.93% argon, and 0.031% carbon dioxide (percentages here are mole % = volume %). The atmosphere contains an average water vapor content with a pressure of 5 mm Hg. On the basis of

TABLE 87   Solubilities of Gases in Various Salt Solutions

Solution	Oxygen	Carbon dioxide	Nitrogen
NaCl solution			
0 g NaCl/kg solution	$0.049^{0,a}$	1.713^0	0.0235^0
	0.0374^{12}	1.117^{12}	0.179^{12}
	0.0288^{24}	0.718^{24}	0.0145^{24}
28.91 NaCl/kg solution	0.041^0	1.489^0	0.152^0
	0.0306^{12}	0.980^{12}	0.0116^{12}
	0.0248^{24}	0.695^{24}	0.695^{24}
36.11 g NaCl/kg solution	0.0380^0	1.439^0	0.0142^0
	0.0291^{12}	0.980^{12}	0.0110^{12}
	0.0236^{24}	0.677^{24}	0.0089^{24}
Ringer's solution	0.0480^0		
	0.0340^{10}		
	0.0310^{20}		
	0.0260^{30}		

Note. Sea water (34.96 salinity) 6.89 ml O_2 liter (= 9.8 mg per liter).
[a]Superscripts are temperatures (°C).

TABLE 88   Vapor Pressure of Water

Temperature	P_{H_2O}	Temperature	P_{H_2O}
0	4.579	20	17.535
1	4.926	21	18.650
2	5.294	22	19.827
3	5.865	23	21.068
4	6.101	24	22.377
5	6.543	25	23.756
6	7.103	26	25.209
7	7.513	27	26.739
8	8.045	28	28.349
9	8.609	29	30.043
10	9.209	30	31.824
11	9.844	31	33.695
12	10.518	32	35.668
13	11.231	33	37.729
14	11.987	34	39.898
15	12.788	35	42.175
16	13.634	36	44.563
17	14.530	37	47.067
18	15.477	38	47.692
19	16.477	39	52.442

containing water vapor, the nitrogen content is 79.02%, oxygen 20.94%, and carbon dioxide 0.04%. On any basis, the atmosphere is composed almost entirely of nitrogen and oxygen with argon and carbon dioxide making up less than 1% of the atmospheric composition.

As discussed earlier, each component in a mixture of gases contributes to the total pressure in direct proportion to its percentage of the composition (Dalton's law, as discussed earlier). The pressure exerted by nitrogen at sea level is (0.7902) (760 mm Hg) = 600.55 Hg. Partial pressures are symbolized as P_{N_2}, where the subscript indicates the gas under discussion. The partial pressure of oxygen in the atmosphere is 159.16 mm Hg, and the partial pressure of carbon dioxide is 0.30 mm Hg. When the total pressure of a gas mixture is 760 mm Hg, the partial pressure of any given gaseous component may be calculated from:

$$P_x = \frac{x}{100} P$$

where P_x is the partial pressure of the gas, P is the total pressure of the gas mixture, and x is the percentage volume of the given gas.

The partial pressure of a gas is dependent on the amount of water vapor present in the gas mixture. The higher the temperature, the more water evaporates per unit time, and such water vapor takes up volume within the gas mixture, thus changing the proportion of gases present. Atmospheric gases are usually dried before measurements are made, and their contents are usually expressed in terms of dry air. To calculate partial pressure of respiratory gases, the water vapor pressure is first subtracted from the total atmospheric pressure. Table 88 gives water vapor pressures at some different temperatures.

For example, consider that during inspiration in humans atmospheric air enters the lungs, which are at a temperature of about 37°C, and the atmospheric air becomes saturated with water vapor. To calculate the partial pressure of oxygen, the water vapor pressure at 37°C is subtracted from the atmospheric pressure: $760 - 47 = 713$ mm Hg. The P_{O_2} is then equal to $(713) (0.2095) = 149.4$ mm Hg. On a similar basis, the P_{CO_2} is zero, and P_{N_2} is 564 mm Hg.

Gas volumes, of course, depend on both temperature and pressure. In order to compare gas volumes, measured volumes are usually converted to normal temperature and pressure. Normal temperature is taken as 0°C, and normal pressure is 760 mm Hg.

When a gas is dissolved in a liquid, the term gas tension is used to indicate the content of gas within the liquid. Gas tensions are dependent on the partial pressure of the gas above the liquid in the atmosphere and are usually expressed in terms of the gas partial pressure.

THE MAMMALIAN RESPIRATORY SYSTEM

Structure

Because of the relative simplicity of the methods of analysis and its amenability to quantitative analysis, the mammalian respiratory system is probably the best understood physiological system. The structure and function of the human respiratory system will be the one principally described here. It is the best understood and is generally similar to other mammalian respiratory systems.

The lungs serve other functions than that of gas exchange. As already noted, they are involved in temperature regulation and water loss. In addition to providing a site for gaseous exchange, the lungs also serve to warm incoming air and to saturate it with water vapor.

Air enters the body through the mouth and nose; the latter possesses mucous membranes that filter foreign particles from the entering air. The air then passes through the pharynx, through the open glottis, through the larynx, and into the trachea—a large tube held open by rings of cartilage that encircle it transversely.

The trachea enters the thoracic cavity and branches into two major air passages, the bronchi, one of which leads to each lung. The bronchi ramify profusely, finally forming smaller tubes, the bronchioles. Except for the smallest terminal bronchioles, all of these tubes have cartilaginous rings. Bronchioles are also equipped with smooth muscle fibers. The terminal bronchioles lead into an expanded portion known as the atrium and from the atrium a number of alveoli open.

The lungs are masses of spongy and elastic tissues and lie in the airtight thoracic cavity. The lungs are enclosed by the viscereal pleura, a layer of connective tissue anatomically contiguous with the pericardium. The pleura is another membranous layer lying next to the thoracic cage. Between the two pleura is a thin layer of fluid that lubricates the lungs and membranes during their movements.

Ribs form the side walls of the thoracic cage, and between the ribs are intercostal muscles that can cause movements of the ribs. The base of the thorax is formed from the diaphragm, a sheet of muscle. The diaphragm is cone shaped in the relaxed condition of the diaphragm muscle fibers.

The intercostal muscles are innervated by intercostal nerves derived from the thoracic region of the spinal cord. The diaphragm is innervated by the phrenic nerves derived from a plexus in the cervical region. These muscles and nerves are the main respiratory apparatus. When breathing is heavy, as in exercise, accessory respiratory muscles of the abdominal wall and upper chest are called into play.

Lungs

The lungs are elastic bodies that can return to their normal shape after a deforming force is removed. The inflation of the lungs is accompanied by an increase in potential energy. The conversion of this potential energy into kinetic energy during deflation provides part of the force needed to expel gas. The lungs may be considered as passive elements in the ventilation process, although their elasticity plays a major role in ventilation. It may be noted that the lungs of mammals are inflated by the development of negative pressures in contrast to the positive pressure systems of frogs and lungfish.

The elasticity of the lungs has been studied by filling them with air or saline solution and measuring the resulting pressure under static conditions. When volume is plotted against pressure, a straight line results whose slope is a measure of the stiffness (compliance); i.e., the change in volume per unit change in pressure per centimeter of water. It is found that the pressure necessary to enlarge the lungs to a given volume is less when the lungs are filled with liquid than when they are filled with air. There is not as much elastic recoil in a liquid-filled lung. Such differences depend on surface tension differences, which in turn are dependent on the nature of the interfaces present. In the liquid–liquid interface condition present when the lungs are filled with a liquid, the surface tension is greatly reduced and depends only on the elasticity of the lungs. When a gas–liquid interface is present, as in the air-filled lung, the compliance includes both the elastic properties of the lungs and the significant surface tension of the interface.

The surface tension is caused by a film of liquid that layers the alveolar surfaces of the lungs. At an interface the attractive forces between molecules are directed downward and sideways more than upward, and this surface force is the surface tension. Laplace showed how the surface tension, T, is related to the pressure, P, and the radius, r, in an object such as a soap bubble ($4T=Pr$). If two bubbles have different radii, the pressure in the larger will be less than that of the smaller. Also, when two such bubbles are connected, the small bubble will empty into the larger. Alveoli have different sizes, and with a uniform surface tension it would be expected that small alveoli would empty into large ones, but this does not normally occur.

The stability of alveoli is produced by the presence of a surface coating, a surfactant, which causes a nonlinear change in surface tension with surface area. As the lungs are filled with air, alveoli that are most inflated have higher surface tensions than do those that are underdistended. This serves to stabilize alveoli of different sizes.

The surface coating of mammalian alveoli is a complex of proteins with dipalmityl lecithin. Whereas surfactants have been most intensively studied in mammals, such substances have also been found in all birds, reptiles, and amphibians studied.

Ventilation

Because the air space in the lungs directly connects with the outside air, the pressure within the lungs (the intrapleural pressure) will be equal to the atmospheric pressure, unless some volume change occurs in the lungs.

Contraction of the inspiratory muscles (the diaphragm and external inter-costal muscles) enlarges the thoracic cavity and causes a reduced pressure between the lungs and the thoracic wall (the intrathoracic pressure). This reduction causes the lungs to expand and reduces the intrapleural pressure. The alveoli and bronchioles expand, and air at atmospheric pressure flows through the upper respiratory tract and into the alveoli and bronchioles, where the pressure has been reduced below atmospheric by the expansion.

The intrapulmonic pressure is the force causing movement of air into and out of the lungs and is the pressure gradient between the lung spaces and the atmosphere. When the diaphragm contracts, the sheet of muscle flattens, lowering the floor of the thoracic cavity and thereby increasing its volume. Under these conditions intrapulmonic pressure is reduced, and air flows into the lungs.

The external intercostal muscles cause a rotation of the ribs upward and laterally and a movement of the sternum forward. These actions increase the circumference of the thoracic cavity and thus enlarge its volume also.

To expire air, the inspiratory muscles relax, and the thoracic cavity returns to its normal volume. The elastic recoil of the lungs aid in restoring them to their deflated volume. These forces increase the intrapulmonic pressure and cause air to move from the lungs, through the upper respiratory tract and into the atmosphere.

These are the ventilation movements responsible for bringing fresh air into the lungs and into contact with the alveolar surfaces and for removing the stale air during exhalation.

The volume of air that can be taken into the lungs can be measured by any of the many forms of spirometers. The vital capacity is the volume of air expired by the most forceful expiration after a maximal inspiration. It is the total moveable air in the lungs. The residual volume is the amount of air remaining in the lungs after the most forceful expiration and amounts to about 1.5 liters in humans. The total lung volume is the sum of the vital capacity and the residual volume and amounts to about 6 liters in humans. The tidal volume is the actual amount of air moved at each cycle of inspiration–expiration. It varies according to the needs of the organism and is about 500 ml in humans at rest. The dead space is a volume of about 150 ml in man where air remains in those parts ot the respiratory tract, such as the bronchi, where no gas exchange can occur. This is illustrated in Fig. 56.

All of these ventilation movements are designed to bring fresh air into the alveoli, where oxygen can diffuse down its concentration gradient into the oxygen-depleted venous blood and where carbon dioxide can diffuse from the blood into the air for elimination to the atmosphere.

It is worth noting that a standardized set of symbols has been developed for describing respiratory activities and gas exchanges and is used for describing circulatory actions as well. These symbols are, however, beyond the scope of this chapter.

Respiration is controlled by the central nervous system. Both the pneumotaxic and apneustic centers are probably innervated by ascending neurons from the medulla. At one time it was thought that stretch reflexes (the Hering–Breuer reflexes) were responsible for the rhythmic respiratory action. Stretch receptors in the lungs respond to the degree of inflation or stretch of the lungs and send impulses through vagal fibers to the respiratory center of the medulla. These impulses inhibit the inspiratory center, and its output to the inspiratory muscles is stopped. There is a time delay in response to muscle stretch, and inspiration can reach completion before the inspiratory center is inhibited. This is a positive feedback control. It is not considered to create the rhythmicity of breathing because the receptors respond only to relatively extreme degrees of

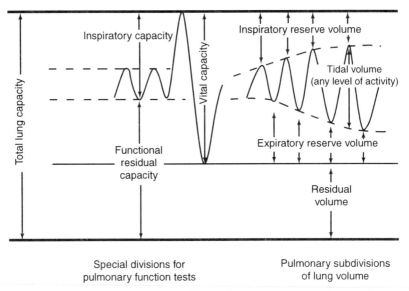

FIGURE 56 Diagrammatic representation of lung volumes and capacities of mammals as measured with a spirometer, with definitions of key functional terms.

stretch, and additionally transection of the vagus nerves does not inhibit this rhythmic action.

Other sensory inputs affect breathing rates. Especially important are chemoreceptors and baroreceptors located in the carotid sinus and aortic arch. Impulses from these receptors are carried by the vagus and glossopharyngeal nerves to the medullary centers. Chemoreceptors of the carotid sinus and aortic arch are sensitive to the P_{O_2} of the blood. They fire continuously at normal blood P_{O_2} levels, and their rate of firing greatly increases when the P_{O_2} is reduced to about 50 mm Hg (normal blood P_{O_2} in the arteries is about 100 mm Hg). Increase in the blood P_{CO_2} increases the sensitivity of the chemoreceptors to lowered oxygen levels. Impulses from the chemoreceptors excite the inspiratory center as well as the cardioexcitatory center of the medulla. Baroreceptors are stretch receptors activated by changes of intravascular pressure. A rise in blood pressure increases the frequency of baroreceptor impulses and inhibits respiration rate. However, these receptors are probably more important to circulatory system control than to normal respiratory activity.

The medulla has receptors that are directly sensitive to changes in the P_{CO_2} level of the cerebrospinal fluid, which in turn is dependent on the P_{CO_2} of the blood. It also appears that the neurons capable of spontaneous discharge and responsible for the basic rhythmic activity of respiration are themselves sensitive to the carbon dioxide levels of blood passing them.

Respiratory control has been analyzed in terms of systems analysis. The respiratory system is, in many respects, part of the excretory system and respiratory control is designed to adequately eliminate CO_2 and also to maintain normal levels of blood CO_2, oxygen, and H^+.

Under conditions of stress accessory muscles of the abdominal wall and upper thorax can be called into activity. Their contractions increase the depth of breathing and thus the amount of air moved into and out of the lungs at each cycle.

TRANSPORT OF RESPIRATORY GASES

Hemoglobin

Once oxygen has diffused from the atmosphere across the respiratory surface and into the blood, it is often transported by means of respiratory pigments. These are required, at least in larger and more active animals, because of the relatively low solubility of oxygen in aqueous solutions. Vertebrate blood plasma can contain maximally about 0.3 ml of O_2 per 100 ml. However, by using transport pigments the concentration of oxygen carried by the blood may amount to 5–30 ml O_2/ml depending on the species.

Oxygen transport pigments are conjugated proteins, that is, proteins complexed with another organic molecule or with one or more metal atoms. Because of the nature of the conjugated group, such transport molecules are colored; hence the term respiratory pigment.

Transport pigments contain metal atoms such as Cu^{2+} or Fe^{3+} to which oxygen can reversibly attach. Respiratory pigments are not oxidized by oxygen; rather, they are oxygenated, that is, they combine reversibly with molecular oxygen. Respiratory pigments are of value not only because they allow the blood to carry a larger amount of oxygen than would otherwise be possible but also because they quickly remove oxygen from solution at the respiratory surface, thus maintaining a concentration gradient down which oxygen can diffuse. In addition, it is of value to carry molecular oxygen, O_2, rather than single oxygen atoms.

Further, the oxygenation process allows the pigment to pick up oxygen at sites of high oxygen tension and to release the oxygen at sites of low oxygen tension (body cells requiring oxygen).

In vertebrates the respiratory pigment is hemoglobin. Hemoglobin has a molecular weight of about 68,000 and is composed of two pairs of polypeptide chains. Each chain carries an iron-containing heme group. The hemoglobin molecule is capable of transporting four oxygen molecules. When four oxygens are attached to hemoglobin the resulting complex is oxyhemoglobin and is said to be fully saturated with oxygen. The oxygen capacity of blood is defined as the total amount of oxygen that can be taken up by a unit volume of the blood and includes that oxygen transported by respiratory pigments as well as that in solution.

At a given pH the amount of oxygen that a given quantity of hemoglobin can pick up depends on the partial pressure of oxygen. The oxygen pressure is usually given in units of mm Hg, and the loading of the hemoglobin is given as the percentage of saturation with oxygen. Such plots are oxygen dissociation curves. At about 40 mm Hg oxygen tension a small reduction in the P_{O_2} will allow a relatively large amount of oxygen to be released by the hemoglobin. Because 40 mm Hg is about the P_{O_2} of body fluids and tissues, hemoglobin is adapted to release its oxygen at pressures close to those of the cells that need it. At higher P_{O_2} levels, which fall in the range of alveolar oxygen concentrations, hemoglobin becomes completely saturated with oxygen.

The term half-saturation pressure is given to the P_{O_2} at which hemoglobin (or any respiratory pigment) is only half-saturated with oxygen. A respiratory pigment with a lower half-saturation pressure has a higher affinity for oxygen when compared with a pigment having a higher half-saturation pressure. It is of interest to compare the muscle oxygen-storage pigment myoglobin with hemoglobin. Myoglobin has a half-saturation pressure of about 6 mm Hg, and that of human hemoglobin is about 24 mm Hg. Myoglobin remains complexed with oxygen until the oxygen levels of the muscle are lowered considerably—a time at which the muscle requires oxygen.

The oxygen dissociation curve of myoglobin is hyperbolic, whereas that for hemoglobin is sigmoid. Myoglobin contains only one chain and one heme group and can combine with only one oxygen molecule. The sigmoid oxygen dissociation curve of hemoglobin results from the combination of hemoglobin with four oxygen molecules. As is desirable in an oxygen storage pigment, myoglobin hangs onto all of its oxygen at oxygen tensions where hemoglobin is 98% dissociated.

The hemoglobin equilibrium with oxygen has been mathematically described as

$$\frac{y}{100} = \frac{KP^n}{1 + KP^n}$$

where y is the percentage saturation with O_2, P is the partial pressure of oxygen, K is the equilibrium constant of the reaction, and n is a measure of the interaction between heme groups. After rearranging and taking the logarithms of both sides:

$$\log \frac{y}{100 - y} = \log K + n \log P$$

A plot of log $[y/(100 - y)]$ against log P yields a straight line whose slope is n. The intercept on the log $[y/(100 - y)]$ axis gives the value of K. For myoglobin, which contains only one heme group, $n = 1$. For hemoglobin, between 10 and 98% saturation, $n = 2.7$.

In hemoglobin the interaction of one heme group with an oxygen molecule influences (increases) the affinity of the other groups for oxygen. Because the three-dimensional structure of hemoglobin shows that the heme groups are relatively separated, it is thought that combination of oxygen with one heme group affects the total protein structure, thus making other heme groups more available for oxygenation.

Oxygen dissociation curves are also affected by the pH and by the blood P_{CO_2}. Low pH or high P_{CO_2} both shift the curve to the right (in most cases). This is the Bohr effect and is important in the functioning of oxygen transport pigment. In active tissues the P_{CO_2} is elevated, and the blood is slightly more acid. Under these conditions the shift of the oxygen dissociation curve to the right under the influence of pH facilitates oxygen unloading and therefore increases the amount of oxygen available to active cells. The mechanisms by which P_{CO_2} and pH affect the dissociation curve appear to be different, although high P_{CO_2} decreases blood pH. Increases in temperature also shift the oxygen dissociation curve to the right.

Carbon Dioxide Transport

Carbon dioxide produced by cells is transported to the lungs or other respiratory surfaces for excretion. Only small amounts of CO_2 are in solution in the blood because of reactions that occur in the plasma and in the erythrocytes of vertebrates.

CO_2 dissolved in water forms carbonic acid, H_2CO_3, a reaction facilitated by the enzyme carbonic anhydrase found in the blood of many animal species. In vertebrates carbonic anhydrase occurs primarily in erythrocytes. Carbonic acid can dissociate into H^+ and HCO_3 and these ions then can enter into the acid–base regulating mechanisms to be discussed in the next section.

Some carbon dioxide (15–20%) reacts with hemoglobin:

$$HbNH_2 + CO_2 \rightleftharpoons HbNHCOOH \rightleftharpoons HbNHCOO\text{-}$$

where the NH_2 represents amino groups of the amino acids of the hemoglobin. The complex is known as carbaminohemoglobin.

At the respiratory surface CO_2 diffuses from the blood to the atmosphere or aqueous medium. Carbonic anhydrase catalyzes the reverse reaction from that given above and forms CO_2 that can be eliminated. The direction of the reaction depends on the P_{CO_2}. Where the CO_2 pressure is low, as in the region of the respiratory exchange surface, H_2CO_3 is split into H_2O and CO_2, and the latter moves down its concentration gradient to the exterior.

It may be noted that the interactions of P_{CO_2} and P_{O_2} levels at different sites in the animal are coordinated and intermeshed in such a way that oxygen diffusion to tissue cells is facilitated just where oxygen is most needed, while oxygen intake from the environment is also facilitated. Similarly, carbon dioxide removal from the tissues to the blood and then from the blood to the external medium is facilitated by the actions involved in oxygen transport. The two systems are interwoven to fill the requirements of the organism.

ACID–BASE BALANCE

When CO_2 diffuses into the blood and forms carbonic acid, the dissociation of the latter forms H^+ and HCO_3^-. The hydrogen ions, unless buffered, would cause dangerously low pH levels in the animal. The hydrogen ions are taken up by proteins of the blood in exchange for metal ions such as K^+ and Na^+. $NaHCO_3$, $KHCO_3$, and phosphates are formed in the blood. Thus, plasma components act to buffer the blood pH and prevent it from decreasing. These reactions also reduce the further formation of HCO_3^- from carbonic acid and keep CO_2 flowing into the system from the tissues (again it may be noted that this is based on the maintenance of adequate concentration gradients. When a given substance is converted to a new compound, the concentration of the latter does not influence the diffusion of the original substance).

Erythrocyte hemoglobin also aids in buffering the blood pH and allows more CO_2 to enter the blood from body tissues. Then CO_2 diffuses into the erythrocytes from the plasma and is converted to H_2CO_3 by erythrocyte carbonic anhydrase. Again, the carbonic acid dissociates to form H^+ and HCO_3^- within the cell.

At the tissue level, hemoglobin gives up its oxygen and may then combine with H^+: $Hb- + H^+ = HbH$. This reaction is of extreme importance in maintaining the pH of the cell at a constant level. The structure of hemoglobin is such that when it gives up oxygen it is converted at the right time and the right place to a substance capable of combining with the hydrogen ions formed as a result of CO_2 diffusion from the tissues.

The HCO_3^- ion concentration within the erythrocyte increases because of the reactions just described, and bicarbonate diffuses out to the plasma. The erythrocyte membrane is not permeable to cations, so in order to preserve electrical neutrality, for every HOC_3^- ion that diffuses into the plasma, a Cl^- moves into the erythrocyte, where it associates with an alkali metal ion, usually Na^+ or K^+. This is known as the chloride or Hamburger shift.

At the respiratory surface all of these reactions reverse because CO_2 can diffuse into the external medium. When hemoglobin combines with oxygen, it releases hydrogen ions (the Haldane effect). The oxygenated hemoglobin associated with the alkali metal ions that were originally associated with the Cl^-. Chloride ions diffuse out of the cell, and HCO_3^- diffuses back into the cell to react with the H^+. Carbonic acid is formed and then rapidly converted by carbonic anhydrase to CO_2 and water. The CO_2 follows its concentration gradient and diffuses out of the cell, through the plasma, into the external environment.

It is to be noted that the operation of this system depends on the presence of proper levels of protein, alkali metal ions, Cl^-, HCO_3^-, and phosphate. One function of the kidney is to maintain proper levels of Na^+ and K^+ in the body fluids. An important need for relatively high levels of these ions arises from the requirement for these substances in the buffering system that maintains blood pH at its proper level even while the acid waste product CO_2 is being transported. The kidney tubules have enzyme systems and buffering mechanisms that trade waste products such as NH_4 and H^+ for ions such as Na^+ and K^+. There is also an exchange of HCO_3^- for Cl^-. The pH is maintained constant while simultaneously needed ions are retained.

Proteins may have many ionizable side groups because of the nature of their constituent amino acids, and a molecule such as hemoglobin is capable of reacting with 20–50 positively charged ions. That is, the buffering capacity of proteins is relatively high. When blood proteins are low in concentration because of disease or metabolic upsets, H^+ begins to accumulate, lowering the blood pH and finally resulting in the condition of acidosis. Low blood pH will, in turn, create low pHs of the body fluids and cells (alkalosis). Unless such a condition is rectified, death will ensue because cells can withstand only relatively small changes in pH. In mammals, for example, changes in the blood pH greater than a few tenths of a pH unit result in death.

Table 89 presents a comparison of the structural characteristics of the lungs of man and the common laboratory species. Based on the majority of characteristics, these species are grouped into three major groups. Note that only the rabbit is in the same class as humans—but differs in other ways which limits its usefulness as a model for humans. Note there really is no ideal or best animal model for inhalation in humans.

MECHANISMS OF TOXICITY

As with exposures by any of the other routes, inhaled chemicals (no matter what their physical state) can cause toxic effects in one or two broad categories—local effects or systemic effects. The broad mechanisms involved and

TABLE 89   Subgross Pulmonary Anatomy Types: Man and Common Laboratory Animals

	Types			
	I	II	III	
Species	Pig (Rat), (Mouse)	Monkey, Cat, Dog, Guinea Pig, Rabbit, Rat, Mouse, Ferret	Human (Rabbit)	
Lobulation	Extremely well developed	Absent	Imperfectly developed	
Plura	Thick	Thin	Thick	
Arterial supply to pleura	Bronchial artery	Pulmonary artery	Bronchial artery	
			Distal	Proximal
General brochovascular	PV++	PV++	PV++	+++
relationships (in	BR++	BR++	BR++	++
comparative	BA++	BA++	BA 2(+)	2(+)
diameters)	PA++	PA++	PA++	++
Intrapulmonary termination of bronchial artery	Distal airway	Distal airway	Distal airway and alveoli	
Terminal bronchioles	Present Predominant distal airway	Absent	Present	
Respiratory bronchioles	Infrequently observed, extremely poor development	Present Very well developed	Present Poorly developed	
Bronchial artery–pulmonary artery shunts	Present (not demonstrated in the pig)	Not demonstrated	Present	

Note. Parentheses indicate that species fits this category to a lesser degree.

the ways in which effects resulting from acute exposures are expressed need to be considered.

First, however, it should be remembered that certain functional peculiarities make the respiratory tract uniquely vulnerable to toxic injury. Although situated deeply within the body, the lung is in immediate contact with the external environment at each breath and this contact is renewed at least 20 times per minute in humans (more often in rodents). During strenuous exercise or labor, the frequency and depth of respiratory effort, and hence air intake, is markedly increased, leading to potentially greater toxic exposure. Second, the alveolar lining cells have a large surface area and thin cytoplasm, with few organelles. This combination of large absorbing surface and modest defensive ability renders the thin, surface epithelial (type I) cells vulnerable to toxic injury. Third, the alveolar surface is extremely large (30 times that of the skin), and its abundant thin-walled capillaries lie in intimate contact with the epithelium. The alveolar surface represents the largest area in the body at which the blood comes into virtually direct contact with the external environment. Consequently, toxic fumes are capable not only of injuring extensive areas of alveolar tissue and adjacent structures but also of initiating rapid absorption and distribution throughout the body to injure specific target organs, or the body as a whole.

Many foreign substances can produce irritation at the point of contact with the respiratory system. Gases and vapors tend to be more chemically reactive and therefore more irritating, but particulates can serve as "carriers" for other phases (liquid or gas) absorbed to their surface.

In the lung, these irritants can interact with pulmonary membranes to produce edema, pleural effusion, and a hyperemic reaction. With the breakdown of the pulmonary barrier, the flow of fluid and protein becomes altered, leading ultimately to the loss of the ability to appropriately oxygenate blood. The inflammatory process is essentially the same within the lung as elsewhere in the body but selected portions may be affected, due to differences in the solubility, boiling point, and volatility of the irritant chemical. The solubility of a compound is probably the most important factor in determining the site of action. Highly soluble materials such as ammonia and hydrogen chloride affect primarily the upper respiratory tract, producing rhinitis and related inflammatory changes. Chemicals of intermediate solubility such as ozone affect both the upper respiratory tract and the pulmonary tissue, while less soluble materials such as nitrogen dioxide and phosgene affect primarily the deep lung.

Irritants can produce changes both at the site of contact and systemically. Those which act only locally at the point of contact are considered primary irritants. These exert little systemic toxicity because they are either metabolized to products which are nontoxic or the local effects far exceed any systemic reaction. Examples of primary irritants are hydrogen chloride and sulfuric acid. Another type of primary irritant is characterized by reactive materials such as the caustic war gases (such as mustard gas; see Chapter 14).

These compounds are extremely toxic if absorbed but produce such a rapid and severe degree of irritation that death due to asphyxia occurs before systemic poisoning can be produced. Secondary irritants are agents which have a significant irritating effect on mucous membranes, but following absorption have a more profound systemic effect. Hydrogen sulfide, acetic acid, and many organic chemicals fall into this category. There are materials which are irritants but also produce systemic injury; hyrogen fluoride, for example, produces severe injury at the point of contact but also produces kidney damage.

Inhalation of a wide variety of particulates produces pulmonary disease. Pneumoconiosis is a term used to designate a fibrotic condition of the lung caused by inhaled dust. The character of the fibrosis depends on the type of dust inhaled, with the more important agents being crystalline silica (silicosis), asbestos (asbestosis), talc, and coal that contains silica (see Kennedy, 1988). Deposition of metals and their compounds in the lung produces a variety of disease states. The pulmonary response to particulates is determined by factors such as (1) the nature of the particles, (2) the site of deposition in the respiratory tract, (3) the amount of deposition in the lung, (4) the exposure period, and (5) individual variation and immunologic status. Lee (1985) described five categories based on the lung tissue reaction to inorganic (mineral) dusts. These include the macrophage reaction produced by so-called nuisance dusts such as soot, iron, and titanium dioxide, foreign body granuloma produced by beryllium and talc, sarcoid-type granuloma normal produced by beryllium, collagenized fibrosis of both the diffuse (from hard metals and asbestos) and nodular (from quartz and silica) forms, and neoplasia produced by nickel and asbestos.

The range of local effects limited to the lungs is illustrated in Table 90.

A broader, but less detailed, characterization of toxic effects resulting from respiratory tract exposure includes the following.

Systemic effects
    Lungs (see Menzel and McClellan, 1980, for a discussion of five categories of actions on lungs)
    Any other possible target organ (see Lu, 1985)
Local effects
    Local irritation
    Cellular damage and edema
    Fibrosis and emphysema
    Immonologic responses
    Upper respiratory tract effects

TABLE 90   Responses of the Lungs to Toxic Injury

Alveoli		Examples
Acute	Epithelial injury	Simple repair O_2
		Exudation and NO_2, SO_2, Cd^{2+} fibrosis
	Endothelial injury	Thrombosis, O_2, O_3
	Interstitial injury	Fibrosis, proteolytic enzymes
Chronic	Granulomatous injury	Tuberculosis beryllium, etc.
	Immunologic injury	Farmer's lung
Bronchi		
Acute	Mucosal ulceration	
	Metaplasia	
Chronic	Atypia	
	Dysplasia	
	Neoplasia	
	(Different patterns of cancer)	
Systemic damage	Central nervous system	
	Target organ toxicity	

Hyperemia
Deciliation (Cobb, 1981)
Goblet cell hyperplasia

ABSORPTION AND DISTRIBUTION

Inhalation occurs when a gaseous or airborne phase of a material is drawn into the respiratory tract. Characteristics of the inhaled material and of the person or animal inhaling it will determine how much material is actually taken in, how deeply it penetrates the tract, and how well it is absorbed.

The respiratory tract provides an enormous (7.5 m^2 in the rat—10 times this in humans) and efficient absorption surface for potentially toxic materials in many forms.

Gases penetrate the respiratory tract epithelium with great rapidity. These substances have small molecular sizes and lipid-to-water partition coefficients, but often their high lipid solubility greatly enhances absorption.

Very little quantitative information is available concerning the pulmonary absorption of organic solids. Although many drugs and other chemicals appear to be absorbed readily when inhaled as sprays, aerosols, or dusts, the observations are based on the appearance of pharmacologic action or appearance of materials in blood or urine; consequently, rates of absorption and relative rates of absorption are not as well known.

An indication of a lipid-like character for the pulmonary membrane has been supplied by a quantitative study with the isolated, perfused dog lung (Taylor et al., 1965). It was shown that the lipid-soluble compound dinitrophenol crosses the pulmonary epithelium more than 100 times faster than a lipid-insoluble substance such as glucose.

Quantitative studies with the rat lung in vivo such as those by Enna and Schanger (1960) suggest a lipid-pore nature for the pulmonary membrane. In this work, 0.1 ml of drug solution was administered to anesthetized rats through a tracheal cannula. After various periods of time, the lungs and trachea were removed and assayed for remaining drug. Although lipid-insoluble substances such as p-aminohippurate and sucrose were absorbed fairly readily, much more rapid rates of absorption were seen with lipid-soluble chemicals such as aniline and procaine amide. A suggestion of the presence of membrane pores was provided by the observation that inulin—a large, lipid-insoluble molecule (mw 5000)—was absorbed at a significant rate, and the smaller sucrose molecule was absorbed even more readily. The reader is referred to Munson and Eger (1971) for a more detailed discussion of absorption of gas-phase materials, which primarily diffuse across the alveolar membrane and enter the circulation.

Chemical moieties may also be inhaled as aerosols, and many toxic substances enter the body in this way. Aerosols are liquid or solid particles so small that they remain suspended in air for a long time instead of sedimenting rapidly under the force of gravity. Table 91 gives sedimentation rate as a function of particle diameter, computed from Stokes' law for the viscous drag on a moving sphere.

Stokes' law is the primary theoretical statement of the behavior of a particle in a gas and is stated as $f = 6\pi nrv$, where f is force in dynes, n is viscosity of air at 20°C and atmospheric pressure and is equal to 1.9×10^{-1} g sec^{-1} cm^{-1}, r is radius of sphere in centimeters, and v is constant velocity of movement when force f is balanced by the viscous drag.

For a sphere moving under the force of gravity, $f =$ mass $\times g$, where $g = 980$ cm sec^{-2}, and assuming unit density,

$$f = 4r^3g/3$$

When the viscous drag opposes the force of gravity so that the rate of fall is constant,

$$6\,nrv = 4r^3g/3$$

$v = D^2g/18n$, where D is the diameter of sphere in centimeters $v = 2.87 \times 10^2 5D^2$.

Particles below about 10 μm in diameter are of interest for humans, though it is frequently overlooked that in the rat (the primary animal model) this cutoff is 3 μm.

There are four types of inhalation exposure when classified by physical type of material—gases, vapors (the gas phase from a material that is primarily a liquid at ambient temperatures), aerosols (though technically this term implies any liquid or solid particle), and dusts. Each of these has specific characteristics and details of exposure atmospheres generation which must be considered.

TABLE 91   Rate of Gravitational Sedimentation in Quiet Air as a Function of Particle Size[a]

Particle diameter (μm)	Sedimentation rate (cm sec^{-1})
100	28.7
50	7.17
25	1.79
10	0.287
5	0.072
1	0.0029

[a]Sedimentation rates are computed from Stokes' law.

Once deposited, a particle may be cleared from the respiratory tract (primarily from the pulmonary region because the physiologic mechanism for clearance from the NP and TB regions—coughing and swallowing—are more straightforward and effective) by various means which include ciliary action (the mucocilliary "elevator"), alveolar macrophages, phagocytosis (into the lymphatic system), and solubility. These clearance mechanisms are, with the exception of solubility, adversely affected by article cytotoxicity and fiber length (above 50 μm, there is no clearance). A mucous blanket, propelled toward the head by ciliary movements, covers the upper respiratory tract down to the terminal bronchioles, and impacted aerosol particles are cleared by this mechanism.

Particles that deposit in the alveolar sacs must first be transported up to the mucous layer to be cleared. Particles in the alveoli are also ingested by phagocytic cells. The efficiency of clearance of solid particles from the lungs is remarkable (not more than a minute fraction of all the mineral dust inhaled during a lifetime is retained in the lungs). However, a small decrease in the clearance capacity of the lungs could cause a marked increase in the amount of retained particulate matter; this may be a factor leading to the development of pneumonoconiosis in miners exposed to silica dusts.

In addition to systemic toxicity, particles deposited in the pulmonary region can have other local biological effects. These include synergism with gases and vapors, irritation, fibrosis, and infection.

Particle size strongly influences the rate at which material is absorbed through the alveolar epithelium, probably because of the greatly increased relative surface area for solubilization as particle diameter becomes smaller. For example, particles of uranium dioxide larger than 3 μm had no toxic effect whatsoever when introduced into the trachea in rats, but the same relatively insoluble material was absorbed into the circulation and caused kidney damage when smaller particles were employed. Figure 57 illustrates the three major mechanisms for particle deposition.

Likewise, lead in aerosol form is extremely well absorbed. Figure 56 presents the aerodynamic diameter of some common environmental aerosols. Active chemical moieties in aerosol form can elicit extremely rapid responses when inhaled, due to the minimal separation between the gas phase and the systemic circulation in the deep lung. Histamine given to a guinea pig or dog as an aerosol can cause bronchiolar constriction and asphyxia within a minute.

Particles larger than 2 μm in diameter probably do not reach the alveolar sacs of humans. Some commercially available nebulizers produce particles 1–3.5 μm in diameter (as will be reviewed under generation systems) so most of the deposition will occur in the large bronchial passages. But for most effective exposure, the smallest bronchi and alveolar ducts should be reached by an agent, so particles smaller than 1 μm in diameter are desirable. A technique that promotes deposition of particles is for the subject to hold their

SCHEMATIC OF DEPOSITION MECHANISMS

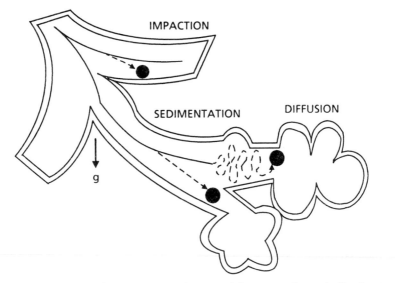

FIGURE 57 Illustration of three major mechanisms of deposition of particles/droplets in a respiratory tract.

breath after inhalation, to maximize the effective time for particle diffusion. Another technique is to add hygroscopic substances to the aerosol; the droplets then become larger as they traverse the moist respiratory tract, and the rate of impaction due to sedimentation is increased.

With aerosols of small particle size, the amount of chemical reaching the alveoli may be large; and because the rate of absorption into the bloodstream is much more rapid at the alveolar sacs than elsewhere in the pulmonary tree, the systemic absorption of the drug may be appreciable.

Vapors have some special characteristics and behaviors which set them apart from simple gases. Because they are the gas phase of materials that are predominantly liquid at ambient temperatures (25°C) and pressures (1 atm), and because, frequently, we seek to generate sufficient concentrations of this gas phase (to meet our experimental needs) by subjecting the parent liquid phase to increased temperatures, careful consideration must be given to keeping the material as a gas phase. Subjecting an airstream saturated with the vapor of a chemical to cooling will, at the least, cause a reduction in vapor-phase concentration (as some of the chemical condenses out as a liquid along the walls of the air handling or exposure system) and may lead to the inadvertent generation of an aerosol as the vapor condenses out as a mist.

There is also a special problem for vapors which are mixtures of chemical moieties. Achieving and maintaining the desired representative concentration of all the components in a vapor mixture (as opposed to a unitary vapor) can be a complex problem.

MECHANICS OF EXPOSURE

The mechanics of performing acute inhalation exposures to state-of-the-art standards can be complex in their entirety but the individual technical components of the problem are rather simple.

As a starting place, remember that there are four sequential components to an exposure system. These are generation systems, exposure chambers, systems for measuring exposure, and systems for cleaning the effluent airstream.

GENERATORS

Optimal generation systems have four major desirable features. These are

Uniform rate of sample delivery
Uniform character of sample delivered
Able to deliver in desired range of concentrations
Safety to operations

For each of our types of exposure (vapor, aerosol, and dust), there are a multitude of systems available. For example, the case of dust generators will be presented here in some detail, with a brief overview of the other two cases.

GENERATION SYSTEMS: NOTES AND CONSIDERATIONS

1. Definitions
   Aerosols (fine particles, solid or liquid, in a stable gaseous suspension; maximum diameter is 1 μm)
   Dusts (solid particles in air—not necessarily a stable suspension)
   Fumes (agglomerates of many fine particles)
   Smokes (stable agglomerates of fine particles in gaseous suspension)
   Mists (liquid particles >40 μm in diameter)
   Fogs (liquid particles 5–40 μm in diameter)

2. Monodisperse vs polydisperse aerosols
   For monodisperse, the standard deviation of geometric diameter about the mean is less than 1.25
3. Factors to be considered in dust generation
   Particle size (and size distribution)
   Particle shape
   Density of material
   Concentrations needed (necessary capacity)

Vapor generation systems are based on the principle of maximizing surface area of the liquid, temperature (within the limits of chemical stability), and airflow across the surface of the liquid as a means of increasing efficiency. Four common generation systems utilizing these principles are

Tube generators (where the parent liquid flows along the inside surface of a tube while an airflow is passed over this surface)
Wick generators (where a liquid phase is passed up some form of porous wick while an airflow is played over it)
Bubble generators (where the airflow is passed through the liquid phase)
Special instrument generators (where a turning tube generator has the internal surface area of the tube maximized by adding ridges or sections and the tube itself, as well as the airflow passing through it, is warmed)

Liquid aerosols only present generation problems and concerns in a couple of special cases. First, if they are extremely volatile, one may actually end up generating a vapor. Second, denser or more viscous liquids require greater energy to overcome surface tension and form droplets of the desired size. There are four widely used generation systems:

Spray nozzle
Ultrasonic generation (uses sound to provide energy to disrupt liquid into droplets)
Spinning discs
Nebulizers

The most common of these aerosol generator designs are shown in Figs. 58 (for solids) and 59 (for liquids).

Drew (1983) has published a review of the most common generation systems. After a stream of test material is generated into an air flow, it is mixed (usually by allowing the mixture to transit a ducting system of sufficient length, with some turbulence) and then introduced into the exposure chamber system in which test animals are contained (or are to be contained). Table 92 presents, for example, guidance for selecting dust (solid aerosol) generators.

DUST GENERATORS

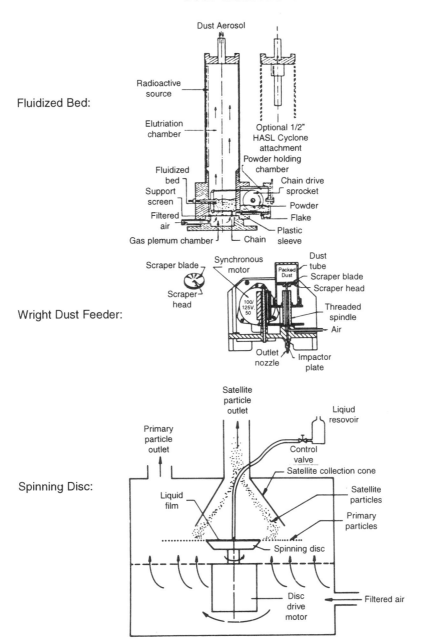

FIGURE 58 The three most common types of dust generators used in acute inhalation testing. Multiple other types exist.

AEROSOL GENERATORS

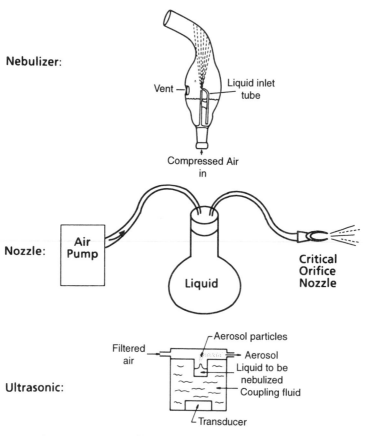

FIGURE 59   Three common types of liquid aerosol generators used in acute inhalation testing.

CHAMBERS

Technically, chamber exposures can be static (there is no airflow through the system; animals are entered into a closed system that contains an atmosphere "precharged" with the desired test material) or dynamic. Only dynamic systems are considered state-of-the-art, with static systems being inadequate for anything other than some minor short-term rank hazard type assessments. Details of the different designs and their characteristic advantages and disadvantages are given in Table 93.

TABLE 92   Generation Methods for Dusts

Device	Monodisperse?	Capacity
Wright dust feeder (the subject material must be compressable and brittle)	No	μg/min to 20 mg/min
Marple fluidized bed (material cannot be sticky; the particle size generated is determined by sample particle size)	Yes	μg/min to 100 mg/min
NBS/vibratory hopper (material cannot be sticky; generates many doubles and triplets)	No	g/min to kg/min
Spinning disc (particle size generated is determined by sample particle size)	Yes	μg/min to mg/min
Pneumatic nebulizer (small particles only—the particle size generated is determined by the sample particle size)	Yes	μg/min to $\sim$2 mg/min
Condensation (certain materials only—very selectively useful)	Yes	μg/min to g/min
Elutreator	Yes	μg/min to g/min

Figures 60 and 52 present the basic designs of whole body and head/nose-only exposure chambers, respectively. These are the major categories of inhalation chambers.

MEASUREMENT OF TEST ATMOSPHERES

While animals are being exposed in a chamber, the test atmosphere must be measured and (if appropriate) characterized. The desirable characteristics for a measurement system include

Accuracy and precision across the range of concentrations (or characteristics) to be measured

Reproducibility

Continuous measurement (failing this, as frequent intermittent measurement as possible)

Direct measurement of the variable of interest (not inference or calculation based on an indirect measurement)

Automatic measurement

Measurement at a number of discrete different locations in the exposure chamber

Achievement all of these characteristics in practice is usually an impossibil-

TABLE 93   Inhalation Chamber Design

Major classifications	Advantages	Disadvantages
Static whole body	Animals not stressed	Limited time of exposure
	Cheap	Rodents only
	Easy to operate	Dermal exposure
		Large volume/animal ratio
		Oral exposure (if dusts)
		No control of atmosphere
		No measurements possible
		Degrading exposure levels
Dynamic whole body	Good atmosphere control	Dermal exposure
	Almost any species	Oral exposure (if dusts)
	Animals not stressed	Only limited measurements possible
	Suitable for long-term exposure	Engineering requirements
		Large amounts of material necessary
Dynamic head only	No dermal exposure	Rodents only
	Little oral exposure	Animals stressed
	Requires little test material	Time-consuming
	Measurements possible	
Mask exposure	Larger animals possible	No small animals
	Measurements possible	Time-consuming
	Requires little test material	Animals stressed
	No dermal exposure	Not suitable for long-term exposure
	Little oral exposure	

Shapes for whole body exposures
  Laskin (animal load limit = 5% of total volume); also called "Rochester" style (misnomer)
  Batelle
  Cube (if static, 500 liters/kg/animal mass/hour of exposure time)
  Cylinders
Heat balance
  Animals act as heat sources
  Variables
    animals
    entering air temperature
    airflow
Chamber distribution
  How to measure
  Dead spaces
  Program
Multiple tiers of animals
  Effects on distribution
  Metabolic excretion
  Pans or no pans
Direction of flow
  Horizontal vs vertical

WHOLE BODY INHALATION CHAMBER DESIGNS

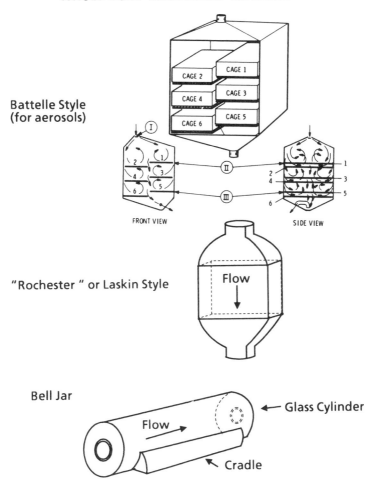

**Battelle Style
(for aerosols)**

CAGE 1
CAGE 2
CAGE 3
CAGE 4
CAGE 5
CAGE 6

I
II
III

FRONT VIEW

SIDE VIEW

"Rochester" or Laskin Style

Flow

Bell Jar

Flow

Glass Cylinder

Cradle

FIGURE 60 The three major designs for whole body type inhalation chambers. The Battelle style is not commonly used for acute studies.

ity. Rather, a set of acceptable compromises are made. The particular problems, concerns, and instruments associated with each of the separate types of exposure (dust, aerosol, and vapor or gas) are again very different. The case for dust measurement is presented in some detail, while that for the other two is reviewed.

DUSTS—MEASUREMENT AND CHARACTERIZATION

Parameters affecting measurement and characterization:

Size-dependent forces (inertia, gravity, diffusion, and electrical charge)
Weight/density
Shape (five basic classes)

Measurement of aerosol concentrations (and characterization of droplet sizes) requires two separate and independent measurements. Such measurements must be performed with sampling in such a way that the droplets in the sample are not altered in either concentration (by deposition on the walls of the sampling device) or in aerodynamic size (by either evaporation or condensation). Concentration sampling is the easier of the two measurements to complete, almost always being done by volumetric sampling into some form of impinger. Droplet size characterization can be done optically (using microscope slides precoated with a film of magnesium oxide) with a laser particle sizer (for low to medium concentrations), or with an impactor if the liquid is not too volatile. Table 94 summarizes available methods.

For gases and vapors, there exists the possibility of doing either continuous (but limited in scope) measurements of concentration of many materials by infrared spectrophotometric or all-inclusive intermittent measurements by either gas chromatography or high-pressure liquid chromatography.

CLEANUP

The last step or phase in the process of properly conducting an inhalation exposure is cleaning up the airstream leaving the exposure system before releasing it into the atmosphere. Also, of course, then properly disposing of the collected waste products that result from such a cleanup.

Depending on the nature of the chemical being evaluated, one or a combination of three methods may be utilized. These are filters, incinerators, or scrubbers (using either water or more exotic fluids such as sulfuric acid or potassium permanganate).

For acute studies, one has much more flexibility in applying these methods than for longer term studies in which logistics limit choices.

Filters can be fibers (such as HEPA or cotton), particulates (such as activated charcoal), or the simple expedient of (for relatively nontoxic materials) a series of cloth bags in a box (in effect, a miniature bag house). A variant on filtration for acutes is to pass the airstream through a glass or metal container packed with glass wool as a filtration medium.

Incineration is only used when the material being tested is gas or volatile,

TABLE 94 Particle Measuring Devices/Techniques

Device	Number of separations	Particle size	Concentration or volume	Particle classification By weight	By number	By volume	Restrictions and error factors
Microscope/micrometer (optical characterization)	None	0.5 μm and above	NA[a]	No	Yes	No	Separation of sizes by film Tedious Time-consuming Small samples only
Image analyzer	None	0.005–20 μm	NA[a]	Indirect	Yes	Yes	Medium-sized samples only
Sierra impactor	10	0.05–25 μm	0.25–25 liter/min	Yes	No	Indirect	Bounce Wall losses Small samples
Mercer impactor	7	0.05–25 μm	100 μg/m^3 to 65 mg/m^{3b}	Yes	No	No	Must be suspendable in polar liquids (but not soluble)
Diffusion battery	10	0.005–0.2 μm	to 2 liters/min	Yes	No	Indirect	Only samples one size range at a time, not 10 simultaneously
Optical particle counter	None	0.2–20 μm	116 particles per second	No	Yes	No	Coincidence Very sensitive to errors due to shape

[a]Utilizes sample collected by other names.
[b]Extendable with multiple apperature tubes and filtering.

is very toxic, and is subject to thermal degradation. This approach is very rarely used for acute studies.

Washing or "scrubbing" the contaminants out of an airstream is an attractive alternative for acute studies. A liquid (usually water or an aqeous solution of sulfuric acid, sodium hydroxide, or potassium permanganate) is used as a filter medium for the contaminated airstream. This can be done by either bubbling the gas stream through a volume of the liquid or passing the gas stream through a spray "curtain."

DOSE QUANTITATION

Measuring (or even expressing) the dose received in an acute inhalation study is a difficult, and, at best, inexact undertaking. Unlike other routes, one starts knowing two variables: how long an animal was exposed and the concentration of material in the atmosphere. One does not know what volume of the atmosphere was inhaled by the animal or how much of the material in the inhaled volume was absorbed.

The traditional approach has been to express and evaluate exposures in terms of concentrations and times of exposure. For acute exposures, Haber's rule generally holds. That is: $ct = K$, where c is the concentration, t is the time of exposure, and K is the constant specific for material. This is a handy relationship for comparing exposures at different concentrations or for different lengths of time, but it obviously has limits as to applicability (very high or very low concentrations, for example).

Just expressing exposure concentrations is more complex than it appears on the surface. First of all, in a dynamic exposure situation, the initial concentration in a chamber is clearly lower than the final concentration. It takes time for the atmosphere to equilibrate to a concentration at or very near the desired target concentration. This equilibration time can be calculated as (Kennedy and Trochimowicz, 1982):

$$C = (w/b) \, [1\text{-evp} \, (bt/a)]$$

where C is the desired chamber concentration, w is the weight of material introduced per unit time, b is the total airflow through chamber, t is the time, and a is the chamber volume.

A second complication to expressing concentration is that for gases and vapors, it is properly expressed as parts per million (ppm). Interconversions can be calculated with the following formulas: $mg/l = gm/m^3$ and $mg/m^3 = (ppm) \, (MW)/24.5$, where MW is molecular weight.

One consideration in model selection is the comparability of doses received with those likely in humans. In the special case of the inhalation route, doses received must be calculated (rather than measured) in a manner somewhat specific to the animal model being employed.

Calculated inhalation dosimetry models, though not extremely accurate, do have some utility in the cases of (a) comparing toxicity via the inhalation route with toxicity via other routes, (b) in risk assessment models and calculations, and (c) in interspecies calculations and extrapolations such as will be discussed later.

These calculations are performed using the formula:

$$E = [RF \times TV \times C \times 60 \times T]/1000$$

where E is the total maximum possible exposure, RF is the respiratory frequency (per minute), TV is the tidal volume in ml, C is the concentration of test agent in mg/liter, and T is the daily exposure time in hours. Note that this formula can also be used to compare total doses received over different lengths of exposure. If exposure is repeated over a period of several days, the result of the above calculation is also multiplied by the number of days of exposure.

Values to be used in this equation for the laboratory species commonly used in inhalation studies and man are the following:

Species	RF	TF	Reference
Rat	85.5	0.86	Baker *et al.* (1979)
Mouse	109	0.18	Attman and Dittmer (1971)
Guinea pig	90	1.8	Attman and Dittmer (1971)
Rabbit	49	15.8	Swenson (1971)
Man	11.7	750.0	Attman and Dittmer (1971)

These values will, in turn, result in hourly exposure values which can be reduced to the following:

Rat	= 4.4118 liters C
Mouse	= 1.1772 liters C
Guinea pig	= 9.720 liters C
Rabbit	= 46.452 liters C
Man	= 526.5 liters C

It must be remembered in using this model that the values obtained will be the maximum average limits on the dose delivered to the test animal. A number of factors that are not included will affect the actual doses delivered systemically, in all cases except one (Item A below) serving to reduce the actual values of doses delivered systemically. These factors include

A. Variations in individual animals (and in the same animal at different ages, weights, and states of exercise) in RF and TV.

B. If the material is a particulate or is water insoluble, the degree of deposition and clearance (respectively) in and from the lungs will vary.

C. The degree of absorption from the lungs into the body will vary from chemical to chemical and is affected by a wide variety of factors [solubility, protein binding metabolism (both in the lung and the liver) etc.].

A note of caution needs to be injected here. These calculations will yield estimates of the amounts inhaled, not necessarily the amounts absorbed. Indeed, they may not accurately reflect the amounts that make it into the lungs of different species. Dosimetry (calculation or determination of systemic exposure) will depend on the species and the nature of the chemical, as discussed in a review by Dahl *et al.* (1991). For example, different species exposed to the same particulate atmosphere will not receive the same doses in comparable regions of the respiratory system because of anatomic and physiologic differences. Rats and mice, for example, have much faster rates of alveolar clearance than dogs.

For reactive gas, such as formaldehyde, the amounts of reactive products are not well predicted across species by applying the appropriate scaling factors, due to marked differences in nasopharynx anatomy in rats versus monkeys. Such differences must be borne in mind when attempting to extrapolate the results of an inhalation test to man.

The absorption of particulates and aerosols across the lung into the system circulation is difficult to model. Before any substance can cross into the circulation, it must first be in solution, whereupon it passes into the circulation by passive diffusion. Thus, particulate materials must first be broken down by chemical or enzymatic reaction. In general, particulates are ingested by macrophages and removed by mucocilliary motion. Species differences in pulmonary xenobiotic metabolism will also play a role in different species. Once a chemical enters the systemic circulation via the lung, its behavior will obviously be no different than if it had been absorbed across the GI tract. There will be a peak plasma, an area under the curve, etc.

The inhalation dosimetry of gases and/or vapors, in contrast to particulates and aerosols, represents a much more defined situation, and an area where species differences are less important. As reviewed by any classic treatise in pharmacokinetics (such as by Goldstein *et al.*, 1974) the blood levels of an inhaled gas are determined solely by the concentration or partial pressure of the gas in the inhaled atmosphere and the blood gas partition coefficient of the gas, such that

$$C_B = S \cdot C_A$$

where C_B is the concentration in blood, C_A is the atmospheric concentration, and S is the solubility in blood or the partition coefficient. In general, the smaller the partition coefficient, the more rapid equilibration will take place, but the lower the blood concentration. Once the blood and the atmospheric gas are in equilibrium, which for some gases may take only a few minutes, but will almost certainly occur for almost all gases within 60 min, blood gas concentrations will not increase regardless of the length of the exposure period. For a more complete review of this area, the reader is referred to Goldstein *et al.* (1974) or Gargas *et al.* (1989).

COMMON TEST DESIGNS

Because inhalation is not an endpoint for study but rather a route of exposure, there are actually a number of different types of acute inhalation studies that are commonly performed. Currently, these basic designs can be sorted into five basic groups. These groups are the limit test, LC50 study, "standard regulatory," acute pulmonary irritation, and pulmonary sensitization. The characteristics of these are summarized in Table 95 as to objectives, species used, length of evaluation of animals after exposure, endpoints evaluated, and maximum concentrations achieved.

The first three of these test types have a lot in common and are largely driven (and their designs constrained) by various regulatory guidelines. Table 96 summarizes the major testing guidelines for acute inhalation studies. Such acute studies are, as the guidelines require, at least initially conducted at relatively high concentrations and are aimed at determining the general range and characteristics of the acute toxicity of a chemical. Figure 61 depicts what actually goes on during the course of the period of exposure. Given the imprecision of all but a few of the generation systems described earlier, it should be readily apparent why measured acute exposures concentrations have as much variability as they do.

Acute exposures of the limit test type are intended only to pass or fail a material on the basis of lethality. The more detailed acute studies may be intended to provide information used in determining exposure levels to be used in longer term studies. (It is common practice to perform studies with 4-hr exposures because this meets the minimum requirements for various guidelines. In the experience of the author (SCG), however, because all longer term studies have a daily exposure of at least 6 hr, it is preferable to have acute studies (other than limit tests) be based on 6-hr exposures. This serves to remove one step in the extrapolation process for setting doses for longer studies.) The clinical signs evoked at these high exposures often allow determination of the nature of the toxic effect induced. The two most common numerical values that come from an acute study are the approximately lethal concentration (ALC) and the LC50. The ALC is defined as the lowest concentration that produces death in at least 1 of a group of exposed animals, while the LC50 is the calculated concentration at which one-half of the exposed

TABLE 95 Acute Inhalation Study Designs

Type	Species	Exposure period	Postexposure observation	Maximum exposure concentration	Objective
Limit test (DOT)	Rat	1 hr	2 Days	2 mg/liter	Labeling requirement
Acute "standard regulatory"	Rat or mouse	At least 4 hr	14 Days	5 mg/liter	Registration requirement (systemic toxicity assessment)
LC$_{50}$	Rat or mouse	6 hr	14 Days	NA	To set doses for longer study
Pulmonary sensitization	Guinea pig	1 hr on 6 alternate days over 2 weeks	Hold 7 days, then challenge observe during challenge exposure	NA	Assessment of delayed pulmonary sensitization potential
Pulmonary irritation	Rat or mouse	1 hr	None	NA	Assessment of potential to cause respiratory irritation.

Note. NA, not applicable.

TABLE 96 Summary of Testing Guidelines—Acute Inhalation Toxicity Tests

Parameter	FIFRA (1984)	TOSCA	DOT	OECD	OECD[a]	MAFF
Test animals						
Species	Rat	Mouse and rat	Rat	Rat	Rat	2 including rat
Age	Young adult	NS	NS	NS	NS	Young adults
Weight (g)	NS (±20% of mean)	125–250	200–300	NS (±20% of mean)	NS (±20% of mean)	NS
Limit test						
Amount (mg/liter)	5	2.0 and 0.2	2	5	[b]	5
Acceptable mortality	None	NS	Less than half	None	[c]	None
LC50 determination	[d]	Suggested	NA	[d]	NA	Required
Minimum No. animals/group	5/sex	5/sex	10	5/sex	5/sex	5/sex
Number of exposure levels (groups)	3	2 (as above)	1 (as above)	At least 3	NS[c]	NS
Untreated controls	NR	NR	NR	NS	NS	NR
Measurement of concentration[e]	At least twice	NS	NS	Yes	NR[f]	Yes
Particle/droplet size[g]	Less than 15 μm	NS	NS	NS	NA	Yes
Exposure system	Dynamic	Dynamic	NS	Dynamic	Dynamic	Dynamic
Length of exposure (hr)	At least 4	At least 4	1 or less	At least 4	7	At least 4
Chamber air changes (per hour)	At least 10	NS	NS	12–15	NS	NS
Observation period	14 Days	At least 14 days	48 Hours	At least 14 days	At least 14 days	At least 14 days
Body weights[h]	Day 0 + weekly[i]	NS	NS	Before exposure	Day 0 + weekly[i]	Day 0 + weekly[i]
Necropsy	All animals	All animals	NS	All animals	All animals	All animals
Histopathology	Gross lesions	Gross lesions	NS	Target organs	Tissue list	Gross lesion

Note. NS, not specified; NR, not required; NA, not applicable.
[a] Inhalation hazard test for volatile substances.
[b] Maximum attainable under conditions of test.
[c] None. If deaths occur, test should be repeated over shorter periods of exposure until no more deaths among the test animals occur.
[d] If limit test fails.
[e] During exposure.
[f] Concentration should be known. Nominal determination is acceptable.
[g] Aerodynamic particle/droplet size for dusts or liquid aerosols in a test atmosphere.
[h] On study days specified, where 0 = day of exposure.
[i] At least weekly after exposure plus at death/termination.

451

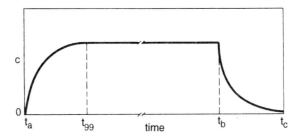

FIGURE 61 The buildup and decay of a toxicant in a chamber. Exposure starts at t_a and stops at t_c, but the flow of the toxicant is terminated at t_b. The duration of exposure is recorded as from t_a to t_b; the extra exposure from t_b to t_c is intended to compensate for the exponential buildup of the toxicant in the chamer from t_a to t_{99}.

population would be expected to die for a given period of exposure. Generally, the exposures are conducted for a single 4- or 6-hr period and the animals are observed for 14 days after treatment.

There has been considerable discussion on what constitutes an appropriate dose or exposure level for an acute inhalation study with particulate materials. The U.S. Environmental Protection Agency's (EPA) recommended maximal exposure level is 5 mg/liter, and that 25% of such particles must be less than 1 μm across. This issue was reviewed by the Inhalation Specialty Section of the Society of Toxicology in 1992. Whatever the EPA may demand, physical and natural laws may intercede. Agglomeration, due to physical and chemical laws, may make it impossible to achieve both 5 mg/liter and a particle size distribution with 25% being less than 1 μm.

Also, particle size will dictate preferred location of deposition, and there is no reason to assume that any one portion of the respiratory system is any more sensitive or important than any other. The committee, therefore, recommended that the limit test concentration for particulate and aerosol substances should be the highest concentration that could be achieved (up to 5 mg/liter) that maintained a particle size between 1 and 4 μm. This would result in deposition along the entire length of the rodent respiratory system, resulting in a more thorough evaluation of the material's inhiliatory toxicity. One such protocol is as follows:

Inhalation study procedure
   1. All involved personnel must be familiarized with the goal of the study, the protocol, and the proper handling practices for the test article. Empty chamber trials (at least one) must be performed in order to establish a reliable system for generating and monitoring the test atmosphere in compliance with the protocol design. Records of these trials will be maintained in the study file.

2. The group of animals (typically rats) will be equally divided between males and females. The animals will be randomly selected from a colony maintained for acute study purposes in general or from animals specifically purchased for the study. The selected animals must be in good health based on physical examination and body weights prior to exposure.

3. The selected animals are uniquely identified with an eartag number which must also be marked on the cage cards.

4. On the day of exposure (Day 0), the selected animals are physically observed and any animals considered unsuitable for test are replaced. Also, the selected animals are weighed. The preexposure observations and the body weights are recorded.

5. The selected animals are placed into the exposure chamber and exposed to the test article atmosphere. Whole body inhalation chambers will be used unless it is deemed necessary to use head-only exposure equipment. At all times, except where specifically precluded by the protocol, a dynamic flow system shall be employed. Because of the variety and complexity of inhalation exposure techniques, which are usually adapted to the properties of a particular test article, this protocol will not attempt to describe these systems. The actual system employed for a project is described in an actual protocol and in detail. The generating system is monitored continuously during the exposure, and any adjustments are noted.

6. The inhalation chamber shall be operated at an overall flow rate that will prevent anoxia of the animals by maintaining a minimum of 19% oxygen in the atmosphere. When the test article or carrier gas (e.g., nitrogen) is expected to displace more than 10% of the chamber atmosphere, oxygen must be used as makeup air in a quantity sufficient to maintain the oxygen content at or above 19%. Otherwise, compressed air (breathing grade) is the preferred carrier gas for generating and makeup air. The flow of air through the chamber is monitored continuously during the exposure and recorded.

7. All components of the generating system that come in contact with the test article are weighed before and after the exposure for the purpose of calculating a nominal concentration. These data and the calculations are recorded and shown.

8. The exposure period shall be for the time period which is specified in the protocol (usually 1–6 hr) or until all the animals in the chamber are dead, whichever occurs first. Exposures are not usually interrupted to remove dead animals unless all animals appear to be dead. Exposures often are interrupted to effect repairs or adjustments of generating equipment, and these interruptions must be noted.

When interruptions represent significant portions ($>5\%$) of the planned exposure period, the exposure period must be extended to compensate or, at the study director's discretion, the exposure can be aborted.

9. Chamber measurement

The chamber temperature is maintained at $22 \pm 2°C$ and the relative humidity at $50 \pm 20\%$. Both these values must be monitored continuously and recorded at least hourly.

Actual chamber concentration of the test article must be taken often enough (at least hourly) to demonstrate a stable atmosphere. Measurements of the particle size must be taken when aerosols or dusts are generated. Calculations of mass median diameter and standard deviation are made.

10. During the exposure period, the animals are observed at 15-min intervals for the first hour and at hourly intervals beyond the first hour. The in-chamber observations need not be individual observations, but can be generalized estimates of number of animals exhibiting a particular sign using these terms: some, most, or all. Once a particular sign is recorded at an interval, it must be recorded at all subsequent intervals until it totally disappears. These observations are recorded.

11. Upon termination of the exposure, the chamber is allowed to clear for at least 30 min or one T_{99} [T_{99} is a calculated value in minutes that represents the theoretical time for a chamber to clear 99% of an airborne contaminant: T_{99} (min) $= 4.6$[(chamber vol. (liter)/air flow (liter/min)] cycle (whichever is greater) at the same airflow as employed during the exposure. This is illustrated in Fig. 59.

12. After the clearing interval, the animals are removed from the chamber and individually observed before being returned to their cages. At this point, animals exposed to a dust or aerosol may be wiped with a damp cloth to remove gross quantities of residue to prevent subsequent oral ingestion of the article during preening. This should be noted if performed. The contaminated cloth must be disposed according to proper procedures.

13. The animals are individually observed each hour for up to 6 hr during the postexposure period and observations recorded.

14. The animals are observed twice daily for mortality and unusual toxic signs and a full recorded physical examination is performed once daily for the 14 days postexposure (Days 1–14). They are weighed individually on Days 1, 2, 3, 4, 7, 11, and 14 (terminus). Observations and body weights are recorded. The observation interval may be extended beyond 14 days if signs of reversible toxicity are persistent

and the study director judges that this will provide useful information.

15. On Day 14 postexposure (or at later termination day), all surviving animals are sacrificed by an appropriate humane method and are subjected to a gross necropsy examination.

16. A concurrent air-only control group, if used, must be exposed under the same conditions as the test group(s). In addition, if any solvent (nonaqueous) is employed to generate the test article atmosphere, a solvent control group must be run at a level comparable to the highest solvent concentration of any test group.

17. When an LC50 evaluation is required because of mortality at the initial dose level, at least two additional groups of animals are exposed to varying levels in order to achieve mortality rates between 10 and 90%, if possible. Upon completion of the study, an LC50 value and 95% confidence interval are calculated. Consideration should be given to whether an LC50 is actually required, however.

Additional parameters which may be evaluated either as part of the main acute inhalation study or as separate specialized studies include respiratory function, morphologic and biochemical changes, and particle deposition/clearance.

Tests on respiratory functions are often carried out because of their greater sensitivity compared to morphologic changes and because of their ability to detect reversible effects. As a result, these tests might be used in studies in humans, thereby allowing a more direct comparison between humans and the experimental animals with respect to their relative susceptibility to the toxic effects of the substance being tested.

Respiratory frequency is a sensitive indicator of local irritation and is often concentration related. Certain gases, e.g., ozone and nitrogen dioxide, increase the frequency, whereas others, e.g., sulfur dioxide and formaldehyde, decrease it. This, and respiratory volume, are thus commonly measured as part of pulmonary irritation or sensitization tests (as discussed later).

The mechanics of respiration can be measured in terms of pulmonary flow resistance and pulmonary compliance. An increase in pulmonary flow resistance can result from bronchoconstriction, swelling of the respiratory mucosa, or an increase in mucous secretion. Pulmonary compliance is decreased by fibrosis, and it is increased in emphysema because of loss of supportive connective tissue.

Respiratory efficiency can be estimated by measuring oxygen and carbon dioxide in the blood or by measuring the rate at which inhaled carbon monoxide is taken into the blood (Cobb, 1981).

Various morphologic changes can result from inhalation exposure to toxicants. These include local irritation, cellular damage, edema, fibrosis, and neoplasms. In addition, toxicants can cause a number of other types of morphologic changes such as inflamation, hyperplasia, edema, and emphysema.

Some examinations are especially useful. For example, lung weight increase is an indicator of vascular congestion, edema, or increase in connective tissue. Washings of the lung can provide information on cell number, type, and morphology as well as on noncellular components, especially the enzyme content. Collagen content can be estimated by determining hydroxyproline or prolylhydroxylase (Cobb, 1981), and with careful study design and conduct, both article deposition and clearance can also be evaluated. There are several techniques for making determinations as to where and how much of the aerosol was deposited in the respiratory tract. This is not always an easy question to answer but the following approaches will be helpful.

MICROSCOPIC

The particles may be light-opaque and/or colored and therefore visible by light microscopy, e.g., carbon or hematite. Certain compounds may be crystalline and can be made visible with polarizing lenses, e.g., silica and talc.

HISTOCHEMICAL

Many agents will react with chemicals to give a colored end product, e.g., iron oxide by the Prussian blue reaction or peroxidase-coupled agents with the diaminobenzidene reaction.

RADIOISOTOPIC

Most compounds can be obtained in a radioactive form (preferably low-energy, beta-emission type for safety). Two procedures which may be used are liquid scintillation counting and autoradiography.

In liquid scintillation counting, pieces of lung or conducting airways are rendered soluble by caustic digestion and emissions are measured in a liquid scintillation counter. This method can also be used with radiation markers emitting gamma particles.

AUTORADIOGRAPHY

Although technically more difficult, this approach achieves more precise localization of the material. Moreover, quantitation can be achieved with morphometric methods. Although space does not permit a full discussion of the subject here, in principle, photographic emulsion of high sensitivity (because of its small grain size) is layered over the tissue sections. The sections are kept in total darkness for several days or weeks and then developed with standard photographic techniques. Black and silver grains identify the site of deposition.

Matched groups of animals can then be used to address the clearance of deposited aerosols.

Pulmonary Irritation

Chemicals irritating the sensory apparatus of the upper respiratory tract can be identified by measuring respiratory rate to detect a reflex-induced decrease (Alarie, 1966; Alarie et al., 1974; Amdur, 1957). The basic design uses an apparatus which detects changes in thoracic body cavity volume and can determine the depth and rate of respiration. The animal, usually a rat or mouse, is placed into a whole body tube (plethysomograph) connected to an inhalation chamber such that only the nose protrudes into the exposure area. Animals are then exposed to various concentrations of the agent and a plot of respiration rate against concentration is made. Dose–response curves and minimum effect levels can be determined, the data usually being expressed in terms of the RD50 (concentration required to lower the respiration rate by 50%). The method, as described below, is quite simple and detects the effects of irritation at concentrations where no associated pathological modifications occur.

This method has been demonstrated for a variety of airborne chemical irritants in numerous species; cats, dogs, mice, rats, rabbits, guinea pigs, and humans. This reflex reaction has been exploited as a quantitative measure for evaluation of sensory irritation to airborne chemicals. It consists of measuring the percentage decrease in respiratory rate during exposure to various concentrations of a given gas, vapor, or aerosol. The animals serve as their own controls because the respiratory rate before exposure offers a base line. A dose–response curve is obtained by plotting the percentage decrease from control values in respiratory rate during the exposure interval against the logarithm of the exposure concentration.

1. The maximum number of animals that can be simultaneously monitored are loaded into a Plexiglas tube which serves as a plethysmograph when the tail end is sealed with a rubber stopper and the head protrudes through a tightly fitted latex dam.

2. Each plethysmograph is then mounted on the side of the exposure chamber such that the animal's head protrudes into the center of the chamber. The exposure chamber consists of a Plexiglas cylinder with Plexiglas covers

on both ends, two large holes on each side for the plethysmographs, and several taps for introduction, sampling, and exhaust of the test air.

3. Each plethysmograph is connected via a pneumatic line to a pressure sensing transducer. If the animal is properly sealed in the plethysmograph, the pressure pulses caused by inspiration and expiration are sensed by the transducer, converted into an electrical signal, amplified, and charted on a recorder.

4. The animals' breathing is monitored for at least 15 min while breathing clean air as a baseline. Then, the test material is introduced in an appropriately controlled manner into the airstream. The exposure lasts 1 hr, unless all animals die, and the animals' breathing is continuously monitored. Also, the test air is appropriately sampled to establish the concentration level. After the 1-hr exposure, the animals are monitored for at least 15 min to allow clearing of the chamber and to observe if the animals' breathing patterns return to baseline values.

5. The data from each exposure are analyzed by counting for each animal the breaths per minute (BPM) during the minute prior to exposure initiation [BPM (-1)] and during the 60th min into the exposure [BPM (60)]. The data are recorded. Then the respiratory rate decrease (%) is calculated for each animal:

$$\text{Decrease } (\%) = \frac{\text{BPM}_{-1} - \text{BPM}_{60}}{\text{BPM}_{-1}} \times 100$$

The decreases for all the animals are then averaged to give the mean response for the dose level.

6. After several different dose level experiments are performed, a dose–response curve can be obtained by plotting the mean breathing rate decrease (%) versus the logarithm of the dose level. The regression line is determined by the method of least squares, easily performed on a calculator. From the regression equation, the RD50 is determined.

PULMONARY SENSITIZATION

The inhalation of certain gases, vapors, or dusts has been known to induce immunologic hypersensitivity reactions within the respiratory tract for some time (Ratner *et al.*, 1927). To assess the sensitizing potencies of various inhaled materials, an animal model for pulmonary hypersensitivity has been developed (Karol, 1980). Guinea pigs are sensitized by exposures designed to simulate those experienced in the occupational setting, i.e., exposure via inhalation and dermal contact. Using toluene diisocyanate (TDI), a dose–response relationship has been detected between exposure concentration of TDI and development of immunologic response. Extension of the animal model to ascertain a "no-response" concentration can enable the setting of threshold limit values for industrial workers to protect against industrial sensitization. Most of the work with this model (but not all) has been done with more potent sensitizers such as isocynates and hydroxyamine.

After induction (preferably by inhalation exposure, but it can also frequently be achieved by dermal exposures such as detailed in Chapter 5), guinea pigs are challenged with low concentrations of test chemical aerosol while restrained in body plethysmographs. Sensitization is evaluated by measuring respiratory rates and tidal volumes during bronchial provocation challenge and comparing the values during challenge with those immediately preceeding challenge when ambient air flowed through the chamber. Respiratory rate increases during inhalation challenge with specific antigen are known to occur in numerous species of animals including rabbits, calves, dogs, monkeys, sheep, guinea pigs, and man (Patterson and Kelly, 1974; also reviewed by Karol *et al.*, 1980).

ALTERNATIVE MODELS

There are many alternative models and test designs for acute inhalation toxicology. The alternatives, unlike other areas of acute toxicology, include some that have as an objective avoiding the high capital cost and technical complications of performing exposures in intact animals.

INTRATRACHEAL INSTILLATION

This is an economical alternative to inhalation exposure to animals. The advantages of these types of exposure include the need for very small amounts of test material, extensive chambers are not required, and the complex technical support needed to generate and maintain exposure conditions is avoided. These make this type of study very inexpensive to conduct. Furthermore, the dose can be delivered very precisely to respiratory tract tissues. However, dose distribution to the respiratory tract tissues does not accurately simulate an inhaled dose and, hence, does not reflect the real-life response very clearly. Inhalation of airborne toxins generally results in a relatively well-distributed dose throughout the respiratory system. Intratracheal instillation tends to lead to a less uniform deposition and to favor the lower portions of the lung due to gravimetric settling of material. Brain *et al.* (1976) exposed rats and hamsters to radioactive particles and examined the distribution following both inhalation and instillation. The resulting distributions were strikingly different with instillation producing heavy deposits in the medium-sized bronchi. Instilled materials seldom reached the alveoli, whereas inhalation led to considerable deposition in the small airways. High local concentrations following instillation can lead to localized tissue damage which would not be seen following more uniform deposition. The use of this technique then is basically limited to situations in which tissue reactions, both of an acute (inflammation) and chronic (neoplasia and fibrosis) nature, to a variety of materials are to be compared side by side.

Isolated Perfused Lung

Lungs isolated from rabbits or rats can be perfused with heparinized blood or a suitable salt solution at a constant pressure and ventilated with positive pressure through the trachea or negative pressure from outside of the lung. A constant blood flow can be maintained over a period of several hours. The system is especially useful in determining nonrespiratory functions of the lung. For example, the levels of the endogenous hormones and vasoactive amines can be readily determined in the exudate. Furthermore, the pulmonary metabolism of a toxicant can be ascertained by adding it to the perfusate and analyzing the exudate for the toxicant and its metabolite (see Anderson and Eling, 1976; Roth, 1980).

Tracheal Explants

The effects of toxic gases and vapors on the trachea can be assessed by removing them from animals, such as rats, that have been exposed to toxicants. When incubated in a tissue culture medium the trachea will continue to secrete mucous glycoproteins. The rate of secretion can be affected by exposure to toxicants. For example, tracheal explants taken from rats exposed to ozone at 0.8 ppm showed an increased rate of secretion, but those from rats exposed to 0.5 ppm ozone or 1.1 mg/m^3 sulfuric acid did not.

Isolated Cells

Various types of cells from the respiratory system have been isolated and cultured. These include the epithelial cells of the trachea and lung tissue as well as endothelial cells. Isolated cultured cells show promise of becoming useful tools in the study of the toxicology of the respiratory system. Reiser and Last (1979), for example, pointed out the importance of pulmonary alveolar macrophages and fibroblasts in the development of fibrosis in chronic silicosis. They also noted the likelihood of involvement of other cell types, the precise role of which awaits further studies with isolated cells. This is the basis of the rabbit alveolar macrophage (RAM) test—a screen for fibrogenicity (Mossman, 1990).

Lung Organ Culture

Placke and Fisher (1987) have developed procedures to culture 1 or 2-mm-thick cross sections of lung lobes for periods of 4–6 weeks. Normal morphology and macromolecular composition are maintained. Eight different, supplemented, serum-free media, mixed with heated liquid agarose, were infused into the airways of hamster and rat lungs. Cross sections were explanted onto squares of porous surgical packing material, placed in medium, and incubated for 4–6 weeks. The ability of each medium to maintain normal lung tissue structure was assessed microscopically by quantitative image analysis and by biochemical analyses. The optimal medium formulation for each species is described. The adult peripheral lung culture system should provide toxicologists with a unique model for mechanistic evaluations and the screening of potential lung toxicants.

COMMON PROBLEMS AND THEIR SOLUTIONS

The inhalation toxicity test is a complex endeavor involving chemical, engineering, and biological skills. As such, there are numerous points in the design and execution of a study which need constant attention or the results will be of little or no use for safety evaluation purposes. A few of the commonly encountered problems should be presented and either generic answers or questions that need to be asked and answered before and during the conduct of such studies be suggested. This section is not complete, in that both entire books could be written on the subject and new types of problems will continue to arise. Those problems discussed here are frequently encountered and do need appropriate attention at all phases of the inhalation experiment.

The reactivity and physical characteristics of the test chemical itself need to be considered. Interaction with containment vessels, transfer lines, exposure chambers, humidity, and air can result in achieved concentrations much lower than desired or exposures to reaction products rather than the intended test chemical. Awareness of potential reactivity and use of equipment that will minimize the potential for reaction, as well as restricting the contact points for the chemical prior to introduction into the breathing zone of the animal, will limit this potential problem. Hydrolysis of chemicals in both the test atmosphere and the aqueous environment of the respiratory tract can occur and the extent and rate of the reaction should be known to fully appreciate the hazard involved in breathing the material. Likewise, care should be taken to limit (and if possible, preclude) physical changes in a test atmosphere. Materials with boiling points close to those in the laboratory, when generated as gases, can sometimes arrive in the test chambers as liquid aerosols due to cooling along the way. Wrapping the pipes connecting the source (generator or tank) and test chamber with a heating tape is a sound precaution in such cases.

Appropriate and accurate chemical analysis is mandatory for relating the quantity and exact nature of chemical inhaled with any effects produced. Inhalation exposures generally involve the introduction of a single agent into the atmosphere which then needs to be measured. Although interfering substances are less likely to exist here than in actual exposure situations (in which chemicals exist potentially among concentrations of other agents), the need to use a specific analytical method is important. Methods that give "real-time" results are most useful so that deviations from desired concentrations can be readily corrected. However, situations arise in which more lengthy analytical procedures are necessary for accuracy. In some cases, the use of more than one method, that is, one (such as IR spectrophotometry) as a rough screen to monitor the chamber concentration and allow for short-term control corrections and a second (such as a GC method) to quantitate exactly for actual concentrations, may be used. Another example of this practice may be seen in studies involving solid particulates, in which the total airborne particulate concentration may be measured gravimetrically every half hour and particle sizing and analytical determination of the particulate trapped on the filter may be done at selected time intervals (often at the beginning, in the middle, and at the end of the exposure period).

When working with mixtures of materials with different boiling points, care needs to be taken not to generate atmospheres which are initially enriched in the more volatile components. Similarly, mixtures of solids (such as drugs in an excepient) must be monitored carefully to ensure that lighter or smaller particles in a mixture are not differentially "generated" into a test atmosphere. Continuing exposures of this type follow the laws of fractional distillation and may produce atmospheres which are both much different from that of the starting mixture and change considerably as the exposure continues [and depletion of the more volatile materials(s) or smaller particles occurs]. This can be prevented by either testing the material as an aerosol and directing the total fluid into the chamber or by flash evaporating the liquid on a heated surface, for example, prior to entry to the chamber.

The problem of actual versus nominal concentration is generally a thing of the past but, particularly for acute studies, experiments continue to report concentrations in terms of material used as a function of air flow to the chamber (nominal concentration). This practice in itself is a problem because the values arrived at by that calculation represent maximum concentrations possible rather than the concentration actually presented to the animal. For certain materials such as gases, the difference between actual and nominal may not be great. However, for particulates, the difference may be almost two orders of magnitude. Specifically, the concentration in the breathing zone of the animal needs to be determined analytically.

With both liquid and solid aerosols, the test material in the breathing zone needs to be present in respirable sizes (for that species) to produce a response. Hence, with such materials, it is important to accurately define the test atmosphere in terms of both chemical concentration and particle (or droplet) size. Experiments using particulates with mass medium diameters much in excess of 3–5 μm really are not measuring the toxicity of the material for rodents. Unless the material produces local irritation of the mucous membranes of the respiratory tract, there is little possibility of the material entering the system (the lower respiratory tract) and doing damage. With materials whose physical form is such that the dusts exist mainly in the form of large nonrespirable particles, the method for testing should involve either concentrating those particles at the respirable end of the size distribution or using physical means to reduce them to that size. This allows the determination of toxicity—what the chemical can do when it enters the lungs. The hazard determination then will involve knowing what portion of the material normally exists in respirable sizes and relating that concentration to the effects seen. For example, you find little toxicity in a test after, with heroic effort, you are able to generate and maintain a respirable test atmosphere of 50 mg/m^3.

Only a very small fraction of the naturally occurring particles of this material are of respirable size and you find much less than 1 mg/m^3 in the workplace. In this situation, the inhalation hazard of this material would be considered quite low. One frequently has to generate and test atmospheres up to the "nuisance dust" level (2 g/m^3) for some regulatory purposes, however.

The type of exposure system chosen can also present problems when one is trying to measure only the effects of materials entering via the lung. As pointed out at the beginning of this chapter, whole body exposures can also involve absorption through the skin and through the gastrointestinal tract (following preening). The contribution of other routes to that amount absorbed via inhalation can be minimized by exposing only the nose of the animal to the test atmosphere. As discussed earlier, this type of exposure is not difficult but does have some limitations that need to be kept in mind—for example, it is difficult to observe the response of an animal while it is restrained in the equipment necessary to accomplish nose-only exposures.

This section has highlighted only some of the basic problems which are frequently encountered in inhalation hazard determinations. The procedures which can be applied to generate and analyze test atmospheres in the wide variety of experimental setups which are used in the field makes the application of common sense and sound scientific principles a necessity in producing information which is genuinely useful for hazard determination purposes.

Further discussion of acute inhalation toxicity testing can be found in Kennedy and Trachimorvicz (1982), Leong (1981), or Cobb (1981).

REFERENCES

Alarie, Y. (1966). Irritating properties of airborne material respiratory tract. *Arch. Environ. Health* **13**, 433–449.

Alarie, Y., Lin, C. K., and Geary, D. L. (1974). Sensory irritation evoked by plastic decomposition products. *Am. Ind. Hyg. Assoc. J.* **35**, 654–661.

Amdur, M. O. (1957). The Influence of Aerosols Upon the Respiratory Response of Guinea Pigs to Sulfur Dioxide. *Am. Ind. Hyg. Assoc. Q.* **18**, 149–155.

Anderson, M. W., and Eling, T. E. (1976). Studies on the uptake, metabolism, and release of endogenous and exogenous chemicals by the use of the isolated perfused ling. *Environ. Health Perspect.* **16**, 77–81.

Attman, P. L., and Dittmer, D. S. (Eds.) (1971). *Respiration and Circulation*, pp. 56–59. FASEB, Bethesda, MD.

Baker, H. J., Lindsey, J. R., and Weisbroth, S. H. (1979). *The Laboratory Rat,* Vol. I, pp. 411–412. Academic Press, New York.

Brain, J. D., Knudson, D. E., Sorokin, S. P., and Davis, M. A. (1976). Pulmonary distribution of particles given by intratracheal instillation or by aerosol inhalation. *Environ. Res.* **11**, 13.

Cobb, L. M. (1981). Pulmonary toxicity, In *Testing for Toxicity* (J. W. Gorrod, Ed.), pp. 255–274. Taylor and Francis, London.

Dahl, A. R., Schlesinger, R. B., D'A. Heck, H., Medinsky, M. A., and Lucier, G. W. (1991). Comparative dosimetry of inhaled materials: Differences among animal species and extrapolation to man. *Fundam. Appl. Toxicol.* **16**, 1–13.

Drew, R. T. (1983). Methods for generation of test atmosphere. In *Chemistry for Toxicity Testing* (C. W. Jameson and D. D. Walters, Eds.), pp. 123–138. Butterworth, Boston.

Enna, S. J., and Schanger, L. S. (1960). Drug absorption from the lung. *Fed. Proc.* **28**, 359.

Gargas, M. L., Burgess, R. J., Voissard, D. E. Cason, G. H., and Anderson, M. E. (1989). Partician coefficient of low molecular weight volatile chemicals in various tissues and liquids. *Toxicol. Appl. Pharmacol.* **798**, 87–99.

Goldstein, A., Aronow, L., and Kalman, S. (1974). The time course of drug action. In *Principles of Drug Action: The Basis of Pharmacology*, 2nd ed., Chap. 4, pp. 338–356. Wiley, New York.

Karol, M. H. (1980). Immunologic response of the respiratory system to industrial chemicals. In *Proceedings of the Inhalation Toxicology and Technology Symposium* (B. K. J. Leong, Ed.), pp. 233–246. Ann Arbor Science, Ann Arbor, MI.

Karol, M. H., Dixon, C., Brady, M., and Alarie, Y. (1980). Immunologic sensitization and pulmonary hypersensitivity by repeated inhalation of aromatic isocyanates. *Toxicol. Appl. Pharmacol.* **53**, 260–270.

Kennedy, G. L. (1988). Techniques for evaluating hazards of inhaled products. In *Product Safety Evaluation* (S. C. Gad, Ed.), pp. 259–289. Dekker, New York.

Kennedy, G. L., and Trochimowicz, H. J. (1982). Inhalation Toxicology. In *Principles and Methods of Toxicology* (A. W. Hayes, Ed.), pp. 185–208. Raven Press, New York.

Last, J. A., and Kaizer, T. (1980). Mucus glycoprotein secretion by tracheal explants: Effect of pollutants. *Environ. Health Perspect.* **35**, 131–137.

Lee, K. P. (1985). Lung response to particulates with emphasis on asbestos and other fibrous dust. *CTC Crit. Rev. Toxicol.* **14**, 33.

Leong, B. K. J. (1981). *Inhalation Toxicology and Technology,* Ann Arbor Science, Ann Arbor, MI.

Lu, F. C. (1985). *Basic Toxicology.* Hemisphere, New York.

Menzel, D. B., and McClellan, R. O. (1980). Toxic responses of the respiratory system. In *Casarett and Doull's Toxicology: The Basic Science of Poisons,* 2d ed. (J. Doull, C. D. Klaassen, and M. O. Amdur, (Eds.), 2nd ed. Macmillan, New York.

Morrow, P. E. (1960). Some physical and physiological factors controlling the fate of inhaled substances. *Health Phys.* **2**, 366–378.

Mossman, B. T. (1990). In vitro studies on the biologic effects of fibers: Correlation with in vivo bioassays. *Environ. Health Perspect.* **88**, 319–322.

Munson, E. S., and Eger, E. I. (1971). Pulmonary disposition of drugs. In *Fundamentals of Drug Metabolism and Drug Disposition* (B. N. La Du, H. G. Mandel, and E. L. Way, Eds.), pp. 106–118. Williams and Wilkins, Baltimore.

Nelson, G. O. (1971). *Controlled Test Atmospheres.* Ann Arbor Science, Ann Arbor, MI.

Parent, R. A. (1991). *Comparative Biology of the Normal Lung.* CRC Press, Boca Raton, FL.

Patterson, R., and Kelly, J. F. (1974). Animal models of the asthmatic state. *Annu. Rev. Med.* **25**, 53–68.

Phalen, R. F. (1976). Inhalation exposure of animals. *Health Perspect.* **16**, 17–24.

Placke, M. E., and Fisher, G. L. (1987). Adult peripheral lung organ culture—A model for respiratory tract toxicology. *Toxicol. Appl. Pharmacol.* **90**, 284–298.

Ratner, B., Jackson, HI.C., and Gruehl, H. L. (1927). Respiratory anaphylaxis. Sensitization, shock, bronchial asthma and death induced in the guinea pig by the nasal inhalation of dry horse dander. *Am. J. Dis. Child* **34**, 23–52.

Reiser, K. M., and Last, J. A. (1979). Silicosis and fibrogenesis: Fact and artifact. *Toxicology* **13**, 51–72.

Roth, J. A. (1980). Use of perfused lung in biochemical toxicology. *Rev. Biochem. Toxicol.* **1**, 287–309.

Swenson, M. J. (Ed.) (1977). *Dukes Physiology of Domestic Animals,* p. 178. Comstock, Ithaca, NY,

Taylor, A. E., Guyion, A. C., and Bishop, V. B. (1965). Permeability of the aveolar membrane to solutes. *Circ. Res.* **16**, 353–362.

Technical Committee, Inhalation Specialty Section, Society of Toxicology (1992). Recommendations for the conduct of acute inhalation limit test. *Fundam. Appl. Toxicol.* **18**, 321–327.

CHAPTER 14

Problems and Issues

Toxicology as a whole, and acute toxicology in particular, is very much a moving target. No author can realistically hope to capture its entire scope in a single volume or to have a book when it is actually published reflect the state of the art. One can, however, try to at least point out any significant areas that have not been adequately addressed and present the problems and forces which are (or should be) causing the field to change. In this last chapter, we will try to draw together all of these miscellaneous points.

The issue of proper animal usage is one of the most compelling ones in acute toxicology. The authors have tried to address most of the considerations involved as they arise through the course of this volume. Several points which are central to the issue remain, however.

USE OF AVAILABLE TOXICOLOGY INFORMATION SOURCES

One of the first and best things that toxicologists can do to reduce animal testing is to make sure that they do not perform studies when the desired information already exists. The first step in developing toxicology evaluation should be to search and review the existing literature.

The first step in any such literature review is to obtain as much of the following information as possible:

Correct chemical identity including molecular formula, Chemical Abstract Service (CAS) number, common synonyms, trade names, and a structural diagram. Goseelin *et al.* (1984) is an excellent source of information on existing commercial products, their components, and uses.

Chemical composition (if a mixture) and major impurities.

Production and use information.

Chemical and physical properties (physical state, vapor pressure, pH, solubility, chemical reactivity, etc.).

Any structurally related chemical substances which are already on the market or in production.

Collection of the previous information is not only important for hazard assessment (high vapor pressure would indicate high inhalation potential just as high and low pH would indicate high irritation potential) but also the prior identification of all product uses and exposure patterns may provide alternative information sources; for example, chemicals formerly used as anesthetics, food additives, or pesticides may have extensive toxicology data obtainable from government or private sources. A great deal of the existing toxicity information (particularly information on acute toxicity) is not available in the published or electronic literature. This is because of both concerns as to its proprietary nature and the widespread opinion that is does not have enough intrinsic scholarly value to merit publication. This is unfortunate because it leads to much replication of effort and expenditure of resources that could be better used elsewhere. It also means that an experienced toxicologist will use an informal search of the unpublished literature by colleagues as a supplement to searches of the published and electronic literature.

There are now numerous published texts that should be considered for use in literature reviewing activities. An alphabetic listing of 19 of the more commonly used sources for acute data is provided in Table 97. Obviously, this is not a complete listing and consists of only the general multipurpose texts that have a wider range of applicability for toxicology. Texts dealing with specialized classes of chemicals, e.g., petroleum hydrocarbons, plastics, or specific target organ toxicity (neurotoxins and teratogens), are generally beyond the scope of this text. Parker (1987) should be consulted for details on the use of these texts. Both Wexler (1982) and Parker (1987) should be consulted for more extensive listings of the literature as it relates to more specialized information beyond the scope of acute toxicology.

TABLE 97   Published Information Sources for Acute Toxicology

Title	Reference
Burger's Medicinal Chemistry	Wolff (1994, 1996)
Chemical Hazards of the Workplace	Proctor and Hughes (1978)
Clinical Toxicology of Commercial Products	Gosselin *et al.* (1984)
Contact Dermatitis	Cronin (1980)
Criteria Documents	NIOSH (various)
Current Intelligence Bulletins (NIOSH)	
Dangerous Properties of Industrial Materials	Sax (1985)
Documentation of the Threshold Limit Values (AIHA)	ACGIH (1986)
Handbook of Toxic and Hazardous Chemicals	Sittig, (1985)
Hygienic Guide Series (AIHA)	AIHA (1980)
Industrial Toxicology	Finkel (1983)
Medical Toxicology	Ellenhorn *et al.* (1997)
Merck Index	Budavari (1989)
Occupational Health Guidelines for Chemical Hazards (NIOSH/OSHA)	Mackinson (1981)
Patty's Industrial Hygience and Toxicology	Clayton and Clayton (1981)
Physician's Desk Reference	Barnhart (1987)
Registry of Toxic Effects of Chemical Substances (RETECS)	NIOSH (1984)
Toxicology: The Basic Science of Poisons	Klaassen (1996)
Toxicology of the Eye	Grant (1993)

In the past decade, the use of on-line literature searches for many toxicologists has changed from an occasional, sporadic activity to a semicontinuous need. Usually nontoxicology-related search capabiliies are already in place in many companies. Therefore, all that is needed is to expand the information source to include some of the databases that cover the types of toxicology information you desire. However, if no capabilities exist within an organization one can approach a university or a private contract laboratory and utilize their on-line system at a reasonable rate. It is even possible to access most of these sources from home using a personal computer. The major available on-line databases are as follows:

A. National Library of Medicine: The National Library of Medicine (NLM) information retrieval service contains the well-known and frequently used Medline, Toxline and Cancerline databases. Databases commonly used by toxicologists for acute data in the NLM service are:

    1. Toxline (Toxicology Information Online) is a bibliographic data-

base covering the pharmacological, biochemical, physiological, environmental, and toxicological effects of drugs and other chemicals. It contains approximately 1.7 million citations, most of which are complete with abstract, index terms, and CAS registry numbers, Toxline citations have publication dates of 1981 to present. Older information is on Toxback 76 (1976–1980) and Toxback 65 (pre-1965 through 1975).

2. Medline (Medical Information Online) is a database containing approximately 800,000 references to biomedical journal articles published since 1980. These articles, usually with an English abstract, are from more than 3000 journals. Coverage of previous years (back to 1966) is provided by back files, searchable on-line, that total approximately 3.5 million references.

3. Toxnet (Toxicology Data Network) is a computerized network of toxicologically oriented databanks. Toxnet offers a sophisticated search and retrieval package which accesses the three subfiles. The two relevant to acute toxicology are the following:

   HSDB (Hazardous Substances Data Bank) is a scientifically reviewed and edited databank containing toxicological information enhanced with additional data related to the environment, emergency situations, and regulatory issues. Data are derived from a variety of sources including government documents and special reports. This database contains records for more than 4100 chemical substances.

   TDB (Toxicology Data Bank) is a peer-reviewed databank focusing on toxicological and pharmacological data, environmental and occupational information, manufacturing and use data, and chemical and physical properties. References have been extracted from a selective list of standard source documents.

4. RTECS (Registry of Toxic Effects of Chemical Substances) is the NLM on-line version of NIOSH's annual compilation of substances with toxic activity. The original collection of data was derived from the 1971 Toxic Substances Lists. RTECS data contain threshold limit values, aquatic toxicity ratings, air standards, NTP carcinogenesis bioassay information, and toxicological/carcinogenic review information. NIOSH is responsible for the file content in RETCS and for providing quarterly updates to NLM. RTECS currently covers toxicity data on more than 61,000 substances.

B. *Merck Index*: The *Merck Index* is now available on-line for up-to-the-minute access to new chemical entities. Parker (1987) should be consulted for guidance as to search strategies and procedures for on-line databases.

CONSIDERATIONS IN ADOPTING NEW TEST SYSTEMS

Conducting toxicological investigations in three or more species of laboratory animals is generally accepted as being a prudent and responsible practice in developing a new chemical entity, especially one that is expected to receive widespread use and to have exposure potential over human lifetimes. Adding a second or a third species to the testing regimen offers an extra measure of confidence to the toxicologist and the other professionals who will be responsible for evaluating the associated risks, benefits, and exposure limitations or protective measures. Although undoubtedly broadening and deepening a compound's profile of toxicity, the practice of enlarging on the number of test species is, as has been demonstrated at multiple points in this book, an indiscriminate scientific generalization. Moreover, such a tactic is certain to generate the problem of species-specific toxicoses; that is, a toxic response or an inordinately low biological threshold for toxicity is evident in one species or strain, while all other species examined are either unresponsive or strikingly less sensitive. The investigator confronting such findings must be prepared to address the all-important question, "Are humans likely to react positively or negatively to the test agent in similar circumstances?"

Assuming that numerical odds prevail and humans automatically fit into the predominant category, whether on the side of being safe or at risk, would be scientifically irresponsible. Far from being an irreconcilable nuisance, however, such a confounded situation can be an opportunity to advance more quickly into the heart of the search for predictive information. This is the case for cross-species extrapolation. a species-specific toxicosis can frequently contribute toward better understanding of the general case if the underlying biological mechanism either causing or enhancing toxicity is defined and especially if it is discovered to uniquely reside in the sensitive species. The purpose of Chapter 12 was to review selected examples of species-specific toxicoses, collected from the author's experiences or the literature, wherein such ancillary research has provided a means for rationally predicting an expectation for, or the probable absence of, human toxic responses.

Mention of species-specific toxicoses usually implies that different metabolic pathways for converting and excreting xenobiotics are involved. Species differences from this standpoint are reviewed elsewhere in this book. Likewise, the design of our current tests appears to serve society reasonably well (i.e., significantly more times than not) in identifying hazards that would be unacceptable. However, the process can just as clearly be improved from the standpoints of both improving our protection of society and doing necessary testing in a manner that uses fewer animals and uses these fewer animals in a more humane manner.

Throughout this volume, the authors have tried to present and review alternatives to existing tests. Alternative designs which still use intact animals but in smaller numbers represent one of three classes of alternatives and have been presented and addressed individually. The other two classes of alternatives are *in vitro* models (which do not use intact higher organisms but do use some form of test system) and mathematical or structure–activity relationship (SAR) approaches (which construct theoretical analogies but require no actual generation or interpretation of new data).

IN VITRO MODELS

In vitro models, at least as screening tests, have been with us in toxicology for some 20 years now. The past 10 to 15 years have seen a great upsurge in interest in such models. This increased interest is due to economic and animal welfare pressures and technological improvements.

Criteria against which an *in vitro* model might be evaluated for its suitability in replacing (partially or entirely) an accepted *in vivo* model are incorporated in the process detailed in Table 98.

In vitro systems per se have a number of limitations which can contribute to their not being acceptable models. Some of these reasons are detailed in Table 99.

At the same time there are substantial potential advantages in using *in vitro* systems. The advantages of using cell or tissue culture in toxicological testing are isolation of test cells or organ fragments from homeostatic and hormonal control, accurate dosing, and quantitation of results. It is important to devise a suitable model system which is related to the mode of toxicity of the compound. Tissue and cell culture have been used in two very different ways in screening studies. First, they have been used to examine a particular aspect of the toxicity of a compound in relation to its toxicity *in vivo*. Second, they have been used as a form of rapid screening to compare the toxicity of a group of compounds.

SAR MODELS

SAR methods have become a legitimate and useful part of toxicology during the past 20 years or so. These methods are various forms of mathematical or statistical models which seek to predict the adverse biological effects of chemicals based on their structure. The prediction may be of either a qualitative irritant/nonirritant) or quantitative (LD_{50}) nature, with the second group usually being denoted as quantitative structure–activity relationship (QSAR) models. It should be obvious at the outset that the basic techniques utilized to

TABLE 98 Multistage Scheme for the Development, Validation, and Transfer of *in Vitro* Test System Technology in Toxicology

---

Stage I. Statement of test objective
  Identify existing test system and its strengths and weaknesses
  Clearly state objectives for alternative test system
  Identify potential alternative test system

Stage II. Define developmental test design
  Identity relevant variables
  Evaluate effects of variables on test system
  Redesign test to optimize test performance
  Understand what the test does in a functional sense
    Is it a simulation of an *in vivo* event?
    Is this simply a response to the presence of the agent?
    Is this a functional step or link in that event?
    Is this an event or a property mechanistically linked to that event or some intermediate stage?
    Is this an effect on some structure or function analogous to the *in vivo* structure or function?

Stage III. Evaluate performance of optimum test
  Develop battery of known positive and negative response materials of diverse structure
  Use optimum test design to evaluate battery of "knowns" under "blind" conditions
  Compare correlation of test results to those of other test systems and to real case of interest—human results

Stage IV. Technology transfer
  Present and publish results through professional media (society meetings and peer reviewed journals)
  Provide hands-on training to personnel from other facilities and facilitate their performing internal evaluations of test methods

Stage V. Validation
  Arrange for test of coded samples in multiple labs (i.e., interlaboratory validation)
  Compare, present, and publish results

Stage VI. Continue to refine and evaluate test system performance and utilization
  Continually strive for an underlying of why the test "works" and its relevance to effects in man
  Remain skeptical. Why should any one of us be the one to make the big breakthrough? Clearly there is some basic flaw in the design or conduct of the study which has given rise to these promising results. Doubt, check, and question; then let your most severe critic review the data; then go to a national meeting and give a presentation; then go back home and doubt, check, and question some more!

---

construct such models are mathematical modeling and reduction of dimensionality methods, as discussed in Gad and Weil (1986).

The concept that the biological activity of a compound is a direct function of its chemical structure is now at least a century old (Crum-Brown and Fraser, 1869). During most of this century, the development and use of SARs were the domain of pharmacology and medicinal chemistry. These two fields are

TABLE 99   Possible Interpretations When *in Vitro* Data Do Not Predict Results
of *in Vivo* Studies

Chemical is not absorbed at all or is poorly absorbed in *in vivo* studies.

Chemical is well absorbed but is subject to first-pass effect in liver.

Chemical is distributed so that less (or more) reaches the receptors than would be predicted on the basis of its absorption.

Chemical is rapidly metabolized to an active or inactive metabolite that has a different profile of activity and/or different duration of action than the parent drug.

Chemical is rapidly eliminated (e.g., through secretory mechanisms).

Species of the two test systems used are different.

Experimental conditions of the *in vitro* and *in vivo* experiments differed and may have led to different effects than expected. These conditions include factors such as temperature or age, sex, and strain of animal.

Effects elicited *in vitro* and *in vivo* differ in their characteristics.

Tests used to measure responses will probably differ greatly for *in vitro* and *in vivo* studies, and the types of data obtained may not be comparable.

The *in vitro* study did not use adequate controls (e.g., pH, vehicle used, volume of test agent given, or samples taken from sham-operated animals).

In vitro data cannot predict the volume of distribution in central or in peripheral compartments.

In vitro data cannot predict the rate constants for chemical movement between compartments.

In vitro data cannot predict whether linear or nonlinear kinetics will occur with specific dose of a chemical *in vivo*.

Pharmacokinetic parameters (e.g., bioavailability, peak plasma concentration, or half-life) cannot be predicted based solely on *in vitro* studies.

In vivo effects of chemical are due to an alteration in the higher-order integration of an intact animal system, which cannot be reflected in a less complex system.

---

responsible for the beginnings of all the basic approaches in SAR work, usually with the effort being called drug design. An introductory medicinal chemistry text (such as Foye, 1974) is strongly recommended as a starting place for SAR.

Having already classified SAR methods into qualitative and quantitative, it should also be pointed out that both of these can be approached on two different levels. The first in on a local level, where prediction of activity (or lack of activity) is limited to other members of a congeneric series or structural near neighbors. The accuracy of predictions via this approach is generally greater but is of value only if one has sufficient information on some of the structures within a series of interest.

The second approach is prediction of activity over a wide range, generally based on the presence or absence of particular structural features (functional groups or "toxicophores").

For toxicology, SARs have a small but important number of uses at present. These can all be generalized as identifying potentially toxic effects, or restated as three main uses:

1. For the selection and design of toxicity tests to address endpoints of possible concern.

2. If a comprehensive or large testing program is to be conducted, SAR predictions can be used to prioritize the test so that the highlighted questions (the answers to which might preclude the need to do further testing) may be addressed first.

3. As an alternative to testing at all. Though in general it is not believed that the state of the art for SAR methods allows such usage, in certain special cases (such as selecting which of several alternative candidate compounds to develop further and then test), this use may be valid and valuable. These cases have been pointed out elsewhere in this volume.

BASIC ASSUMPTION

Starting with the initial assumption that there is a relationship between structure and biological activity, one can proceed to more readily testable assumptions.

First, the dose of chemical is subject to a number of modifying factors (such as membrane selectivities and selective metabolic actions) which are each related in some manner to chemical structure. Indeed, absorption, metabolism, pharmacologic activity, and excretion are each subject to not just structurally determined actions but also (in many cases) stereospecific differential handlings.

Given these assumptions, actual elucidation of SARs requires the following:

1. Knowledge of the biological activities of existing structures
2. Knowledge of structural features which serve to predict activity (also called molecular parameters of interest)
3. One or more models which relate 2 to 1 with some degree of reliability

MOLECULAR PARAMETERS OF INTEREST

Which structural and physicochemical properties of a chemical are important in predicting its toxicologic activity is open to considerable debate. The reader is referred to Gad and Weil (1986) for a discussion on the subject.

There are now several sets of systems available to study the three-dimensional structural aspects of molecules and their interactions. The first are the various molecular modeling sets, which can actually be very useful for some simpler problems. The second are the molecular design and analysis packages which are available for mainframe computers. Lastly, molecular graphics software packages have become available recently for such microcomputers as the Apple IIe, MacIntosh, and IBM. Use of such forms of graphic structural examination as a tool or method in SAR analysis has been discussed by Cohen *et al.* (1974) and Gund *et al.* (1980). Such methods are generally called topological methods.

SAR MODELING METHODS

A detailed review of even the major methodologies available for SAR/QSAR modeling in toxicology is beyond the scope of this book. The reader is directed to one of the several very readable introductory articles (Chu, 1980) or books (Olson and Christoffersen, 1979; Topliss, 1983; Goldberg, 1983) for somewhat detailed presentations.

All the current major SAR methods used in toxicology can be classified based on what kinds of compound-related structural data they use and what method is used to correlate this structural data with the existing biological data.

The more classical approaches use physiochemical data (such as molecular weight, free energies, etc.) as a starting point. The major approaches to it are by manual pattern recognition methods, cluster analysis, or regression analysis. It is this last, in the form of Hansch or linear-free energy relationships (LFER), which actually launched all SAR work (other than that on limited congeneric cases) into the realm of a useful approach. Indeed, still foremost among the QSAR methods is the model proposed by Hansch and co-workers (Hansch, 1971). It was the major contribution of this group to propose the incorporation of earlier observations of the importance of the relative lipophilicity to biologic activity into the formal LFER approach to provide a general QSAR model for biological effects.

There are a number of approaches for using structural and substructural data and correlating these to biological activities. Such approaches are generally classified as regression analysis methods, pattern recognition methods, and miscellaneous other (such as factor analysis, principal components, and probalistic analysis).

The regression analysis methods which use structural data have been, as we will see when we survey the state of the art in toxicology, the most productive and useful. "Keys" or fragments of structure are assigned weights as predictors of an activity, usually in some form of the Free–Wilson model (Free and Wilson, 1964) which was developed at virtually the same time as the Hansch. According to this method, the molecules of a chemical series are structurally decomposed into a common moiety (or core) that may be substituted in multiple positions. A series of linear equations are constructed.

The favorite aspects of Free–Wilson models are the following:

Any set of quantitative biological data may be employed as the dependent variable.

No independently determined substituent constants are required.

The molecules comprising a sample of interest may be structurally dismembered in any desired or convenient manner.

Multiple sites of variable substitution are readily handled by the model.

There are also several limitations; a substantial number of compounds with varying substituent combinations are required for a meaningful analysis, the derived substituent contributions give no reasonable basis for extrapolating predictions from the substituent matrix analyzed, and the model will break down if nonlinear dependence on substituent properties is important or if there are interactions between the substituents.

Pattern recognition methods comprise yet another approach to examining structural features and/or chemical properties for underlying patterns that are associated with differing biological effects. Accurate classification of untested molecules is again the primary goal. This is carried out in two stages. First, a set of compounds, designated the training set, is chosen for which the correct classification is known. A set of molecular or property description features is generated for each compound. A suitable classification algorithm is then applied to find some combination and weight of the descriptors that allow perfect classification. Many different statistical and geometric techniques for this purpose have been used and were presented in earlier chapters. The derived classification function is then applied in the second step to compounds not included in the training set to evaluate test performance in terms of accuracy of prediction. In published work these have generally been other compounds of known classification. Performance is judged by the percentage of correct predictions. Stability of the classification function is usually tested by repeating the procedure several times with slightly altered, but randomly varied, sets or samples.

The main difficulty with these methods is in "decoding" the QSAR in order to identify particular structural fragments responsible for the expression of a particular toxicity. Also, even if identified as "responsible" for activity, far harder questions for the model to answer are whether the structural fragment so identified is "sufficient" for activity, whether it is always "necessary" for activity, and to what extent its expression is modified by its molecular environment. Most pattern recognition methods use as weighting factors either the presence or absence of a particular fragment or feature (coded 1 or 0) or the

TABLE 100   Existing SAR Models for Acute Toxicology Endpoints

Endpoint	Prediction		Reference
	Quantitative	Qualitative	
Sensitization			Dupuis and Benezra (1982)
LD$_{50}$		X	Enslein et al. (1983a)
Teratogenicity	X		Enslein et al. (1983b)
Biological oxygen demand		X	Enslein et al. (1984)
Dermal irritation		X	K. Enslein (personal communication)

frequency of occurrence of a feature. They may be made more sophisticated by coding the spatial relationship between features. Enslein (1984) has published a good, brief description of the problems involved in applying these methods in toxicology.

APPLICATIONS IN TOXICOLOGY

SAR methods have been developed to predict a number of toxicological endpoints (mutagenesis, carcinogenesis, dermal sensitization, lethality LD$_{50}$ values, biological oxygen demands, and teratogenicity) with varying degrees of accuracy, and models for the prediction of other endpoints are under development. Some of these existing models are presented by category of use in Table 100.

It should be expected that qualitative models are more "accurate" than quantitative ones, and that the more possible mechanisms associated with an endpoint, the less accurate (or more difficult) a prediction.

SAFETY FACTORS, POTENCY PREDICTORS, AND PROTECTING SOCIETY

In the whole process involved in toxicity or safety testing and in all discussions about it and how the resulting testing is used, it must always be kept in mind that the major objective is to produce information so that individuals and society are not subject to undue risk of harm or injury. All other considerations must come second to this one. As scientists we wish to do the best job possible, which means having as little uncertainty about our results and the process as possible. As has been shown, this can be done to a great extent but not entirely. Acute toxicity studies have three major limitations or precautions associated with them in a broad manner:

1. The data may be misleading in predicting the type of toxicity produced by the compound when administered for a prolonged period.

2. Biochemical, hematological, and pathological studies, with few exceptions, have been observed to have limited value in acute toxicity studies.

3. Acute toxicity studies may have little predictive value when there is a wide range between therapeutic doses and acute lethal doses. In such cases, adequate subacute studies may give a better estimate of tolerated and toxic doses.

The classical approach to providing the desired protection against hazard in the face of various degrees of uncertainty is the use of safety factors. As Weil (1972) stated,

> In summary, for evaluation of safety for man, it is necessary to: (1) design and conduct appropriate toxicologic tests, (2) statistically compare the data from treated and control animals, (3) delineate the minimum effect and maximum no ill-effect levels (NIEL) for these animals, and (4) if the material is to be used, apply an appropriate safety factor, e.g., (a) 1/100 (NIEL) for some effects or (b) 1/500 (NIEL), if the effect was a significant increase in cancer in an appropriate test.

This approach has served society reasonably well over the years once the experimental work has identified the potential hazards and quantitated the observable dose–response relationships. The safety factor approach, however, has not generally been accepted or seriously entertained by regulatory agencies. But until such times as the most elegant risk assessment procedures can instill greater public confidence, the use of the safety factor approach should perhaps not be abandoned so readily for more "mathematically precise" methodologies.

For acute animal toxicity data the traditionally employed safety factors are as follows:

1. If our starting point is a dose or exposure level where we have appropriate data saying there is no effect in a model system, a suitable level for human exposure would be 1/10th this level (unless the data are from dogs or primates, in which case 1/5th is generally used).

2. If we have been unable to establish a "clean" no-observable-effect level, an additional 1/10th safety factory is added. This would make the safety factor 1/100th for all model systems except dogs and primates. It should be remembered that the effects that are referred to here are not severe ones, such as death. Severe effects in the lowest dose studied make it inappropriate (and very risky) to use the safety factor approach, or any other kind of extrapolation approach, because safety factors are really there to bridge the gaps between species, strains, and other uncertainties of relative relationships—not to make up for poor data which are completely indeterminate.

MIXTURES

As was pointed out at the beginning of this book, none of our past or current systems for predicting effects works well in one particular case—that of mixtures. What we have data on are either pure materials or fairly simple mixtures with a fixed ratio of components. While predicting or using analogy over a limited range for single structures based on current data can generally be performed with reasonable comfort, the interactions between mixture components as both total amounts and relative proportions vary is beyond our current understanding, especially because many commercially or environmentally encountered mixtures are very complex, containing in some cases hundreds of components. Also, frequently we are faced with a desire to explore mixtures with a range of amounts of the same components, or with alterations (substitutions) in components.

There can be four general categories of interactions between components—additivity (effect A + effect $B = A + B$), antagonism (effect A and effect $B = A - B$), synergism (effect A and effect $B = AB$), or a combined effect which is qualitatively very different from that of the individual components. Such interactions may also be very time (temporally) dependent.

Our current understanding of human health and the real-world effect of toxicants is a reflection of what is called the multiple causation theory of disease. This holds that each input into the status of an individual's physiological and psychological condition (whether that input is a xenobiotic chemical or a "susceptibility factor," as was discussed in the earlier chapter on animals) is a component cause of that status.

Pozzani et al. (1959) published data on the toxicity of 36 simple (two-component or "binary") mixtures of vapors to rats and found that in only two of the cases did the results differ by more than 1.96 standard errors of the estimate from the predictions of Finney's (1952) model for additive joint. This model calculates the harmonic mean of the LD_{50} of mixture components as

$$1/\text{predicted } LD_{50} = P_A/LD_{50} \text{ of component } A + P_B/LD_{50} \text{ of component } B$$

where P_A and P_B are the proportions of components A and B in the mixture. Smyth et al. (1969) later found much the same result of the oral LD_{50}'s of 27 pairs of chemicals in rats, and, indeed, for many binary (two-component) mixtures the system works well (and is not limited to LD_{50}'s). But most mixtures of concern are multicomponent. It has been proposed that some form of multiple logistic regression model be used for such extrapolations.

An alternative approach to studying the interactions of mixture components is to assume that response be called Y, that its response can be linearized, and that for Drug $A = Y_A = \alpha_A + \beta_A \log Z$ and Drug $B = Y_B = \alpha_B + \beta_B \log Z$.

When $\beta_A = \beta_B = \beta$, the potency of β is relative or linear and you have parallel potencies.

Given this model, methods to estimate p (relative potency) and n (interaction component) have been proposed. If $p = 1$, the joint effect is additive. If it is less than 1.0 then the effect is synergistic. To study interactions, what must first be done is to determine approximately equipotent doses of components. Interaction studies would then center around evaluating effects at a joint (two-agent) dose with equipotent component portions, from which we could determine if the interaction was greater (synergism), the same (additivity), or less (antagonism) than twice the dose of either component alone. This approach could then be extended in steps to more complicated mixtures.

As was pointed out in Chapter 10, mixtures present problems in dosing/exposing intact animals while ensuring that a truly representative sample of the mixture is being administered. But this problem is even worse in the case of *in vitro* tests systems, which usually require maintenance of a narrow range of conditions in an aqueously based media to survive. How does one ensure that what gets into the media and from there to the *in vitro* system is the complete mixture of interest?

SPECIAL CASES

At least four special cases of acute toxicity testing have not been addressed in this volume but should be at least briefly reviewed. The four areas are important but generally are of interest to more limited audiences than addressed by the rest of this text.

Military Agent Toxicology

Chemical agents have been used as weapons or as crowd control agents on a widespread basis since the beginning of the 20th century. Though their use as weapons is now prohibited by treaty, there remains ample evidence that they continue to be used, and that multiple parties retain the capability to use them. This requires the development of protective devices and antidotes as defensive measures. The testing of the agents themselves and of any protective gear and antidotes is clearly a specialized form of acute toxicology.

A search of the MEDLINE database from 1967 through 1987 revealed 170 articles on the area, indicating that it is still of significant interest. The United States spent approximately 6 or 7 billion dollars from 1983 through 1987 working on its chemical warfare deterrent program (Connor, 1984). The actual chemical agents involved in such work (now called "surety compounds" in the United States) are divided into three major classes: riot control (which include vomiting and tear compounds and is generally for use in police operations), casualty (which include blister, blood, choking, and nerve), and incapacitating agents (both CNS stimulants and CNS depressants) with the two last categories being for use in military operations. Poziomek (1984) has addressed some of the special concerns in working with such compounds. A text on this subject has been published (Compton, 1988). Use by terrorists in Japan and the near use in the Gulf War have kept interest current.

Combustion Toxicology

The field of evaluating the potential health hazards of the decomposition products formed when plastics are heated is a relatively new one. Though early work on simple pyrolysis product toxicity has been around for perhaps 45 years, the oldest true references to combustion toxicology go back only to the early 1950s (Zapp, 1951). Yet today it has become a high priority area within toxicology. It has it own journals (*Journal of Combustion Toxicology* and *Journal of Fire Science*), annual conferences, study committees (both in industry and government), and stands on the verge of becoming the subject of federal regulation. Why?

There are currently approximately 5,575,000 unintentional fires annually in the United States alone, of which only 10% require action by fire departments. More than 9000 people are estimated to die each year in these fires and, as will be demonstrated later, there is good reason to believe that more than half of these deaths are due not to the flames themselves but rather to the gases, vapors, and smokes generated by these fires. We also have a good deal of data to suggest that those dying due to the products they inhale is increasing annually. Recent large fires with multiple toxic inhalant-caused deaths (such as the MGM Grand, Stoeffers, and Sao Paulo, Brazil high-rise fires) have renewed the concern of the public but should be recognized as not being unique. Just for perspective, one should remember four earlier large fires with similar patterns;

Newport, Kentucky, night club (1978)
Maury County, Tennessee, jail (1977)
Coconut Grove night club (1942)
Cleveland Clinic (1929)

As our society (not just in this country but throughout the world) has progressed, we have turned more and more to synthetic polymers for use in our clothes, furnishings, appliances, wall coverings, furniture, carpets, and homes. Not only are these materials less expensive, but in many cases they are more durable, lighter, and stronger than the natural products that were used in earlier days, and, especially with the addition of fire and flame retardants, their fire performance in buildings is superior. But the problem arises that when they burn, they can generate gas-phase decomposition products which are considerably more toxic than the old natural products (that is, primarily wood). This concern is widespread (international, in fact), as demonstrated by the multitude of reviews of the problems (Autian 1970; Birky, 1977; Bott *et al.*, 1969; Einhorn, 1977; Forestier, 1975; Hilado, 1978; Jouany & Raoul, 1975; Raftery, 1974; Reinke and Reinhardt, 1973; Reploh *et al.*, 1966; Rumberg, 1977; Sand and Hofmann, 1977; Terril *et al.*, 1977; Vasileve and Ilichkin, 1975; Wooley, 1973) from around the world.

Wood itself generates a multitude of decomposition products when burned. When the combustion is incomplete, the major product in terms of toxicity is carbon monoxide (CO), which acts by competing with oxygen for binding to hemoglobin. When so bound carboxyhemoglobin is formed. Because CO has a greater affinity than oxygen for the hemoglobin structure, it competes favorably and it is difficult for oxygen to displace.

The body depends on hemoglobin (in the form of a complex with oxygen called oxyhemoglobin) to transport oxygen to its tissues. If too much hemoglobin (50% or more) is tied up as carboxyhemoglobin then the results, in progressive order, are drowsiness, unconciousness, and finally death.

The major concern, however, is that the synthetic polymers will either generate a greater amount of carbon monoxide (than wood) under fire conditions or that they will generate quantitatively worse toxic materials (hereafter called, for the purposes of this section, toxicants) than wood. The initial concern was largely centered on the generation of hydrogen cyanide or of isocyanates, particularly by the various nitrogen-containing polymers. Cyanide is of such great concern because it causes death (by a mechanism called histotoxic hypoxia, which involves interfering with the cytochrome system in cells, therefore starving the body of oxygen on a molecular level) at very low levels ($1 \ \mu g/ml$ being a lethal level in the blood).

This brings us to the final point to be raised in the consideration of why combustion toxicology has become such a pressing issue. This is the matter of current and (more important) future regulations on polymers based on the real or perceived hazard posed by their combustion gases. Currently, the International Organization for Standardization and the city and state of New York regulate what may be used in buildings based on the results of mandatory combustion toxicity tests. The French regulate purely on the basis of having allowable limits on the amounts of N and Cl present in the structure of a building (believing that in so doing they are limiting the amounts of HCN and HCl which may be released in a fire). In an effort stretching over 6 years a committee gathered by the National Bureau of Standards has produced a "standard" test and protocol which several agencies (e.g., FAA and CPSC) are considering for use as the basis for the federal regulation of polymers in certain uses. The state of New York currently bases its regulation on the University of Pittsburgh's test system.

What must be kept firmly in mind and hand are the limits of these tests and their results. The fact that although combustion product toxicity is an important consideration, it should not be the only (or even the most important) factor in regulation. The use of combustion toxicity data must be tempered with the knowledge of ignition temperatures and of what portions of the fuel load they would comprise in a fire. The test system employed and results to date are the subject of a book in preparation, though Kaplan *et al.* (1983) did adequately address the then current test systems. A current and comprehensive address is of the subject Gad and Anderson (1990).

Medical Devices

The medical device industry in the United States and worldwide is immense in its economic impact (sales in 1993 were $93 billion worldwide and $38 billion in the United States, $24 billion in the European Community, and $17 billion in Japan; in 1994, the United States medical equipment trade surplus was $4.3 billion), scope (between 84,000 and 130,000 different devices are produced in the United States by ~7700 different manufacturers employing approximately 282,000 people; it is believed that ~1000 of these manufacturers are development stage companies without products yet on the market), and importance to the health of the world's citizens (Gad, 1997). The assessment of the safety to patients of the multitude of items produced by this industry is dependent on schemes and methods which are largely particular to these kinds of products; not as rigorous as those employed for foods, drugs, and pesticides; and are in a state of flux. Regulation of such devices is, in fact, relatively new. It is only with the Medical Device Amendments (to the Food, Drug, and Cosmetics Act) of 1976 that devices have come to be explicitly regulated at all, and with the Safe Medical Devices Act of 1990 and the Medical Device Amendments of 1992 that the regulation of devices for biocompatability became rigorous.

The basic tests used in evaluating devices for safety (or "biocompatability," as it is called in the device industry) are fairly set and largely familiar to us. These studies are the following:

Sensitization assay: Estimates the potential for sensitization of a test mate-
    rial and/or the extracts of a material using it in an animal and/or
    human.
Irritation tests: Estimates the irritation potential of test materials and
    their extracts, using appropriate site or implant tissue such as skin and
    mucous membrane in an animal model and/or human.

Cytotoxicity: With the use of cell culture techniques, this test determines the lysis of cells (cell death), the inhibition of cell growth, and other toxic effects on cells caused by test materials and/or extracts from the materials.

Acute systemic toxicity: Estimates the harmful effects of either single or multiple exposures to test materials and/or extracts, in an animal model, during a period of less than 24 hr.

Hemocompatibility: Evaluates any effects of blood contacting materials on hemolysis, thrombosis, plasma proteins, enzymes, and the formed elements using an animal model.

Pyrogenicity, material-mediated: Evaluates the material-mediated pyrogenicity of test materials and/or extracts.

Hemolysis: Determines the degree of red blood cell lysis and the separation of hemoglobin caused by test materials and/or extracts from the materials *in vitro*.

Implantation tests: Evaluates the local toxic effects on living tissue, at both the gross level and microscopic level, to a sample material that is surgically implanted into appropriate animal implant site or tissue (e.g., muscle or bone) for 7–90 days.

Mutagenicity (Genotoxicity): The application of mammalian or nonmammalian cell culture techniques for the determination of gene mutations, changes in chromosome structure and number, and other DNA or gene toxicities caused by test materials and/or extracts from materials.

Subchronic toxicity: The determination of harmful effects from multiple exposures to test materials and/or extracts during a period of 1 day to less than 10% of the total life of the test animal (e.g., up to 90 days in rats).

Chronic toxicity: The determination of harmful effects from multiple exposures to test materials and/or extracts during a period of 10% to the total life of the test animal (e.g., over 90 days in rats).

Carcinogenesis bioassay: The determination of the tumorigenic potential of test materials and/or extracts from either single or multiple exposures, over a period of the total life (e.g., 2 years for rat, 18 months for mouse, or 7 years for dog).

Pharmacokinetics: To determine the metabolic processes of absorption, distribution, biotransformation, and elimination of toxic leachables and degradation products of test materials and/or extracts.

Reproductive and developmental toxicity: Most, as is readily apparent, are by nature acute studies.

All but a few of these have previously been described in this volume. The exceptions are cytotoxicity, hemolysis, and pyrogenicity.

Materials for medical and paramedical applications should be tested or evaluated at three levels: (1) toxicity test on the various ingredients used to manufacture the basic resin, (2) toxicity evaluation of the final plastic or elastomeric material, and (3) evaluation of the final device. Each of these levels would, of course, require a battery of tests. Often, toxicity information on individual ingredients may be known and thus lengthy test procedures on these substances would not be required. In other cases, however, with introduction of new chemical compounds, there must be sufficient toxicity testing to establish a broad toxicity profile for the specific ingredient. Special tests may also be needed such as carcinogenic and mutagenic studies on the test substance because these latter two problems are becoming recognized as important health hazards to the public. The information derived from the group of toxicity tests becomes important because it can guide the manufacturer in developing safe handling and other safety features for the workers who may come in contact with the toxic agent.

In most instances, the final material will not contain the monomer, catalysts, or other reactive ingredients used to manufacture the final resin. There is, however, the possibility that residues of the reactive chemicals might still be adequate to produce one or more types of toxic responses.

One of the first groups in this country to develop a standardized toxicity testing program of items for medical application was the American Pharmaceutical Manufacturers Association in the early 1960s. Their objective was to develop acceptable testing methods for plastic items to be used with drug products that would be injected into humans. The testing program took on an official status when it became part of the United States Pharmacopeia and National Formulary. Even though these tests are for materials that may have contact with drug products, the same test methods are appropriate as an initial test or screening for all types of materials for which acute toxicity information is desired. Details of these tests are available from the official compendia.

Common to all of the guidelines promulgated by various organizations is the designation for testing methods based on usage classification. An example of usage classification identified by the HIMA/PMA guideline is presented below. It should be kept in mind that some devices could be placed into either one or more of the classification types; thus, the prescribed testing suggestion for each type category would be applicable.

Type I: Internal devices
   Short term: Devices that are introduced into the body (actually pene-
      trate the surface of the body or penetrate the wall of a passage lead-
      ing to the interior of the body) for a period of 30 days or less, such
      as intravenous catheters, hypodermic needles, and drainage tubes.
   Long term: Devices that are introduced into the body and are left *in*

situ for a period longer than 30 days, such as vascular prostheses, heart valves, metallic clips for ligation, and orthopedic prostheses.

Type II: Topical devices

Devices that contact the skin, for example, gloves, orthopedic casts, dressings, and tapes.

Devices that contact mucous membranes, for instance, urinary catheters, endotracheal tubes and cuffs, and intravaginal devices.

Type III: Indirect devices—Devices that are not introduced into the body or contact the body but serve as a means of delivering medication, collecting body fluids, administering blood or blood constituents, or dialyzing and oxygenating blood, such as hypodermic syringes, infusion and transfusion assemblies, oxygenators, and dialyzers.

Type IV: Nonpatient contact devices—Devices that do not touch the body but physically come into contact with those devices that do contact the body, such as dressing trays and operating room table covers.

Many of these devices are cast into their molded shape using a thermoplastic process. Polymeric materials having thermoplastic properties may be recast in various shapes subject to the thermal variation of their environment. Several questions must be addressed about the component material making up this device. These include the following:

What is the basic formulation of the polymeric material?

What is the probability that nonpolymerized monomer may be present in the formulation?

Were additional chemicals added during the molding process, such as mold release agent?

What impact does temperature alteration have on the thermal plasticizing process?

Were solvents employed during the molding process resulting in solvent residues remaining in the component?

What type of cleaning agents were used in the final cleaning process prior to packaging of the component?

Is the product to be gas sterilized and, if so, is there a potential for ethylene oxide residues to be present?

What manufacturing controls were employed during the fabrication of the device to ensure that material contamination may not inadvertently render the device pyrogenic?

Are there potential storage conditions for the device prior to its use that result in aggregation of the base polymer?

As can be appreciated from this line of reasoning, the initial focus is on the component material comprising the test device. The more clearly these questions can be addressed and answered, the more appropriately safety can be ascertained.

Once information has been gained about the use, classification, and specific component material or materials comprising the medical device, the initial phase of safety evaluation begins, consisting of toxicity screening of those components. This screening phase may be conducted directly on the component material or on various solvent extracts for the detection of potential extractables having biological activity. The various screen approaches that can be taken for component materials and extracts according to use category are presented in Table 101. As evidenced from the table, test methods selected for initial screen consist of both *in vitro* and *in vivo* test procedures. Those tests identified are general in nature and reconducted to focus on more compre-

TABLE 101   Test Methods for Medical Devices

Category	Tests on material	Tests on extracts
Type I: Internal devices		
Short term	Tissue culture	Tissue culture
	Implantation (short)	Acute toxicity
		Intracutaneous irritation
	Blood compatibility	Sensitization
Long term	Tissue culture	Tissue culture
	Implantation	Acute toxicity
	(short)	Intracutaneous irritation
	Implantation (long)	Sensitization
	Blood compatibility	
Type II: Topical devices	Skin contact	Tissue culture
	Tissue culture	Acute toxicity
	Skin irritation	Intracutaneous irritation
	Inhalation toxicity	Ocular irritation
		Sensitization
Mucous membrane contact	Tissue culture	Tissue culture
	Mucous membrane	Acute toxicity
	irritation	Intracutaneous irritation
		Sensitization
Type III: Indirect devices	Tissue culture Im-	Tissue culture
	plantation (short)	Acute toxicity
	Blood compatibility	Intracutaneous irritation
		Subchronic toxicity
		Sensitization
Type IV: Nonpatient contact	Tissue culture	Tissue culture
devices	Skin irritation	Intracutaneous irritation
		Ocular irritation

Note: Conducting suitable, simulated usage tests should be considered where applicable in Type I and II categories.

hensive biological indicators of safety assessment. Gad (1997) provides a current and comprehensive review of issues associated with the testing of devices.

A series of *in vitro* and *in vivo* biologic tests have been developed for the assessment of new biomaterials. These tests are listed in Table 102. Each of the tests is given a numerical value depending on the biologic response. From these individual values, a cumulative toxicity index (CTI) may be calculated. The index can range from a "0" (no response in any of the tests) to 1500 (highest response in each of the individual tests). In general, materials that have a value of 100 or less are considered good candidates for biomedical applications. Autian (1977) has reviewed and evaluated these tests. The tests alluded to can be considered an "acute toxicity screening program," which can also be applied to food-packaging systems if so desired. The addition of an *in vitro* test such as the Ames test would assist in making a judgment that leachable constituents in the material may have carcinogenic activities, and as such a version of this approach is used in evaluating polymers in other uses, as referred to in the following section. Appropriate "in use" tests must then be considered to establish the safety of the final item. Depending on the specific device, there may also be the need for long-term animal studies to confirm the safety of the device during the period of actual use.

Bear *et al.* (1983) have published the results of differential and comparative testing results of a number of device materials in cell culture test systems for the special case of thermally degraded polymers.

Polymers—Special Issues

Many of the concerns with the toxicity associated with the polymers used in medical devices are also relevant to polymers used in other ways—particularly

TABLE 102   Primary Acute Toxicity Screening Tests for Materials
(Autian, 1977)

Tests directly on material
    Tissue culture–agar overlay
    Rabbit muscle implant (1 week)
    Hemolysis (rabbit blood)

Tests on extracts[a]—Extracting conditions: One hour in an autoclave at 121°C
    Tissue culture–agar overlay
    Intracutaneous injection in rabbits
    Systemic toxicity in mice
    Cell growth inhibition on aqueous extract

Note: From Autian. (1977).
[a]Extraction media can be saline, polyethylene glycol 400, cottonseed oil, or
    "artificial saliva."

in home furnishings such as carpet materials. If infants chew or suck on these materials, will they be adversely affected by materials being extracted in the process?

The approaches taken to answering these questions are primarily those used for medical devices. Extraction studies are performed with water or artificial saliva, and the resulting extract is evaluated in *in vivo* and/or *in vitro* test systems.

REFERENCES

American Conference of Governmental Industrial Hygienists (ACGIH) (1986). *Documentation of the Threshold Limit Values,* 5th ed. ACGIH, Cincinnati, OH.

American Industrial Hygiene Association (AIHA) (1980). *Hygienic Guide Series,* Vols. I and II. AIHA, Akron, OH.

Autian, J. (1970). Toxicologic aspects of flammability and combustion of polymeric materials. *J. Fire Flammability* 1, 239–268.

Autian, J. (1977). Toxicological evaluation of biomaterials: Primary acute toxicity screening program. *Artif. Org.* 1, 53–60.

Barnhart, E. R. (1987). *Physicians Desk Reference.* Medical Economics, Oradell, NJ.

Bear, M. P., Johnson, D. S., and Schneider, F. S. (1983). Differential cytotoxicity testing of medical device materials. In *Safety Evaluation and Regulation of Chemicals* (F. Homburger, Ed.). Karger, Basel.

Birky, M. (1977). Hazard characteristics of combustion products in fires: The state-of-the-art review. NBSIR-77-1234, pp. 50.

Bott, B., Firth, J. G., and Jones. T. A. (1969). Evolution of toxic gases from heated plastics. *Br. Polymer J.* 1, 203–204.

Budavari, M. (1989). *The Merck Index,* 10th ed. Merck, Rahway, NJ.

Chu, K. C. (1980). The quantitative analysis of structure–activity relationships. In *Burger's Medicinal Chemistry* (M. E. Wolff, Ed), Vol. I. pp. 393–418. Wiley, New York.

Clayton, D. G., and Clayton, F. E. (1981). *Patty's Industrial Hygiene and Toxicology,* (3rd rev. ed., Vol. 2A, 2B, and 2C. Wiley, New York.

Cohen, J. L., Lee, W., and Lien, E. J. (1974). Dependence of toxicity on molecular structure: Group theory analysis. *J. Pharm Sci.* 63, 1068–1072.

Compton, J. A. F. (1988). *Military Chemical and Biological Agents.* Telford Press, Caldwell, NJ.

Connor, G. A. (1984). DOD program to deter chemical warfare. In *Toxicology Laboratory Design and Management for the 1980's and Beyond* (A. S. Tegeris, Ed.), pp. 237–242. S Karger, Basel.

Cronin, E. (1980). *Contact Dermatitis.* Churchill Livingstone, Edinburgh, UK.

Crum-Brown, A., and Fraser, T. (1869). *Trans R Soc Edinburgh* 25, 693.

Dupuis, G., and Benezra, C. (1982). *Allergic Contact Dermatitis to Simple Chemicals—A Molecular Approach.* Dekker, New York.

Einhorn, I. N. (1977). Methodology for the study of toxicology in combustion: Application to PUC. *J. Macromol. Sci. Chem.* 8, 1519–1528.

Ellenhorn, M. J., Echonwald, S., Ordog, G., and Wasserberger, J. (1997). *Ellenhorn's Medical Toxicology.* Williams and Wilkens, Baltimore.

Enslein, K. (1984). Estimation of toxicological endpoints by structure–activity relationships. *Pharmacol. Rev.* 36, 131–134.

Enslein, K., Lander, T. R., Tomb, M. E., and Landis, W. G. (1983a). Mutagenicity (Ames): A structure–activity model. *J. Teratogen. Carcinogen. Mutagen.* **3**, 503–514.

Enslein, K., Lander, T. R., Tomb, M. E., and Craig, P. N. (1983b). *A Predictive Model for Estimating Rat Oral LD50 Values.* Princeton Scientific, Princeton, NJ.

Enslein, K., Tomb, M. E., and Lander, T. R. (1984). Structure–activity models of biological oxygen demand. In *QSAR in Environmental Toxicology* (K. L. E. Kaiser, Ed.), Reidel, Dordrecht.

Finkel, A. J. (1983). *Hamilton and Hardy's Industrial Toxicology,* 4th ed. Wright, Boston.

Finney, D. J. (1952). *Probit Analysis,* 2nd ed. Cambridge Univ. Press, New York.

Forestier, M. (1975). Combustion products of synthetic materials. *Rev. Tech. Feu.* **16**, 24–26.

Foye, W. O. (1974). *Principles of Medicinal Chemistry.* Lea & Febiger, Philadelphia.

Free, S. M., and Wilson, J. W. (1964). A mathematical contribution to structure–activity studies. *J. Med. Chem.* **7**, 395–399.

Gad, S. C. (1997). *Safety Assessment of Medical Devices.* Dekker, New York.

Gad, S. C., and Anderson, R. S. (1990). *Combustion Toxicology.* CRC Press, Boca Raton, FL.

Gad, S. C., and Weil C. S. (1986). *Statistics and Experimental Design for Toxicologists.* Telford Press, Caldwell, NJ.

Goldberg, L. (1983). *Structure–Activity Correlations as a Predictive Tool in Toxicology.* Hemisphere, New York.

Goseelin, R. E., Smith, R. P., and Hodge, H. C. (1984). *Clinical Toxicology of Commercial Products,* 5th ed. Williams and Wilkens, Baltimore.

Grant, W. M. (1993). *Toxicology of the Eye,* Charles C Thomas, Springfield, IL.

Gund, P., Andosf, J. D., Rhodes, J. B., and Smith, G. M. (1980). Three-dimensional molecular modeling and drug design. *Science* **208**, 1425–1431.

Hansch, C. (1971). *Drug Design,* (E. J. Ariens, Ed.), Vol. I, Chap. 2. Academic Press, New York.

Hilado, C. J. (1978). Toxicity of pyrolysis gases from materials. *Sample Q.* **9**, 14–15.

Jouany, J., and Raoul, P. (1975). Fire hazard evaluation of both synthetic and natural materials. *Soc. Plast. Eng. Tech. Pap.* **21**, 114–117.

Kaplan, H. L., Grand, A. F., and Hartzell, G. E. (1983). *Combustion Toxicology,* pp. 174. Technomics, Lancaster, PA.

Klaassen, C. D., Doull, J., and Amdur, M. O. (1996). *Casarett and Doull's Toxicology: The Basic Science of Poisons,* 3rd ed. Macmillan, New York.

Mackinson, F. (1981). *Occupational Health Guidelines for Chemical Hazards,* DHHS No. 81–123, Department of Health and Human Services (NIOSH)/Department of Labor (OSHA) Government Printing Office, Washington, DC.

National Institute for Occupational Safety and Health, *NIOSH Current Intelligence Bulletins.* Department of Health, Education and Welfare, Cincinnati, OH.

National Institute for Occupational Safety and Health, *NIOSH Criteria for a Recommended Standard for Occupational Exposure to · · ·* Department of Health, Education and Welfare, Cincinnati, OH.

National Institute for Occupational Safety and Health (NIOSH) (1984). *Registry of Toxic Effects of Chemical Substances,* 11th ed., Vols. 1–3. Department of Health and Human Services DHHS No. 83–107 (1983) and RTECS Supplement DHHS 84–101. DHHS, Washington, DC.

National Library of Medicine, Office of Inquiries and Publications Management, 8600 Rockville Pike, Bethesda, MD, 20209.

Olson, E. C., and Christoffersen, R. E. (1979). *Computer Assisted Drug Design.* ACS, Washington, DC.

Parker, C. M. (1987). Available toxicology information source and their use. In *Handbooks for Product Safety Evaluation* (S. C. Gad, Ed.), pp. 23–41. Dekker, New York.

Poziomek, E. J. (1984). Toxicity evaluation of surety compounds. In *Toxicology Laboratory Design and Management for the 80's and Beyond* (A. S. Tegeris, Ed.), pp. 243–249. S. Karger, Basel.

Pozzani, U. C., Weil, C. S., and Carpenter, C. P. (1959). The toxicological basis of threshold limit values. 5. The experimental inhalation of vapor mixtures by rats, with notes upon the relationship between single dose inhalation and single dose oral data. *Am. Ind. Hygiene Assoc. J.* **20**, 364–369.

Proctor, N. H., and Hughes, J. P. (1978). *Chemical Hazards of the Workplace.* Lippincott, Philadelphia.

Raftery, M. M. (1974). Smoke and toxicity hazards of plastics in fires. *Nehorlavost. Plast. Hmot.,* 130–139.

Reinke, R. E., and Reinhardt, C. F. (1973). Fires, toxicity and plastics. *Mod. Plast.* **50**, 94–95, 97–98.

Reploh, H., Klosterkoetter, W., and Einck—Rosskamp, P. (1966). Toxicity of carbonization products of synthetics. *Arch. Hyg. Bakteriol.* **150**, 393–405.

Rumberg, E. (1971). Disintegration products and smoke generation from fire action on plastics. *Ver. Deut. Ing.* **113**, 20–24.

Sand, H. E., and Hofmann, H. T. (1977). Evaluation of health hazards posed by thermal decomposition products of flammable materials. *Oesterr. Kunstst. Z.* **8**, 37–41.

Sax, N. I. (1985). *Dangerous Properties of Industrial Materials,* 6th ed. Van Nostrand Reinhold, New York.

Sittig, M. (1985). *Handbook of Toxic and Hazardous Chemicals.* Noyes, Park Ridge, NJ.

Smyth, H. F., Weil, C. S., West, J. F., and Carpenter, C. P. (1969). An explanation of joint toxic action: Twenty-seven industrial chemicals intubated in rats in all possible pairs. *Toxicol. Appl. Pharmacol.* **14**, 340–347.

Terril, J. B., Montgomery, R. R., and Reinhardt, C. F. (1977). Devising a screening test for toxic fire gases. *Fire Techol.* **13**, 95–104.

Topliss, J. G. (1983). *Quantitative Structure–Activity Relationships of Drugs.* Academic Press, New York.

United States Pharmacopeia (USP) (1990). *The United States Pharmacopeia.* United States Pharmacopeial Convention, Rockville, MD.

Vasilev, G. A., and Ilichkin, V. S. (1975). Evaluation of the toxicity of volatile products from the combustion of polymer materials. *Gig. Sanit.* **5**, 87–91.

Weil, C. S. (1972). Statistics vs. safety factors and scientific judgement in the evaluation of safety for man. *Toxicol. Appl. Pharmacol.* **21**, 454–463.

Wexler, P. (1982). *Information Resources in Toxicology,* pp. 333. Elsevier, New York.

Wolff, M. E. (1994). *Burger's Medicinal Chemistry,* Part II. Wiley, New York.

Wolff, M. E. (1996). *Burger's Medicinal Chemistry,* Part III. Wiley, New York.

Wooley, W. D. (1973). Toxic products from plastics materials in fires. *Plast. Polym.* **41**, 280–286.

Zapp, J. A. (1951). The toxicity of fire, Medical Division Spec. Rep. No. 4. Chemical Corps., Army Chemical Center, Maryland.

Common Regulatory and Toxicological Acronyms

AALAS	American Association Laboratory Animal Science
ABT	American Board of Toxicology
ACT	American College of Toxicology
ACGIH	American Conference of Governmental Industrial Hygienists
CRF	Code of Federal Regulations
CIIT	Chemical Industries Institute of Toxicology
CPSC	Consumer Product Safety Commission
DOT	Department of Transportation
EPA	Environmental Protection Agency
FDA	Food and Drug Administration
FDC	Food Drug and Cosmetic Act
FHSA	Federal Hazardous Substances Act
FIFRA	Federal Insecticides, Fungicides and Rodenticides Act
id	Intradermal
ip	Intraperitoneal
IRLG	Interagency Regulatory Liaison Group
iv	Intravenous
JMAFF	Japanese Ministry of Agriculture, Forestry, and Fishery
LD_{50}	Lethal dose 50: The dose calculated to kill 50% of a subject population, median lethal dose
MSDS	Material safety data sheet
MTD	Maximum tolerated dose
NAS	National Academy of Science
NIOSH	National Institute Occupational Safety and Health
NOEL	No-observable-effect level
OECD	Organization for Economic Cooperation and Development
PMN	Premanufacturing notice

po	Per os (orally)
RCRA	Resources Conservation and Recovery Act
RTECS	Registry of Toxic Effects of Chemical Substances
SARA	Superfund/Amendments and Reauthorization Act
sc	Subcutaneous
SNUR	Significant New Use Regulations
SOT	Society of Toxicology
TLV	Threshold limit value
TSCA	Toxic Substances Control Act
USP	United States Pharmacopeia

Table for Calculation of Median Effective Dose by Moving Average

n = 2, K = 3

r value	f	σf
0,0,1,2	1.00000	0.50000
0,0,2,2	0.50000	0.00000
0,1,1,2	0.50000	0.70711
0,1,2,2	0.00000	0.50000
1,0,1,2	1.00000	1.00000
1,0,2,2	0.00000	1.00000
1,1,1,2	0.00000	1.73205
0,0,2,1	1.00000	1.00000
0,1,1,1	1.00000	1.73205
0,1,2,1	0.00000	1.00000

n = 3, K = 3

r value	f	σf
0,0,2,3	0.83333	0.33333
0,0,3,3	0.50000	0.00000
0,1,1,3	0.83333	0.47140
0,1,2,3	0.50000	0.47140

n = 4, K = 3

r value	f	σf
2,0,3,4	0.50000	0.57735
2,0,4,4	0.00000	0.57735
2,1,1,4	1.00000	0.70711
2,1,2,4	0.50000	0.81650
2,1,3,4	0.00000	0.91287
2,2,2,4	0.00000	1.00000
3,0,2,4	1.00000	1.15470
3,0,3,4	0.00000	1.41421
3,1,1,4	1.00000	1.41421
3,1,2,4	0.00000	1.82574
0,0,3,3	1.00000	0.47140
0,0,4,3	0.66667	0.22222
0,1,2,3	1.00000	0.60858
0,1,3,3	0.66667	0.52116
0,1,4,3	0.33333	0.35136
0,2,2,3	0.66667	0.58794
0,2,3,3	0.33333	0.52116

n = 5, K = 3

r value	f	σf
0,1,2,5	0.90000	0.31623
0,1,3,5	0.7000	0.31623
0,1,4,5	0.50000	0.28284
0,1,5,5	0.30000	0.20000
0,2,2,5	0.70000	0.34641
0,2,3,5	0.50000	0.34641
0,2,4,5	0.30000	0.31623
0,2,5,5	0.10000	0.24495
0,3,3,5	0.30000	0.34641
0,3,4,5	0.10000	0.31623
1,0,3,5	0.87500	0.30778
1,0,4,5	0.62500	0.26700
1,0,5,5	0.37500	0.15625
1,1,2,5	0.87500	0.39652
1,1,3,5	0.62500	0.40625
1,1,4,5	0.37500	0.38654
1,1,5,5	0.12500	0.33219

n = 4, K = 3

r value	f	σf
0,1,3,3	0.16667	0.33333
0,2,2,3	0.16667	0.47140
1,0,2,3	0.75000	0.51539
1,0,3,3	0.25000	0.37500
1,1,1,3	0.75000	0.71807
1,1,2,3	0.25000	0.80039
2,0,2,3	0.50000	1.11803
0,0,3,2	0.75000	0.37500
0,1,2,2	0.75000	0.80039
0,1,3,2	0.25000	0.51539
0,2,2,2	0.25000	0.71807
0,1,3,1	0.50000	1.11803

n = 4, K = 3

r value	f	σf
0,0,2,4	1.00000	0.28868
0,0,3,4	0.75000	0.25000
0,0,4,4	0.50000	0.00000

n = 4, K = 3

r value	f	σf
0,2,4,3	0.00000	0.38490
0,3,3,3	0.00000	0.47140
1,0,3,3	1.00000	0.70711
1,0,4,3	0.50000	0.35355
1,1,2,3	1.00000	0.91287
1,1,3,3	0.50000	0.79057
1,1,4,3	0.00000	0.70711
1,2,2,3	0.50000	0.88976
1,2,3,3	0.00000	0.91287
2,0,3,3	1.00000	1.41421
2,0,4,3	0.00000	1.15470
2,1,2,3	1.00000	1.82574
2,1,3,3	0.00000	1.82574
2,2,2,3	0.00000	2.00000
0,0,4,2	1.00000	0.57735
0,1,3,2	1.00000	0.91287
0,1,4,2	0.50000	0.57735
0,2,2,2	1.00000	1.00000

n = 5, K = 3

r value	f	σf
1,2,2,5	0.62500	0.44304
1,2,3,5	0.37500	0.46034
1,2,4,5	0.12500	0.45178
1,3,3,5	0.12500	0.48513
2,0,3,5	0.83333	0.41388
2,0,4,5	0.50000	0.39087
2,0,5,5	0.16667	0.34021
2,1,2,5	0.83333	0.53142
2,1,3,5	0.50000	0.56519
2,1,4,5	0.16667	0.58134
2,2,2,5	0.50000	0.61237
2,2,3,5	0.16667	0.67013
0,0,4,4	0.87500	0.33219
0,0,5,4	0.62500	0.15625
0,1,3,4	0.87500	0.45178
0,1,4,4	0.62500	0.38654
0,1,5,4	0.37500	0.26700
0,2,2,4	0.87500	0.48513

(Continues)

Table for Calculation of Median Effective Dose by Moving Average (*Continued*)

r value	f	σf	r value	f	σf	r value	f	σf
	n = 4, K = 3			n = 4, K = 3			n = 5, K = 3	
0,1,1,4	1.00000	0.35355	0,2,3,2	0.50000	0.81650	0,2,3,4	0.62500	0.46034
0,1,2,4	0.75000	0.38188	0,2,4,2	0.00000	0.57735	0,2,4,4	0.37500	0.40625
0,1,3,4	0.50000	0.35355	0,3,3,2	0.00000	0.70711	0,2,5,4	0.12500	0.30778
0,1,4,4	0.25000	0.25000	1,0,4,2	1.00000	1.15470	0,3,3,4	0.37500	0.44304
0,2,2,4	0.50000	0.40825	1,1,3,2	1.00000	1.82574	0,3,4,4	0.12500	0.39652
0,2,3,4	0.25000	0.38188	1,1,4,2	0.00000	1.41421	1,0,4,4	0.83333	0.43744
0,2,4,4	0.00000	0.28868	1,2,2,2	1.00000	2.00000	1,0,5,4	0.50000	0.23570
0,3,3,4	0.00000	0.35355	1,2,3,2	0.00000	1.82574	1,1,3,4	0.83333	0.59835
1,0,2,4	1.00000	0.38490	0,2,3,1	1.00000	1.82574	1,1,4,4	0.50000	0.52705
1,0,3,4	0.66667	0.35136	0,2,4,1	0.00000	1.15470	1,1,5,4	0.16667	0.43744
1,0,4,4	0.33333	0.22222	0,3,3,1	0.00000	1.41421	1,2,2,4	0.83333	0.64310
1,1,1,4	1.00000	0.47140	0,1,4,1	1.00000	1.41421	1,2,3,4	0.50000	0.62361
1,1,2,4	0.66667	0.52116				1,2,4,4	0.16667	0.59835
1,1,3,4	0.33333	0.52116		n = 5, K = 3		1,3,3,4	0.16667	0.64310
1,1,4,4	0.00000	0.47140				2,0,4,4	0.75000	0.64348
1,2,2,4	0.33333	0.58794	0,0,3,5	0.90000	0.24495	2,0,5,4	0.25000	0.47598
1,2,3,4	0.00000	0.60858	0,0,4,5	0.70000	0.20000	2,1,3,4	0.75000	0.88829
2,0,2,4	1.00000	0.57735	0,0,5,5	0.50000	0.00000	2,1,4,4	0.25000	0.85239

Note. This portion reprinted from *Biometrics* with permission of Trustees.

Table for Calculation of Median Effective Dose by Moving Average

r value	f	σf	r value	f	σf	r value	f	σf
	n = 5, K = 3			n = 6, K = 3			n = 6, K = 3	
2,2,2,4	0.75000	0.95607	1,4,4,6	0.00000	0.36878	0,3,6,5	0.00000	0.26833
2,2,3,4	0.25000	0.98821	2,0,3,6	1.00000	0.33541	0,4,4,5	0.20000	0.36000
0,0,5,3	0.83333	0.34021	2,0,4,6	0.75000	0.32596	0,4,5,5	0.00000	0.32249
0,1,4,3	0.83333	0.58134	2,0,5,6	0.50000	0.29580	1,0,4,5	1.00000	0.40311
0,1,5,3	0.50000	0.39087	2,0,6,6	0.25000	0.23717	1,0,5,5	0.75000	0.31869
0,2,3,3	0.83333	0.67013	2,1,2,6	1.00000	0.40311	1,0,6,5	0.50000	0.17678
0,2,4,3	0.50000	0.56519	2,1,3,6	0.75000	0.42573	1,1,3,5	1.00000	0.48734
0,2,5,3	0.16667	0.41388	2,1,4,6	0.50000	0.43301	1,1,4,5	0.75000	0.44896
0,3,3,3	0.50000	0.61237	2,1,5,6	0.25000	0.42573	1,1,5,5	0.50000	0.39528
0,3,4,3	0.16667	0.53142	2,1,6,6	0.00000	0.29580	1,1,6,5	0.25000	0.31869
1,0,5,3	0.75000	0.47598	2,2,2,6	0.75000	0.45415	1,2,2,5	1.00000	0.51235
1,1,4,3	0.75000	0.85239	2,2,3,6	0.50000	0.48734	1,2,3,5	0.75000	0.50156
1,1,5,3	0.25000	0.64348	2,2,4,6	0.25000	0.50621	1,2,4,5	0.50000	0.48088
1,2,3,3	0.75000	0.98821	2,2,5,6	0.00000	0.43301	1,2,5,5	0.25000	0.44896
1,2,4,3	0.25000	0.88829	2,3,3,6	0.25000	0.53033	1,2,6,5	0.00000	0.40311
1,3,3,3	0.25000	0.95607	2,3,4,6	0.00000	0.48734	1,3,3,5	0.50000	0.50621
			3,0,3,6	1.00000	0.44721	1,3,4,5	0.25000	0.50156
	n = 6, K = 3		3,0,4,6	0.66667	0.43885	1,3,5,5	0.00000	0.48734
			3,0,5,6	0.33333	0.44721	1,4,4,5	0.00000	0.51235
0,0,3,6	1.00000	0.22361	3,0,6,6	0.00000	0.44721	2,0,4,5	1.00000	0.53748

(*Continues*)

Table for Calculation of Median Effective Dose by Moving Average (*Continued*)

n = 6, K = 3			n = 6, K = 3			n = 6, K = 3		
r value	f	σf	r value	f	σf	r value	f	σf
0,0,4,6	0.83333	0.21082	3,1,2,6	1.00000	0.53748	2,0,5,5	0.66667	0.42455
0,0,5,6	0.66667	0.16667	3,1,3,6	0.66667	0.57090	2,0,6,5	0.33333	0.30225
0,0,6,6	0.50000	0.00000	3,1,4,6	0.33333	0.61464	2,1,3,5	1.00000	0.64979
0,1,2,6	1.00000	0.26874	3,1,5,6	0.00000	0.64979	2,1,4,5	0.66667	0.59835
0,1,3,6	0.83333	0.27889	3,2,2,6	0.66667	0.60858	2,1,5,5	0.33333	0.55998
0,1,4,6	0.66667	0.26874	3,2,3,6	0.33333	0.68313	2,1,6,5	0.00000	0.53748
0,1,5,6	0.50000	0.23570	3,2,4,6	0.00000	0.74536	2,2,2,5	1.00000	0.68313
0,1,6,6	0.33333	0.16667	3,3,3,6	0.00000	0.77460	2,2,3,5	0.66667	0.66852
0,2,2,6	0.83333	0.29814	4,0,3,6	1.00000	0.67082	2,2,4,5	0.33333	0.66852
0,2,3,6	0.66667	0.30732	4,0,4,6	0.50000	0.70711	2,2,5,5	0.00000	0.68313
0,2,4,6	0.50000	0.29814	4,0,5,6	0.00000	0.80622	2,3,3,5	0.33333	0.70097
0,2,5,6	0.33333	0.26874	4,1,2,6	1.00000	0.80622	2,3,4,5	0.00000	0.74536
0,2,6,6	0.16667	0.21082	4,1,3,6	0.50000	0.89443	3,0,4,5	1.00000	0.80622
0,3,3,6	0.50000	0.31623	4,1,4,6	0.00000	1.02470	3,0,5,5	0.50000	0.65192
0,3,4,6	0.33333	0.30732	4,2,2,6	0.50000	0.94888	3,0,6,5	0.00000	0.67082
0,3,5,6	0.16667	0.27889	4,2,3,6	0.00000	1.11803	3,1,3,5	1.00000	0.92195
0,3,6,6	0.00000	0.22361	5,0,3,6	1.00000	1.34164	3,1,4,5	0.50000	0.90830
0,4,4,6	0.16667	0.29814	5,0,4,6	0.00000	1.61245	3,1,5,5	0.00000	0.92195
0,4,5,6	0.00000	0.26874	5,1,2,6	1.00000	1.61245	3,2,2,5	1.00000	1.02470
1,0,3,6	1.00000	0.26833	5,1,3,6	0.00000	1.94936	3,2,3,5	0.50000	1.01242
1,0,4,6	0.80000	0.25612	5,2,2,6	0.00000	2.04939	3,2,4,5	0.00000	1.11803
1,0,5,6	0.60000	0.21541	0,0,4,5	1.00000	0.26833	3,3,3,5	0.00000	1.16190
1,0,6,6	0.40000	0.12000	0,0,5,5	0.80000	0.25612	4,0,4,5	1.00000	1.61245
1,1,2,6	1.00000	0.32249	0,0,6,5	0.60000	0.12000	4,0,5,5	0.00000	1.61245
1,1,3,6	0.80000	0.33704	0,1,3,5	1.00000	0.34641	4,1,3,5	1.00000	1.94936
1,1,4,6	0.60000	0.33226	0,1,4,5	0.80000	0.36000	4,1,4,5	0.00000	2.04939
1,1,5,6	0.40000	0.30724	0,1,5,5	0.60000	0.30724	4,2,2,5	1.00000	2.04939
1,1,6,6	0.20000	0.25612	0,1,6,5	0.40000	0.21541	4,2,3,5	0.00000	2.23607
1,2,2,6	0.80000	0.36000	0,2,2,5	1.00000	0.36878	0,0,5,4	1.00000	0.29580
1,2,3,6	0.60000	0.37736	0,2,3,5	0.80000	0.40200	0,0,6,4	0.75000	0.23717
1,2,4,6	0.40000	0.37736	0,2,4,5	0.60000	0.37736	0,1,4,4	1.00000	0.43301
1,2,5,6	0.20000	0.36000	0,2,5,5	0.40000	0.33226	0,1,5,4	0.75000	0.42573
1,2,6,6	0.00000	0.26833	0,2,6,5	0.20000	0.25612	0,1,6,4	0.50000	0.29580
1,3,3,6	0.40000	0.39799	0,3,3,5	0.60000	0.39799	0,2,3,4	1.00000	0.48734
1,3,4,6	0.20000	0.40200	0,3,4,5	0.40000	0.37736	0,2,4,4	0.75000	0.50621
1,3,5,6	0.00000	0.34641	0,3,5,5	0.20000	0.33704	0,2,5,4	0.50000	0.43301
0,2,6,4	0.25000	0.32596	2,3,4,4	0.00000	1.11803	1,3,5,3	0.00000	0.92195
0,3,3,4	0.75000	0.53033	3,0,5,4	1.00000	1.67332	1,4,4,3	0.00000	1.02470
0,3,4,4	0.50000	0.48734	3,0,6,4	0.00000	1.34164	2,0,6,3	1.00000	1.34164
0,3,5,4	0.25000	0.42573	3,1,4,4	1.00000	2.09762	2,1,5,3	1.00000	1.94936
0,3,6,4	0.00000	0.33541	3,1,5,4	0.00000	1.94936	2,1,6,3	0.00000	1.67332
0,4,4,4	0.25000	0.45415	3,2,3,4	1.00000	2.28035	2,2,4,3	1.00000	2.23607
0,4,5,4	0.00000	0.40311	3,2,4,4	0.00000	2.23607	2,2,5,3	0.00000	2.09762
1,0,5,4	1.00000	0.53748	3,3,3,4	0.00000	2.32379	2,3,3,3	1.00000	2.32379
1,0,6,4	0.66667	0.30225	0,0,6,3	1.00000	0.44721	2,3,4,3	0.00000	2.28035

(*Continues*)

Table for Calculation of Median Effective Dose by Moving Average (Continued)

n = 6, K = 3			n = 6, K = 3			n = 6, K = 3		
r value	f	σf	r value	f	σf	r value	f	σf
1,1,4,4	1.00000	0.68313	0,1,5,3	1.00000	0.64979	0,1,6,2	1.00000	0.80622
1,1,5,4	0.66667	0.55998	0,1,6,3	0.66667	0.44721	0,2,5,2	1.00000	1.02470
1,1,6,4	0.33333	0.42455	0,2,4,3	1.00000	0.74536	0,2,6,2	0.50000	0.70711
1,2,3,4	1.00000	0.74536	0,2,5,3	0.66667	0.61464	0,3,4,2	1.00000	1.11803
1,2,4,4	0.66667	0.66852	0,2,6,3	0.33333	0.43885	0,3,5,2	0.50000	0.89443
1,2,5,4	0.33333	0.59835	0,3,3,3	1.00000	0.77460	0,3,6,2	0.00000	0.67082
1,2,6,4	0.00000	0.53748	0,3,4,3	0.66667	0.68313	0,4,4,2	0.50000	0.94868
1,3,3,4	0.66667	0.70097	0,3,5,3	0.33333	0.57090	0,4,5,2	0.00000	0.80622
1,3,4,4	0.33333	0.66852	0,3,6,3	0.00000	0.44721	1,1,6,2	1.00000	1.61245
1,3,5,4	0.00000	0.64979	0,4,4,3	0.33333	0.60858	1,2,5,2	1.00000	2.04939
1,4,4,4	0.00000	0.68313	0,4,5,3	0.00000	0.53748	1,2,6,2	0.00000	1.61245
2,1,6,4	0.00000	0.80622	1,2,5,3	0.50000	0.90830	0,3,5,1	1.00000	1.94936
2,2,3,4	1.00000	1.11803	1,2,6,3	0.00000	0.80622	0,3,6,1	0.00000	1.34164
2,2,4,4	0.50000	1.00000	1,3,3,3	1.00000	1.16190	0,4,4,1	1.00000	2.04939
2,2,5,4	0.00000	1.02470	1,3,4,3	0.50000	1.01242	0,4,5,1	0.00000	1.61245
2,3,3,4	0.50000	1.04881						

n = 10, K = 3			n = 10, K = 3			n = 10, K = 3		
r value	f	σf	r value	f	σf	r value	f	σf
0,0,5,10	1.0	0.16667	1,1,5,10	0.88889	0.21631	2,2,7,10	0.50000	0.26021
0,0,6,10	0.9	0.16330	1,1,6,10	0.77778	0.21419	2,2,8,10	0.37500	0.24694
0,0,7,10	0.8	0.15275	1,1,7,10	0.66667	0.20621	2,2,9,10	0.25000	0.24296
0,0,8,10	0.7	0.13333	1,1,8,10	0.55556	0.19166	2,2,10,10	0.12500	0.22140
0,0,9,10	0.6	0.10000	1,1,9,10	0.44444	0.16882	2,3,3,10	0.87500	0.27043
0,0,10,10	0.5	0.00000	1,1,10,10	0.33333	0.13354	2,3,4,10	0.75000	0.28106
0,1,4,10	1.0	0.19149	1,2,3,10	1.00000	0.22529	2,3,5,10	0.62500	0.28603
0,1,5,10	0.9	0.19436	1,2,4,10	0.88889	0.23457	2,3,6,10	0.50000	0.28565
0,1,6,10	0.8	0.19149	1,2,5,10	0.77778	0.23843	2,3,7,10	0.37500	0.27990
0,1,7,10	0.7	0.18257	1,2,6,10	0.66667	0.23715	2,3,8,10	0.25000	0.28260
0,1,8,10	0.6	0.16667	1,2,7,10	0.55556	0.23064	2,3,9,10	0.12500	0.27081
0,1,9,10	0.5	0.14142	1,2,8,10	0.44444	0.21842	2,3,10,10	0.00000	0.25345
0,1,10,10	0.4	0.10000	1,2,9,10	0.33333	0.19945	2,4,4,10	0.62500	0.29204
0,2,3,10	1.0	0.20276	1,2,10,10	0.22222	0.17151	2,4,5,10	0.50000	0.29756
0,2,4,10	0.9	0.21082	1,3,3,10	0.88889	0.24034	2,4,6,10	0.37500	0.29789
0,2,5,10	0.8	0.21344	1,3,4,10	0.77778	0.24968	2,4,7,10	0.25000	0.30619
0,2,6,10	0.7	0.21082	1,3,5,10	0.66667	0.25391	2,4,8,10	0.12500	0.30117
0,2,7,10	0.6	0.20276	1,3,6,10	0.55556	0.25331	2,4,9,10	0.00000	0.29166
0,2,8,10	0.5	0.18856	1,3,7,10	0.44444	0.24784	2,5,5,10	0.37500	0.30369
0,2,9,10	0.4	0.16667	1,3,8,10	0.33333	0.23715	2,5,6,10	0.25000	0.31732
0,2,10,10	0.3	0.13333	1,3,9,10	0.22222	0.22050	2,5,7,10	0.12500	0.31799
0,3,3,10	0.9	0.21602	1,3,10,10	0.11111	0.19637	2,5,8,10	0.00000	0.31458
0,3,4,10	0.8	0.22361	1,4,4,10	0.66667	0.25926	2,6,6,10	0.12500	0.32340

(Continues)

Table for Calculation of Median Effective Dose by Moving Average (*Continued*)

n = 10, K = 3			n = 10, K = 3			n = 10, K = 3		
r value	f	bf	r value	f	of	r value	f	of
0,3,5,10	0.7	0.22608	1,4,5,10	0.55556	0.26392	2,6,7,10	0.00000	0.32543
0,3,6,10	0.6	0.22361	1,4,6,10	0.44444	0.26392	3,0,5,10	1.00000	0.23809
0,3,7,10	0.5	0.21602	1,4,7,10	0.33333	0.25926	3,0,6,10	0.85714	0.23536
0,3,8,10	0.4	0.20276	1,4,8,10	0.22222	0.24968	3,0,7,10	0.71429	0.22695
0,3,9,10	0.3	0.18257	1,4,9,10	0.11111	0.23457	3,0,8,10	0.57143	0.21695
0,3,10,10	0.2	0.15275	1,4,10,10	0.00000	0.21276	3,0,9,10	0.42857	0.18962
0,4,4,10	0.7	0.23094	1,5,5,10	0.44444	0.26907	3,0,10,10	0.28571	0.15587
0,4,5,10	0.6	0.23336	1,5,6,10	0.33333	0.26963	3,1,4,10	1.00000	0.27355
0,4,6,10	0.5	0.23094	1,5,7,10	0.22222	0.26565	3,1,5,10	0.85714	0.27941
0,4,7,10	0.4	0.22361	1,5,8,10	0.11111	0.25690	3,1,6,10	0.71429	0.28057
0,4,8,10	0.3	0.21082	1,5,9,10	0.00000	0.24287	3,1,7,10	0.57143	0.28074
0,4,9,10	0.2	0.19149	1,6,6,10	0.22222	0.27076	3,1,8,10	0.42857	0.26877
0,4,10,10	0.1	0.16330	1,6,7,10	0.11111	0.26736	3,1,9,10	0.28571	0.25517
0,5,5,10	0.5	0.23570	1,6,8,10	0.00000	0.25926	3,1,10,10	0.14286	0.23536
0,5,6,10	0.4	0.23336	1,7,7,10	0.00000	0.26450	3,2,3,10	1.00000	0.28965
0,5,7,10	0.3	0.22608	2,0,5,10	1.00000	0.20833	3,2,4,10	0.85714	0.30278
0,5,8,10	0.2	0.21344	2,0,6,10	0.87500	0.20465	3,2,5,10	0.71429	0.31122
0,5,9,10	0.1	0.19436	2,0,7,10	0.75000	0.19320	3,2,6,10	0.57143	0.31857
0,5,10,10	0.0	0.16667	2,0,8,10	0.62500	0.17237	3,2,7,10	0.42857	0.31536
0,6,6,10	0.3	0.23094	2,0,9,10	0.50000	0.10534	3,2,8,10	0.28571	0.31122
0,6,7,10	0.2	0.22361	2,0,10,10	0.37500	0.07365	3,2,9,10	0.14286	0.30278
0,6,8,10	0.1	0.21082	2,1,4,10	1.00000	0.23936	3,2,10,10	0.00000	0.28965
0,6,9,10	0.0	0.19149	2,1,5,10	0.87500	0.22902	3,3,3,10	0.85714	0.31018
0,7,7,10	0.1	0.21602	2,1,6,10	0.75000	0.24116	3,3,4,10	0.71429	0.32546
0,7,8,10	0.0	0.20276	2,1,7,10	0.62500	0.23246	3,3,5,10	0.57143	0.33926
1,0,5,10	1.0	0.18518	2,1,8,10	0.50000	0.21651	3,3,6,10	0.42857	0.34291
1,0,6,10	0.88889	0.18186	2,1,9,10	0.37500	0.19151	3,3,7,10	0.28571	0.34574
1,0,7,10	0.77778	0.17151	2,1,10,10	0.25000	0.17678	3,3,8,10	0.14286	0.34480
1,0,8,10	0.66667	0.15270	2,2,3,10	1.00000	0.25345	3,3,9,10	0.00000	0.34007
1,0,9,10	0.55556	0.12159	2,2,4,10	0.87500	0.26393	3,4,4,10	0.57143	0.34588
1,0,10,10	0.44444	0.06172	2,2,5,10	0.75000	0.26842	3,4,5,10	0.42857	0.35589
1,1,4,10	1.00000	0.21276	2,2,6,10	0.62500	0.26717	3,4,6,10	0.28571	0.36488
3,4,7,10	0.14286	0.37017	5,3,4,10	0.60000	0.46667	9,0,6,10	0.00000	1.77951
3,4,8,10	0.00000	0.37192	5,3,5,10	0.40000	0.48990	9,1,4,10	1.00000	1.77951
3,5,5,10	0.28571	0.37104	5,3,6,10	0.20000	0.52068	9,1,5,10	0.00000	2.18581
3,5,6,10	0.14286	0.38223	5,3,7,10	0.00000	0.54569	9,2,3,10	1.00000	2.02759
3,5,7,10	0.00000	0.38978	5,4,4,10	0.40000	0.49889	9,2,4,10	0.00000	2.33333
3,6,6,10	0.00000	0.39555	5,4,5,10	0.20000	0.53748	9,3,3,10	0.00000	2.38048
4,0,5,10	1.00000	0.27778	5,4,6,10	0.00000	0.56960	0,0,6,9	1.00000	0.21276
4,0,6,10	0.83333	0.27592	5,5,5,10	0.00000	0.57735	0,0,7,9	0.88889	0.19637
4,0,7,10	0.66667	0.27027	6,0,5,10	1.00000	0.41667	0,0,8,9	0.77778	0.17151
4,0,8,10	0.50000	0.26058	6,0,6,10	0.75000	0.45644	0,0,9,9	0.66667	0.13354
4,0,9,10	0.33333	0.24637	6,0,7,10	0.50000	0.43301	0,0,10,9	0.55556	0.06172

(*Continues*)

Table for Calculation of Median Effective Dose by Moving Average (*Continued*)

r value	ƒ	σf	r value	ƒ	σf	r value	ƒ	σf
	n = 10, K = 3			n = 10, K = 3			n = 10, K = 3	
4,0,10,10	0.16667	0.22680	6,0,8,10	0.25000	0.45262	0,1,5,9	1.00000	0.24287
4,1,4,10	1.00000	0.31914	6,0,9,10	0.00000	0.47871	0,1,6,9	0.88889	0.23457
4,1,5,10	0.83333	0.32710	6,1,4,10	1.00000	0.47871	0,1,7,9	0.77778	0.22050
4,1,6,10	0.66667	0.33178	6,1,5,10	0.75000	0.52705	0,1,8,9	0.66667	0.19945
4,1,7,10	0.50000	0.33333	6,1,6,10	0.50000	0.52042	0,1,9,9	0.55555	0.16882
4,1,8,10	0.33333	0.33178	6,1,7,10	0.25000	0.54962	0,1,10,9	0.44444	0.12159
4,1,9,10	0.16667	0.32710	6,1,8,10	0.00000	0.58333	0,2,4,9	1.00000	0.25926
4,1,10,10	0.00000	0.31914	6,2,3,10	1.00000	0.50690	0,2,5,9	0.88889	0.25690
4,2,3,10	1.00000	0.33793	6,2,4,10	0.75000	0.56519	0,2,6,9	0.77778	0.24968
4,2,4,10	0.83333	0.35428	6,2,5,10	0.50000	0.57130	0,2,7,9	0.66667	0.23715
4,2,5,10	0.66667	0.36711	6,2,6,10	0.25000	0.60953	0,2,8,9	0.55556	0.21842
4,2,6,10	0.50000	0.37679	6,2,7,10	0.00000	0.65085	0,2,9,9	0.44444	0.19166
4,2,7,10	0.33333	0.38356	6,3,3,10	0.75000	0.57735	0,2,10,9	0.33333	0.15270
4,2,8,10	0.16667	0.38756	6,3,4,10	0.50000	0.59512	0,3,3,9	1.00000	0.26450
4,2,9,10	0.00000	0.38889	6,3,5,10	0.25000	0.64280	0,3,4,9	0.88889	0.26736
4,3,3,10	0.83333	0.36289	6,3,6,10	0.00000	0.69222	0,3,5,9	0.77778	0.26565
4,3,5,10	0.66667	0.38356	6,4,4,10	0.25000	0.65352	0,3,6,9	0.66667	0.25926
4,3,6,10	0.50000	0.40062	6,4,5,10	0.00000	0.71200	0,3,7,9	0.55556	0.24784
4,3,7,10	0.33333	0.41450	7,0,5,10	1.00000	0.55556	0,3,8,9	0.44444	0.23064
4,3,8,10	0.16667	0.42552	7,0,6,10	0.66667	0.57013	0,3,9,9	0.33333	0.20621
4,4,4,10	0.00000	0.43390	7,0,7,10	0.33333	0.61195	0,3,10,9	0.22222	0.17151
	0.50000	0.48025	7,0,8,10	0.00000	0.67586	0,4,4,9	0.77778	0.27076
4,4,5,10	0.33333	0.42913	7,1,4,10	1.00000	0.63828	0,4,5,9	0.66667	0.26963
4,4,6,10	0.16667	0.44675	7,1,5,10	0.66667	0.66975	0,4,6,9	0.55556	0.26392
4,4,7,10	0.00000	0.46148	7,1,6,10	0.33333	0.72293	0,4,7,9	0.44444	0.25331
4,5,5,10	0.16667	0.45361	7,1,7,10	0.00000	0.79349	0,4,8,9	0.33333	0.23715
4,5,6,10	0.00000	0.47466	7,2,3,10	1.00000	0.67586	0,4,9,9	0.22222	0.21419
5,0,5,10	1.00000	0.33333	7,2,4,10	0.66667	0.72293	0,4,10,9	0.11111	0.18186
5,0,6,10	0.80000	0.33333	7,2,5,10	0.33333	0.78829	0,5,5,9	0.55556	0.26907
5,0,7,10	0.60000	0.33333	7,2,6,10	0.00000	0.86780	0,5,6,9	0.44444	0.26392
5,0,8,10	0.40000	0.33333	7,3,3,10	0.66667	0.73981	0,5,7,9	0.33333	0.25391
5,0,9,10	0.20000	0.33333	7,3,4,10	0.33333	0.81901	0,5,8,9	0.22222	0.23843
5,0,10,10	0.00000	0.33333	7,3,5,10	0.00000	0.90948	0,5,9,9	0.11111	0.21631
5,1,4,10	1.00000	0.38297	7,4,4,10	0.00000	0.92296	0,5,10,9	0.00000	0.18518
5,1,5,10	0.80000	0.39440	8,0,5,10	1.00000	0.83333	0,6,6,9	0.33333	0.25926
5,1,6,10	0.60000	0.40552	8,0,6,10	0.50000	0.88192	0,6,7,9	0.22222	0.24968
5,1,7,10	0.40000	0.41633	8,0,7,10	0.00000	1.01379	0,6,8,9	0.11111	0.23457
5,1,8,10	0.20000	0.42687	8,1,4,10	1.00000	0.95743	0,6,9,9	0.00000	0.21276
5,1,9,10	0.00000	0.43716	8,1,5,10	0.50000	1.02740	0,7,7,9	0.11111	0.24034
5,2,3,10	1.00000	0.40552	8,1,6,10	0.00000	1.16667	0,7,8,9	0.00000	0.22529
5,2,4,10	0.80000	0.42688	8,2,3,10	1.00000	1.01379	1,0,6,9	1.00000	0.23936
5,2,5,10	0.60000	0.44721	8,2,4,10	0.50000	1.10554	1,0,7,9	0.87500	0.22060
5,2,6,10	0.40000	0.46667	8,2,5,10	0.00000	1.25830	1,0,8,9	0.75000	0.19376
5,2,7,10	0.20000	0.48534	8,3,3,10	0.50000	1.13039	1,0,9,9	0.62500	0.15468
5,2,8,10	0.00000	0.50332	8,3,4,10	0.00000	1.30171	1,0,10,9	0.50000	0.08838

(*Continues*)

Table for Calculation of Median Effective Dose by Moving Average (*Continued*)

r value	f	σf	r value	f	σf	r value	f	σf
	$n = 10, K = 3$			$n = 10, K = 3$			$n = 10, K = 3$	
5,3,3,10	0.80000	0.43716	9,0,5,10	1.00000	1.66667	1,1,5,9	1.00000	0.27323
1,1,6,9	0.87500	0.26363	2,3,6,9	0.57143	0.34194	4,1,6,9	0.80	0.42016
1,1,7,9	0.75000	0.24869	2,3,7,9	0.42857	0.33423	4,1,7,9	0.60	0.40596
1,1,8,9	0.62500	0.22738	2,3,8,9	0.28571	0.32261	4,1,8,9	0.40	0.39486
1,1,9,9	0.50000	0.19766	2,3,9,9	0.14286	0.30838	4,1,9,9	0.20	0.38713
1,1,10,9	0.37500	0.15468	2,3,10,9	0.00000	0.28966	4,1,10,9	0.00	0.38297
1,2,4,9	1.00000	0.29167	2,4,4,9	0.71429	0.34960	4,2,4,9	1.00	0.46667
1,2,5,9	0.87500	0.28877	2,4,5,9	0.57143	0.35496	4,2,5,9	0.80	0.46053
1,2,6,9	0.75000	0.28144	2,4,6,9	0.42857	0.35400	4,2,6,9	0.60	0.45743
1,2,7,9	0.62500	0.26933	2,4,7,9	0.28571	0.34960	4,2,7,9	0.40	0.45743
1,2,8,9	0.50000	0.25173	2,4,8,9	0.14286	0.34318	4,2,8,9	0.20	0.46053
1,2,9,9	0.37500	0.22738	2,4,9,9	0.00000	0.33333	4,2,9,9	0.00	0.46667
1,2,10,9	0.25000	0.19376	2,5,5,9	0.42857	0.36034	4,3,3,9	1.00	0.47610
1,3,3,9	1.00000	0.29756	2,5,6,9	0.28571	0.36234	4,3,4,9	0.80	0.47944
1,3,4,9	0.87500	0.30055	2,5,7,9	0.14286	0.36246	4,3,5,9	0.60	0.48571
1,3,5,9	0.75000	0.29938	2,5,8,9	0.00000	0.35952	4,3,6,9	0.40	0.49477
1,3,6,9	0.62500	0.29398	2,6,6,9	0.14286	0.36867	4,3,7,9	0.20	0.50649
1,3,7,9	0.50000	0.28413	2,6,7,9	0.00000	0.37192	4,3,8,9	0.00	0.52068
1,3,8,9	0.37500	0.26933	3,0,6,9	1.00000	0.31914	4,4,4,9	0.60	0.49477
1,3,9,9	0.25000	0.24869	3,0,7,9	0.83333	0.29310	4,4,5,9	0.40	0.51242
1,3,10,9	0.12500	0.22060	3,0,8,9	0.66667	0.26254	4,4,6,9	0.20	0.53216
1,4,4,9	0.75000	0.30512	3,0,9,9	0.50000	0.22567	4,4,7,9	0.00	0.55377
1,4,5,9	0.62500	0.30557	3,0,10,9	0.33333	0.18703	4,5,5,9	0.20	0.54045
1,4,6,9	0.50000	0.30190	3,1,5,9	1.00000	0.36340	4,5,6,9	0.00	0.56960
1,4,7,9	0.37500	0.29398	3,1,6,9	0.83333	0.35000	5,0,6,9	1.00	0.47871
1,4,8,9	0.25000	0.28144	3,1,7,9	0.66667	0.33487	5,0,7,9	0.75	0.43800
1,4,9,9	0.12500	0.26363	3,1,8,9	0.50000	0.31672	5,0,8,9	0.50	0.41248
1,4,10,9	0.00000	0.23936	3,1,9,9	0.33333	0.30089	5,0,9,9	0.25	0.40505
1,5,5,9	0.50000	0.30760	3,1,10,9	0.16667	0.26692	5,0,10,9	0.00	0.41667
1,5,6,9	0.37500	0.30557	3,2,4,9	1.00000	0.38889	5,1,5,9	1.00	0.54645
1,5,7,9	0.25000	0.29938	3,2,5,9	0.83333	0.38423	5,1,6,9	0.75	0.52457
1,5,8,9	0.12500	0.28887	3,2,6,9	0.66667	0.37816	5,1,7,9	0.50	0.51707
1,5,9,9	0.00000	0.27323	3,2,7,9	0.50000	0.37060	5,1,8,9	0.25000	0.52457
1,6,6,9	0.25000	0.30512	3,2,8,9	0.33333	0.36571	5,1,9,9	0.00000	0.54645
1,6,7,9	0.12500	0.30055	3,2,9,9	0.16667	0.34731	5,2,4,9	1.00000	0.58333
1,6,8,9	0.00000	0.29167	3,2,10,9	0.00000	0.33793	5,2,5,9	0.75000	0.57509
1,7,7,9	0.00000	0.29756	3,3,3,9	1.00000	0.39674	5,2,6,9	0.50000	0.58035
2,0,6,9	1.00000	0.27355	3,3,4,9	0.83333	0.39997	5,2,7,9	0.25000	0.59875
2,0,7,9	0.85714	0.25170	3,3,5,9	0.66667	0.40190	5,2,8,9	0.00000	0.62915
2,0,8,9	0.71429	0.22283	3,3,6,9	0.50000	0.40254	5,3,3,9	1.00000	0.59512
2,0,9,9	0.57143	0.18786	3,3,7,9	0.33333	0.40572	5,3,4,9	0.75000	0.59875
2,0,10,9	0.42857	0.12834	3,3,8,9	0.16667	0.39707	5,3,5,9	0.50000	0.61520
2,1,5,9	1.00000	0.31226	3,3,9,9	0.00000	0.35573	5,3,6,9	0.25000	0.64348
2,1,6,9	0.85714	0.30094	3,4,4,9	0.66667	0.40965	5,3,7,9	0.00000	0.68211
2,1,7,9	0.71429	0.28531	3,4,5,9	0.50000	0.41759	5,4,4,9	0.50000	0.62639

(*Continues*)

Table for Calculation of Median Effective Dose by Moving Average (*Continued*)

n = 10, K = 3			n = 10, K = 3			n = 10, K = 3		
r value	f	σf	r value	f	σf	r value	f	σf
2,1,8,9	0.57143	0.26753	3,4,6,9	0.33333	0.42793	5,4,5,9	0.25000	0.66471
2,1,9,9	0.42857	0.23934	3,4,7,9	0.16667	0.42703	5,4,6,9	0.00000	0.71200
2,1,10,9	0.28571	0.20146	3,4,8,9	0.00000	0.39674	5,5,5,9	0.00000	0.72169
2,2,4,9	1.00000	0.33333	3,5,5,9	0.33333	0.43509	6,0,6,9	1.00000	0.63828
2,2,5,9	0.85714	0.32970	3,5,6,9	0.16667	0.44125	6,0,7,9	0.66667	0.58443
2,2,6,9	0.71429	0.32261	3,5,7,9	0.00000	0.41944	6,0,8,9	0.33333	0.58443
2,2,7,9	0.57143	0.31430	3,6,6,9	0.00000	0.42673	6,0,9,9	0.00000	0.63828
2,2,8,9	0.42857	0.29838	4,0,6,9	1.00	0.38297	6,1,5,9	1.00000	0.72860
2,2,9,9	0.28571	0.27725	4,0,7,9	0.80	0.35100	6,1,6,9	0.66667	0.69979
2,2,10,9	0.14286	0.25170	4,0,8,9	0.60	0.32028	6,1,7,9	0.33333	0.71722
2,3,3,9	1.00000	0.34007	4,0,9,9	0.40	0.29120	6,1,8,9	0.00000	0.77778
2,3,4,9	0.85714	0.34318	4,0,10,9	0.20	0.26432	6,2,4,9	1.00000	0.77778
2,3,5,9	0.71429	0.34305	4,1,5,9	1.00	0.43716	6,2,5,9	0.66667	0.76712
6,2,6,9	0.33333	0.79866	0,4,10,8	0.125	0.20465	2,1,8,8	0.66667	0.32341
6,2,7,9	0.00000	0.79349	0,5,5,8	0.625	0.30369	2,1,9,9	0.50000	0.28328
6,3,3,9	1.00000	0.79349	0,5,6,8	0.500	0.29756	2,1,10,8	0.33333	0.23497
6,3,4,9	0.66667	0.79866	0,5,7,8	0.375	0.28603	2,2,5,8	1.00000	0.41944
6,3,5,9	0.33333	0.84376	0,5,8,8	0.250	0.26842	2,2,6,8	0.83333	0.39890
6,3,6,9	0.00000	0.85346	0,5,9,8	0.125	0.22902	2,2,7,8	0.66667	0.37634
6,4,4,9	0.33333	0.85827	0,5,10,8	0.000	0.20833	2,2,8,8	0.50000	0.35136
6,4,5,9	0.00000	0.88192	0,6,6,8	0.375	0.29204	2,2,9,8	0.33333	0.32341
7,0,6,9	1.00000	0.95743	0,6,7,8	0.250	0.28106	2,2,10,8	0.16667	0.29163
7,0,6,9	1.00000	0.95743	0,6,7,8	0.250	0.28106	2,2,10,8	0.16667	0.29163
7,0,7,9	0.50000	0.88976	0,6,8,8	0.125	0.26393	2,3,4,8	1.00000	0.43390
7,0,8,9	0.00000	1.01379	0,6,9,8	0.000	0.23936	2,3,5,8	0.83333	0.42174
7,1,5,9	1.00	1.09291	0,7,7,8	0.125	0.27043	2,3,6,8	0.66667	0.40783
7,1,6,9	0.50	1.06066	0,7,8,8	0.000	0.25345	2,3,7,8	0.50000	0.40062
7,1,7,9	0.00	1.10924	1,0,7,8	1.00000	0.28966	2,3,8,8	0.33333	0.37634
7,2,4,9	1.00	1.16667	1,0,8,8	0.85714	0.25170	2,3,9,8	0.16667	0.35813
7,2,5,9	0.50	1.16070	1,0,9,8	0.71429	0.20146	2,3,10,8	0.00000	0.33793
7,2,6,9	0.00	1.30171	1,0,10,8	0.57143	0.12834	2,4,4,8	0.83333	0.42783
7,3,3,9	1.00	1.19024	1,1,6,8	1.00000	0.33333	2,4,5,8	0.66667	0.42269
7,3,4,9	0.50	1.20761	1,1,7,8	0.58714	0.30838	2,4,6,8	0.50000	0.43033
7,3,5,9	0.00	1.36422	1,1,8,8	0.71429	0.27725	2,4,7,8	0.33333	0.40783
7,4,4,9	0.00	1.38444	1,1,9,8	0.57143	0.23934	2,4,8,8	0.16667	0.39890
8,0,6,9	1.00	1.77951	1,1,10,8	0.42857	0.18786	2,4,9,8	0.00000	0.38888
8,0,7,9	0.00	2.02759	1,2,5,8	1.00000	0.35952	2,5,5,8	0.50000	0.44445
8,1,5,9	1.00	2.18581	1,2,6,8	0.58714	0.34318	2,5,6,8	0.33333	0.42269
8,1,6,9	0.00	2.33333	1,2,7,8	0.71429	0.32261	2,5,7,8	0.16667	0.42147
8,2,4,9	1.00	2.33333	1,2,8,8	0.57143	0.29839	2,5,8,8	0.00000	0.41944
8,2,5,9	0.00	2.51661	1,2,9,8	0.42857	0.26753	2,6,6,8	0.16667	0.42873
8,3,3,9	1.00	2.38048	1,2,10,8	0.28571	0.22283	2,6,7,8	0.00000	0.43390
8,3,4,9	0.00	2.60342	1,3,4,8	1.00000	0.37192	3,0,7,8	1.00000	0.40552
0,0,7,8	1.000	0.25345	1,3,5,8	0.58	0.36246	3,0,8,8	0.80000	0.34692

(*Continues*)

Table for Calculation of Median Effective Dose by Moving Average (*Continued*)

\(n = 10, K = 3 \)			\(n = 10, K = 3 \)			\(n = 10, K = 3 \)		
r value	f	σf	r value	f	σf	r value	f	σf
0,0,8,8	0.875	0.22140	1,3,6,8	0.71429	0.34960	3,0,9,8	0.60000	0.28378
0,0,9,0	0.750	0,17678	1,3,7,8	0.57143	0.33423	3,0,10,8	0,40000	0.21208
0,0,10,8	0.625	0.07365	1,3,8,8	0.42857	0.31430	3,1,6,8	1.00000	0.46667
0,1,6,8	1.000	0.29166	1,3,9,8	0.28571	0.28531	3,1,7,8	0.80000	0.42729
0,1,7,8	0.875	0.27081	1,3,10,8	0.14286	0.25170	3,1,8,8	0.60000	0.38941
0,1,8,8	0.750	0.24296	1,4,4,8	0.85714	0.36867	3,1,9,8	0.40000	0.35352
0,1,9,8	0.625	0.19151	1,4,5,8	0.71429	0.36234	3,1,10,8	0.20000	0.32028
0,1,10,8	0.500	0.10534	1,4,6,8	0.57143	0.35400	3,2,5,8	1.00000	0.50332
0,2,5,8	1.000	0.31458	1,4,7,8	0.42857	0.34194	3,2,6,8	0.80000	0.47647
0,2,6,8	0.875	0.30117	1,4,8,8	0.28571	0.32261	3,2,7,8	0.60000	0.45274
0,2,7,8	0.750	0.28260	1,4,9,8	0.14286	0.30094	3,2,8,8	0.40000	0.43267
0,2,8,8	0.625	0.24694	1,4,10,8	1.00000	0.27355	3,2,10,8	0.20000	0.41676
0,2,9,8	0.500	0.21651	1,5,5,8	0.57143	0.26034	3,2,10,8	0.00000	0.40552
0,2,10,8	0.375	0.17237	1,5,6,8	0.42857	0.35496	3,3,4,8	1.00000	0.52068
0,3,4,8	1.000	0.32543	1,5,7,8	0.28571	0.34305	3,3,5,8	0.80000	0.50368
0,3,5,8	0.875	0.31799	1,5,8,8	0.14286	0.32970	3,3,6,8	0.60000	0.49044
0,3,6,8	0.750	0.30619	1,5,9,8	0.00000	0.31226	3,3,7,8	0.40000	0.48129
0,3,7,8	0.625	0.27990	1,6,6,8	0.28571	0.34960	3,3,8,8	0.20000	0.47647
0,3,8,8	0.500	0.26021	1,6,7,8	0.14286	0.34318	3,3,9,8	0.00000	0.47610
0,3,9,8	0.375	0.23246	1,6,8,8	0.00000	0.33333	3,4,4,8	0.80000	0.51242
0,3,10,8	0.250	0.19320	1,7,7,8	0.00000	0.34007	3,4,5,8	0.60000	0.50824
0,4,4,8	0.875	0.32340	2,0,7,8	1.00000	0.33793	3,4,6,8	0.40000	0.50824
0,4,5,8	0.750	0.31732	2,0,8,8	0.83333	0.29163	3,4,7,8	0.20000	0.51242
0,4,6,8	0.625	0.29789	2,0,9,8	0.66667	0.23497	3,4,8,8	0.00000	0.52068
0,4,7,8	0.500	0.28565	2,0,10,8	0.50000	0.15713	3,5,5,8	0.40000	0.51691
0,4,8,8	0.375	0.26717	2,1,6,8	1.00000	0.38888	3,5,6,8	0.20000	0.52949
0,4,9,8	0.250	0.24116	2,1,7,8	0.83333	0.35813	3,5,7,8	0.00000	0.54569
3,6,6,8	0.00000	0.55377	6,3,6,8	0.00000	1.38444	1,2,7,7	0.83333	0.39707
4,0,7,8	1.00000	0.50690	6,4,4,8	0.50000	1.26930	1,2,8,7	0.66667	0.36571
4,0,8,8	0.75000	0.42898	6,4,5,8	0.00000	1.42400	1,2,9,7	0.50000	0.31672
4,0,9,8	0.50000	0.36324	7,0,7,8	1.00000	2.02759	1,2,10,7	0.33333	0.26254
4,0,10,8	0.25000	0.31732	7,0,8,8	0.00000	2.02759	1,3,5,7	1.00000	0.41944
4,1,6,8	1.00000	0.58333	7,1,6,8	1.00000	2.33333	1,3,6,7	0.83333	0.42703
4,1,7,8	0.75000	0.53033	7,1,7,8	0.00000	2.38048	1,3,7,7	0.66667	0.40572
4,1,8,8	0.50000	0.49301	7,2,5,8	1.00000	2.51661	1,3,8,7	0.50000	0.37060
4,1,9,8	0.25000	0.47507	7,2,6,8	0.00000	2.60342	1,3,9,7	0.33333	0.33487
4,1,10,8	0.00000	0.47871	7,3,4,8	1.00000	2.60342	1,3,10,7	0.16667	0.29310
4,2,5,8	1.00000	0.62915	7,3,5,8	0.00000	2.72845	1,4,4,7	1.00000	0.42673
4,2,6,8	0.75000	0.59219	7,4,4,8	0.00000	2.76887	1,4,5,7	0.83333	0.44125
4,2,7,8	0.50000	0.57130	0,0,8,7	1.00000	0.28965	1,4,6,7	0.66667	0.42793
4,2,8,8	0.25000	0.56826	0,0,9,7	0.85714	0.23536	1,4,7,7	0.50000	0.40254
4,2,9,8	0.00000	0.58333	0,0,10,7	0.71429	0.15587	1,4,8,7	0.33333	0.37816
4,3,4,8	1.00000	0.65085	0,1,7,7	1.00000	0.34007	1,4,9,7	0.16667	0.35000
4,3,5,8	0.75000	0.62639	0,1,8,7	0.85714	0.30278	1,4,10,7	0.00000	0.31914

(*Continues*)

Table for Calculation of Median Effective Dose by Moving Average (*Continued*)

n = 10, K = 3			n = 10, K = 3			n = 10, K = 3		
r value	f	σf	r value	f	σf	r value	f	σf
4,3,6,8	0.50000	0.61802	0,1,9,7	0.71429	0.25517	1,5,5,7	0.66667	0.43509
4,3,7,8	0.25000	0.62639	0,1,10,7	0.57143	0.18962	1,5,6,7	0.50000	0.41759
4,3,8,8	0.00000	0.65085	0,2,6,7	1.00000	0.37192	1,5,7,7	0.33333	0.40190
4,4,4,8	0.75000	0.63191	0,2,7,7	0.85714	0.34480	1,5,8,7	0.16667	0.38423
4,4,5,8	0.50000	0.64010	0,2,8,7	0.71429	0.31122	1,5,9,7	0.00000	0.36423
4,4,6,8	0.25000	0.66926	0,2,9,7	0.57143	0.26877	1,6,6,7	0.33333	0.40965
4,4,7,8	0.00000	0.69222	0,2,10,7	0.42857	0.21695	1,6,7,7	0.16667	0.39997
4,5,5,8	0.25000	0.68971	0,3,5,7	1.00000	0.38978	1,6,8,7	0.00000	0.38889
4,5,6,8	0.00000	0.71200	0,3,6,7	0.85714	0.37017	1,7,7,7	0.00000	0.39674
5,0,7,8	1.00000	0.67586	0,3,7,7	0.71429	0.34574	2,0,8,7	1.00000	0.40552
5,0,8,8	0.66667	0.56534	0,3,8,7	0.57143	0.31536	2,0,9,7	0.80000	0.32028
5,0,9,8	0.33333	0.51984	0,3,9,7	0.42857	0.28074	2,0,10,7	0.60000	0.21208
5,0,10,8	0.00000	0.55556	0,3,10,7	0.28571	0.22695	2,1,7,7	1.00000	0.47610
5,1,6,8	1.00000	0.77778	0,4,4,7	1.00000	0.39555	2,1,8,7	0.80000	0.41676
5,1,7,8	0.66667	0.70175	0,4,5,7	0.85714	0.38223	2,1,9,7	0.60000	0.35352
5,1,8,8	0.33333	0.68393	0,4,6,7	0.71429	0.36488	2,1,10,7	0.40000	0.28378
5,1,9,8	0.00000	0.72860	0,4,7,7	0.57143	0.34291	2,2,6,7	1.00000	0.52068
5,2,5,8	1.00000	0.83887	0,4,8,7	0.42857	0.31857	2,2,7,7	0.80000	0.47647
5,2,6,8	0.66667	0.78480	0,4,9,7	0.28571	0.28057	2,2,8,7	0.60000	0.43267
5,2,7,8	0.33333	0.78480	0,4,10,7	0.14286	0.23536	2,2,9,7	0.40000	0.48941
5,2,8,8	0.00000	0.83887	0,5,5,7	0.71429	0.37104	2,2,10,7	0.20000	0.34692
5,3,4,8	1.00000	0.86780	0,5,6,7	0.57143	0.35589	2,3,5,7	1.00000	0.54569
5,3,5,8	0.66667	0.83065	0,5,7,7	0.42857	0.33927	2,3,6,7	0.80000	0.51242
5,3,6,8	0.33333	0.84539	0,5,8,7	0.28571	0.31122	2,3,7,7	0.60000	0.48129
5,3,7,8	0.00000	0.90948	0,5,9,7	0.14286	0.37941	2,3,8,7	0.40000	0.45274
5,4,4,8	0.66667	0.84539	0,5,10,7	0.00000	0.23809	2,3,9,7	0.20000	0.42729
5,4,5,8	0.33333	0.87410	0,6,6,7	0.42857	0.34588	2,3,10,7	0.00000	0.40552
5,4,6,8	0.00000	0.94933	0,6,7,7	0.28571	0.32546	2,4,4,7	1.00000	0.55377
5,5,5,8	0.00000	0.96225	0,6,8,7	0.14286	0.30278	2,4,5,7	0.80000	0.52949
6,0,7,8	1.00000	1.01379	0,6,9,7	0.00000	0.27355	2,4,6,7	0.60000	0.50824
6,0,8,8	0.50000	0.84984	0,7,7,7	0.14286	0.31018	2,4,7,7	0.40000	0.49044
6,0,9,8	0.00000	0.95743	0,7,8,7	0.00000	0.28965	2,4,8,7	0.20000	0.47647
6,1,6,8	1.00000	1.16667	1,0,8,7	1.00000	0.33793	2,4,9,7	0.00000	0.46667
6,1,7,8	0.50000	1.05409	1,0,9,7	0.83333	0.26692	2,5,5,7	0.60000	0.51691
6,1,8,8	0.00000	1.16667	1,0,10,7	0.66667	0.18793	2,5,6,7	0.40000	0.50824
6,2,5,8	1.00000	1.25830	1,1,7,7	1.00000	0.35573	2,5,7,7	0.20000	0.50368
6,2,6,8	0.50000	1.17851	1,1,8,7	0.83333	0.34731	2,5,8,7	0.00000	0.50332
6,3,7,8	0.00000	1.30171	1,1,9,7	0.66667	0.30089	2,6,6,7	0.20000	0.51242
6,3,4,8	1.00000	1.30171	1,1,10,7	0.50000	0.22567	2,6,7,7	0.00000	0.52068
6,3,5,8	0.5000	1.24722	1,2,6,7	1.00000	0.39674	3,0,8,7	1.00000	0.50690
3,0,9,7	0.75000	0.39198	5,3,7,7	0.00000	1.36422	1,3,7,6	0.80000	0.50649
3,0,10,7	0.50000	0.27003	5,4,4,7	1.00000	1.38444	1,3,8,6	0.60000	0.45743
3,1,7,7	1.00000	0.59512	5,4,5,7	0.50000	1.29636	1,3,9,6	0.40000	0.40596
3,1,8,7	0.75000	0.51454	5,4,6,7	0.00000	1.42400	1,3,10,6	0.20000	0.35100

(*Continues*)

Table for Calculation of Median Effective Dose by Moving Average (*Continued*)

n = 10, K = 3			n = 10, K = 3			n = 10, K = 3		
r value	ƒ	σƒ	r value	ƒ	σƒ	r value	ƒ	σƒ
3,1,9,7	0.50000	0.44488	5,5,5,7	0.00000	1.44338	1,4,5,6	1.00000	0.56960
3,1,10,7	0.25000	0.39198	6,0,8,7	1.00000	2.10818	1,4,6,6	0.80000	0.53216
3,2,6,7	1.00000	0.65085	6,0,9,7	0.00000	1.77951	1,4,7,6	0.60000	0.49477
3,2,7,7	0.75000	0.58999	6,1,7,7	1.00000	2.44949	1,4,8,6	0.40000	0.45743
3,2,8,7	0.50000	0.54327	6,1,8,7	0.00000	2.33333	1,4,9,6	0.20000	0.42016
3,2,9,7	0.25000	0.51454	6,2,6,7	1.00000	2.66667	1,4,10,6	0.00000	0.38297
3,2,10,7	0.00000	0.50690	6,2,7,7	0.00000	2.60342	1,5,5,6	0.80000	0.54045
3,3,5,7	1.00000	0.68211	6,3,5,7	1.00000	2.78887	1,5,6,6	0.60000	0.51242
3,3,6,7	0.75000	0.63533	6,3,6,7	0.00000	2.76887	1,5,7,6	0.40000	0.48571
3,3,7,7	0.50000	0.60403	6,4,4,7	1.00000	2.82427	1,5,8,6	0.20000	0.46053
3,3,8,7	0.25000	0.58999	6,4,5,7	0.00000	2.84800	1,5,9,6	0.00000	0.43716
3,3,9,7	0.00000	0.59512	0,0,9,6	1.00000	0.31914	1,6,6,6	0.40000	0.49477
3,4,4,7	1.00000	0.69222	0,0,10,6	0.83333	0.22680	1,6,7,6	0.20000	0.47944
3,4,5,7	0.75000	0.65683	0,1,8,6	1.00000	0.38889	1,6,8,6	0.00000	0.46667
3,4,6,7	0.50000	0.63191	0,1,9,6	0.83333	0.32710	1,7,7,6	0.00000	0.47610
3,4,7,7	0.25000	0.63533	0,1,10,6	0.66667	0.24637	2,0,9,6	1.00000	0.47871
3,4,8,7	0.00000	0.65085	0,2,7,6	1.00000	0.43390	3,0,10,6	0.75000	0.31732
3,5,5,7	0.50000	0.64818	0,2,8,6	0.83333	0.38756	2,1,8,6	1.00000	0.58333
3,5,6,7	0.25000	0.65683	0,2,9,6	0.66667	0.33178	2,1,9,6	0.75000	0.47507
3,5,7,7	0.00000	0.68211	0,2,10,6	0.50000	0.26058	2,1,10,6	0.50000	0.36324
3,6,6,7	0.00000	0.69222	0,3,6,6	1.00000	0.46148	2,2,7,6	1.00000	0.65085
4,0,8,7	1.00000	0.67586	0,3,7,6	0.83333	0.42552	2,2,8,6	0.75000	0.56826
4,0,9,7	0.66667	0.50917	0,3,8,6	0.66667	0.38356	2,2,9,6	0.50000	0.49301
4,0,10,7	0.33333	0.40062	0,3,9,6	0.50000	0.33333	2,2,10,6	0.25000	0.42998
4,1,7,7	1.00000	0.79349	0,3,10,6	0.33333	0.27027	2,3,6,6	1.00000	0.69222
4,1,8,7	0.66667	0.67586	0,4,5,6	1.00000	0.47466	2,3,7,6	0.75000	0.62639
4,1,9,7	0.33333	0.61864	0,4,6,6	0.83333	0.44675	2,3,8,6	0.50000	0.57130
4,1,10,7	0.00000	0.63828	0,4,7,6	0.66667	0.41450	2,3,9,6	0.25000	0.53033
4,2,6,7	1.00000	0.86780	0,4,8,6	0.50000	0.37679	2,3,10,6	0.00000	0.50690
4,2,7,7	0.66667	0.77778	0,4,9,6	0.33333	0.33178	2,4,5,6	1.00000	0.71200
4,2,8,7	0.33333	0.74536	0,4,10,6	0.16667	0.27592	2,4,6,6	0.75000	0.66926
4,2,9,7	0.00000	0.77778	0,5,5,6	0.83333	0.45361	2,4,7,6	0.50000	0.61802
4,3,5,7	1.00000	0.90948	0,5,6,6	0.66667	0.42913	2,4,8,6	0.25000	0.59219
4,3,6,7	0.66667	0.83887	0,5,7,6	0.50000	0.40062	2,4,9,6	0.00000	0.58333
4,3,7,7	0.33333	0.82402	0,5,8,6	0.33333	0.36711	2,5,5,6	0.75000	0.68971
4,2,8,7	0.00000	0.86780	0,5,9,6	0.16667	0.32710	2,5,6,6	0.50000	0.64010
4,4,4,7	1.00000	0.92296	0,5,10,6	0.00000	0.27778	2,5,7,6	0.25000	0.62639
4,4,5,7	0.66667	0.86780	0,6,6,6	0.50000	0.40825	2,5,8,6	0.00000	0.62915
4,4,6,7	0.33333	0.86780	0,6,7,6	0.33333	0.38356	2,6,6,6	0.25000	0.63191
4,4,7,7	0.00000	0.92296	0,6,8,6	0.16667	0.35428	2,6,7,6	0.00000	0.65085
4,5,5,7	0.33333	0.88192	0,6,9,2	0.00000	0.31914	3,0,9,6	1.00000	0.63828
4,5,6,7	0.00000	0.94933	0,7,7,6	0.16667	0.36289	3,0,10,6	0.66667	0.40062
5,0,8,7	1.00000	1.01379	0,7,8,6	0.00000	0.33793	3,1,8,6	1.00000	0.77778
5,0,9,7	0.50000	0.75462	1,0,9,6	1.00000	0.38297	3,1,9,6	0.66667	0.61864

(*Continues*)

Table for Calculation of Median Effective Dose by Moving Average (*Continued*)

$n = 10, K = 3$			$n = 10, K = 3$			$n = 10, K = 3$		
r value	ʃ	ʃσ	r value	ʃ	ʃσ	r value	ʃ	ʃσ
5,0,10,7	0.00000	0.83333	1,0,10,6	0.80000	0.26432	3,1,10,6	0.33333	0.50917
5,1,7,7	1.00000	1.19024	1,1,8,6	1.00000	0.46667	3,2,7,6	1.00000	0.86780
5,1,8,7	0.50000	1.00692	1,1,9,6	0.80000	0.38713	3,2,8,6	0.66667	0.74536
5,1,9,7	0.00000	1.09291	1,1,10,6	0.60000	0.29120	3,2,9,6	0.33333	0.67586
5,2,6,7	1.00000	1.30171	1,2,7,6	1.00000	0.52068	3,2,10,6	0.00000	0.67586
5,2,7,7	0.50000	1.16070	1,2,8,6	0.80000	0.46053	3,3,6,6	1.00000	0.92296
5,2,8,7	0.00000	1.25830	1,2,9,6	0.60000	0.39486	3,3,7,6	0.66667	0.82402
5,3,5,7	1.00000	1.36422	1,2,10,6	0.40000	0.32028	3,3,8,6	0.33333	0.77778
5,3,6,7	0.50000	1.25277	1,3,6,6	1.00000	0.55377	3,3,9,6	0.00000	0.79349
3,4,5,6	1.00000	0.94933	0,6,7,5	0.40000	0.46667	3,3,9,5	0.00000	1.19024
3,4,6,6	0.66667	0.86780	0,6,8,5	0.20000	0.42688	3,4,6,5	1.00000	1.42400
3,4,7,6	0.33333	0.83887	0,6,9,5	0.00000	0.38297	3,4,7,5	0.50000	1.25277
3,4,8,6	0.00000	0.86780	0,7,7,5	0.20000	0.43716	3,4,8,5	0.00000	1.30171
3,5,5,6	0.66667	0.88192	0,7,8,5	0.00000	0.40552	3,5,5,5	1.00000	1.44388
3,5,6,6	0.33333	0.86780	1,0,10,5	1.00000	0.41667	3,5,6,5	0.50000	1.29636
3,5,7,6	0.00000	0.90948	1,1,9,5	1.00000	0.54645	3,5,7,5	0.00000	1.36422
3,6,6,6	0.00000	0.92296	1,1,10,5	0.75000	0.40505	3,6,6,5	0.00000	1.38444
4,0,9,6	1.00000	0.95743	1,2,8,5	1.00000	0.62915	4,0,10,5	1.00000	1.66667
4,0,10,6	0.50000	0.57735	1,2,9,5	0.75000	0.52457	4,1,9,5	1.00000	2.18581
4,1,8,6	1.00000	0.16667	1,2,10,5	0.50000	0.41248	4,1,10,5	0.00000	2.23607
4,1,9,6	0.50000	0.91287	1,3,7,5	1.00000	0.68211	4,2,8,5	1.00000	2.51661
4,1,10,6	0.00000	0.95743	1,3,8,5	0.75000	0.59875	4,2,9,5	0.00000	2.60342
4,2,7,6	1.00000	1.19024	1,3,9,5	0.50000	0.51707	4,3,7,5	1.00000	2.72845
4,2,8,6	0.50000	1.10554	1,3,10,5	0.25000	0.43800	4,3,8,5	0.00000	2.84800
4,2,9,6	0.00000	1.16667	1,4,6,5	1.00000	0.71200	4,4,6,5	1.00000	2.84800
4,3,6,6	1.0	1.28019	1,4,7,5	0.75000	0.64348	4,4,7,5	0.00000	3.00000
4,3,7,6	0.5	1.22474	1,4,8,5	0.50000	0.58035	4,5,5,5	1.00000	2.88675
4,3,8,6	0.0	1.19024	1,4,9,5	0.25000	0.52457	4,5,6,5	0.00000	3.07318
4,4,5,6	1.0	1.32288	1,4,10,5	0.00000	0.47871	0,1,10,4	1.00000	0.47871
4,4,6,6	0.5	1.29099	1,5,5,5	1.00000	0.72169	0,2,9,4	1.00000	0.58333
4,4,7,6	0.0	1.28019	1,5,6,5	0.75000	0.66471	0,2,10,4	0.75000	0.45262
4,5,5,6	0.5	1.31233	1,5,7,5	0.50000	0.61520	0,3,8,4	1.00000	0.65085
4,5,6,6	0.0	1.32288	1,5,8,5	0.25000	0.57509	0,3,9,4	0.75000	0.54962
5,0,9,6	1.0	2.23607	1,5,9,5	0.00000	0.54645	0,3,10,4	0.50000	0.53301
5,0,10,6	0.0	1.66667	1,6,6,5	0.50000	0.62639	0,4,7,4	1.00000	0.69222
5,1,8,6	1.0	2.60342	1,6,7,5	0.25000	0.59875	0,4,8,4	0.75000	0.60953
5,1,9,6	0.0	2.18581	1,6,8,5	0.00000	0.58333	0,4,9,4	0.50000	0.52042
5,2,7,6	1.0	2.84800	1,7,7,5	0.00000	0.59512	0,4,10,4	0.25000	0.45644
5,2,8,6	0.0	2.51661	2,1,9,5	1.00000	0.72860	0,5,7,4	0.75000	0.64280
5,3,7,6	0.0	2.72845	2,1,10,5	0.66667	0.51985	0,5,8,4	0.50000	0.57130
5,4,5,6	1.0	3.07318	2,2,8,5	1.00000	0.83887	0,5,9,4	0.25000	0.52705
5,4,6,6	0.0	2.84800	2,2,9,5	0.66667	0.68393	0,5,10,4	0.00000	0.41667
5,5,5,6	0.0	2.88675	2,2,10,5	0.33333	0.56534	0,6,6,4	0.75000	0.65352
0,0,10,5	1.0	0.33333	2,3,7,5	1.00000	0.90948	0,6,7,4	0.50000	0.59512

(*Continues*)

Table for Calculation of Median Effective Dose by Moving Average (*Continued*)

r value	ƒ	σƒ	r value	ƒ	σƒ	r value	ƒ	σƒ
	$n = 10, K = 3$			$n = 10, K = 3$			$n = 10, K = 3$	
0,1,9,5	1.0	0.43716	2,3,8,5	0.66667	0.78480	0,6,8,4	0.25000	0.56519
0,1,10,5	0.8	0.33333	2,3,9,5	0.33333	0.70175	0,6,9,4	0.00000	0.47871
0,2,8,5	1.0	0.50332	2,3,10,5	0.00000	0.67586	0,7,7,4	0.25000	0.57735
0,2,9,5	0.8	0.42687	2,4,6,5	1.00000	0.94933	0,7,8,4	0.00000	0.50690
0,2,10,5	0.6	0.33333	2,4,7,5	0.66667	0.84539	1,1,10,4	1.00000	0.63828
0,3,7,5	1.0	0.54569	2,4,8,5	0.33333	0.78480	1,2,9,4	1.00000	0.77778
0,3,8,5	0.8	0.48534	2,4,9,5	0.00000	0.77778	1,2,10,4	0.66667	0.58443
0,3,9,5	0.6	0.41633	2,5,5,5	1.00000	0.96225	1,3,8,4	1.00000	0.79349
0,3,10,5	0.4	0.33333	2,5,6,5	0.66667	0.87410	1,3,9,4	0.66667	0.71722
0,4,6,5	1.0	0.56960	2,5,7,5	0.33333	0.83065	1,3,10,4	0.33333	0.58443
0,4,7,5	0.8	0.52068	2,5,8,5	0.00000	0.83887	1,4,7,4	1.00000	0.85346
0,4,8,5	0.6	0.46667	2,6,6,5	0.33333	0.84539	1,4,8,4	0.66667	0.79866
0,4,9,5	0.4	0.40552	2,6,7,5	0.00000	0.86780	1,4,9,4	0.33333	0.69979
0,4,10,5	0.2	0.33333	3,0,10,5	1.00000	0.83333	1,4,10,4	0.00000	0.63828
0,5,5,5	1.0	0.57735	3,1,9,5	1.00000	1.09291	1,5,6,4	1.00000	0.88192
0,5,6,5	0.8	0.53748	3,1,10,5	0.50000	0.75462	1,5,7,4	0.66667	0.84376
0,5,7,5	0.6	0.48990	3,2,8,5	1.00000	1.25830	1,5,8,4	0.33333	0.76712
0,5,8,5	0.40000	0.44721	3,2,9,5	0.50000	1.00692	1,5,9,4	0.00000	0.72860
0,5,9,5	0.20000	0.39440	3,2,10,5	0.00000	1.01379	1,6,6,4	0.66667	0.85827
0,5,10,5	0.00000	0.33333	3,3,7,5	1.00000	1.36422	1,6,7,4	0.33333	0.79866
0,6,6,5	0.60000	0.49889	3,3,8,5	0.50000	1.16070	1,6,8,4	0.00000	0.77778
1,7,7,4	0.00000	0.79349	0,4,10,3	0.33333	0.57013	2,5,8,3	0.0	2.51661
2,1,10,4	1.00000	0.95743	0,5,7,3	1.00000	0.90948	2,6,6,3	1.0	2.76887
2,2,9,4	1.00000	1.16667	0,5,8,3	0.66667	0.78829	2,6,7,3	0.0	2.60342
2,2,10,4	0.50000	0.84984	0,5,9,3	0.33333	0.66975	0,3,10,2	1.0	1.01379
2,3,8,4	1.00000	1.30171	0,5,10,3	0.00000	0.55556	0,4,9,2	1.0	1.16667
2,3,9,4	0.50000	1.05409	0,6,6,3	1.00000	0.92296	0,4,10,2	0.5	0.88192
2,3,10,4	0.00000	1.01319	0,6,7,3	0.66667	0.81901	0,5,8,2	1.0	1.25830
2,4,7,4	1.00000	1.38444	0,6,8,3	0.33333	0.72293	0,5,9,2	0.5	1.02740
2,4,8,4	0.50000	1.17851	0,6,9,3	0.00000	0.63828	0,5,10,2	0.0	0.83333
2,4,9,4	0.00000	1.16667	0,7,7,3	0.33333	0.73981	0,6,7,2	1.0	1.30171
2,5,6,4	1.00000	1.42400	0,7,8,3	0.00000	0.67586	0,6,8,2	0.5	1.10554
2,5,7,4	0.50000	1.24722	1,2,10,3	1.0	1.01379	0,6,9,2	0.0	0.95743
2,5,8,4	0.00000	1.25830	1,3,9,3	1.0	1.19024	0,7,7,2	0.5	1.13039
2,6,6,4	0.50000	1.26930	1,3,10,3	0.5	0.88976	0,7,8,2	0.0	1.01379
2,6,7,4	0.00000	1.30171	1,4,8,3	1.0	1.30171	1,3,10,2	1.0	2.02759
3,1,10,4	1.00000	1.79951	1,4,9,3	0.5	1.06066	1,4,9,2	1.0	2.33333
3,2,9,4	1.00000	2.33333	1,4,10,3	0.0	0.95743	1,4,10,2	0.0	1.77951
3,2,10,4	0.00000	2.10818	1,5,7,3	1.0	1.36422	1,5,8,2	1.0	2.51661
3,3,8,4	1.00000	2.60342	1,5,8,3	0.5	1.16070	1,5,9,2	0.0	2.18581
3,3,9,4	0.00000	2.44949	1,5,9,3	0.0	1.09291	1,6,7,2	1.0	2.60342
3,4,7,4	1.00000	2.76887	1,6,6,3	1.0	1.38444	1,6,8,2	0.0	2.33333
3,4,8,4	0.00000	2.66667	1,6,7,3	0.5	1.20761	1,7,7,2	0.0	2.38048

(*Continues*)

Table for Calculation of Median Effective Dose by Moving Average (*Continued*)

$n = 10, K = 3$			$n = 10, K = 3$			$n = 10, K = 3$		
r value	f	σf	r value	f	σf	r value	f	σf
3,5,6,4	1.00000	2.84800	1,6,8,3	0.0	1.16667	0,4,10,1	1.0	0.77951
3,5,7,4	0.00000	2.78887	1,7,7,3	0.0	1.19024	0,5,9,1	1.0	2.18581
3,6,6,4	0.00000	2.82427	2,2,10,3	1.0	2.02759	0,5,10,1	0.0	1.66667
0,2,10,3	1.00000	0.67586	2,3,9,3	1.0	2.38048	0,6,8,1	1.0	2.33333
0,3,9,3	1.00000	0.79349	2,3,10,3	0.0	2.02759	0,6,9,1	0.0	1.77951
0,3,10,3	0.66667	0.61195	2,4,8,3	1.0	2.60342	0,7,7,1	1.0	2.38048
0,4,8,3	1.00000	0.86780	2,4,9,3	0.0	2.33333	0,7,8,1	0.0	2.02759
0,4,9,3	0.66667	0.72293	2,5,7,3	1.0	2.72845			

Table for Calculation of Median Effective Dose by Moving Average

			$d = 0.30103^a$	
r value	f	σf	$d(f + 0.5)$	$2.306\ d\sigma_f$
0,0,5	1.0	(0)	0.45154	(0)
0,1,5	0.8	0.20000	0.39134	0.13884
0,2,5	0.6	0.24495	0.33113	0.17004
0,3,5	0.4	0.24495	0.27093	0.17004
0,4,5	0.2	0.20000	0.21072	0.13884
0,5,5	0.0	(0)	0.15052	(0)
1,0,5	1.0	(0)	0.45154	(0)
1,1,5	0.75	0.25769	0.37629	0.17888
1,2,5	0.5	0.33072	0.30103	0.22958
1,3,5	0.25	0.35904	0.22577	0.24924
1,4,5	0.0	0.35355	0.15052	0.24543
2,0,5	1.0	(0)	0.45154	(0)
2,1,5	0.66667	0.36004	0.35120	0.24993
2,2,5	0.33333	0.49065	0.25086	0.34060
2,3,5	0.0	0.57735	0.15052	0.40078
3,0,5	1.0	(0)	0.45154	(0)
3,1,5	0.5	0.58630	0.30103	0.40700
3,2,5	0.0	0.86603	0.15052	0.60118
4,0,5	1.0	(0)	0.45154	(0)
4,1,5	0.0	1.41421	0.15052	0.98171
0,1,4	1.0	0.35355	0.45154	0.24543
0,2,4	0.75	0.35904	0.37629	0.24924
0,3,4	0.5	0.33072	0.30103	0.22958
0,4,4	0.25	0.25769	0.22577	0.17888
0,5,4	0.0	(0)	0.15052	(0)
1,1,4	1.0	0.47140	0.45154	0.32723
1,2,4	0.6667	0.47791	0.35120	0.33175
1,3,4	0.3333	0.47791	0.25086	0.33175
1,4,4	0.0	0.47140	0.15052	0.32723

[a]Calculation by moving average interpolation for $N = 5$, $K = 2$, and $d = 0.30103$ from the formula: $\text{Log } m = \log D_a + \dfrac{d(K - 1)}{2} + df = \log D_a + d(f + 0.5)$; in this case, $2.306\ \sigma \log m = 2.306\ d\sigma_f$.

Table for Calculation of Median Effective Dose

r value	*σf*	*σf*	$d(f + 0.5)$	2.306 $d\sigma_f$
			$d = 0.30103^a$	
2,1,4	1.0	0.70711	0.45154	0.49086
2,2,4	0.5	0.72887	0.30103	0.50596
2,3,4	0.0	0.86603	0.15052	0.60118
3,1,4	1.0	1.41421	0.45154	0.98171
3,2,4	0.0	1.73205	0.15052	1.20235
0,2,3	1.0	0.57735	0.45154	0.40078
0,3,3	0.66667	0.49065	0.35120	0.35060
0,4,3	0.33333	0.36004	0.25086	0.24993
0,5,3	0.0	(0)	0.15052	(0)
1,2,3	1.0	0.86603	0.45154	1.20235
1,3,3	0.5	0.72887	0.30103	0.50596
1,4,3	0.0	0.70711	0.15052	0.49806
2,2,3	1.0	1.73205	0.45154	1.20235
2,3,3	0.0	1.73205	0.15052	1.20235
0,3,2	1.0	0.86602	0.45154	0.60118
0,4,2	0.5	0.58630	0.30103	0.40700
0,5,2	0.0	(0)	0.15052	(0)
1,3,2	1.0	1.73205	0.45154	1.20235
1,4,2	0.0	1.41421	0.15052	0.98171
0,4,1	1.0	1.41421	0.45154	0.98171
0,5,1	0.0	(0)	0.15052	(0)

[a]Calculation by moving average interpolation for $N = 4$, $K = 2$, and $d = 0.30103$ from the formula: Log $m = \log D_a + \dfrac{d(K - 1)}{2} + df = \log D_a + d(f + 0.5)$; $2.447_\sigma = 2.447_{\sigma f}(d)$.

Table for Calculation of Median Effective Dose

r value	f	σf	d(f + 1)	2.179 dσf	r value	f	σf	d(f + 1)	2.179 dσf
			d = 0.30103[a]					d = 0.30103[a]	
0,0,3,5	0.9	0.24495	0.57196	0.16067	0,2,4,4	0.375	0.40625	0.41392	0.26648
0,0,4,5	0.7	0.20000	0.51175	0.13119	0,2,5,4	0.125	0.30778	0.33866	0.20189
0,0,5,5	0.5	0.0	0.45154	0.0	0,3,3,4	0.375	0.44304	0.41392	0.29061
0,1,2,5	0.9	0.31623	0.57196	0.20743	0,3,4,4	0.125	0.39652	0.33866	0.26010
0,1,3,5	0.7	0.31623	0.51175	0.20743	1,0,4,4	0.83333	0.43744	0.55189	0.28694
0,1,4,5	0.5	0.28284	0.45154	0.18553	1,0,5,4	0.50	0.23570	0.45154	0.15461
0,1,5,5	0.3	0.20000	0.39134	0.13119	1,1,3,4	0.83333	0.59835	0.55189	0.39248
0,2,2,5	0.7	0.34641	0.51175	0.22723	1,1,4,4	0.50	0.52705	0.45154	0.34572
0,2,3,5	0.5	0.34641	0.45154	0.22723	1,1,5,4	0.16667	0.43744	0.35120	0.28694
0,2,4,5	0.3	0.31623	0.39134	0.20743	1,2,2,4	0.83333	0.64310	0.55189	0.42184
0,2,5,5	0.1	0.24495	0.33113	0.16067	1,2,3,4	0.50	0.62361	0.45154	0.40905
0,3,3,5	0.3	0.34641	0.39134	0.22723	1,2,4,4	1.16667	0.59835	0.35120	0.39248
0,3,4,5	0.1	0.31623	0.33113	0.20743	1,3,3,4	0.16667	0.64310	0.35120	0.42184
1,0,3,5	0.875	0.30778	0.56443	0.20189	2,0,4,4	0.75	0.64348	0.52680	0.42209
1,0,4,5	0.625	0.26700	0.48917	0.17514	2,0,5,4	0.25	0.47598	0.37629	0.31222
1,0,5,5	0.375	0.15625	0.41392	0.10249	2,1,3,4	0.75	0.88829	0.52680	0.58267
1,1,2,5	0.875	0.39652	0.56443	0.26010	2,1,4,4	0.25	0.85239	0.37629	0.55912
1,1,3,5	0.625	0.40625	0.48917	0.26648	2,2,2,4	0.75	0.95607	0.52680	0.62713
1,1,4,5	0.375	0.38654	0.41392	0.25355	2,2,3,4	0.25	0.98821	0.37629	0.64821
1,1,5,5	0.125	0.33219	0.33866	0.21790	3,0,4,4	0.5	1.27475	0.45154	0.83616
1,2,2,5	0.625	0.44304	0.48917	0.29061	3,1,3,4	0.5	1.76777	0.45154	1.15956
1,2,3,5	0.375	0.46034	0.41392	0.30196	3,2,2,4	0.5	1.90394	0.45154	1.24888
1,2,4,5	0.125	0.45178	0.33866	0.29634	0,0,5,3	0.83333	0.34021	0.55189	0.22316

Index					Index				
1,3,3,5	0.125	0.48513	0.33866	0.31822	0,1,4,3	0.83333	0.58134	0.55134	0.38133
2,0,3,5	0.83333	0.41388	0.55189	0.27148	0,1,5,3	0.50000	0.39087	0.45154	0.25639
2,0,4,5	0.50000	0.39087	0.45154	0.25639	0,2,3,3	0.83333	0.67013	0.55189	0.43957
2,0,5,5	0.16667	0.34021	0.35120	0.22316	0,2,4,3	0.50000	0.56519	0.45154	0.37073
2,1,2,5	0.83333	0.53142	0.55189	0.34858	0,2,5,3	0.16667	0.41388	0.35120	0.27148
2,1,3,5	0.50	0.56519	0.45154	0.37073	0,3,3,3	0.50000	0.61237	0.45154	0.40168
2,1,4,5	0.16667	0.58134	0.35120	0.38133	0,3,4,3	0.16667	0.53142	0.35120	0.34858
2,2,2,5	0.50	0.61237	0.45154	0.40168	1,0,5,3	0.75	0.47598	0.52680	0.31222
2,2,3,5	0.16667	0.67013	0.35120	0.43957	1,1,4,3	0.75	0.85239	0.52680	0.55912
3,0,3,5	0.75	0.63122	0.52680	0.41404	1,1,5,3	0.25	0.64348	0.37629	0.42209
3,0,4,5,	0.25	0.67892	0.37629	0.44533	1,2,3,3	0.75	0.98821	0.52680	0.64821
3,1,2,5	0.75	0.80526	0.52680	0.52820	1,2,4,3	0.25	0.88829	0.37629	0.58267
3,1,3,5	0.25	0.91430	0.37629	0.59973	1,3,3,3	0.25	0.95607	0.37629	0.62713
3,2,2,5	0.25	0.98028	0.37629	0.64301	2,0,5,3	0.5	0.86602	0.45154	0.56806
4,0,3,5	0.5	1.32288	0.45154	0.86774	0,1,5,2	0.75	0.67892	0.52680	0.44533
4,1,2,5	0.5	1.64831	0.45154	1.08776	0,2,4,2	0.25	0.91430	0.37629	0.59973
0,0,4,4	0.875	0.33219	0.56443	0.21790	0,2,5,2	0.25	0.63122	0.37629	0.41404
0,0,5,4	0.625	0.15625	0.48917	0.10249	0,3,3,2	0.75	0.98028	0.52680	0.64301
0,1,3,4	0.875	0.45178	0.56443	0.29634	0,3,4,2	0.25	0.80526	0.37625	0.52820
0,1,4,4	0.625	0.38654	0.48917	0.25355	1,1,5,2	0.5	1.27475	0.45154	0.83616
0,1,5,4	0.375	0.26700	0.41392	0.17514	1,2,4,2	0.5	1.76777	0.45154	1.15956
0,2,2,4	0.875	0.48513	0.56443	0.31822	1,3,3,2	0.5	1.90394	0.45154	1.24888
0,2,3,4	0.625	0.46034	0.48917	0.30196	0,2,5,1	0.5	1.32288	0.45154	0.86774
					0,3,4,1	0.5	1.65831	0.45154	1.08776

[a]Calculation by moving average interpolation for $N = 5$, $K = 3$, and $d = 0.30103$ from the formula: Log $m = \log D_a + d(K - 1)/2 + df = \log D_a + d(f + 1)$; in this case, $2.179^a \log m = 2.179_{of}(d)$.

Table for Calculation of Median Effective Dose

r value	f	σf	$d(f + 0.5)$	$2.306\, d\sigma_f$
			$d = 0.30103$[a]	
0,0,4	1.0	(0)	0.45154	(0)
0,1,4	0.75	0.25000	0.37629	0.18416
0,2,4	0.5	0.28868	0.30103	0.21265
0,3,4	0.25	0.25000	0.22577	0.18416
0,4,4	0.0	(0)	0.15052	(0)
1,0,4	1.0	(0)	0.45154	(0)
1,1,4	0.66667	0.35138	0.35120	0.25883
1,2,4	0.33333	0.44444	0.25086	0.32738
1,3,4	0.0	0.47140	0.15052	0.34724
2,0,4	1.0	(0)	0.45154	(0)
2,1,4	0.5	0.57735	0.30103	0.42529
2,2,4	0.0	0.81650	0.15052	0.60145
3,0,4	1.0	(0)	0.45154	(0)
3,1,4	0.0	1.41421	0.15052	1.04174
0,1,3	1.0	0.47140	0.45154	0.34724
0,2,3	0.66667	0.44444	0.35120	0.32738
0,3,3	0.33333	0.35138	0.25086	0.25883
0,4,3	0.0	(0)	0.15052	(0)
1,1,3	1.0	0.70711	0.45154	0.52087
1,2,3	0.5	0.6770	0.30103	0.49869
1,3,3	0.0	0.70711	0.15052	0.52087
2,1,3	1.0	1.41421	0.45154	1.04174
2,2,3	0.0	1.63299	0.15052	1.20289
0,2,2	1.0	0.81650	0.45154	0.60145
0,3,2	0.5	0.57735	0.30103	0.42529
0,4,2	0.0	(0)	0.15052	(0)
1,2,2	1.0	1.63299	0.45154	1.20289
1,3,2	0.0	1.41421	0.15052	1.04174
0,3,1	1.0	1.41421	0.45154	1.04174
0,4,1	0.0	(0)	0.15052	(0)

[a]Calculation by moving average interpolation for $N = 4$, $K = 2$, and $d = 0.30103$ from the formula: $\text{Log } m = \log D_a + \dfrac{d(K - 1)}{2} + df = \log D_a + d(f + 0.5)$; $2.447_\sigma = 2.447_{\sigma f}(d)$.

Table for Calculation of Median Effective Dose

			$d = 0.30103^a$	
r value	f	σf	df	$3.182\ d\sigma_f$
		$N = 4$		
0,4	0.5	(0)	0.15052	(0)
1,4	0.33333	0.22222	0.10034	0.21286
2,4	0.0	0.57735	0.0	0.55303
0,3	0.66667	0.22222	0.20069	0.21286
1,3	0.5	0.34355	0.15052	0.33866
2,3	0.0	1.15470	0.0	1.10606
0,2	1.0	0.57735	0.30103	0.55303
1,2	1.0	1.15470	0.30103	1.1060
		$N = 5$		$2.776d\sigma_f$
0,5	0.5	(0)	0.1505	(0)
1,5	0.375	0.15625	0.11289	0.13057
2,5	0.16667	0.34021	0.05017	0.28430
0,4	0.625	0.15625	0.18814	0.13057
1,4	0.5	0.23570	0.15052	0.19696
2,4	0.25	0.47599	0.07526	0.39776
0,3	0.83333	0.34021	0.25086	0.28430
1,3	0.75	0.47599	0.22577	0.39776
2,3	0.5	0.86603	0.15052	0.72371

[a]Calculation by moving average interpolation for $N = 4$ or 5, $K = 1$, and $d = 0.30103$ from the formula: $\text{Log}\ m = \log D_a + \dfrac{d(K-1)}{2} + df = \log D_a + df$ in this case.

Table for Calculation of Median Effective Dose

r value	f	σf	d = 0.30103[a]		r value	f	σf	d = 0.30103[a]	
			d(f + 1)	2.262 dσf				d(f + 1)	2.262 dσf
0,0,2,4	1.00000	0.28868	0.60206	0.19657	0,1,4,3	0.33333	0.35136	0.40137	0.23925
0,3,4	0.7500	0.25000	0.52680	0.17023	0,2,2,3	0.66667	0.58794	0.50172	0.40035
0,0,4,4	0.50000	0.35355	0.45154	0.0	0,2,3,3	0.33333	0.52116	0.40137	0.35487
0,1,1,4	1.00000	0.38188	0.60206	0.24074	0,2,4,3	0.00000	0.38490	0.30103	0.26209
0,1,2,4	0.75000	0.35355	0.52680	0.26003	0,3,3,3	0.00000	0.47140	0.30103	0.26209
0,1,3,4	0.50000	0.25000	0.45154	0.24074	1,0,3,3	1.00000	0.70711	0.60206	0.48149
0,1,4,4	0.25000	0.40825	0.37629	0.17023	1,0,4,3	0.50000	0.35355	0.45154	0.24074
0,2,2,4	0.50000	0.38188	0.45154	0.27799	1,1,2,3	1.00000	0.91287	0.60206	0.62160
0,2,3,4	0.25000	0.28868	0.37629	0.26003	1,1,3,3	0.50000	0.79057	0.45154	0.53832
0,2,4,4	0.00000	0.35355	0.30103	0.19657	1,1,4,3	0.00000	0.70711	0.30103	0.48149
0,3,3,4	0.00000	0.38490	0.30103	0.24074	1,2,2,3	0.50000	0.88976	0.45154	0.60586
1,0,2,4	1.00000	0.35136	0.60206	0.26209	1,2,3,3	0.00000	0.91287	0.30103	0.62160
1,0,3,4	0.66667	0.22222	0.50172	0.23925	2,0,3,3	1.00000	1.41421	0.60206	0.96298
1,0,4,4	0.33333	0.47140	0.40137	0.15132	2,0,4,3	0.00000	1.15470	0.30103	0.78627
1,1,1,4	1.00000	0.52116	0.60206	0.32099	2,1,2,3	1.00000	1.82574	0.60206	1.24320
1,1,2,4	0.66667	0.52116	0.50172	0.35487	2,1,3,3	0.00000	1.82574	0.30103	1.24320
1,1,3,4	0.33333	0.47140	0.40137	0.35487	2,2,2,3	0.00000	2.00000	0.30103	1.36186
1,1,4,4	0.00000	0.58794	0.30103	0.32099	0,0,4,2	1.00000	0.57735	0.60206	0.39313
1,2,2,4	0.33333	0.58794	0.40137	0.40035	0,1,3,2	1.00000	0.91287	0.60206	0.62160

[a]Calculation by moving average interpolation for N = 4, K = 3, and d = 0.30103 from the formula: $\log m = \log D_a = \dfrac{d(k-1)}{2+\delta f}$.

Table for Calculation of Median Effective Dose

r value	f	σf	d(f+1)	2.179 dσf
		$d = 0.30103^a$		
1,2,3,4	0.00000	0.60858	0.30103	0.41440
2,0,2,4	1.00000	0.57735	0.60206	0.39313
2,0,3,4	0.50000	0.57735	0.45154	0.39313
2,0,4,4	0.00000	0.57735	0.30103	0.39313
2,1,1,4	1.00000	0.70711	0.60206	0.48149
2,1,2,4	0.50000	0.81650	0.45154	0.55598
2,1,3,4	0.00000	0.91287	0.60206	0.62160
2,2,2,4	0.00000	1.00000	0.30103	0.68093
3,0,2,4	1.00000	1.15470	0.60206	0.78627
3,0,3,4	0.00000	1.41421	0.30103	0.96298
3,1,1,4	1.00000	1.41421	0.60206	0.96298
3,1,2,4	0.00000	1.82574	0.30103	1.24320
0,0,3,3	1.00000	0.47140	0.60206	0.32099
0,0,4,3	0.66667	0.22222	0.50172	0.15132
0,1,2,3	1.00000	0.60858	0.60206	0.41440
0,1,3,3	0.66667	0.52116	0.50172	0.35487

r value	f	σf	d(f+1)	2.179 dσf
		$d = 0.30103^a$		
0,1,4,2	0.50000	0.57735	0.45154	0.39313
0,2,2,2	1.00000	1.00000	0.60206	0.68093
0,2,3,2	0.50000	0.81650	0.45154	0.55598
0,2,4,2	0.00000	0.57735	0.30103	0.39313
0,3,3,2	0.00000	0.70711	0.30103	0.48149
1,0,4,2	1.00000	1.15470	0.60206	0.78627
1,1,3,2	1.00000	1.82574	0.60206	1.24320
1,1,4,2	0.00000	1.41421	0.30103	0.96298
1,2,2,2	1.00000	2.00000	0.60206	1.36186
1,2,3,2	0.00000	1.82574	0.30103	1.24320
0,2,3,1	1.00000	1.82574	0.60206	1.24320
0,2,4,1	0.00000	1.15470	0.80103	0.78627
0,3,3,1	0.00000	1.41421	0.30103	0.96298
0,1,4,1	1.00000	1.41421	0.60206	0.96298

[a]Calculation by moving average interpolation for $N = 4$, $K = 3$, and $d = 0.30103$ from the formula: $\log m = \log D_a = \dfrac{d(k - 1)}{2 + \delta f}$.

Vehicles

Common name: **Acetone**
Chemical name: 2-Propanone
Molecular weight: 58.08
Formula: C_3H_6O
Density: 0.780 g/ml
Volatility: High
Solubility/miscibility: Miscible with water, ethanol, DMFO, vegetable oils.
Biological considerations: Orally, will produce transient ($\sim$4 hr) neurobe-havioral intoxication. Repeated dermal use will lead to defatting of skin at application site. Oral LD_{50} (rats) = 10.7 ml/kg. Higher doses can cause systemic acidosis.
Chemical compatibility/stability considerations: Highly flammable, color-less liquid.
Uses (routes): Dermal and oral. Not preferred for oral—volume of instil-lation should be limited to 5 ml/kg by the oral route.

Common name: **Carboxyl methyl cellulose; CMC**
Chemical name: NA
Molecular weight: 21,000–500,000
Formula: R_nOCH_2COOH
Density: 1.59 g/ml
Volatility: NA
Solubility/miscibility: Soluble in both hot and cold water.
Biological considerations: Practically inert polymer.
Chemical compatibility/stability considerations: White granules; stable in pH range 0.2–10.
Uses (routes): Orally, as a 0.1 to 5% mixture with water.

Common name: **Corn oil/Mazola**
Chemical name: NA
Molecular weight: NA
Formula: Mixture of natural products
Density: 0.916–0.921 g/ml
Volatility: Low
Solubility/miscibility: Miscible with chloroform and ether. Slightly soluble in ethanol.
Biological considerations: Orally, serves as energy source (and therefore can alter food consumption and/or body weight). Prolonged oral administration has been associated with enhanced carcinogenesis.
Chemical compatibility/stability considerations: Thickens upon prolonged exposure to air.
Uses (routes): Oral, dermal, vaginal, rectal, and subcutaneous.

Common name: **DMFO**
Chemical name: *N,N*-dimethylformamide
Molecular weight: 73.09
Formula: $HCON(CH_3)_2$
Density: 0.945 g/ml
Volatility: Low
Solubility/miscibility: Miscible with water and most common organic solvents.
Biological considerations: Oral LD_{50} (rats) 7.6 ml/kg. Not cytotoxic to primary cells in culture.
Chemical compatibility/stability considerations: Colorless to very slightly yellow liquid.
Uses (routes): Carrier for oral, dermal, intraperitoneal, or intravenous at concentrations up to 1%.

Common name: **DMSO/dimethyl sulfoxide**
Chemical name: Sulfinylbis (methane)
Molecular weight: 78.13
Formula: C_2H_6OS
Density: 1.100 g/ml
Volatility: Medium
Solubility/miscibility: Soluble in water, ethanol, acetone, and ether.
Biological considerations: Oral LD_{50} (rats) = 17.9 ml/kg. Repeated dermal exposure can defat skin. Repeated oral exposure can produce corneal opacities. Not cytotoxic to cells in primary culture. Intraperitoneal LD_{50} (mice) = 11.6 ml/kg.
Chemical compatibility/stability considerations: Very hydroscopic liquid.

Uses (routes): All, as a carrier at up to 5% to enhance absorption.

Common name: **Ethanol; EtOH**
Chemical name: Ethyl alcohol
Molecular weight: 46.07
Formula: C_2H_6O
Density: 0.789 g/ml
Volatility: High, but declines when part of mixture with water.
Solubility/miscibility: Miscible with water, acetone, and most other vehicles.
Biological considerations: Orally, will produce transient neurobehavioral intoxication. Oral LD_{50} (rats) = 13.0 ml/kg. Intravenous LD_{50} (mice) = 5.1 ml/kg.
Chemical compatibility/stability considerations: Flammable colorless liquid.
Uses (routes): Dermal and oral, though can be used in lower concentrations for most other routes. Volume of oral instillation should be limited to 5 ml/kg.

Common name: **Glycerol; Glycerin**
Chemical name: 1,2,3-propanetriol
Molecular weight: 92.09
Formula: $C_3H_8O_3$
Density: 1.264 g/ml
Volatility: Low
Solubility/miscibility: Miscible with water and ethanol. Soluble in water and ether.
Biological considerations: Oral LD_{50} (rats) greater than 20 ml/kg. Can serve as an energy source.
Chemical compatibility/stability considerations: Syrupy liquid, absorbs moisture from air. Contact with strong oxidizing agents (such as potassium permanganate) may cause an explosion.
Uses (routes): Oral, dermal, vaginal, rectal, and intravenous (as part of an aqueous solution).

Common name: **Gum arabic; acacia**
Chemical name: NA
Molecular weight: Estimated 240,000–580,000
Formula: Mixture of natural products
Density: 1.35–1.49 g/ml
Volatility: NA
Solubility/miscibility: Insoluble in ethanol. Soluble to twice its weight (2× g) in water (×ml). Soluble in glycerol and propylene glycol.

Biological considerations: Virtually biologically inert.

Chemical compatibility/stability considerations: None

Uses (routes): Orally, as diluent or viscosity increases in solvents.

Common name: **Lactose (milk sugar)**.

Chemical name: 4.0. β-D-galactopyranosyl-D-glucose

Molecular weight: 342.30

Formula: $C_{12}H_{22}O_{11}$

Density: NA

Volatility: None

Solubility/miscibility: One gram soluble in 5 ml water; slightly soluble in alcohol.

Biological considerations: White powder. Energy source.

Chemical compatibility/stability considerations: None

Uses (routes): Orally, as a diluent for materials which may be excessively irritant if given pure.

Common name: **Methyl cellulose/methocel**

Chemical name: Cellulose methyl ether

Molecular weight: 40,000–180,000

Formula: NA

Density: Depends on concentration

Volatility: NA

Solubility/miscibility: Soluble in cold water, insoluble in hot water. Forms stable aqueous solution at room temperature. Insoluble in alcohol or ether.

Biological considerations: Can act as a laxative.

Chemical compatibility/stability considerations: White granules or grayish white powder. Aqueous solutions are neutral to litmus. Combustible.

Uses (routes): Orally, as a 0.1 to 5% mixture with water. Acts to increase viscosity of suspension, thereby reducing settling rate and improving hemogeneity.

Common name: **Methyl ethyl ketone; MEK**

Chemical name: 2-Butanone

Molecular weight: 72.10

Formula: C_4H_8O

Density: 0.805 g/ml

Volatility: Medium

Solubility/miscibility: 22.6% soluble in water, miscible with methanol and oils. Soluble in alcohol and ether.

Biological considerations: Oral LD_{50} (rats) = 6.86 ml/kg. Repeated dermal use can lead to defatting of skin. CNS depressent by inhalation.

Chemical compatibility/stability considerations: Flammable, colorless liquid.
Uses (routes): Dermal

Common name: **Mineral oil; liquid petrolatum**
Chemical name: NA
Molecular weight: NA (mixture)
Formula: A mixture of light hydrocarbons from petroleum
Density: 0.83–0.90 g/ml
Volatility: Very low
Solubility/miscibility: Insoluble in water and ethanol. Soluble in ether and oils.
Biological considerations: Laxative. Aspiration may cause lipoid pneumonia.
Chemical compatibility/stability considerations: NA
Uses (routes): Oral, vaginal, rectal, and dermal. Suspending agent.

Common name: **Olive oil**
Chemical name: NA
Molecular weight: NA
Formula: Mixture of natural products
Density: 0.909–0.915 g/ml
Volatility: Very low
Solubility/miscibility: Slightly soluble in ethanol, miscible with ether.
Biological considerations: Can serve as an energy source.
Chemical compatibility/stability considerations: Pale yellow or light greenish yellow oil. Becomes rancid upon exposure to air.
Uses (routes): Oral

Common name: **Peanut oil/arachis oil**
Chemical name: NA
Molecular weight: NA
Formula: Mixture of natural products
Density: 0.910–0.915 g/ml
Volatility: Low
Solubility/miscibility: Miscible with ether and other oils. Slightly soluble in ethanol. Soluble in ether.
Biological considerations: Orally, serves as an energy source.
Chemical compatibility/stability considerations: Clouds at low room temperatures. Thickens upon prolonged exposure to air.
Uses (routes): Oral, dermal, vaginal, rectal, subcutaneous, and intramuscular.

Common name: **Petrolatum/Vaseline/petroleum jelly**

Chemical name: NA
Molecular weight: NA
Formula: Mixture of petroleum fractions
Density: 0.820–0.869 g/ml
Volatility: None
Solubility/miscibility: Practically insoluble in water, glycerol, or ethanol.
Biological considerations: Practically inert.
Chemical compatibility/stability considerations: Yellowish, white, or light amber semisolid.
Uses (routes): Dermal, vaginal, and rectal.

Common name: **Polyethylene glycol-400 (Carbowax)**
Chemical name: NA
Molecular weight: 400 (approximate average, range 380–420)
Formula: $H(OCH_2CH_2)_nOH$
Density: 1.128 g/ml
Volatility: Very low
Solubility/miscibility: Highly soluble in water. Soluble in alcohol and many organic solvents.
Biological considerations: Employed as water-soluble emulsifying/dispersing agents. Oral LD_{50} (mice) = 23.7 ml/kg. Oral LD_{50} (rats) = 30 ml/kg.
Chemical compatibility/stability considerations: Does not hydrolyze or deteriorate on storage and will not support mold growth. Clear, viscous liquid.
Uses (routes): For oral administration as a vehicle full strength or mixed with water. Total dosage of PEG-400 should not exceed 5–10 ml.

Common name: **Propylene glycol**
Chemical name: Propane-1,2-diol; 1,2-propanediol
Molecular weight: 76.09
Formula: $C_3H_8O_2$
Density: 1.036 g/ml
Volatility: Low
Solubility/miscibility: Miscible with water and acetone. Soluble in ether and ethanol.
Biological considerations: Orally, causes transient (24 hr!) neurobehavioral intoxication. Oral LD_{50} (rats) = 25 ml/kg. Subcutaneous LD_{50} (mice) = 20.0 ml/kg.
Chemical compatibility/stability considerations: None
Uses (routes): Oral, dermal, vaginal, rectal, subcutaneous, and intradermal.

Common name: **Saline**
Chemical name: Physiological saline
Molecular weight: 18.02
Formula: 0.9% NaCl in water (weight to volume)
Density: As water
Volatility: Low
Solubility/miscibility: As water
Biological considerations: No limitations—preferable to water in paren-
    teral applications.
Chemical compatibility/stability considerations: None
Uses (routes): All except dermal and perocular.

Common name: **Tween 80/Polysorbate 80**
Chemical name: Sorbitan mono-9-octadecenoate poly(oxy-1,2-ethanediyl)
    derivatives.
Molecular weight: NA (mixture)
Formula: A complex mixture of polyoxyethylene ethers of mixed partial
    oleic esters of sorbital anhydrides.
Density: 1.06–1.10 g/ml
Volatility: High
Solubility/miscibility: Generally very soluble or miscible in water. Soluble
    in ethanol, corn oil, and olive oil. Insoluble in mineral oil.
Biological considerations: Surfactant. May cause micelle formation, with
    encumbent effects on bioavailability if included at concentrations of
    1% or higher. May be associated with irritation if given intravenously
    or intramuscularly. Dogs have the peculiarity that Tweens injected par-
    entherally induce the spontaneous systemic release of histamine. This
    response is particularly striking with iv injection, and therefore
    Tweens should not be components of iv vehicles in dogs.
Chemical compatibility/stability considerations: Acts as detergent in
    polar/nonpolar mixed solvent systems.
Uses (routes): Wetting agent (at 0.1 to 0.5%) in the preparation of sus-
    pensions. Most commonly used in water.

Common name: **Water**
Chemical name: Hydrogen oxide
Molecular weight: 18.02
Formula: H_2O
Density: 1.000 g/ml
Volatility: Low
Solubility/miscibility: Miscible with MEK, ethanol, and acetone.
Biological considerations: No limitations except higher volumes via the iv

route can disturb systemic electrolyte balance and cause hemolysis and hematuria.

Chemical compatibility/stability considerations: None

Uses (routes): All—the vehicle and solvent of first choice.

References

American Pharmaceutical Association (APhA) (1986). *Handbook of Pharmaceutical Excipients.* AphA, Washington, DC.

Hawley, G. G. (1971). *The Condensed Chemical Dictionary.* Van Nostrand Reinhold, New York.

Windholz, M. (1983). *The Merck Index,* 10th ed., Merck, Rahway, NJ.

Definition of Terms and Lexicon of Clinical Observations

Movement

Anesthetized	The absence of or reduced response to external stimuli, accompanied with a loss of righting reflex.
Ataxia	Incoordination of muscular action involving locomotion, including loss of coordination and unsteady gait.
Hyperactivity	An abnormally high level of motor activity.
Hypersensitivity	An abnormally strong reaction to external stimuli such as noise or touch.
Hypoactivity	An abnormally low level of motor activity.
Lethargy	A state of deep and prolonged depression stupor from which it is possible to be aroused, followed by an immediate relapse.
Low carriage	The animal's torso is carried very close to the ground during movement.
Prostrate	Animal assumes a recumbent position due to loss of strength or exhaustion and may slow intermittent uncoordinated movements.
Righting reflex	The ability of an animal, when placed on its back, to regain a position on all fours.
Unsteady gait	An erratic manner or style of walking.
Catalepsy	A condition characterized by a waxy rigidity of the muscles such that the animal tends to remain in any position in which it is placed.
Paralysis	Inhibition or loss of motor function; may be characterized by affected portion of the body.

Respiration

Audible respiration	An abnormal respiratory sound heard while listening to the breathing of the animal (e.g., wheezing and rales).
Bradypnea	An abnormal slowness of the respiration rate.

Dyspnea	"Shortness of breath"; difficult or labored breathing.
Gasping	Spasmodic breathing with the mouth open, or laborious respiration with the breath caught convulsively.
Hyperpnea	Deep and rapid breathing.
Cheyne–Stokes respiration	Breathing characterized by rhythmic waning and waxing of the depth of respiration, with regularly recurring periods of apnea: seen especially in coma resulting from affection of the nervous centers.
Hypopnea	Shallow and slow breathing.
Irregular respiration	No definite cycle or rate of breathing.
Labored respiration	Forced or difficult, usually irregular breathing.
Tachypnea	An excessive rapidity of the respiration rate.

Condition of skin and fur

Alopecia	Deficiency of hair (baldness).
Cyanosis	Visible skin and/or mucous membranes turn dusky blue due to lack of oxygenation of the blood.
Necrosis	Actual tissue destruction, masses of dead/destroyed tissue.

Urogenital region

Anuria	An absence of or sharp decline in urine excretion.
Diarrhea	An abnormal frequency and liquidity of fecal discharge.
Polyuria	An abnormally sharp increase in the amount of urine excretion.

Convulsions and tremors

Convulsions	Transient, self-sustaining electrical dysrhythmias which have a tendency to recur. Convulsions are generally associated with a finite period of unconsciousness and have a muscular involvement manifested as disorganized limb movements.
Clonic	This is often seen as a "paddling" motion of the forelegs of the animal.
Tonic	Muscular contraction, keeping limbs in a fixed position, generally extended to the rear.
Torsion	Postural incoordination or rolling. This is generally associated with the vestibular (ear canal) system.
Fasciculation	Rapid, often continuous contraction of a bundle of skeletal muscle fibers which does not produce a purposeful movement (twitching).
Tremor	Fine oscillating muscular movements which may or may not be rhythmic.

Condition of eyes

Blepharospasm	A twitching or spasmodic contraction of the orbicularis occuli muscle.
Chemosis	Edema of conjunctiva(e)—The conjunctival tissue responds to noxious stimuli by swelling.

Chromodacryorrhea	The presence of reddish conjunctival exudate; no blood cells present in exudate (i.e., not true "bloddy tears").
Conjunctivitis	Inflammation of conjunctiva (mucous membrane which lines the eyelids and is reflected into the eyeball).
Exophthalmos	An abnormal protrusion of the eyeball from the orbit.
Lacrimation	The secretion of tears.
Miosis	Constriction of the pupil.
Mydriasis	Dilation of the pupil.
Nystagmus	An abnormal involuntary movement of the eyes. It may be rotational or horizontal or vertical plane.
Ocular exudate	Secretion (usually transparent and yellow) directly from the eye.
Opacity	A loss of transparency of the eyeball.
Pinpoint pupils	Ultimate state of miosis.
Ptosis	Refers to a dropping of the upper eyelid, thought to be due to impaired conduction in the third cranial nerve.

Miscellaneous

Analgesia	The absence of (or reduced response to) painful stimuli.
Hunched posture	The drawing-in of both ends of the body and extremities with a sharp arching of the back.
Kyphosis	Humpback—an abnormal curvature and dorsal prominence of the vertebrae column.
Nasal discharge	Fluid secretion from the nostrils.
Piloerection	Body hair stands on end; dilation of the pupils usually accompanies piloerection.
Salivation	Excessive secretion of saliva from the mouth.
Straub tail	Condition, especially in mice, in which the animal carries its tail in an erect (vertical or nearly vertical) position. This sign is commonly associated with chemicals (e.g., morphine) that bind to opiate receptors.

Reflexes

Corneal reflex	Closure of the eyelids in response to a corneal touch (e.g., with a soft brush bristle).
Grip strength (or Screen grip)	Measure of the grip strength of the forelimbs or hindlimbs; may be evaluated quantitatively or by subjective estimate or impairment (rodents only).
Pinna reflex	Twitch of the outer ear in response to a gentle touch.
Preyer's reflex (auditory startle response)	Involuntary movement of the outer ears produced by an auditory stimulus (especially in rats).
Pupillary reflex	Contraction of the pupil in response to light stimulation of the retina.
Righting reflex	The ability to land on (when dropped) or regain normal stance on all four limbs.
Startle reflex	Response to sharp sound, touch, or other startling stimulus; response may range from "absent," to "normal," to "hyperreactive," including exaggerated jerking, jumping, frantic attempts to escape, and even convulsions.

INDEX

NATIONAL UNIVERSITY
LIBRARY   SAN DIEGO